Handbook of
Pathophysiology

Handbook of Pathophysiology

Ramona Browder Lazenby, EdD, MSN, FNP-BC, CNE
Professor
Auburn University Montgomery School of Nursing
Auburn University Montgomery
Montgomery, Alabama

FOURTH EDITION

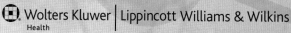

Wolters Kluwer | Lippincott Williams & Wilkins
Health
Philadelphia • Baltimore • New York • London
Buenos Aires • Hong Kong • Sydney • Tokyo

Acquisitions Editor: Hilarie Surrena
Product Manager: Eric Van Osten
Editorial Assistant: Laura Scott
Production Director: Helen Ewan
Senior Designer: Joan Wendt
Illustration Coordinator: Brett MacNaughton
Manufacturing Coordinator: Karin Duffield
Prepress Vendor: MPS Limited, A Macmillan Company

4th Edition

Library of Congress Cataloging-in-Publication Data
Lazenby, Ramona Browder.
Handbook of pathophysiology. —4th ed./Ramona Browder Lazenby.
    p. ; cm.
Rev. ed. of: Handbook of pathophysiology/Elizabeth J. Corwin. 3rd ed. c2008.
Includes bibliographical references and index.
Summary: "This pathophysiology handbook is ideally suited for easy reference in the classroom or clinical environment. The book presents a summary of physiology concepts for each body system, followed by an overview of important pathophysiology concepts related to 'alterations' in that body system. These pathophysiology concepts provide the necessary foundation for understanding the disease or injury states that are presented next in the chapter"—Provided by publisher.
ISBN 978-1-60547-725-1 (pbk. : alk. paper) 1. Physiology, Pathological—Handbooks, manuals, etc. I. Corwin, Elizabeth J. Handbook of pathophysiology. II. Title.
[DNLM: 1. Pathologic Processes—Handbooks. 2. Physiological Phenomena—Handbooks. QZ 39]
RB113.C785 2011
616.07—dc22
                                                                                            2010025906

RRS1101

To all my students who have said,
and actually meant: "I LOVE Patho."

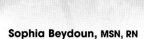

Sophia Beydoun, MSN, RN
Nursing Instructor
Nursing Department
Henry Ford Community College
Dearborn, Michigan

Barbara Coles, BS, MS, PhD
Associate Department Head, Natural
   Science, Health and PE Department
Wake Technical Community College
Raleigh, North Carolina

Deb Filer, PhD, RN, CNE
Associate Professor
Nursing Department
St. Catherine University
St. Paul, Minnesota

Sheila Grossman, PhD, FNP-BC
Professor & FNP Specialty Track
   Coordinator
Fairfield University School of Nursing
Fairfield, Connecticut

Lorie Judson, RN, PhD
Associate Director/Undergraduate Chair
California State University, Los Angeles
   School of Nursing
Los Angeles, California

Lori Knight, CHIM
Instructor, Health Information
   Management
SIAST Wascana Campus
Regina, Saskatchewan
Canada

DeAnn Mitchell, PhD, RN
Professor of Nursing
Tarrant County College
Fort Worth, Texas

Mary Ellen Morrissey, RN, MSN
Assistant Professor
Nursing Department
Salem State College
Salem, Massachusetts

Cheryl Neudauer, PhD, MEd
Science Division Coordinator
Biology Department
Minneapolis Community & Technical
   College
Minneapolis, Minnesota

Deborah Pool, MS, RN, CCRN
Department Chair
Maricopa Nursing Program
Glendale Community College
Glendale, Arizona

As a nurse educator for over 20 years, I learned rather early that a foundational knowledge of basic pathophysiology made other concepts make better sense. Understanding the normal anatomy and physiology of the body lays a foundation to understanding the pathophysiology behind various disease processes. The understanding of pathophysiology then helps make sense of why certain medications and other therapeutic interventions are effective in treating different health alterations. An understanding of pathophysiology is vital to safe and effective patient care.

I truly believe pathophysiology is the most important course in the curriculum. Every semester that I teach it to nursing students, I begin class the same way: "I love pathophysiology and I want you to love it as much as I do." Then, I have them repeat "We love patho!" in unison. It does not take students long to sense my passion for pathophysiology and I would like to believe that my passion is contagious. Although it may not be the most important course, historically students who have a good understanding of pathophysiology tend to have a better understanding of pharmacology and other therapeutic interventions. This text is designed to present an overview of the more common health alterations. While no one book can contain all the information, hopefully this information will stimulate further research on the reader's part. In the clinical setting this text will serve as a quick reference for the pathophysiology, clinical manifestations, diagnostic tools, possible complications, and treatments of many disease processes.

CONTENT ORGANIZATION

The format of this edition of the *Handbook of Pathophysiology* continues to follow the same outline as in the previous books, with section headings of Physiologic Concepts, Pathophysiologic Concepts, and Conditions of Disease or

Injury. The text is organized this way because I believe not only that a solid understanding of physiology is essential to understanding pathophysiology, but also that understanding both physiology and pathophysiology is required in order for the symptoms and treatment of any disease to make sense.

NEW TO THIS EDITION

This edition of the text includes 20 chapters, with expanded discussions of cutting-edge research and knowledge in cell biology, cancer, and genetics. All of the chapters in this edition have been updated and expanded, based upon the most recent scientific studies and information available. In addition, more tables have been added as a quick reference.

Pediatric and Geriatric Considerations are highlighted at the end of each chapter. As in the previous editions, they are included to alert the reader to variations in both normal and pathophysiologic processes in children and older adults. Many of these features have been expanded to include pearls gleaned from practice.

SPECIAL FEATURES

Each chapter includes features designed to assist the reader's understanding of pathophysiology.

- **Key Words** are indicated in boldface type and are defined in the text in order to help readers quickly master what can sometimes be a difficult vocabulary.
- **Figures,** especially chosen or created for the *Handbook,* are used throughout the text to visually explain concepts that are not easily grasped by words alone.
- **Geriatric Considerations** at the end of each chapter alert readers to the important differences in the physiologic and pathophysiologic systems and conditions of disease or injury in the older adults.
- **Pediatric Considerations** highlight developmental, physiologic, and pathophysiologic differences in both wellness and illness in children.

Ramona Browder Lazenby, EdD, MSN, FNP-BC, CNE

ACKNOWLEDGMENTS

It would be impossible to acknowledge everyone who has contributed to my growth as a person and a professional. First and foremost is my husband, John, who has always supported anything and everything I have pursued. Thank you to my dean who has allowed me to continue teaching pathophysiology despite my administrative role. Also, to my colleagues at Auburn Montgomery School of Nursing who constantly encourage each other as we all strive for excellence. Finally, a great big thank you to all the students who I have had the privilege of teaching. Your enthusiasm and desire for knowledge has kept me motivated to continue my lifelong learning—and of course hearing you say "We love patho" stirs more passion for the content.

CONTENTS

UNIT FOUR
Oxygen Balance and Deficiencies

UNIT FIVE
Nutrition, Elimination, and Reproductive Function and Dysfunction

Fundamental Mechanisms of Health and Disease

CHAPTER

Cell Structure and Function

The cell is the building block of each living organism. Each cell is a self-contained system that undergoes the functions of energy production and usage, respiration, reproduction, and excretion. Cells join together to form tissues, tissues join to form organs, and organs form body systems. To understand how the organs and systems of the body work, one must first understand the cell. This understanding requires an investigation of the individual structures that make up the cell and of the separate function each structure carries out to serve the whole.

● Physiologic Concepts

CELL STRUCTURES

A cell is made up of internal structures separated from each other by semi-permeable membranes. These internal structures are bound together inside one cell membrane to form a single unit. Although cells differ as to their function in the body, all cells contain the same internal structures. The inside of each cell can be divided into two main compartments: the cytoplasm and the nucleus. All internal structures reside in the cytoplasm or the nucleus (Table1-1).

TABLE 1-1 Cell Structures (Fig. 1-1)	
Structure	**Description/Function**
Cytoplasm	
Mitochondria	Energy source
Endoplasmic reticulum	Protein synthesis
Ribosomes	Protein synthesis
Golgi apparatus	Secretes synthesized protein
Lysosomes	Digestive enzymes
Cytoskeleton (microtubules, microfilaments)	Support; movement of substances
Microtubules	Chromosome separation during cell division; maintain structural integrity
Nucleus	Control center
Deoxyribonucleic acid (DNA)	Genetic material
Cell Membrane	Semipermeable barrier surrounding each cell
	Composed of phospholipids bilayer
Phospholipid Bilayer	Consist of polar head with phosphate and nonpolar head
	Diffusion of lipid-soluble substances
Integral Proteins	Extend through the membrane
	Glucose or lipid bound on extracellular side
	Receptor molecules for hormones
	Facilitate cell communication
	Channels for movement of ions
	Some are enzymes to catalyze reactions
	Necessary for nonlipid substances to enter the cell

MOVEMENT THROUGH THE MEMBRANE

Lipid-soluble substances, such as oxygen, carbon dioxide, alcohol, and urea, move across the lipid bilayer by simple diffusion. Other substances that are not lipid soluble, such as most small ions, glucose, amino acids, and proteins, move between the extracellular fluid and the intracellular compartments through pores provided by the integral proteins or through carrier-mediated transport systems. Carrier-mediated transport also originates in the integral proteins. The extracellular fluid consists of the fluid between the cells, called the **interstitial fluid**, and the blood. The fluid inside the cell is called the **intracellular fluid**.

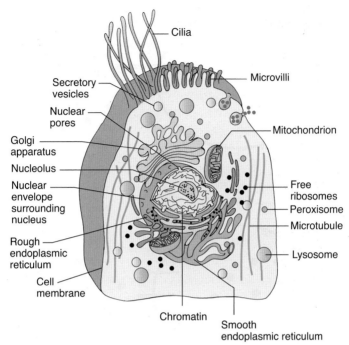

FIGURE 1-1 Cell structure with major components. (From Porth, C. & Matfin, G [2009]. *Pathophysiology, concepts of altered health states* [8th edition]. Philadelphia: Lippincott Williams & Wilkins.)

Simple Diffusion through the Cell Membrane

Simple diffusion occurs through random movement of molecules from an area of higher concentration to an area of lower concentration until equilibrium is reached (Fig. 1-2). This process does not require energy, but can result in the movement of a substance across a membrane. However, the substance cannot accumulate in higher concentration on one side of the membrane compared to the other.

Osmosis

The movement of water across a semipermeable membrane from an area of lower particle concentration to an area of higher concentration is called osmosis. The drive for water to move in one direction or the other is described as the **osmotic pressure**. The osmotic pressure of a solution depends on the number of particles or ions present in the water solution and the **hydrostatic pressure** (mechanical water force against cell membranes). The more ions are

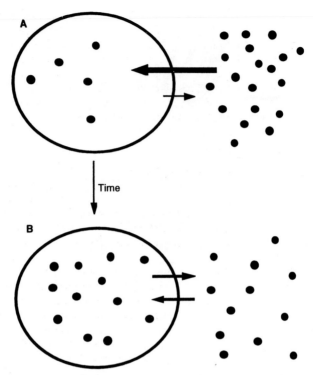

FIGURE 1-2 Simple diffusion across a membrane. Molecules randomly diffuse from an area of high concentration to an area of low concentration (A) until equilibrium is reached (B).

present in the solution, the lesser is the water concentration and the greater the osmotic pressure (i.e., the pressure for water to diffuse into the solution). Osmosis continues until equilibrium is reached or hydrostatic pressure opposes the flow.

Simple Diffusion through Protein Pores

Small ions, such as hydrogen, sodium, potassium, and calcium, are too electrically charged to diffuse through the lipid membrane of the cell. Instead, they diffuse through the pores provided by the integral proteins. Selectivity of the protein channels is based on the shape and size of the channel and the electrical nature of the ion.

Many protein channels are gated; they can be open or closed to an ion. Whether the gate is open or closed usually depends on the electrical potential across the gate (i.e., the voltage-gated sodium channel), or on binding to the gate by a ligand that causes it to open or close. An example of ligand gating is when acetylcholine binds to proteins on the neuromuscular junction, thereby opening gates to many small molecules, especially sodium and, to a lesser extent, calcium ions. Diffusion through a gate continues until the concentrations on either side of the membrane are equal or the gate is closed. Several human diseases are related to dysfunction of transmembrane protein channels. Cystic fibrosis is the best-known human disease caused by a defective transmembrane protein that results in abnormal ion movement through a pore.

Mediated Transport

For many substances like glucose and amino acids, simple diffusion is impossible. These molecules are too charged to pass through the lipid portion of the membrane or too large to pass through a pore. Instead, these substances, called substrates, are transported across the membrane with the assistance of a **carrier**. This type of movement is called mediated transport and may require energy derived from the splitting of adenosine triphosphate (ATP) (see Energy Production section).

Active transport is mediated transport that requires energy (Fig. 1-3A). With active transport, energy is used by the cell to maintain a substance at higher concentration on one side of the membrane than the other. Examples of substances moved by active transport include sodium, potassium, calcium, and the amino acids. Each of these substances is actively transported, with the assistance of a carrier, in one direction against a concentration gradient. It then moves down its concentration gradient by simple diffusion in the opposite direction.

Facilitated diffusion is mediated transport that does not require energy, but cannot concentrate a substance (Fig. 1-3B). Simple diffusion continues at some level in all carrier-mediated systems. Facilitated diffusion is similar to simple diffusion in that no energy is used by the cell to transport a substance; therefore, the substance cannot be transported against its concentration gradient. With facilitated diffusion, a molecule that is limited in its ability to cross the cell membrane on its own is assisted (facilitated) by a carrier to cross the membrane. For example, insulin increases the transport of glucose into most cells.

The Sodium–Potassium Pump

An important example of active transport is the pumping of sodium and potassium across cell membranes. This transport depends on an integral carrier protein known as the sodium–potassium pump. Associated with the pump is an enzyme that splits ATP and provides the energy needed for the pump to function. This enzyme is known as the sodium–potassium ATPase. The sodium–potassium pump transports sodium ions out of the cells to the extracellular region where the concentration is approximately 14 times that inside

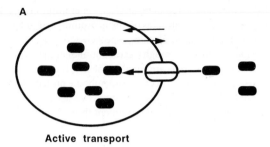

Active transport

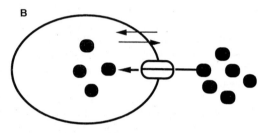

Facilitated diffusion

FIGURE 1-3 Carrier transport. Active transport (A) requires energy to provide a final difference in concentration; facilitated diffusion (B) does not require energy, but cannot concentrate a substance. Simple diffusion continues at some level in all carrier-mediated systems.

the cell. Potassium ions are moved into the cell where the concentration is approximately 35 times greater than outside the cell. This transport causes greater sodium concentration in the extracellular fluid (142 mEq/L) compared to the intracellular fluid (14 mEq/L), and greater potassium concentration in the intracellular fluid (140 mEq/L) compared to the extracellular fluid (4 mEq/L). The sodium–potassium pump carries three sodium molecules out of the cell for every two potassium molecules it carries in.

The Effects of Pumping Sodium and Potassium

Because sodium and potassium are cations (carrying a positive charge), the transport of three sodium ions out of the cell and only two potassium ions into the cell creates an electrical gradient across the cell membrane. It is this electrical **membrane potential** that allows nerve and muscle function and action potentials to occur (see Chapter 8).

The sodium–potassium pump is essential in controlling cell volume. The presence of intracellular proteins and other organic substances that cannot cross the cell membrane increases intracellular osmotic pressure and creates a tendency for water to diffuse into the cell. This diffusion of water, if unlimited, would cause the cell to swell and eventually burst. However, with the active transport of three sodium ions out of the cell, the osmotic pressure inside the cell is reduced and the diffusion of water into the cell is contained.

Coupled Transport

Many substances are transported coupled to the active transport of sodium. These substances include glucose, amino acids, hydrogen ions, and calcium. The energy required for the transport of these other substances is indirectly supplied through the splitting of ATP by the sodium–potassium ATPase. This type of transport is called secondary active transport.

Coupled transport can be in the same direction as sodium transport (cotransport) or it may occur in the direction opposite to that of sodium transport (countertransport). Both types of transport depend on the diffusion of sodium down its concentration gradient, which in turn depends on the active transport of sodium by the sodium–potassium pump. In cotransport, sodium attaches to a carrier that assists it in moving down its concentration gradient, from outside the cell to inside; the other substance attaches to the same carrier, also on the outside of the cell, and as sodium is moved into the cell, the coupled substance moves with it. In countertransport, the coupled substance binds to the sodium carrier on the inside of the cell membrane with sodium on the outside. Therefore, when sodium is delivered to the inside of the cell, the other substance is delivered to the outside.

Calcium Transport

Calcium can move by simple diffusion through the cell membrane, be transported by coupled transport with sodium, or be moved by primary active transport through a calcium pump. There are two known calcium pumps. One is part of an integral protein present in the cell membrane, which moves calcium out of the cell. The other is an intracellular pump, which pumps calcium out of the cytoplasm into intracellular compartments such as the sarcoplasmic reticulum. This results in sequestering calcium inside the cell. Both pumps keep free intracellular calcium concentration low. The calcium pumps serve as ATPases, which derive energy needed to pump the calcium against its concentration gradient by the splitting of ATP.

Characteristics of Carriers

Active transport and facilitated diffusion require carriers. All carriers are affected by the properties of specificity, saturation, and competition.

Specificity of carriers means that only certain substrates will be transported by any one carrier. The carrier and its specific substrate appear to fit together like a lock and a key.

Saturation of carriers means that at a certain concentration of substrate, all carriers will be filled and transport will level off. Additional substrate will not increase transport across the membrane.

Competition of carriers occurs when there is more than one substrate transported by the same carrier. The multiple substrates compete with each other for the limited number of carrier sites available. Many drugs, naturally occurring and synthetic, compete with endogenous hormones and neurotransmitters for various carrier molecules.

Endocytosis and Exocytosis

When large substances cannot enter the cell by diffusion or mediated transport, endocytosis (engulfment) of the substance by the cell membrane occurs. **Pinocytosis** is the engulfment of, fluids and small particles by vesicles and is important in the transport of proteins to the cytoplasm. **Phagocytosis** involves the engulfment and degradation of microorganisms such as bacteria. Both processes require energy. Only cells of the immune system (i.e., macrophages and neutrophils) perform phagocytosis.

Exocytosis involves the transport of intracellular substances such as debris into the extracellular spaces. It also plays a role in the release of substances synthesized in the cell such as hormones.

ENERGY PRODUCTION

Cells must produce energy for their own use. Cells extract energy from chemical bonds of food molecules by combining the food molecules with oxygen inside the mitochondria of the cell. The food molecules include glucose from carbohydrate metabolism, amino acids from protein metabolism, and fatty acids and glycerol from fat metabolism.

The process whereby the food molecules are combined with oxygen, leading to the production of energy, is called oxidative phosphorylation. This process requires several enzymes, working in sequential fashion in the mitochondria. The net result is the synthesis of the energy-rich molecule ATP. ATP is composed of the nitrogen base adenosine, the sugar ribose, and three phosphate molecules bound together. As the major source of cellular energy, ATP contains two high-energy bonds both of which contain approximately 12 kcal of potential energy.

Oxidative Phosphorylation of Glucose

Glycolysis, an anaerobic (without oxygen) process occurring in the cytoplasm is the initial step in the **oxidative phosphorylation** of glucose that occurs in the mitochondria. During glycolysis, cytoplasmic enzymes convert glucose into pyruvic acid. This process requires two molecules of ATP and produces four molecules of ATP: a result of two net molecules. In times of oxygen deprivation, glycolysis plays a limited but important role in supplying the cell with ATP (see Anaerobic Glycolysis section).

If oxygen is present (aerobic), the molecules of pyruvic acid move into the mitochondria where they enter the citric acid cycle, also called the Krebs cycle (Fig. 1-4) and are converted by enzymes present there into a compound called acetyl coenzyme A (acetyl CoA). This process produces two more ATP molecules. Acetyl CoA is then enzymatically converted to carbon dioxide and hydrogen. The carbon dioxide diffuses out of the mitochondria and out of the cell, where it is picked up by the blood supplying that cell. It is then carried to the lungs and exhaled from the body. The hydrogen atoms remaining in the mitochondria begin the process of oxidative phosphorylation, during which they are combined with molecules of oxygen through an elaborate electron transport chain present in the mitochondrial membrane. The result of this process is to produce a tremendous amount of energy in the form of 36 ATP molecules. From the metabolism of one molecule of glucose, therefore, a total of 38 net ATP molecules are formed (36 from oxidative phosphorylation and 2 from glycolysis).

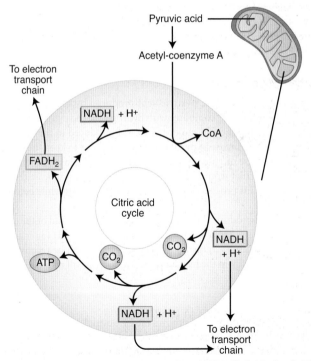

FIGURE 1-4 Kreb's or citric acid cycle. (From Porth, C. & Matfin, G [2009]. *Pathophysiology, concepts of altered health states* [8th edition]. Philadelphia: Lippincott Williams & Wilkins.)

Oxidative Phosphorylation of Fatty Acids and Glycerol

The cell also uses free fatty acids and glycerol in oxidative phosphorylation to produce ATP. Glycerol is a three-carbon carbohydrate, which undergoes glycolysis in the cytoplasm and enters the Krebs cycle as acetyl CoA. Free fatty acids diffuse directly into the mitochondria where they are acted on by enzymes and transformed into acetyl CoA. This acetyl CoA also enters the Krebs cycle. The breakdown of one molecule of fat results in 463 molecules of ATP. Fat has a five times greater weight per mole than glucose. Thus, gram for gram, the metabolism of fat provides about three times as much ATP as glucose metabolism. Therefore, fat is a more efficient form of energy storage than carbohydrate.

Oxidative Phosphorylation of Amino Acids

Amino acids enter the mitochondria after removal of the nitrogen molecule (deamination). After deamination, amino acids enter the Krebs cycle at various points. Some, such as alanine, enter as pyruvic acid; others enter as later intermediates. Where the amino acids enter the Krebs cycle determines how many hydrogen atoms they add to the electron transfer chain and thus how many ATP molecules are synthesized.

Anaerobic Glycolysis

If oxygen is unavailable, the pyruvic acid produced by glycolysis does not enter the Krebs cycle, but combines with hydrogen in the cytoplasm to form lactic acid. Although the two molecules of ATP produced in the breakdown of one molecule of glucose to pyruvic acid are available to keep the cell alive, this is a wasteful use of glucose because it results in the loss of the other 36 molecules of ATP that would have been produced had pyruvic acid entered the Krebs cycle. This process can only continue for a short while before glucose is depleted.

The lactic acid produced by anaerobic glycolysis diffuses out of the cell and into the bloodstream. This can create a decrease in plasma pH (an increase in plasma acidity). With the return of oxygen, lactic acid will be reconverted to pyruvic acid, primarily in the liver, and the Krebs cycle will resume.

ENERGY USAGE

ATP formed in the mitochondria moves into the cytoplasm by a combination of simple and facilitated diffusion. When needed by the cell, ATP can be broken down rapidly into adenosine diphosphate (ADP) by enzymatic splitting of the bond between the last two phosphates. This results in the release of energy, which is used by the cell to perform its duties of solute transport, protein synthesis, reproduction, and movement.

Although it is through ATP synthesis and breakdown that energy is transferred in the cell, very little ATP is stored in the cell. Instead, energy is stored in the form of substrates for ATP—as carbohydrates, fats, proteins, and their metabolic products. The other essential component for ATP production, oxygen, is continually delivered to all cells by the combined efforts of the cardiovascular and respiratory systems.

CELL TYPES

Epithelial Cells

The tissue that lines most internal and external structures of the body is made up of epithelial cells. These cells are packed together, providing support for overlying structures. Epithelial tissue also acts as a protective barrier and a medium for absorption, secretion, and excretion. Examples of epithelial tissue include the skin (epidermis), the covering on all internal organs and tubules, the microvilli of the intestine, and the cilia lining the respiratory passageways. Glandular cells that secrete substances into ducts (exocrine glands) or into the bloodstream (endocrine glands) are made of epithelial tissue. Sensory organs also contain epithelial cells. Epithelial layers are usually one (simple epithelium) to two (stratified and pseudostratified epithelia) cells thick.

Connective Tissue Cells

Connective tissue is represented by many different cell types, including fibroblasts, adipose (fat) cells, mast cells, blood cells, and cells of the blood-forming organs. Connective tissue holds different tissues together by the accumulation of protein and gel-like substances secreted from the fibroblasts into the spaces surrounding the cells. Protein substances secreted include collagen, a thick, white fiber that acts to provide structural support; elastin, a stretchy protein that allows tissues to give when stretched; and reticular fibers, thin flexible strands that allow organs to accommodate increases in volume. Tissue gel consists primarily of hyaluronic acid, which intersperses throughout the interstitial spaces to retain water and provide support and protection.

Adipose tissue and endothelial cells provide nourishment and support for the fibroblasts. Mast cells contain granules filled with histamine and other vasoactive substances. Mast cell degranulation is an important step in initiating an inflammatory reaction.

Hematopoietic tissue is considered connective tissue. Hematopoietic tissue includes bone marrow, blood cells, and lymphatic tissue. The basement membrane found along the interface between connective tissue and an adjacent tissue is also considered a connective tissue layer. This membrane bonds, supports, and allows for tissue repair.

Muscle Cells

Muscle cells are highly differentiated (specialized) cells that have the ability to contract and cause movement or increased tension. Groups of muscle cells form one of the three types of muscle tissue: skeletal, smooth, or cardiac.

Muscle cells are composed of the proteins actin and myosin. Cross-bridges located between the actin and myosin connect and swing when stimulated in the proper sequence (see Chapter 10). This causes the muscle as a whole to contract and do work or produce tension. All types of muscles require an increase in intracellular calcium to contract. Different muscles may use different sources of calcium and thus have slightly different methods of contraction stimulation.

Skeletal muscle is attached to bones by tendons. When stimulated by motor neuron impulses, skeletal muscle voluntarily contracts. Skeletal muscle uses calcium released from intracellular compartments to initiate contraction. Mature skeletal muscle does not undergo further cell division. Skeletal muscle may even be considered a paracrine endocrine organ because it secretes cytokines such as interleukin-8 (IL-8), a peptide that induces angiogenesis (new capillary formation).

Cardiac muscle, found in the heart, contracts spontaneously because of an intrinsic ability to depolarize and fire action potentials. Cardiac muscle is innervated by the nerves of the autonomic nervous system: the sympathetic and parasympathetic nerves. These inputs can increase or decrease the inherent rate or strength of cardiac contraction. Cardiac contraction involves entry of calcium into the muscle cell from the extracellular fluid and from an intracellular compartment, the sarcoplasmic reticulum. During embryogenesis, cardiac muscle cells become highly differentiated and do not undergo further cell division. Cardiac muscle is also an endocrine organ in that it secretes the hormone atrial natriuretic peptide (ANP) that acts on the kidney to participate in the control of blood volume.

Smooth muscle is found throughout the body, including the vascular system, the genitourinary tract, and all parts of the gut. Its function is often considered involuntary. Smooth muscle is innervated by the autonomic nervous system, which can increase or decrease the rate of contraction. When stretched, smooth muscle responds with an increase in contraction. Smooth muscle relies primarily on calcium entry from the extracellular fluid to initiate contraction. Mature smooth muscle cells can undergo cell division.

STEM CELLS

In general, as body cells become differentiated (specialized), they become less able to reproduce and thus eventually die. **Stem cells** are undifferentiated (nonspecialized) cells that have the ability to reproduce indefinitely and act as progenitors of other, specialized body cells. As specialized cells die, they can be replaced by new cells arising from local stem cells. When stem cells divide into two, one cell retains stem cell characteristics and the other daughter cell proceeds through the process to become differentiated.

Stem cells may come from adult sources (intestinal stem cells, hematopoietic stem cells, and epidermal stem cells) or may be derived from human embryos. Human embryo–derived stem cells in particular are highly undifferentiated and have the potential to differentiate into approximately 200 different tissues of the body.

Both adult stem cells and embryonic stem cells may provide therapies for some currently untreatable diseases. For example, one application of stem cell therapy currently under investigation is to repair an infarcted heart. This involves transplanting stem cells into the infarcted area of the heart in order to increase or preserve the number of cardiac muscle cells, improve vascular supply, and improve the contractile function of the injured myocardium. Cancer stem cells have been identified in some types of cancer such as that of breast and prostate and acute myeloid leukemia. It is anticipated that continuing research will reveal cancer treatments that will eliminate the proliferating cells.

Obstacles to using stem cells include a potential for tumorigenicity, immunological rejection of transplanted cells, and the risk of transmitting an infection. The harvesting of embryonic stem cells is of ethical concern for some and is an obstacle to their use in the United States at this time.

● Cellular Adaptation

Cells are continually exposed to changing conditions and potentially damaging stimuli. If these changes and stimuli are minor or brief, the cell adapts. Cellular adaptations include atrophy, hypertrophy, hyperplasia, and metaplasia. Prolonged or intense stimuli can cause cell injury or death (Fig. 1-5).

ATROPHY

Atrophy is a decrease in the size of a cell or tissue when confronted with adverse conditions. Atrophy may be an adaptive response to a decrease in the workload of a cell or tissue, thus decreasing the cells' oxygen and nutrient requirements. Atrophied cells have reduced organelles, fewer mitochondria, myofilaments, and endoplasmic reticulum structures and decreased intracellular vesicle and contractile protein. Atrophy is adaptive, and in most cases, is reversible.

Atrophy may be the result of disuse, denervation, loss of endocrine stimulation, inadequate nutrition, or ischemia. A classical example of disuse muscle atrophy is the individual on prolonged bed rest. The absence of skeletal muscle weight bearing will cause decreased muscle size. Denervation atrophy may be seen in the individual with a paralyzed extremity. The inability to actively move the extremity can cause disuse atrophy. Atrophy can also occur as a result

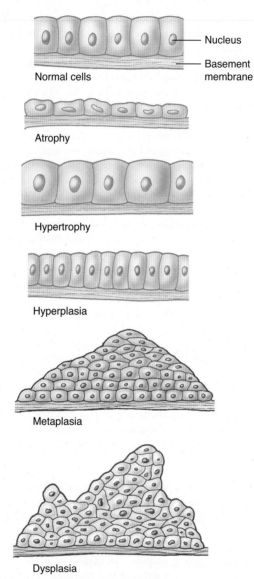

Normal cells

Nucleus

Basement membrane

Atrophy

Hypertrophy

Hyperplasia

Metaplasia

Dysplasia

FIGURE 1-5 Cellular adaptation. Atrophy (decreased cell size), hypertrophy (increased cell size), hyperplasia (increased cell number), metaplasia (change in type), dysplasia (change in size, shape and organization).
(From Porth, C. & Matfin, G [2009]. *Pathophysiology, concepts of altered health states* [8th edition]. Philadelphia: Lippincott Williams & Wilkins.)

of decreased hormonal or neural stimulation of a cell or tissue, which is seen in the breasts of women after menopause or in skeletal muscle after spinal cord transection. Atrophy of fat and muscle occurs in response to a nutritional deficiency and is seen in malnourished or starving people. Atrophy may also occur as a result of insufficient blood supply to cells, which cuts off vital nutrient and oxygen supply.

HYPERTROPHY

Hypertrophy is the increase in the size of a cell or tissue as an adaptive response to an increased workload. The cell's demand for oxygen and nutrients increases, causing an increase in synthesis of actin and myosin filaments, cell enzymes, protein, and ATP. Growth of intracellular structures including the mitochondria, the endoplasmic reticulum, intracellular vesicles, and the contractile proteins occurs. Hypertrophy is primarily seen in cells that cannot adapt to increased work by increasing their numbers through mitosis such as cardiac and skeletal muscle cells. Factors initiating hypertrophy may include ATP depletion, mechanical forces, hormonal factors, and activation of cell-degradation products. The three main types of hypertrophy are physiologic, pathologic, and adaptive or compensatory.

Physiologic hypertrophy occurs as a result of a healthy increase in the workload of a cell. Common examples include the increase of muscle mass through exercise and the growth of the uterus during pregnancy. *Pathologic* hypertrophy occurs in response to a disease state, for example, hypertrophy of the left ventricle in response to long-standing hypertension and an increase in the workload of the heart. There is a point, however, at which continued hypertrophy will no longer be effective. *Compensatory* hypertrophy occurs when cells grow to take over the role of other cells that have died. For example, the loss of one kidney causes the cells of the remaining kidney to undergo hypertrophy, resulting in a substantial increase in the size of the remaining kidney.

HYPERPLASIA

Hyperplasia is the increase in cell number occurring in an organ as a result of increased mitosis. It is an adaptive process associated with activation of genes that control cell proliferation and intracellular messengers that control replication and growth. Hyperplasia is seen in cells stimulated by an increased workload, by hormonal signals, or by signals produced locally in response to a decrease in tissue crowding. It can only occur in cells that undergo mitosis, such as liver, kidney, and connective tissue cells. Hyperplasia is a vital component in wound healing and blood vessel proliferation. Hyperplasia may be physiologic or pathologic.

Physiologic hyperplasia may be hormonal or compensatory. *Hormonal* hyperplasia occurs monthly in uterine endometrial cells during the follicular stage of the menstrual cycle. *Compensatory* hyperplasia occurs when cells of a tissue reproduce to make up for a previous decrease in cells. An example of compensatory hyperplasia is that which occurs in liver cells after surgical removal of sections of liver tissue.

Pathologic hyperplasia can occur with excessive hormonal stimulation, which is seen in acromegaly, a connective tissue disease characterized by growth hormone excess. Excessive estrogen production may cause endometrial hyperplasia and abnormal menstrual bleeding while increased androgen may lead to benign prostatic hyperplasia.

METAPLASIA

Metaplasia is the change in a cell from one subtype to another. It usually occurs in response to some continual irritation or injury that results in chronic inflammation of the tissue. By undergoing metaplasia, cells that are better able to withstand chronic irritation and inflammation replace the original tissue. Although metaplastic cells are not cancer cells, the irritants that cause the initial change may be carcinogenic, and metaplasia is a sign of significant cellular irritation.

The most common example of metaplasia is the change in the cells of the respiratory passages from ciliated columnar epithelial cells to stratified squamous epithelial cells in response to years of cigarette smoking. The ciliated cells, essential for the removal of dirt, microorganisms, and toxins in the respiratory passages, are easily injured by cigarette smoke. Stratified epithelial cells are better able to survive smoke damage. Unfortunately, they do not assume the vital protective role of ciliated cells.

DYSPLASIA

Dysplasia is a derangement in cell growth that results in cells that differ in shape, size, and appearance from their predecessors. Dysplasia appears to occur in cells exposed to chronic irritation and inflammation. Although this cell change is not cancerous, dysplasia indicates a dangerous situation and the possibility that a cancerous condition may occur. Dysplasia is abnormal, but adaptive, and possibly reversible.

The most common sites of dysplasia are the respiratory tract (especially the squamous cells present as a result of metaplasia) and the cervix. Cervical dysplasia usually results from infection of the cells with the human papilloma virus (HPV). Dysplasia is usually rated on a scale to reflect its degree, from minor to severe.

CELL INJURY

Cell injury occurs when a cell can no longer adapt to stimuli that is too long in duration or too severe in nature. Cell injury may cause alterations in shape, size, protein synthesis, genetic makeup, and transport properties. The potential for a cell to recover is dependent on the extent and type of injury. Cellular injury may be the result of physical agents, chemical injury, radiation injury, nutritional imbalances, or injury from biological agents. Physical agents may include forceful impact, temperature extremes, or electrical injuries. Chemical injuries include drugs, lead toxicity, carbon monoxide, ethanol and mercury toxicity while radiation injury may be the result of ionizing, nonionizing, or ultraviolet (UV) radiation. Nutritional injury can be the result of excesses or deficiencies. Unfortunately, biologic agents may range from viruses to parasites and have the potential to replicate and continue the injurious process.

Biochemical mechanisms common to all types of cell injury include free radical formation, ATP depletion, altered membrane permeability, and calcium alterations. Free radicals are unstable and damage cells by chain reactions that have the potential to create more free radicals. Reactions with carbohydrates, lipids, and proteins can inactivate enzymes, damage cell membranes, and injure nucleic acids that compose DNA. Depletion of ATP causes failure of the sodium–potassium pump and the sodium–calcium exchange. This results in increased intracellular calcium and sodium and decreased potassium. The resulting cellular swelling causes vacuolation (formation of vacuoles) in the cytoplasm, mitochondrial and lysosomal swelling, and eventually, damage to the outer membrane. As calcium continues to accumulate, membrane damage continues and increases permeability.

Hypoxia (decreased oxygen concentration in the tissues) is the most common cause of cellular injury, and can be the result of decreased environmental oxygen, altered hemoglobin or hematocrit function, decreased red blood cell production, diseases or poisoning. Decreased oxygen in the blood is called *hypoxemia*. Ischemia, or reduced blood flow, is the most common cause of hypoxia. Causes of hypoxia include respiratory diseases and anything that affects blood flow, such as myocardial infarct, hemorrhagic shock, blood clots, various poisons, and some toxins released from microorganisms.

Although a small amount of oxygen is carried in a dissolved state in the blood, most oxygen is carried bound to an iron-based protein called hemoglobin, present in the red blood cell. Cells and tissues become hypoxic when there is inadequate intake of oxygen by the respiratory system, inadequate delivery of oxygen by the cardiovascular system, or a lack of hemoglobin.

Oxygen is required by the mitochondria for oxidative phosphorylation and the production of ATP. Without oxygen, this process cannot occur. Although some ATP will be produced through anaerobic glycolysis, this is an inefficient source of ATP and cannot support the cellular energy requirements if there is a prolonged period of hypoxia.

When cells are deprived of ATP, they can no longer maintain cellular functions, including the transport of sodium and potassium through the sodium–potassium pump. Without sodium–potassium pumping, cells begin to accumulate sodium as it diffuses into the cell down its concentration and electrical gradients. The electrical potential across the membrane begins to decrease as intracellular sodium, a positive ion, accumulates. Osmotic pressure inside the cell increases, drawing water into the cell. Ischemic cells (those deprived of oxygen or blood supply) begin to swell, resulting in dilation of the endoplasmic reticulum, decreased mitochondrial function, and increased permeability of intracellular membranes.

Another consequence of hypoxia is the production of lactic acid, which occurs during anaerobic glycolysis. Increased lactic acid causes cellular and blood pH levels to decrease. Decreased intracellular pH (increased acidity) causes damage to the nuclear structures, the cellular membranes, and the microfilaments. An alteration in pH can also affect the electrical potential across the membrane.

The effects of hypoxia are reversible if oxygen is returned within a certain period of time, the amount of which varies and depends on the tissue. However, cell swelling can lead to bursting of lysosomal vesicles, release of their enzymes, and lysis (bursting) of the cell. Cell death is marked by higher than normal levels of intracellular enzymes in the general circulation.

CELL DEATH

The two main categories of cell death are necrosis or apoptosis. Necrotic cell death occurs when injurious stimuli to a cell are too intense or prolonged. It is characterized by cell swelling and rupture of internal organelles, most obviously the mitochondria, and by marked stimulation of the inflammatory response. The second category of cell death, apoptosis, is programmed cell death, a process in which an orderly sequence of molecular steps occurs, leading to cellular disintegration. Apoptosis is not characterized by swelling or inflammation, but rather the dying cell shrinks on itself and is engulfed by neighboring cells. Apoptosis is responsible for keeping cell numbers relatively constant and is a mechanism by which unwanted cells, aged cells, dangerous cells, or cells carrying a mistake in DNA transcription can be eliminated. It is an active process, in which the cell itself participates, and draws its name from a Greek word meaning "fallen apart." Interference with apoptosis may contribute to carcinogenesis.

Thymidine phosphorylase (TP), a platelet-derived endothelial cell growth factor, has been discovered to protect cells from undergoing apoptosis by stimulating nucleoside metabolism and angiogenesis. The use of drugs that specifically target TP has been recommended to improve the effects of conventional chemotherapy by enhancing the apoptosis of mutated cells.

Causes of Necrotic Cell Death

Common causes of necrotic cell death include prolonged hypoxia, infection leading to the production of toxins and free radicals, and disruption in membrane integrity, the ultimate result of which is cellular bursting. Typically, the immune and inflammatory responses often stimulated by necrosis lead to further injury and death of neighboring cells. Necrotic cell death can be widespread in the body without causing death of the individual.

Causes of Apoptosis

Programmed cell death begins during embryogenesis and continues throughout the lifetime of an organism. Stimuli that initiate apoptosis include hormonal cues, antigen stimulation, immune peptides, and membrane signals that identify aging or mutated cells. Viral infection of a cell will often turn on apoptosis, ultimately leading to the death of the virus and the host cell. This is one way living organisms have evolved to fight viral infection. Certain viruses (e.g., the Epstein–Barr virus responsible for mononucleosis) have in turn evolved to produce specialized proteins that deactivate the apoptosis response. Deficiencies in apoptosis have been implicated in the development of cancer and in neurodegenerative diseases of unknown origin, including Alzheimer disease and amyotrophic lateral sclerosis (Lou Gehrig disease). Antigen-stimulated apoptosis of immune cells (T and B cells) is essential for the development and maintenance of immune self-tolerance.

Results of Cell Death

Dead cells liquefy or coagulate and are removed from the area or isolated from the rest of the tissue by immune cells in the process of phagocytosis. If mitosis is possible and the area of necrosis is not too large, new cells of the same type fill in the empty space. Scar tissue will form in the vacated space if cell division is impossible or if the area of necrosis is extensive.

Gangrene refers to the death of a large mass of cells. Gangrene may be classified as dry or wet. Dry gangrene spreads slowly with few symptoms and is frequently seen in the extremities, often as a result of prolonged hypoxia. Wet gangrene is a rapidly spreading area of dead tissue, often of internal organs, and is associated with bacterial invasion of the dead tissue. It exudes a strong odor and is usually accompanied by systemic manifestations. Wet gangrene may develop from dry gangrene. Gas gangrene is a special type of gangrene that occurs in response to an infection of the tissue by a type of anaerobic bacteria called *Clostridium*. It is seen most often after significant trauma. Gas gangrene rapidly spreads to neighboring tissue as the bacteria release deadly toxins that kill neighboring cells. Muscle cells are especially susceptible and release characteristic hydrogen sulfide gas when affected. This type of gangrene may prove fatal.

WOUND REPAIR

Destroyed or injured tissues are repaired by regeneration of the same type of cells or by deposition of connective tissue that forms scar tissue. The goal of both types of repair is to fill in the areas of damage in order to return structural integrity to the tissue.

Tissue regeneration and scar formation begin with inflammatory reactions (see Chapter 4). Platelets control bleeding and white blood cells digest and remove dead tissue in the area. Growth factors and immune peptides (cytokines) (see Chapter 3) are released that draw healing cells to the area. Other factors are produced to stimulate mitosis or scar tissue formation.

Types of Wound Repair

Tissues that heal cleanly and quickly are said to heal by primary intention. Large wounds that heal slowly and with a great deal of scar tissue heal by secondary intention.

Delayed Healing and Repair

Tissue repair can be delayed if the host is compromised in any way by malnutrition, systemic disease such as diabetes, or a poorly functioning immune system. Healing can also be poor or delayed if there is reduced blood flow to the injured tissue or if an infection develops.

● Conditions of Disease or Injury

POISONING

Various poisons have the potential to cause hypoxia. Cyanide poisoning occurs as a result of the chemical reaction between cyanide and the final substrate in the electron transport chain. Without this final step, oxidative phosphorylation ceases and ATP is not produced in the mitochondria. Cyanide blocks the use of intracellular oxygen and circulating oxyhemoglobin. Cyanide is present in the seeds of many fruits such as apricots and some apple seeds. Laetrile, an unproven therapy for cancer, is made from the pits of apricots and contains enough cyanide to be fatal.

Carbon monoxide is colorless and odorless until mixed with a pollutant. Poisoning occurs when carbon monoxide is inhaled and binds to oxygen sites on the hemoglobin molecule. The affinity of hemoglobin for carbon monoxide is 300 times greater than that for oxygen so that even small amounts of carbon monoxide quickly result in a high percentage of carboxyhemoglobin (COHb). Exposure to carbon monoxide decreases the binding and transport of oxygen in the blood, causing cellular and tissue hypoxia. The fetus is at an even greater risk because fetal COHb levels may be up to 15% greater than maternal levels. Carbon monoxide is a product of cigarette smoke, defective heating systems, automobile exhaust, and other environmental substances. The most common cause of inadvertent carbon monoxide poisoning is smoke inhalation.

Lead is a heavy metal and even small amounts can easily reach the toxic level. Absorption occurs via the lungs and the gastrointestinal (GI) tract. GI absorption is greater with calcium, vitamin D, zinc, or iron deficiencies. Approximately 85% of lead is stored in bone with the other 15% settling in the blood and soft tissue. Lead is eliminated by the kidneys. It competes with calcium, inactivates enzymes, interferes with nerve transmission and impairs brain development. A cardinal sign of lead toxicity is anemia as it competes with the enzyme necessary for hemoglobin synthesis. Other organs affected include the GI tract, kidneys, and the nervous system. Large doses of lead also cause red blood cell lysis with resultant severe hypoxia. Some sources of lead include lead-based paint, glazed pottery making, printing shops, plastic blinds, plumbing, and engine repair.

Mercury is a neurotoxin and has the potential to damage the kidneys and the GI tract. Inhaled mercury vapor is carried by the blood and accumulates in the brain. Sources of mercury exposure may include dental amalgams, fish consumption, and vaccines. The major source of mercury toxicity is fish consumption such as contaminated tuna and swordfish. The greatest risk is for young children and pregnant and nursing women because the developing brain is more susceptible to damage from mercury. Most vaccines are now free of the preservative thimerosal that contains ethyl mercury.

Clinical Manifestations

- Cyanide poisoning:
  - Choking sensation with accelerated respirations, then gasping
  - Cherry-red appearance
  - Odor of bitter almonds
  - Altered mental status
  - Lactic acidosis
  - Cardiovascular instability
  - Brown-tinged blood with hydrogen cyanide poisoning
- Carbon monoxide poisoning:
  - Accelerated respirations
  - Ringing in the ears
  - Headache
  - Giddiness
  - Malaise

- Dizziness
- Confusion
- Nausea
- Weakness
- Vomiting
- Respirations quickly cease and unconsciousness develops
- Elevated COHb levels
- Lead poisoning:
  - Headaches
  - Irritability
  - Fatigue
  - Abdominal cramping
  - Constipation
  - Vomiting
  - Weight loss
  - Tremors
  - Paresthesia
  - Neuritis
  - Hyperactivity
  - Anorexia
  - Lead line on gums
  - Muscle cramps
  - Joint pain
- Mercury poisoning (symptoms vary with cause):
  - Impaired peripheral vision
  - Tremors
  - Neuromuscular changes
  - Muscular atrophy
  - Headaches
  - Skin rash
  - Dermatitis
  - Memory loss
  - Disturbance in sensation

Complications

- Altered consciousness progressing to coma and death if prolonged cerebral (brain) hypoxia occurs.

- Organ failure, including adult respiratory distress syndrome, cardiac failure, or kidney failure, may occur if hypoxia is prolonged.
- Carbon monoxide poisoning: acute myocardial injury with increased long-term mortality.

Treatment

- Prompt removal from the source of poisoning.
- Increase oxygen in inspired air through a mask or mechanical ventilation.
- For cyanide poisoning, nitrates and sodium thiosulfate therapy.
- For carbon monoxide poisoning, hyperbaric (high pressure) oxygen treatments.
- For lead poisoning, emetics to induce vomiting in acute poisoning.
- For chronic lead poisoning conditions, various chelating agents (which remove lead from the circulation).
- For mercury poisoning, chelation therapy.

TEMPERATURE EXTREMES

Extreme heat or cold has the potential to injure or kill cells. Exposure to very cold temperatures injures cells in two ways. First, cold exposure causes constriction of the blood vessels that deliver nutrients and oxygen to the extremities. This constriction occurs as the body attempts to preserve its core (central) temperature, initially at the expense of the fingers, toes, ears, and nose. Decreased blood flow causes cellular and tissue ischemia. Sluggish blood flow also increases the risk of clot formation, which further blocks tissue oxygenation. The second effect of exposure to very cold temperature is the formation of ice crystals in the cells. These crystals directly damage the cells and can lead to cell lysis (bursting). Prolonged exposure to the cold can lead to hypothermia.

Clinical Manifestations of Cold Exposure and Hypothermia

- Numbness or tingling of the skin or extremities.
- Pale or blue skin that is cool to the touch.
- Shivering early on, then lack of shivering as condition worsens.
- Decreased level of consciousness, drowsiness, and confusion.

Complications of Cold Exposure and Hypothermia

- Blood clotting, characterized by pain and a decrease in pulse downstream from the clot. If blood flow is inadequate for an extended time, gangrene may result.
- Frostbite.
- Ventricular dysrhythmia.

Treatment for Cold Exposure and Hypothermia

- Prevention.
- Transport immediately to a hospital for active rewarming. Any individual who appears dead who may have suffered hypothermia needs to be evaluated at a medical facility and rewarmed to 32°C before being confirmed dead.
- During transport to a clinical facility, wet clothing should be removed and the patient should be covered with blankets. Active rewarming is discouraged until the patient reaches the treatment facility. Warm humidified air or oxygen may be administered during transport.
- For a blood clot, drugs to dissolve the clot may be necessary.
- For gangrene, antibiotics and possible amputation are required.
- Cardiopulmonary resuscitation may be necessary if the patient is in ventricular fibrillation.

Local exposure to very high temperatures can cause burn injuries, which directly kill cells or indirectly injure or kill cells by causing coagulation of blood vessels or the breakdown of cell membranes (see Chapter 5). Systemically, an increased core temperature, known as hyperthermia, can result in nerve damage, coagulation of cell proteins, and even death. Hyperthermia may be the result of excessive environmental heat, accelerated heat production or impaired dissipation of heat. Hyperthermia may be accidental, associated with stroke or head injury, or therapeutic, although this is still a controversial topic. Accidental hyperthermia includes heat cramps, heat exhaustion, heat stroke, drug reaction, and malignant hyperthermia.

Heat cramps are the result of prolonged sweating that leads to excessive sodium loss. Severe cramps in the abdomen and extremities occur due to the sodium loss. With heat exhaustion, prolonged elevated core temperature → (leads to) profound vasodilation and sweating → dehydration → decreased plasma volume → hypotension → decreased cardiac output → tachycardia.

Heat stroke is the result of a thermoregulatory center that is unable to function, causing an extremely elevated core temperature of >40° C. It is potentially life-threatening and damage is most likely the result of cytokine release.

A fever that begins with the administration of a medication and subsides when the medication is discontinued is most likely a drug fever. Drugs such as exogenous thyroid hormone, amphetamines, anticholinergics, tricyclic antidepressants, and vaccines may interfere with heat dissipation, alter temperature regulation in the hypothalamus, act as pyrogens, or induce an immune response.

Malignant hyperthermia is an inherited disorder that can be triggered by general anesthesia or depolarizing muscle relaxants. Altered calcium function results in increased muscle work, increased oxygen consumption, and elevated lactic acid levels. Acidosis and elevated body temperature may result in tachycardia, hypotension, cardiac dysrhythmias, and, if untreated, cardiac arrest.

Clinical Manifestations of Heat Exposure and Hyperthermia

- Heat cramps
  - Tender muscles
  - Sweaty skin
  - Normal or slightly elevated body temperature
  - Fever
  - Rapid pulse
  - Increased blood pressure
- Heat exhaustion
  - Thirst
  - Fatigue
  - Nausea
  - Oliguria
  - Giddiness
  - Weakness
  - Dizziness
  - Confusion
  - Fainting
  - Moist skin
  - Elevated temperature
  - May also exhibit signs of heat cramps
  - Delirium
- Heat stroke
  - Cerebral edema
  - CNS degeneration
  - Dendrite swelling
  - Renal tubular necrosis
  - Death
- Malignant hyperthermia
  - Elevated body temperature
  - Tachycardia
  - Hypotension
  - Unconsciousness
  - Absent reflexes
  - Fixed pupils
  - Apnea
  - Oliguria or anuria

Treatment for Heat Exposure and Hyperthermia

- Prevention
  - Remove from the heat source
  - Avoid outside activities during extreme heat
  - Increase fluid intake
  - Proper clothing for the temperature
  - Oral saline solution for heat cramps
- Malignant hyperthermia
  - Stop anesthesia
  - 100% O_2
  - Dantrolene sodium
  - Cooling blanket
  - Contact Malignant Hyperthermia Association of the United States for more information

RADIATION INJURY

Radiation is the transmission of energy through the emission of rays or waves. Radiation energy may be in the visible range of light, or it may be higher or lower energy than visible light. High-energy radiation (including UV radiation) is called ionizing radiation because it has the capability of knocking electrons off atoms or molecules, thereby ionizing them. Low-energy radiation is called non-ionizing radiation because it cannot displace electrons off atoms or molecules.

Effects of Ionizing Radiation

Ionizing radiation may injure or kill cells directly by destroying the cell membrane and causing intracellular swelling and cell lysis. As cells are killed or injured, the inflammatory response is stimulated, causing capillary leakiness, interstitial edema, white blood cell accumulation, and tissue scarring. Ionizing radiation may also act indirectly on cells by damaging the bonds between the base pairs of the DNA molecules, leading to mistakes in DNA replication or transcription. These mistakes may be repaired; if not, damage may cause programmed cell death or subsequent cancer as a result of the loss of genetic control over cell division.

Ionizing radiation also can cause the production of free radicals, either directly or as a result of cell injury and inflammation. A free radical is a highly reactive atom or molecule with an unpaired electron. The free radical seeks out reactions whereby it may gain back an electron. Sequential reactions may occur, where a series of free radicals are produced. Once produced, a free radical can engage in an energy-rich collision with another molecule, destroying intramolecular bonds. This may ultimately damage the cell membrane, the endoplasmic reticulum, or the DNA of a susceptible cell. It is thought that DNA errors resulting from free radical damage may be involved in the development of some cancers. It is also hypothesized that the free radical production that occurs during the normal metabolism of lipids may damage the endothelial cells lining the blood vessels, leading to atherosclerosis.

Free radicals also accumulate in response to infectious agents and hypoxia. For example, during a period of reduced blood flow, lack of oxygen causes cellular injury or death. If blood flow is restored, free radical production is stimulated by the white blood cells that swarm to the area as part of the inflammatory response; this accumulation of free radicals leads to serious reperfusion injury and a worsening of tissue damage. Free radicals also are produced as a result of exposure to cigarette smoke and are present in many pesticides.

Normally, cells have in place mechanisms to eradicate free radicals or to minimize their effects. Vitamins E, C, and beta-carotene are known as free radical scavengers and are believed to protect cells against the damaging effects of free radicals.

UV radiation can cause sunburn and increase the risk of skin cancer. UV radiation most likely damages the skin by reactive oxygen species and by damaging the melanin-producing process in the skin. It also damages DNA.

Cells Susceptible to Ionizing Radiation

Cells most susceptible to damage by ionizing radiation are cells that undergo frequent divisions, including cells of the GI tract, the integument (skin and hair), and the blood-forming cells of the bone marrow.

Ionizing radiation is emitted by the sun, in x-rays, and in substances undergoing radioactive decay, including substances found in the soil and rocks and those produced by nuclear weapons and reactors. Ionizing radiation is also emitted by substances used in medical diagnosis and treatment.

Clinical Manifestations of Ionizing Radiation

- Skin redness or breakdown.
- With high doses, vomiting and nausea caused by GI damage.
- Anemia if the bone marrow is destroyed.
- Cancer may develop years after the exposure as a result of the production of chromosomal breaks, deletions, or translocations.

Treatment

- Damage caused by low doses will be repaired by the cells and does not require treatment.
- Cancers should be treated with radiation therapy, chemotherapy, immunotherapy, or surgery.

Effects of Nonionizing Radiation

Nonionizing radiation includes microwave and ultrasound radiation. The energy of this radiation is too low to break DNA bonds or damage the cell membrane, but may increase the temperature of a system, causing alterations in transport functions. Nonionizing radiation does not appear to cause health hazards, but research in this area is ongoing.

INJURY CAUSED BY MICROORGANISMS

Microorganisms infectious to humans include prions, bacteria, viruses, mycoplasmas, rickettsiae, chlamydiae, fungi, and protozoa. Some of these organisms infect humans through direct access, such as inhalation, whereas others infect through transmission by an intermediate vector, such as an insect bite.

Cells of the body may be destroyed directly by the microorganism or by a toxin released from the microorganism, or may be indirectly injured as a result of the immune and inflammatory reactions stimulated in response to the microorganism (see Chapter 4). In addition, as described earlier, infection of a cell by a microorganism may so destabilize the cell that it undergoes apoptosis.

Prions

Prions are protein particles that appear to have no genetic master plan. Prions may be inherited or may be the result of converted normal protein. Research is still being conducted to gain understanding of how prions replicate and reproduce. Without reproductive and metabolic functions, antimicrobial agents have not been found to be effective. In humans, a prion-associated disease is Creutzfeldt–Jakob that causes a slowly progressive neuronal degradation with resulting ataxia, dementia, and eventually, death.

Bacteria

Bacteria are free-living, one-celled organisms that reproduce on their own, but use animal hosts for nutrient access. Bacteria contain no nuclei. They consist of cytoplasm surrounded by a rigid cell wall made out of a specific substance called peptidoglycan. Inside the cytoplasm is the genetic material, both DNA and RNA, and the intracellular structures needed for energy metabolism. Bacteria reproduce asexually by DNA replication and simple cell division. Some bacteria synthesize a capsule that surrounds the cell wall, making it less susceptible to the host's immune system. Other bacteria secrete proteins that reduce their susceptibility to standard antibiotics. Bacteria can be aerobic or anaerobic. Bacteria often release toxins specifically damaging to the host.

Laboratories frequently classify bacteria as gram-positive or gram-negative. Gram-positive bacteria release toxins (exotoxins) that damage host cells. Gram-negative bacteria contain in their cell walls proteins that stimulate the inflammatory response (endotoxins). They may also secrete exotoxins. Gram-positive bacteria stain purple with a standard laboratory dye. Gram-negative bacteria stain red with a second laboratory dye.

Examples of human disease caused by bacteria include staphylococcal and streptococcal infections, gonorrhea, syphilis, cholera, plague, salmonellosis, shigellosis, typhoid fever, Legionnaire disease, diphtheria, *Haemophilus influenzae* infection, pertussis, tetanus, and Lyme disease. In a subset of especially difficult-to-treat bacteria are the mycobacteria. These microorganisms cause tuberculosis and leprosy. Studies have shown that human susceptibility to some bacterial infections, including those caused by *Mycobacterium* and *Salmonella*, is genetically controlled. Other superimposing variables that influence bacterial infectivity include host nutritional status, co-infections, exposure to environmental microbes, and previous vaccinations.

Spirochetes

Spirochetes are a special type of gram-negative bacteria with a distinct helical shape. Depending on the specific genus, spirochetes have the potential to infect animals and/or humans. Lyme disease and syphilis are caused by two different genera.

Viruses

Viruses, unlike bacteria, require a host to reproduce. A virus consists of a single strand of DNA or RNA that is contained within a protein coat called a capsid. Viruses must bind to the host cell membrane, enter the cell, and then move into the host cell nucleus to reproduce. Once inside the nucleus, viral DNA can become incorporated into the host cell DNA, thus ensuring that viral genes will be passed to each daughter cell during mitosis. Once in the DNA, the virus begins to take over the functions of the cell. RNA viruses also begin to control cell function after their translation into proteins.

Examples of human disease caused by viruses include encephalitis, yellow fever, German measles, rubella, mumps, poliomyelitis, hepatitis, and many viral respiratory infections. Certain types of viruses can enter the host DNA and remain latent for years, producing infections occasionally or not at all. Viruses that remain latent include all those of the herpes family, including the herpes viruses responsible for varicella (chickenpox), zoster (shingles), cytomegalovirus, mononucleosis, and the herpes simplex viruses 1 and 2, which produce oral cold sores and genital herpes.

Retroviruses

A unique type of virus is the retrovirus. These viruses are RNA viruses that can incorporate into the host DNA as a result of the action of the enzyme reverse transcriptase that changes the viral RNA into DNA. Retroviruses carry reverse transcriptase as part of their structure.

Examples of human disease caused by retroviruses include acquired immunodeficiency syndrome (AIDS), caused by the human immunodeficiency virus (HIV), and a form of leukemia, HTLV-I. Retroviruses also may remain dormant for long periods of time.

Mycoplasmas

Mycoplasmas are unicellular microorganisms similar in action to bacteria but much smaller and without the peptidoglycan cell wall. Because many antibiotics (e.g., the penicillins) act by destroying the peptidoglycan cell wall, mycoplasmas are insensitive to these antibiotics.

Examples of human disease caused by mycoplasmas include mycoplasma pneumonia, upper respiratory tract infections, and some genital infections.

Rickettsiae

Rickettsiae require a host to asexually reproduce. They contain RNA and DNA inside a rigid peptidoglycan cell wall. Rickettsiae are transmitted to humans through the bite of the flea, tick, or louse. Examples of human disease caused by rickettsiae include typhus and Rocky Mountain spotted fever.

Chlamydiae

Chlamydiae are unicellular organisms that reproduce asexually inside a host cell. They transmit directly to humans and undergo cycles of replication. Human diseases caused by chlamydiae include a sexually transmitted urogenital infection and pneumonia.

Fungi

Fungi include yeast and molds. Fungi contain a nucleus and are surrounded by a rigid cell wall. Fungi usually do not cause disease in healthy humans, and some fungi are considered normal human flora. Most fungal infections are superficial, but some may be deep, causing infection of vital organs and tissues.

Superficial fungal infections in humans include oral (thrush) and vaginal candidiasis (yeast infections) and infections of the skin such as ringworm (tinea corporis), athlete's foot (tinea pedis), and jock itch. Onychomycosis refers to fungal infection of the toenails and fingernails.

Deep fungal infections are common in individuals who are immunocompromised. These infections are considered to be opportunistic (produced by organisms that only proliferate if the immune response is poor). Deep, opportunistic fungal infections in humans include the respiratory infections histoplasmosis and coccidioidomycosis, which are common in individuals with AIDS. Systemic and brain fungal infections may also occur.

Parasites

The term parasite refers to protozoa, helminths, and arthropods.

Protozoans are unicellular organisms capable of causing infections. Infection is passed directly between individuals through contaminated food or water, or through an insect vector. Examples of human disease caused by protozoans include malaria and the intestinal disease giardiasis.

Helminths are worms that require a host to sexually reproduce. Transmission to humans occurs through ingestion or penetration of the skin. Examples of human disease caused by helminths include roundworm (nematodes) and tapeworm (cestodes). Helminths are a significant problem in developing countries.

Arthropods are ticks and mosquitoes that act as vectors to carry diseases to humans. Examples of human disease carried by arthropods include bubonic plague (caused by a bacillus) and typhus (caused by a rickettsia). Other arthropods infect and damage body surfaces by their bite or burrowing. Arthropods that infect body surfaces include lice, scabies, chiggers, and fleas.

Clinical Manifestations

Clinical manifestations of infection depend on the specific agent involved, the site of the infection, and the health of the host.

Infection by bacteria, viruses, and mycoplasmas often results in:

- Regional lymph node enlargement
- Fever (usually low-grade with a viral infection)
- Body aches
- Skin rash or eruption, especially with viral infections
- Site-specific responses, such as pharyngitis, cough, otitis media

Infection by chlamydia often results in:

- Urethritis (inflammation of the urethra) in males
- Cervicitis (inflammation of the cervix), often with a mucopurulent discharge and itching or burning during urination

Infection by rickettsia often results in:

- Skin rash
- Fever and chills
- Headache
- Myalgia (muscle aches)
- Thrombus formation in any organ

Infection by fungi often results in:

- Itching and redness of skin or scalp with superficial infections
- Discoloration and thickening with superficial nail infections
- Creamy white vaginal discharge with a yeast infection
- White plaques on inside of mouth with oral thrush
- Signs of pneumonia with deep infections or in an immunocompromised host

Infection with parasites often results in:

- Diarrhea with intestinal parasites
- Fever with malaria
- Itching and rash with skin infections

Treatment

- Bacteria and mycoplasmas are treated with antibiotics, preferably after culturing the infection to determine what the infecting microorganism is and to what antibiotic it is sensitive.
- Certain viral infections may be treated with antiviral agents. Other viral infections usually are left to resolve naturally with care taken that a subsequent bacterial infection does not infect the original site or elsewhere.
- Rickettsiae are usually treated with the antibiotic tetracycline.
- Fungi are treated with topical antifungals, such as nystatin for superficial skin infections and amphotericin B for systemic infections. Oral antifungals are available for treating nail infections, which previously were resistant to treatment. These new therapies, including terbinafine and itraconazole, have a high cure rate, even with sporadic dosing regimens. Pentamidine is used for *Pneumocystis carinii*.
- Parasitic infections of the GI tract are treated with specific agents, including metronidazole (Flagyl) for giardiasis. Malaria is treated with various antimalarial drugs. Prophylactic (preventative) therapy is recommended for individuals traveling to areas where malaria is common. Plague is treated with various antibiotics, including tetracycline. Skin infections are treated with various topical agents.

G *GERIATRIC CONSIDERATION*

- Wound healing in the elderly may be delayed due to:
  - reduced blood flow
  - reduced tissue oxygenation caused by systemic diseases such as diabetes mellitus or atherosclerosis

- reduced immune function
- poor nutrition
- medications that may delay the normal healing process
- increased risk for heat-related problems due to poor circulation

---

P PEDIATRIC CONSIDERATION

- Children are at an increased risk of suffering lead poisoning because lead is absorbed more rapidly through their intestine and they are attracted to lead's sweet taste in paint. Children are also closer to and more frequently sitting on the ground where lead tends to accumulate in the soil and dust. Pediatric lead exposure may lead to learning disabilities and behavioral problems.

- Fetal cells rapidly undergo cellular replication and division and are highly susceptible to the damaging effects of ionizing radiation. Infants and young children also experience periods of rapid cellular growth and proliferation and are at risk of genetic damage from ionizing radiation. Studies suggest that there are no apparent health risks to fetuses exposed to nonionizing radiation (i.e., when a pregnant woman uses an electric blanket or video display terminal), at least in moderation.

- Infants and children are a greater risk for overheating.

SELECTED BIBLIOGRAPHY

Akerstrom, T., Steensberg, A., Keller, P., Keller, C., Penkowa, M., & Pedersen, B. K. (2005). Exercise induces interleukin-8-expression in human skeletal muscle. *Journal of Physiology*, 563, 507–516.

Andrew, A. S., Jewell, D. A., Mason, R. A., Whitfield, M. L., Moore, J. H., & Karagas, M. R. (2008). Drinking-water arsenic exposure modulates gene expression in human lymphocytes from a U. S. population. *Environmental Health Perspectives*, 116(4), 524–531.

Anderson-Pompa, K., Foster, A., Parker, L., Wilks, L., & Cheek, D. J. (2008). Genetics and susceptibility to malignant hyperthermia. *Critical Care Nurse*, 28(6), 32–37.

Baker, J. P. (2008). Mercury, vaccines, and autism: One controversy, three histories. *American Journal of Public Health*, 98(2), 244–253.

Balk, S. J., Forman, J. A., Johnson, C. L., & Roberts, J. R. (2007). Safeguarding kids from environmental hazards. *Comtemporary Pediatrics*, 24(3), 64–78.

Cescon, D. W., & Juurlink, D. N. (2009). Discoloration of skin and urine after treatment with hydroxocobalamin for cyanide poisoning. *Canadian Medical Association Journal*, 180(2), 251.

Copstead, L. C., & Banasik, J. L. (2010). *Pathophysiology*. St. Louis: Saunders Elsevier.

Cyngiser, T. A. (2008). Creutzfeldt–Jakob disease: A disease overview. *American Journal of Electroneurodiagnostic Technology*, 48, 199–208.

Davani, S., Deschaseaux, F., Chalmers, D., Tiberghien, P., & Kantelip, J. -P. (2005). Can stem cells mend a broken heart? *Cardiovascular Research*, 65, 305–316.

De Wardener, H. E., He, F. J., & Macgregor, G. A. (2004). Plasma sodium and hypertension. *Kidney International*, 66, 2454–2466.

Eliopoulos, C. (2010). *Gerontological nursing* (7th ed.). Philadelphia: Wolters Kluwer Health/Lippincott Williams & Wilkins.

Guyton, A. C., & Hall, J. E. (2005). *Textbook of medical physiology* (11th ed.). Philadelphia: W.B. Saunders.

Jenkins, J., Grady, P. A., & Collins, F. S. (2005). Nurses and the genomic revolution. *Journal of Nursing Scholarship*, 37(2), 98–101.

Huether, S. E., & McCance, K. L. (2008). *Understanding pathophysiology* (4th ed.). St. Louis: Mosby Elsevier.

Loo, D. S. (2007). Onychomycosis in the elderly: Drug treatment options. *Drugs Aging*, 24(4), 293–302.

Martin-Rendon, E., Brunskill, S., Doree, C., Hyde, C., Mathur, A., Stanworth, S., et al. (2008). Stem cell treatment for acute myocardial infarction. *Cochran Database of Systemic Reviews*, 2008, Issue 4. Art. No.: CD006536. DOI: 10.1002/14651858. CDC006536.pub2.

Miller, A. T., Saadai, P., Greenstein, A., & Divino, C. M. (2008). Postprocedural necrotizing fasciitis: A 10-year retrospective review. *The American Surgeon*, 74(5), 405–409.

Morris, K., (2008). George Daley: Individualising stem-cell research. *Lancet*, 372(9656), 2107.

Ng, D. K., Chan, C., Soo, M., & Lee, R. S. (2007). Low-level chronic mercury exposure in children and adolescents: Meta-analysis. *Pediatrics International*, 49, 80–87.

Patton, K. T., & Thibodeau, G. A. (2010). *Anatomy and physiology* (7th ed.). St. Louis: Mosby.

Porth, C. M., & Matfin, G. (2009). *Pathophysiology: Concepts of altered health states* (8th ed.). Philadelphia: Lippincott Williams & Wilkins.

Reinisch, C. E. (2008). Carbon monoxide poisoning: Implications for patient and family care in the emergency department. *Clinical Scholars Review*, 1(1), 46–49.

Tabloski, P. A. (2010). *Gerontological nursing* (2nd ed.). Upper Saddle River, NJ: Pearson.

Toi, M., Rahman, M. A., Bando, H., & Chow, L. W. C. (2005). Thymidine phosphorylase and platelet-derived endothelial cell growth factor in cancer biology and treatment. *Lancet Oncology*, 6, 158–166.

Viktorsson, K., Lewensohn, R., & Zhivotovsky, B. (2005). Apoptotic pathways and therapy resistance in human malignancies. *Advanced Cancer Research*, 94, 143–196.

von Zglinicki, T., Saretzki, G., Ladhoff, J., d'Adda di Fagagna, F., & Jackson, S. P. (2005). Human cell senescence as a DNA damage response. *Mechanisms of Ageing and Development*, 126, 111–117.

Genetics

Genetics is the study of genes. Genes are biological units that direct the synthesis of specific proteins. Genes are located inside chromosomes that contain the deoxyribonucleic acid (DNA) that transmits hereditary characteristics. Genes are passed from parent to offspring and determine identity and function at the most basic cellular level. Transmission of genetic information is a balance between ensuring that genes are passed error-free between the generations and allowing enough diversity for the adaptation and survival of the species. Sometimes mistakes (mutations) are made that advance the species—for example, mutations have resulted in several malaria-protective genes that offer evolutionary advantage, but in most cases mutations cause significant disability or death.

Genomics, the study of multiple genes and how they interact with the environment, offers insight into the study of complex diseases. Since the initiation of the Human Genome Project (HGP), specific genes for diseases such as cystic fibrosis, diabetes, Huntington disease, and some inheritable types of breast and colon cancer have been identified. It is anticipated that additional research will be helpful in identifying the most effective cancer treatment with the least potential for toxicity.

● The Human Genome Project

In 1987, the United States Congressional advisory committee recommended a multidisciplinary, scientific, and technological endeavor aimed at sequencing the human genome (all DNA contained in an organism). This recommendation resulted in the HGP that began in 1989 and offered insight into the link between genes and numerous diseases.

APPLICATIONS

According to the National Institute of Health, this 13-year project has resulted in the identification of over 1800 genes linked to diseases and the development of approximately 1000 genetic tests.

The project has further prompted extensive research into the use of gene therapy in which viruses are used to carry genes into the cells. For example, in two separate studies gene transfer therapy was found to be effective in halting retinal degeneration and improving visual acuity in young adults with Leber's congenital amaurosis (optic neuropathy). Gene therapy is designed to replace missing or defective genes. As a result of the HGP, the HapNap project is now focusing on various diseases worldwide. As research continues, the focus will be on genomic scanning to prevent and/or diagnose early, perfecting gene therapy, and gaining more insight into drug discovery based on specific gene targets. Some predict that within 20 years, patients entering a medical facility will be subjected to a genomic scanning for pathogenic and "epistatic" genes. Epistasis refers to the tendency of some genes to interact and cross over with genes other than their allelic partners. Epistasis appears to affect certain diseases positively or negatively and has the potential to result in variable intensities of disease in different ethnicities and individuals.

One area of genomics that has progressed more slowly than anticipated is that involving drug discovery based on specific gene targets unveiled by the HGP. Progress in this area has been slow for a number of reasons. First, the complexity of the human physiologic system has proven to be a bit daunting, perhaps accounting for the fact that most of the highly effective drugs on the market today, such as aspirin, act on multiple gene systems rather than on single-gene disorders. The tendency of genes to experience epistatic interactions has also hindered the pace of drug production through gene targeting.

ETHICAL IMPLICATIONS

Results of the HGP will have enormous ethical implications for prenatal testing and selective abortion of defective embryos. Ethical implications are also involved in testing concerned adults who seek to know the likelihood of their developing a specific disease, such as Huntington disease, in the future. This is especially troubling if the identified disease is one for which there is no treatment or cure, or if testing involves children. For adults and children with disease-causing mutations, future childbearing choices, the ability to purchase health insurance or life insurance, and the ability to find future employment are important considerations. The HGP has dedicated funding and time to explore the ethical factors involved in gene mapping. In the fall of 2005, a study was initiated by the National Human Genome Research Institute among healthy adult volunteers to sequence 100 to 300 genes that have been associated with various disease phenotypes. The aim is to provide information to individuals on potential genetic risk factors and to evaluate how this enormous amount of information is handled by the patients and their families.

● Physiologic Concepts

GENES

There are approximately 25,000 genes in the human genome, with each gene containing a few hundred to a few thousand base pairs of DNA. This is a much smaller number of genes than expected, given the complexity of the human genome. The DNA of a given gene includes coding portions, called exons, and noncoding portions. The coding portions of a gene carry the information needed to make a protein, often an enzyme. Enzymes and other proteins control the synthesis and function of each and every cell or tissue of the body. The function of the millions of molecules of noncoding DNA is unclear. Many genes grouped together make up the chromosomes.

CHROMOSOMES

Chromosomes are made up of molecules of DNA, complexed with proteins called histones. Chromosomes carry the genetic blueprint of an individual. All human somatic (body) cells contain 23 pairs of chromosomes, one pair from each parent, for a total of 46 chromosomes. Of the 23 pairs of chromosomes, 22 are the same in both sexes. The 23rd pair consists of the sex chromosome, X or Y. The female has two X chromosomes and the male has one X and one Y. Each human sex cell, an egg or a sperm, contains 23 unpaired chromosomes. Each chromosome is nearly identical (approximately 99.9%) across the human species in the genetic information it contains. The remaining variations are subtle but enough to make each one of us unique.

GENE ACTIVATION

Although each somatic cell contains the same 23 pairs of chromosomes, only certain genes are activated in any given cell; therefore, only certain proteins or enzymes are produced by that cell. Which genes are activated in which cell is determined during embryologic development and throughout life by circulating growth factors, hormones, and chemical cues produced by a given cell and its neighboring cells. In addition, methylation of certain regions of a gene (adding a CH_3 group) can turn off, or silence, that gene. Demethylating the region can activate that gene and lead to the production of the protein for which it codes. In general, cells that have similar genes turned on and off perform similar functions and group together as tissues.

It has recently become clear that many genes can code for more than one protein, a finding that helps explain how so few genes can result in so many different proteins. Recent research suggests that a process known as "alternative splicing" is responsible for this phenomenon. Alternative splicing refers to different combinations of exons on one gene that become active at different times, with each combination resulting in the production of one protein.

DNA

Each chromosome is composed of hundreds of thousands of molecules of DNA. DNA is made up of phosphoric acid, a sugar molecule called deoxyribose, and one of four possible nitrogen bases: adenine, guanine, cytosine, or thymine. DNA molecules line up in the cell in the form of a double helix (Fig. 2-1) DNA, in which the phosphoric acid and the deoxyribose sugar form

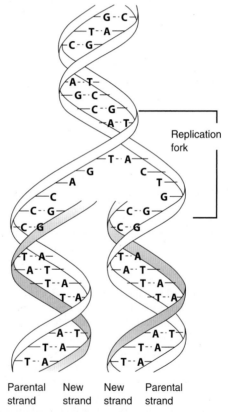

Parental   New   New   Parental
strand   strand strand strand

FIGURE 2-1 DNA. Replicating helix. DNA is composed of sugar phosphates paired with pyrimidine bases of thymine (T) and cytosine (C) and purine bases of adenine (A) and guanine (G). (From Porth, C. & Matfin, G [2009]. *Pathophysiology, concepts of altered health states* [8th edition]. Philadelphia: Lippincott Williams & Wilkins.)

the backbone of the helix. The base pairs from two molecules of DNA lie between the two strands of the helix, opposing each other. Adenine always bonds across the helix with thymine, and cytosine always bonds with guanine. The bonds are loose, so that the helixes can separate when cell division occurs or when protein synthesis is initiated.

● Cellular Reproduction

All cells reproduce during embryonic development, which allows for the growth of the embryo and differentiation (specialization) of the cells making up tissues and organs. After birth and throughout adulthood, many cells continue to reproduce. Cells that reproduce throughout a lifetime include cells of the bone marrow, skin, and digestive tract. Liver and kidney cells reproduce when replacement of lost or destroyed cells is required. Special cells, called stem cells, are capable of reproducing indefinitely. Other cells, including nerve, skeletal muscle, and cardiac muscle cells, do not reproduce significantly after the first few months following birth. Damage to these tissues generally cannot be repaired by the growth of new cells (although nearby stem cells may differentiate into replacement cells). To reproduce, a cell has to replicate its genetic material and then split in two. Replication and division of a cell occur during the cell cycle.

REPLICATION

To replicate, the DNA double helix uncoils and each strand of DNA serves as a template for a new strand. In the formation of a new strand of DNA, each adenine will bind only with a thymine and each cytosine will pair only with guanine. Therefore, only one strand, acting as a mirror-image template for the other, is needed to replicate the entire double helix.

Replication of the chromosome pairs and the DNA occurs in the nucleus of the cell. Various enzymes participate in DNA replication, which results in each chromosome being exactly copied or duplicated. The duplication is checked and double-checked by several proofreading enzymes to ensure that no mistakes are made. If a mistake is identified, proofreading or other enzymes remove the error and correct it, or the cell may initiate its own death in a process called **apoptosis**. If a mistake is not repaired, and the cell does not undergo apoptosis, a mutation in the DNA will exist.

THE CELL CYCLE

The cell cycle (Fig. 2-2) refers to a sequence of stages that a cell goes through during its lifetime. During embryogenesis, all cells go through all stages, as

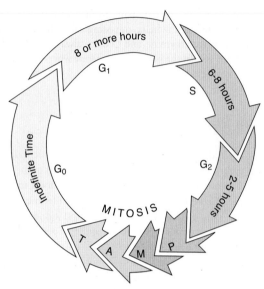

FIGURE 2-2 Cell cycle. Cell division occurs during the reproductive stage and includes prophase (P), metaphase (M), anaphase (A), and telophase (T). Cell growth occurs in three phases: G_1, S, and G_2. Cells that do not reproduce remain in the G_0 or resting phase. (From Porth, C. & Matfin, G [2009]. *Pathophysiology, concepts of altered health states* [8th edition]. Philadelphia: Lippincott Williams & Wilkins.)

do adult cells that continue to reproduce. The rate at which a cell goes through its cell cycle depends on the given cell and the growth factors, hormones, and chemicals to which it is exposed. Cells that do not continue to reproduce after embryogenesis remain in a resting stage and do not cycle through the other stages. The cell cycle is divided into two parts: interphase and mitosis.

Interphase

When not actively dividing, a cell is said to be in interphase. There are three standard stages of interphase: G_1, S, and G_2. A fourth stage, G_0, is a specialized resting stage. In these designations, the G stands for gap, referring to a time period that the cell uses to check and recheck the preceding steps.

G_1 is the stage during which a cell prepares for DNA replication by synthesizing new proteins and activating cytoskeletal components. During this stage, the cell monitors its environment to determine if the time is right for DNA replication. This stage is considered a checkpoint for the cell because if conditions are not right, the cell will not progress further through its cycle. A cell will be stimulated to progress through G_1 when certain genes, including proto-oncogenes, are activated. **S** is the next stage, during which replication (copying) of the DNA occurs; DNA replication is described in Chapter 1. The third stage, G_2, is the stage before cell division, during which the cell again undergoes protein synthesis, this time in preparation for division. This stage is also a checkpoint because if the DNA has not been copied correctly, the cell has a second opportunity to stop its progression through the cycle before mitosis occurs. If an error has occurred, either it is repaired, and the cell re-enters the cell cycle, or the cell is stimulated to undergo apoptosis, i.e., programmed cell death. Genes that are activated at this stage to stop the progression of the cell through its cycle are known as tumor suppressor genes.

G_0 is a resting stage in which a cell in G_1 that has not committed itself to DNA replication may pause. A cell may stay in Go indefinitely, but once a cell is stimulated to leave the Go stage, it will progress through the other stages, unless its progress is restricted at a subsequent checkpoint. The progression through interphase is a lengthy 10- to 22-hour process.

Mitosis

Mitosis (the **M** stage) is the stage of cell division (Fig. 2-3). Mitosis is a shorter event than interphase; it lasts approximately 1 hour. During mitosis, the cell that has duplicated during interphase splits into two daughter cells each of which contains the 23 pairs of chromosomes. Mitosis consists of the substages of prophase, metaphase, anaphase, and telophase.

Prophase

Prophase is the stage in which protein structures (centrioles) present in the cytoplasm of the cell begin to move toward opposite sides or poles of the cell. This stretches the nuclear membrane and causes it to break apart. The chromosomes are now in the cytoplasm rather than isolated in the nucleus.

Metaphase

Metaphase is the stage during which the chromosomes visibly become two sets of pairs lined up next to each other in the center of the cell. Microtubules extend from the centrioles to each chromosome pair.

Anaphase

Anaphase is the stage during which the microtubules begin to pull the chromosome pairs apart. One chromosome goes toward one centriole pole and the other goes toward the other centriole pole.

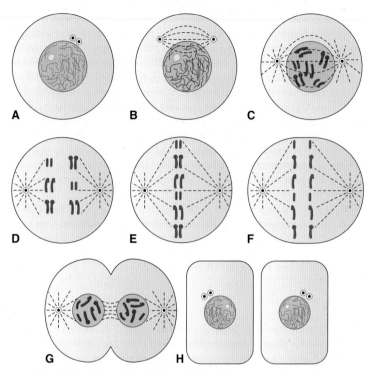

FIGURE 2-3 Mitosis. Nondividing cells (A, H); prophase (B, C, D); metaphase (E); anaphase (F); telophase (G). (From Porth, C. & Matfin, G [2009]. *Pathophysiology, concepts of altered health states* [8th edition]. Philadelphia: Lippincott Williams & Wilkins.)

Telophase

Telophase is the stage during which the cell splits down the middle and a new nuclear membrane develops around each of the two new cells, including the 23 pairs of chromosomes (46 in total) present in each cell.

Control of the Cell Cycle

Cells that continually go through the cell cycle (i.e., cells of the gut and bone marrow) do so at an intrinsic rate that can be increased or decreased by internal and external cues. External cues that turn on the cell cycle may include neural or hormonal stimulation, or may come from cell products released in response to tissue injury and activation of the inflammatory and immune systems. Brakes on the cell cycle may also include neural and hormonal stimulation and proteins synthesized by cells in response to activation of certain regulator genes, including the tumor suppressor genes. Uncontrollable cell growth and cancer (see Chapter 3) may occur with the destruction or inactivation of regulator genes or by excessive stimulation and activation of proto-oncogenes.

Another mechanism that serves to limit cell replication involves structures present on the chromosomes themselves, known as telomeres. A **telomere** is the end region of a chromosome that shortens with each replication. When the telomere shortens to a threshold length, after a certain number of cell cycles, it shuts off cellular replication. Shutting off cellular replication leads to replicative senescence, the characteristic that ensures normal somatic cells do not divide indefinitely. However, a few cells, including cancer cells and germ line cells, contain the enzyme telomerase; telomerase adds telomere sections back onto the chromosome. Telomerase stabilizes telomere length, which results in immortalizing these cells. Telomerase is discussed further in Chapter 3.

MEIOSIS

Meiosis is the process during which germ cells of the ovary (primary oocytes) or testicle (primary spermatocytes) give rise to mature eggs or sperm (Fig. 2-4). Meiosis involves DNA replication in the germ cell, followed by two cell divisions rather than one, which results in four daughter cells, each with 23 (unpaired) chromosomes. In males, all four daughter cells are viable and continue to differentiate into mature sperm. In females, only one viable daughter cell (egg) is formed; the other three cells become nonfunctional polar bodies. During fertilization, genetic information contained in the 23 chromosomes of the egg joins with genetic information contained in the 23 chromosomes of the sperm. This results in an embryro with a total of 46 chromosomes (two pairs of 23).

An interesting phenomenon occurs during DNA replication in the first meiotic stage. At this time, pieces of DNA may shift between the matched chromosome pairs, in a process called crossing over. Crossing over increases the genetic variability of the offspring, and is one reason why siblings within a family may vary considerably in genotype and phenotype.

Control of Cellular Replication and Division

Some cells, such as liver, bone marrow, and gut cells, undergo replication and mitosis frequently. Other cells, such as nerve and cardiac muscle cells, do not replicate or divide except during fetal development or in the neonatal period. Growth factors, hormones, and other cell products turn cell division on or off and determine whether and how frequently a cell will replicate and divide. These factors may affect the replication and division of the cell that produces them, or they may circulate and affect a different cell. Physical factors such as crowding can also influence cell division.

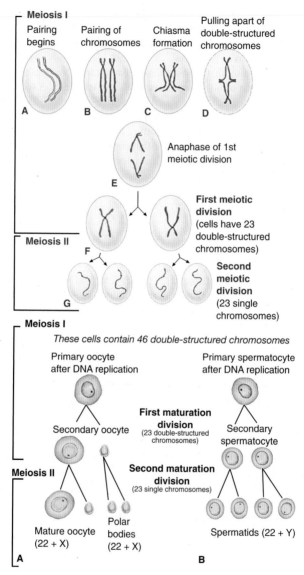

FIGURE 2-4 Meiosis. (Top) Phase 1 involves homologous chromosome pairing, crossing over, and separation of double-stranded chromosomes. During phase II, double-structured chromosomes separate and form four single strands. (Bottom) Meiosis I and II in female and male gametes. (From Porth, C. & Matfin, G [2009]. *Pathophysiology, concepts of altered health states* [8th edition]. Philadelphia: Lippincott Williams & Wilkins.)

● Protein Synthesis

Protein synthesis is an ongoing process in all cells. Protein synthesis occurs when sections of DNA are turned on, which causes the cell to begin making a certain protein. Although each cell contains identical DNA on the 46 chromosomes, some cells have different sections of DNA turned on at a given time compared to other cells. Sections of DNA that turn on and off in different cells are called genes. There are approximately 20,000 to 40,000 genes in the human body distributed among the 46 chromosomes. Each gene contains 90 to 3000 DNA molecules. Each gene codes for a particular protein or enzyme. Turning on or off different genes causes a cell to make different proteins compared to other cells.

Although genes controlling protein synthesis are present in the nucleus, proteins are made in the cytoplasm on specialized structures called ribosomes. The message from the activated gene in the nucleus must be carried to the ribosomes. This is accomplished by making a copy of the gene in the nucleus and transporting the copy to the ribosomes, where it is then translated into a protein.

TRANSCRIPTION OF DNA INTO MESSENGER RNA

To transcribe or make a copy of a gene, the area of the double helix on the chromosome where that gene is contained must unravel. Once unraveled, a special enzyme, called an RNA polymerase, attaches to a certain section at the start of the gene, called the promoter or controlling sequence. When the RNA polymerase attaches to this site, the gene is copied as a mirror image, in a manner similar to that described for DNA replication. The product is a similar molecule called ribonucleic acid (RNA). RNA, like DNA, contains phosphoric acid, but unlike DNA, it contains the sugar ribose instead of deoxyribose and the base uracil instead of thymine. When the gene is copied as RNA, each cytosine base in the gene becomes a guanine in the copy, each guanine becomes a cytosine, each thymine becomes an adenine, and each adenine becomes a uracil. The entire gene is transcribed by this procedure. After the gene is copied, the RNA polymerase will reach a special sequence on the DNA (called the termination sequence) and the process will stop. The RNA copy is released from the gene and moves into the cytoplasm. The RNA copy that carries the DNA message out of the nucleus is called the **messenger RNA** (mRNA). The mRNA then moves through the cytoplasm to the ribosomes (Fig. 2-5).

Adenine, guanine, cytosine, and uracil are carried as mRNA to the ribosomes in groups of three, called triplets or codons. Each triplet codes for one amino acid. There are 20 amino acids used in the human body that combine in various ways to make up all the proteins of the body. The long strand of mRNA triplets can be snipped at any point before the molecule leaves the nucleus, allowing different proteins to be made from one original gene.

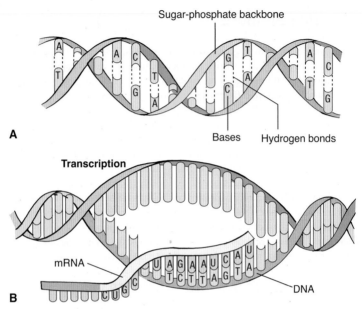

FIGURE 2-5 Messenger RNA (mRNA) transcription. As a DNA molecule separates, RNA nucleotides attach to the exposed DNA base and bind to form mRNA. This process is controlled by RNA polymerase. (From Porth, C. & Matfin, G [2009]. *Pathophysiology, concepts of altered health states* [8th edition]. Philadelphia: Lippincott Williams & Wilkins.)

TRANSFER RNA

Before the ribosomes make the protein from the mRNA template, another type of RNA, called **transfer RNA (tRNA)**, binds to the mRNA by connecting mirror-image bases (called anticodons) to each triplet of mRNA bases. At the opposite end of the anticodon is the amino acid coded for by those three bases. There are at least 20 types of tRNA, each one carrying a certain amino acid on one end and the anticodon for that amino acid on the other end.

THE TRANSLATION OF MESSENGER RNA INTO PROTEIN

When the mRNA has found its matching tRNA, both molecules bind onto the ribosome, which is composed partly of a third type of RNA—**ribosomal RNA**. The amino acid carried by the tRNA is added to a chain of amino acids growing on the ribosome until the ribosome is signaled to stop adding to the chain by a special codon known as a stop codon. The protein is then complete and is freed from the ribosome.

CONTROL OF PROTEIN SYNTHESIS

Regulatory proteins block or activate the promoter section of each gene in the cell, determining which genes will be turned on, transcribed into mRNA, and made into a protein. If a regulatory protein blocks the promoter region of a gene, protein synthesis will not occur from that gene. If a regulatory protein binds to, or near, the promoter area in such a way that it makes the area accessible to the RNA polymerase, it will activate the gene's transcription into mRNA. This type of protein would be considered a transcription factor or enhancer; if, on the other hand, a regulatory protein blocked the promoter area of a gene so that it was not transcribed into mRNA, the regulator protein would be a repressor.

Production and activation of regulatory proteins appear to be linked to other genes responding to feedback signals, chemical cues, and hormones such as thyroid hormone and growth hormone. These signals result in the production of proteins with repressor or activator functions. Other factors that alter the function of the histones responsible for folding and exposing different portions of the DNA may also affect DNA transcription. Methylation (adding a CH_3 complex) or acetylation of the histones associated with a gene, or methylation of the promoter region of a particular gene, may block that gene from being transcribed. This blocking of transcription results in silencing that gene and is an example of "epigenetics," a term coined to describe reversible changes in the genetic material that lead to changes in gene expression.

● Genotype and Phenotype

Precise genetic information carried in the chromosomes of the offspring is termed the genotype. Physical representation of genetic information (tall or short, dark or light) is called the phenotype.

SINGLE-GENE INHERITANCE

Some traits of the phenotype (e.g., eye color) are determined by a single gene. A gene that determines a specific trait is called an **allele**. For each single-gene trait, there are two controlling alleles: one on the chromosome delivered from the mother and one on the chromosome delivered from the father.

HETEROZYGOUS AND HOMOZYGOUS ALLELES

If an individual has two identical alleles (e.g., two alleles coding for brown eyes), the individual is said to be homozygous for the trait. If an individual has different alleles coding for a trait (e.g., one allele for brown eyes and one for blue), the individual is said to be heterozygous for the trait. One allele is usually dominant over the other, for instance, brown eyes over blue, but alleles are occasionally codominant (equally expressed). If a person is heterozygous for a single-gene trait, the phenotype will depend on which, if either, of the alleles is dominant. If the alleles are codominant, for example, those coding for the A and B red blood cell antigens, the individual will express both alleles (i.e., AB blood type).

MULTIFACTORIAL INHERITANCE

Most phenotypic characteristics are influenced by several genes. Height, intelligence, and personality characteristics are among the traits termed multifactorial. They are inherited in a more complicated manner and usually involve many contributing genes present on the same or different chromosomes. The expression of these genes may be influenced by nongenetic (environmental) factors such as nutrition, family support, and exposure to various toxins or microorganisms. Ultimately, however, all human characteristics, including susceptibility to disease, are to some extent affected by our genes, even those characteristics clearly influenced by the environment. For example, research has identified genotypes associated with elevated C-reactive protein (CRP) that has been linked to an increased risk for ischemic heart disease.

● Genetic Testing

Genetic testing, called cytogenetics, involves looking at the overall structure and the number of chromosomes. Genetic testing can be performed on any cell of the body, but is typically done by withdrawing white blood cells in a venous blood sample. For prenatal testing, fetal cells may be gathered during the processes of amniocentesis, at about 16 weeks of gestation, or during chorionic villi sampling, typically between 8 and 12 weeks of gestation. Even genetic testing of preimplantation embryos, obtained during in vitro fertilization procedures, is possible and allows clinicians to test for single-gene disorders at the earliest stage of existence. Analysis of fetal chromosomes accounts for a large percentage of all tests.

For cytogenetic analysis, chemicals typically are added to the cultured cells to arrest the chromosomes during metaphase. The chromosomes are then spread out with members of a pair lined up together. The chromosomes are counted and the structures of the chromosomes under study are compared to control samples. The spread of 23 chromosome pairs is called the **karyotype**; the process is called karyotyping. The 23rd chromosome pair in males will show two chromosomes that are dissimilar in shape, the X and the Y. Females have two X chromosomes. An example of a normal male karyotype is shown in Figure 2-6.

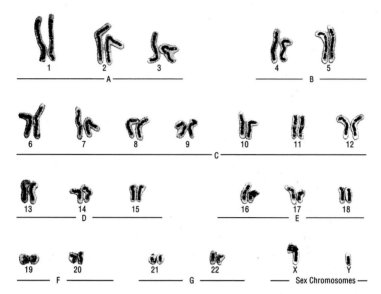

FIGURE 2-6 Karyotype of a normal human boy. (Courtesy of the Prenatal Diagnostic and Imaging Center, Sacramento, CA. Frederick W. Hansen, MD, Medical Director. In Porth, C. (2005). Pathophysiology: Concepts of altered health states (7th ed.). Philadelphia: Lippincott Williams & Wilkins.)

AMNIOCENTESIS

Amniocentesis is performed by inserting a needle through the abdominal wall of a pregnant woman into the amniotic sac that surrounds the fetus. Amniotic fluid, into which fetal cells have been shed, is withdrawn. Chromosomes present in the fluid sample are then cultured and fixed, and their number and shape are analyzed for genetic integrity. This test is usually done at approximately 16 weeks' gestation and the results are available in approximately 2 weeks. Performance of amniocentesis earlier in gestation has been attempted with mixed results. Because of the high cost and risks associated with the procedure, research is under way to find a minimally invasive procedure with greater accuracy and lower risks. Preliminary findings from a study conducted in Hong Kong have supported the use of digital molecular counting of maternal plasma to identify several monogenic disorders.

CHORIONIC VILLI SAMPLING

Chorionic villi sampling involves gathering cells of the chorion, the outer border of the fetal membranes. The cells are gathered by placing a needle through the woman's lower abdomen or cervix between 8 and 12 weeks of pregnancy.

The cells do not need to be cultured, so the chromosomal analysis is available in approximately 1 to 2 days. Chorionic villi sampling earlier than 8 to 12 weeks' gestation is possible, although after sporadic reports of limb or other abnormalities occurring after early testing, this particular procedure was discontinued.

EMBRYOSCOPY

Direct visualization of the embryo can be achieved in the first trimester via insertion of a scope through the cervix and into the uterus. Developmental progress and structural anomalies can be identified. The possibility of managing genetic disorders using targeted gene or stem cell therapy exists.

Genetic Imprinting

Genetic imprinting has been helpful in explaining why a mutation of the same chromosome may result in two totally different syndromes. By marking paternal and maternal genes, it was discovered that the parental origin of a gene determined the outcome. For example, a mutation on maternal chromosome 15 resulted in Angelman syndrome while a mutation of paternal chromosome 15 resulted in Prader–Willi syndrome.

Genetic Engineering

Genetic engineering refers to the experimental manipulation of the genome to produce certain characteristics. One technique of genetic engineering is gene splicing, which involves snipping a certain gene out of one cell and inserting it into another cell or into an attenuated (nonvirulent) virus. The cell or virus may then be administered to an individual who suffers from a lack of that particular gene. This has been performed in clinical trials involving the gene for cystic fibrosis. The goal of gene splicing is that the genetically engineered gene will insert itself into the host's DNA, allowing the host to produce the missing protein or enzyme coded for by that gene. Treatments for genetic hearing loss that are currently being researched include injection of normal genes and injection of stem cells to replace lost or damaged hair cells and nerves in the ear.

Another procedure that takes advantage of the ability to manipulate genes is recombinant DNA technology. With this technology, a piece of DNA extracted from one organism can be inserted into another organism such as a single-celled bacterium. If the DNA incorporates into the bacterium's own genome, it will start directing the bacterium to produce large amounts of a specific protein. In this way, valuable proteins can be produced for mass distribution. Examples of substances produced by recombinant DNA include growth hormone, insulin, clotting factors, and various vaccines.

● Pathophysiologic Concepts

MUTATION

A mutation is an error in the DNA sequence. Mutations can occur spontaneously, or after the exposure of a cell to radiation, certain chemicals, or various viral agents.

Most mutations will be identified and repaired by enzymes working in the cell. Other times, a mutation may lead to apoptosis. If a mutation is not identified or repaired, or if the cell does not undergo programmed death, that mutation will be passed on in all subsequent cell divisions. Mutations may result in a cell becoming cancerous. Mutations in the gametes (the egg or sperm) may lead to congenital defects in an offspring.

CONGENITAL DEFECTS

Congenital defects, also called birth defects, include genotypic and phenotypic errors occurring during embryogenesis and fetal development. Some congenital defects, such as cleft palate and limb abnormalities, may be apparent at birth, whereas other congenital defects, such as an abnormal or absent kidney and certain types of heart disease, may not be recognized immediately. Congenital defects may result from genetic mistakes made during meiosis of the sperm or egg, or from environmental insults experienced by the fetus during gestation. Examples of genetic mistakes include chromosomal breaks, unstable DNA, and mistakes in chromosome number. Environmental insults during gestation that are known to increase the likelihood of a congenital defect include maternal exposure to alcohol, certain drugs, and viruses. Environmental insults may lead to a genotypic or phenotypic error.

Chromosomal Breaks

During mitosis and meiosis, pieces of chromosomes may break off, be added inappropriately to other chromosomes, or be deleted entirely. If deletions or additions occur during meiosis in the egg or sperm, a congenital defect or death of the embryo may result. During fetal development and throughout the life of an individual, mistakes may occur during mitosis in somatic cells. If deletions or additions of chromosomes occur during mitosis, the affected cell line will usually die out.

Hereditary Unstable DNA

Inheritance patterns of some genetic disorders are not easily explained. Recent evidence suggests that occasionally genes coding for a certain trait may not be passed down in a stable fashion from parents to offspring, but instead may have their effect magnified in succeeding generations of offspring. Other genes may be expressed only in certain members of a family, even though all members of the family may carry the gene. Whether an individual in the family expresses the trait coded for by these genes may depend on the individual's sex, the sex of the parent donating the unstable gene, or environmental conditions.

Fragile X Syndrome

A particularly striking finding concerning hereditary unstable DNA is that some diseases occur when a certain group of repeating codons (a set of three DNA bases grouped together) expands. For instance, the genetic disorder known as fragile X syndrome, one of the most common causes of inherited mental retardation, results from a mutation in the fragile X mental retardation 1 (*FMR1*) gene on the X chromosome. Because of a break or weakness in the long arm of the X chromosome the gene cannot make the necessary protein. The incidence is approximately 1 in 1500 males and 1 in 2500 females. Females may not express the disease condition, but they can pass it on to the offspring. Males usually express the disease since they only have one X chromosome. Features include:

- mental retardation
- macroorchidism (large testes)
- elongated face
- prominent ears, jaw, forehead
- hyperextensible joints
- macrocephaly
- pale blue eyes
- unusual speech patterns
- behavioral anomalies
- autistic type behavior or socially engaging
- heart murmur

Fragile X syndrome results when the DNA codon CCG, normally repeated approximately 40 times in a gene near the top of the long arm of the X chromosome, begins to expand and is repeated excessively. Carriers of the disorder show 70 to 200 repeats on the chromosome, but are cognitively and behaviorally normal. However, offspring of the carriers can show the region expanding to greater than 200 repeats of the codon. The degree of mental retardation corresponds to the length of the repeated codon. The degree to which the syndrome is expressed in any one family member depends on whether the expanded codon is inherited from the mother or the father, and whether the offspring is male or female, with the male offspring being more likely and more severely affected. The tendency for the pattern to repeat is caused by a fragility of the chromosome.

Errors in Chromosome Number

Any change from the normal human chromosome number of 46 chromosomes is called aneuploidy. An aneuploidy in which there are only 45 chromosomes is called a monosomy. An aneuploidy in which there are 47 chromosomes is called a trisomy. Having more than 47 chromosomes is possible but rare.

Monosomy

If any chromosome other than the X or Y is lost, the embryo will spontaneously abort. However, the loss of one of the sex chromosomes may result in a viable offspring. Usually the Y chromosome is lost, resulting in 44 somatic chromosomes and one sex chromosome, for a total of 45 chromosomes (often expressed 45, X/O, to indicate no Y chromosome). The resulting disorder is called Turner syndrome. Monosomy of any chromosome is a major cause of spontaneous abortion in the first trimester.

Trisomy

A trisomy occurs when somatic or sex chromosomes do not separate properly during meiosis. This is called nondisjunction. Most trisomies cause spontaneous abortion of the embryo, but rarely live births may result. Trisomies that may result in live births include trisomies of the sex chromosomes and trisomies of chromosomes 8, 13, 18, and 21 (Down syndrome).

Teratogenesis

Teratogenesis is an error in fetal development that results in a structural or functional deficit (e.g., a deficit in brain function). Environmental stimuli that cause congenital defects are called **teratogenic agents**. Teratogenic agents can lead to genetic mutations or errors in phenotype. Common manifestations of teratogenic exposure include congenital heart disease, abnormal limb development, mental retardation, blindness, hearing loss, and abnormalities in growth. Some teratogenic agents, including x-rays and some viruses, are known to cause chromosomal breakage, additions, and deletions. Many drugs, including the anticoagulant warfarin sodium (Coumadin) and the anti-acne medication isotretinoin (Accutane), can also be teratogenic. Other identified tetragens include tobacco, high consumption of caffeine, cocaine, and alcohol.

Alcohol

The most common teratogenic drug used in the United States is alcohol. Fetal alcohol spectrum disorder (FASD) is the result of maternal alcohol consumption during pregnancy. Fetal alcohol syndrome (FAS), the most clinically recognized form of FASD is one of the leading causes of mental retardation in the United States. Although it is difficult to pinpoint the exact incidence, it is estimated to have an occurrence rate of 5.2 per 1000 live births in the United States. Alcohol at any dose is capable of causing neurologic deficits and facial deformities ranging from mild to severe. Alcohol can adversely affect several cellular functions associated with fetal development, including DNA synthesis, protein synthesis, glucose uptake, and the development of neural signaling pathways. Human infants who experience a complex group of congenital effects as a result of exposure to alcohol may be diagnosed as suffering from FAS (Fig. 2-7). Features include:

- microcephaly
- low birth weight
- mental retardation
- small palpebral fissure
- epicanthal folds
- retrognathia (receded upper jaw)
- growth retardation
- hyperactivity

FAS is 100% preventable.

The TORCH Group of Teratogens

Several different microorganisms are known to be teratogenic in humans and can cause congenital defects if the fetus is exposed to them in utero. Many of

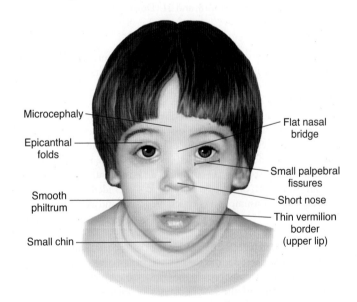

FIGURE 2-7 Fetal alcohol syndrome clinical features. (From Porth, C. & Matfin, G [2009]. *Pathophysiology, concepts of altered health states* [8th edition]. Philadelphia: Lippincott Williams & Wilkins.)

these are described under the acronym TORCH, in which each letter stands for a particular microorganism that may infect the embryo or fetus.

T for toxoplasmosis

O for other infections such as syphilis, hepatitis B, mumps, gonorrhea, and varicella (chicken pox or shingles)

R for rubella

C for cytomegalovirus

H for the herpes simplex virus 2

Effects of Teratogenic Agents

A newborn infected during gestation with any of the TORCH group of microorganisms may show microcephaly, hydrocephaly, mental retardation, or loss of hearing or sight. Congenital heart defects are common, especially with rubella. Radiation exposure may increase the risk that the child will later develop cancer. Certain drugs (e.g., thalidomide, sedatives, antiseizure medications, and sleeping pills) may affect the growth of the embryo or fetus. Angiotensin-converting enzyme inhibitors, used to treat hypertension, may cause the embryo not to develop normal kidneys. Whether an embryo or fetus will be affected by any teratogenic agent depends on several factors, which include the timing and dose of exposure, and maternal and paternal health and nutritional status.

Timing of Exposure to a Teratogen.

Because most organs and tissues are formed during the first trimester, teratogenic agents are most likely to cause structural defects at this time. This is especially true of rubella infection and exposure to drugs that interfere with development. Although the fetus is vulnerable to teratogens between the third and ninth week of gestation, the peak susceptibility period is between the fourth and fifth week. The nervous system is always susceptible to a teratogen because it continues to develop even after birth. Infants exposed to an infectious agent in the third trimester or during the birth process are at increased risk of developing the disease. This is true for neonatal infection by hepatitis B virus or HIV. Primary maternal infection with the herpes simplex virus near the time of labor is associated with the occurrence of neonatal herpes and increased neonatal morbidity and mortality.

Dose of a Teratogen.

The dose of exposure is important in determining the likelihood that a teratogenic agent will cause a congenital defect. Levels of radiation used in most diagnostic techniques or low concentrations of a drug may not produce any discernible effect on the fetus. Higher doses of radiation or a drug may adversely affect the fetus.

Maternal Health and Nutritional Status.

Maternal health and nutritional status also play a role in determining teratogen effect. Infants born to women with diabetes or seizure disorders are at higher risk of fetal anomalies, the latter perhaps due to the effects of both the seizures themselves on fetal growth and the medications used to treat the disorder. Maternal diets low in folic acid have been associated with the development of neural tube defects such as spina bifida. Because most adults do not ingest adequate amounts of folic acid, folic acid supplementation (usually found in a One-A-Day or prenatal vitamin) is recommended for all women for at least 3 months before conception. Folic acid is required for the full functioning of the DNA proofreading enzymes responsible for checking and rechecking DNA replication, which may explain its protective effect against certain congenital malformations.

Paternal Health and Chemical Exposures.
Studies on the effect of diet, chemical exposure, or drug usage in fathers suggest that teratogenic effects may also be passed through damaged sperm. Some studies suggest that paternal (and maternal) cigarette smoking may be associated with increased risk of childhood leukemia in the offspring. Paternal occupational hazards, such as exposure to paint fumes, may increase the risk of spontaneous abortion.

● Conditions of Disease or Injury

SINGLE-GENE DISORDERS

Single-gene disorders (Mendelian inheritance) are caused by a single-gene mistake on the DNA strand. There are approximately 4500 known single-gene disorders, some of which are identified in Table 2-1. Single-gene disorders may be assessed by obtaining a comprehensive family history and preparing a three-generation pedigree, which is the most efficient way to assess hereditary influences on disease. A three-generation pedigree also offers the best chance of determining the likelihood that other members of the family may be at risk for certain genetic diseases.

Causes of Single-Gene Disorders

Single-gene disorders may result from a mistake in the copying of a single code letter. For example, the codon CCG can be transcribed incorrectly to CGG during DNA replication. Because each codon codes for a specific amino acid in a protein, these mistakes usually make the gene incapable of correctly directing the production of its protein.

How important it is to transcribe exactly each letter of each codon is apparent when one considers that, although there are approximately three billion code letters used in the human genome, a mistake in the copying of a single codon is what causes several of the disorders in Table 2-1. For example, sickle cell disease results when one A (adenine) in one gene is replaced by a T (thymine). The fatal neurologic disorder Huntington disease, the congenital bone disease osteogenesis imperfecta, and the metabolic disorders

TABLE 2-1   Some Disorders of Single-Gene Inheritance and Their Significance

Disorder	Significance
Autosomal Dominant	
Achondroplasia	Dwarfism, shortened limbs relative to trunk
Adult polycystic kidney disease	Kidney failure, hypertension, liver problems, heart valve problems
Huntington disease	Neurodegenerative disorder, death typically occurs before 55 years of age
Familial hypercholesterolemia	Premature atherosclerosis, other cardiovascular problems
Marfan syndrome	Connective tissue disorder with abnormalities of skeletal, ocular, and cardiovascular systems
Neurofibromatosis (NF)	Neurogenic tumors; fibromatous skin tumors, pigmented skin lesions, and ocular nodules in NF-1; bilateral acoustic neuromas in NF-2
Osteogenesis imperfecta	Molecular defect of collagen, brittle bones
Spherocytosis	Disorder of red blood cells
von Willebrand disease	Bleeding disorder
Autosomal Recessive	
Color blindness	Abnormal color perception
Cystic fibrosis	Disorder of membrane transport of ions in exocrine glands, causing lung and pancreatic disease
Glycogen storage diseases	Excess accumulation of glycogen in the liver and hypoglycemia (von Gierke disease); glycogen accumulation in striated muscle in myopathic forms
Oculocutaneous albinism	Hypopigmentation of skin, hair, and eyes as the result of inability to synthesize melanin
Phenylketonuria (PKU)	Lack of phenylalanine hydroxylase with hyperphenylalaninemia and impaired brain development
Sickle cell disease	Red blood cell defect

table continues on page 60

TABLE 2-1	Some Disorders of Single-Gene Inheritance and Their Significance (*continued*)
Disorder	**Significance**
Tay–Sachs disease	Deficiency of hexosaminidase A; accumulation of abnormal lipids in the brain leading to severe mental and physical deterioration beginning in infancy; death typically occurs before 4 years of age
X-Linked Recessive	
Burton-type hypogammaglobulinemia	Immunodeficiency
Hemophilia A	Bleeding disorder
Duchenne dystrophy	Progressive atrophy of skeletal muscle
Fragile X syndrome	Mental retardation

phenylketonuria and Tay–Sachs disease also occur as a result of miscopying a single codon.

Codon meanings will also be destroyed and single-gene disorders may result if DNA bases are added or deleted inadvertently. Other single-gene disorders may result from a codon being repeated excessively, as described earlier for the X-linked disorder fragile X syndrome.

The Inheritance Pattern of Single-Gene Disorders

Single-gene disorders may be passed on as dominant or recessive genes. For a disease passed by a dominant gene to be expressed phenotypically, only one gene is required for the disease. For a disease passed by a recessive gene to be expressed phenotypically, either both the maternal and paternal chromosomes must carry the recessive gene or the individual must develop a spontaneous mutation during embryogenesis. Individuals who carry one defective recessive gene causing a particular disease are called carriers for the disease. Although they will not usually express the disease clinically, the gene may pass to their offspring. If their offspring receive a second defective gene from the other parent, they will be homozygous for the recessive gene and will express the disease as shown in Figure 2-8. In this example the capital D is normal, and the lowercase d is the defective gene.

Sex-Linked Single-Gene Disorders

Some single-gene disorders are considered sex-linked disorders because they are passed on the X or Y sex chromosomes. Most sex-linked disorders are passed on the X chromosome and are recessive traits. These disorders are usually seen in males because any woman carrying the defective gene on one

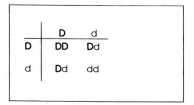

FIGURE 2-8 Inheritance of a single-gene recessive trait. D (dominant gene); d (recessive gene); DD (affected gene); and Dd (carrier gene).

X chromosome will most likely carry the healthy gene on her other X chromosome. A male has a 50% chance of inheriting the defective X chromosome if his mother is a carrier. Because his other sex chromosome is a Y, the recessive gene would be expressed as shown in Figure 2-9 (the X chromosome carrying the defective gene is shown in bold letters). A female may rarely inherit a defective X chromosome from her mother and father. She would then be homozygous for the defective gene and express the disorder.

Clinical Manifestations

- Clinical manifestations depend on the specific altered or missing gene.

Diagnostic Tools

- Prenatal amniocentesis or chorionic villi sampling may identify a single-gene defect.
- Karyotyping of cells from an adult or child may confirm a clinical diagnosis of a single-gene defect.

Treatment

- Treatment for each disease may be supportive if no cure is available, as is the case for Huntington disease, phenylketonuria, fragile X syndrome, or sickle cell disease.

	X	**X**
X	XX	X**X**
Y	XY	**X**Y

FIGURE 2-9 Inheritance of a sex-linked recessive gene.

- Treatment may involve replacing the missing protein or enzyme if possible. This has been tried for persons with hemophilia A.
- Gene splicing may allow the insertion of a correct copy of a defective gene into the host genome. Gene splicing has been tried in individuals suffering from cystic fibrosis and muscular dystrophy.

MULTIFACTORIAL DISORDERS

Multifactorial disorders are polygenic in nature; they are caused by multiple genes, each having a small, additive effect. If the additive effects reach a threshold level, the disorder will be expressed. The severity of any combination of genetic errors in any one person cannot be predicted.

Some multifactorial disorders may be apparent at birth; others may develop during adulthood. Examples of multifactorial diseases apparent at birth include cleft palate, congenital heart disease, anencephaly, and clubfoot. Multifactorial disorders expressed in later childhood or adulthood include hypertension, hyperlipidemia, diabetes mellitus, most autoimmune diseases, many cancers, and schizophrenia. Multifactorial disorders that develop during adulthood are usually strongly influenced by environmental factors.

Causes of Multifactorial Disorders

Multifactorial disorders result from the additive effects of many gene errors. Multifactorial disorders may also result from the less-than-optimum expression of many different genes and not from any particular error. Environmental influences may increase or decrease the likelihood of a multifactorial disorder being expressed and the degree to which it is expressed.

Predicting the Occurrence of a Multifactorial Disease

Whether an individual will develop a multifactorial disease cannot be accurately predicted. However, with complete mapping of the genome it may become possible to identify who is most likely to develop a disease. This would influence risk behavior and preventive screening measures.

For example, individuals with type 2 diabetes mellitus often have a strong family history of the disease, but not every member of the family will develop the disease. A strong predictor of developing type 2 diabetes is obesity, a clear example of the interdependency of genetics and environment. Similarly, various genes have been shown to contribute to the risk of developing cancer. However, whether an individual will develop cancer depends on a variety of personal behaviors, including exercise, smoking, and diet.

Ethical concerns abound for individuals at risk of developing certain multifactorial disorders. For example, certain high-paying jobs that expose workers to potential carcinogens may not be offered to an individual with a high risk of developing cancer.

Clinical Manifestations

- Each disorder has unique clinical manifestations ranging from nonexistent to mild to severe.

Diagnostic Tools

- In families at high risk for a multifactorial disease, genetic mapping may indicate which members of the family are likely to develop the disease and which are not.

Treatment

- Preventative measures based on risk factors.
- An individual at known risk for developing a multifactorial disorder based on genetic mapping or family history may modify his or her diet, toxin exposure, and exercise level to reduce additive environmental factors.
- An individual at known risk for developing a multifactorial disorder based on genetic mapping or family history may consider not having children of his or her own.

DOWN SYNDROME

Down syndrome, also known as Trisomy 21, is seen in 1 in 700 to 800 live births in the United States, making it the most common chromosomal disorder seen in live births. In 95% of cases, Down syndrome is caused by nondisjunction of maternal chromosome number 21 during meiosis. The incidence of Down syndrome related to nondisjunction increases with maternal age. Down syndrome occurs in 1 in approximately 1300 infants born to mothers younger than 25 years of age, but increases to 1 in 100 infants born to mothers 45 years of age and older. Less than 5% of Down cases can be traced to an extra paternal chromosome. A third, uncommon cause of Down syndrome is a translocation of all or part of one of the normally duplicated chromosome 21 onto a different chromosome—most commonly chromosome 13, 14, 15, 18, or 22, but other chromosomes may also be targeted. Children with Down syndrome have variable levels of mental retardation and can often be positively influenced by early child intervention programs. Figure 2-10 illustrates the karyotype of a child with Down syndrome.

Clinical Manifestations

- Variable levels of mental retardation.
- Upward slanting of the eyes with epicanthal folds.
- Short hands with only one crease on the palm (a simian crease) and stubby digits.

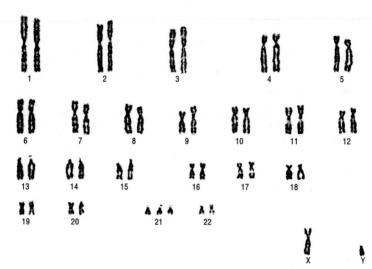

FIGURE 2-10 Trisomy 21 in the karyotype of a child with Down syndrome (note the extra chromosome on 21). All other chromosomes are normal. (Rubin, E., & Farber, J. L. (2005). Pathology (4th ed.). Philadelphia: Lippincott Williams & Wilkins.)

- Low-set ears.
- Short stature.
- Protruding tongue.
- Abundant neck skin.
- Poor muscle tone.

Diagnostic Tools

- Prenatal genetic testing (amniocentesis or chorionic villi sampling).
- Maternal blood tests are available that can screen for fetuses at increased risk of having Down syndrome. In one test, called the quad test, four circulating maternal substances are measured during the second trimester of pregnancy. When considered together, they can predict up to 75% of Down syndrome cases in women under age 35 and up to 85% to 90% of Down syndrome cases in women age 35 years and older. These substances are:
  - Unconjugated estriol (uE3). uE3 is produced by the placenta. It is reduced by about 25% in maternal sera from pregnancies affected by Down syndrome compared to unaffected pregnancies.
  - Alpha-fetoprotein (AFP). AFP is the major serum protein of the fetus. It migrates from the fetal to the maternal circulation. Levels of AFP are reduced in the maternal serum of women carrying a Down syndrome fetus.

AFP levels are also used to detect fetal neural tube defects and anencephaly; maternal AFP levels are increased with these defects.

- Human chorionic gonadotropin (hCG). hCG is produced during pregnancy, first by the trophoblast and then by the placenta. Levels in maternal serum are higher in pregnancies with Down syndrome fetuses than in unaffected pregnancies.

  - Inhibin A. Inhibin A is a glycoprotein produced during pregnancy mainly by the placenta. Among women carrying a Down syndrome fetus, inhibin A is increased.

- The maternal serum marker pregnancy-associated plasma protein A (PAPP-A) typically increases with gestational age. In the case of Down syndrome, the levels are decreased in the first trimester.

- Ultrasound screening in the prenatal period may demonstrate physical suggestions of Down syndrome, especially involving abnormalities in nuchal thickness.

- Genetic karyotyping after birth can confirm a clinical diagnosis of Down syndrome.

Complications

- Congenital heart or other organ defects.
- Risk of childhood leukemia related to the observation that some forms of leukemia may be related to defects on chromosome 21.
- Development of Alzheimer disease in the fourth or fifth decade of life related to the observation that Alzheimer disease may occur partially as a result of a defect on chromosome 21.
- Hearing problems.
- Intestinal problems.
- Celiac disease.
- Eye problems such as cataracts.
- Thyroid dysfunction.
- Skeletal problems.

Approximately 20% of fetuses with Down syndrome are spontaneously aborted between 10 and 16 weeks' gestation. Many others do not implant or are miscarried before 6 to 8 weeks' gestation.

Treatment

- Surgery may be required if another congenital defect is present.
- Early intervention programs may limit the degree of mental retardation.
- Physical therapy, occupational therapy, speech therapy to facilitate functioning at the highest level possible.

TURNER SYNDROME

Turner syndrome is a monosomy of the sex chromosomes. Infants born with Turner syndrome have 45 chromosomes: 22 pairs of somatic chromosomes and 1 sex chromosome, usually the X (45,X/O). This disorder is common in spontaneously aborted fetuses during the first trimester, and is present in approximately 1 in 2500 to 3000 female live births. The damaged or missing X chromosome is most often of paternal origin and may be related to advanced age. Because the ovaries do not develop, the individual is sterile.

Clinical Manifestations

Clinical manifestations may be nonexistent, mild, or moderate and include (Fig. 2-11):

- Short stature.
- Webbing of the neck.
- Pigmented nevi.
- Wide chest.
- Congenital heart defects.
- Fibrous ovaries.
- Lack of secondary sex characteristics and amenorrhea with associated sterility.

Diagnostic Tools

- Prenatal genetic testing.
- Genetic karyotyping after birth can confirm the clinical diagnosis.

Complications

- Congenital heart defects may accompany the sex chromosome monosomy.
- Increased risk of childhood bone fractures and adult osteoporosis due to lack of estrogen.
- Some may demonstrate signs of learning disability.

Treatment

- Surgery may be required if a congenital heart defect is present.
- Estrogen replacement for a female may increase growth and allow development of secondary sex characteristics.
- Growth hormone replacement may also stimulate skeletal growth.
- Counseling to assist with the issue of infertility may be desired. There are incidents of successful pregnancies after in vitro fertilization.

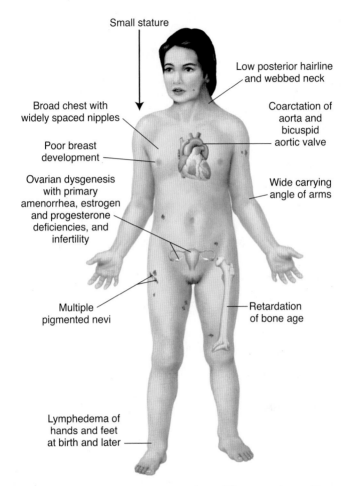

FIGURE 2-11 Characteristic manifestations of Turner syndrome. (From Porth, C. & Matfin, G [2009]. *Pathophysiology, concepts of altered health states* [8th edition]. Philadelphia: Lippincott Williams & Wilkins.)

KLINEFELTER SYNDROME

Klinefelter syndrome is a polysomic disorder characterized by one or more extra X chromosomes in a genotypic male (47,X/X/Y; 47,X/X/X/Y). As one of the most common genetic abnormalities, it occurs in approximately 1 in 600 live births. Klinefelter syndrome may result from nondisjunction of the male or female X chromosome during the first meiotic division, at approximately equal rates in males and females. The risk is slightly increased with advanced maternal age.

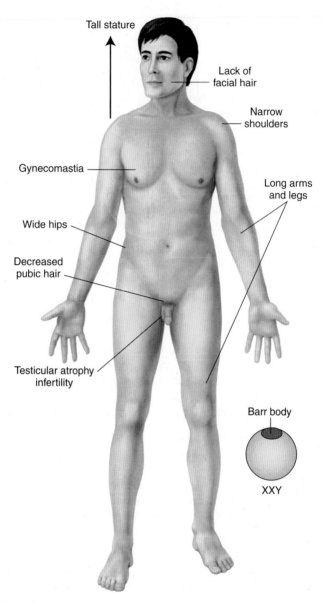

FIGURE 2-12 Characteristic manifestations of Klinefelter Syndrome. (From Porth, C. & Matfin, G [2009]. *Pathophysiology, concepts of altered health states* [8th edition]. Philadelphia: Lippincott Williams & Wilkins.)

Clinical Manifestations

- Infant may appear normal at birth, but show a decrease in male secondary sex characteristics during puberty (Fig. 2-12).
- Gynecomastia (breast enlargement) and other female patterns of fat deposit.
- Small testes.
- Infertility and sexual dysfunction.
- Sparse facial and body hair.
- Tall stature in adult life because decreased levels of testosterone do not contribute to epiphyseal bone plate closure.
- Delayed speech.
- Reduced mental functioning, especially with increasing number of X chromosomes.

Treatment

- Testosterone replacement.
- Physical therapy.
- Infant stimulation programs.
- Speech therapy.
- Counseling may be required.

 GERIATRIC CONSIDERATION

The National Institute of Health is now interested in identifying genes related to healthy aging. To this point research has been focused on identifying disease-associated genes. The challenge now is to identify a phenotype focused on positive attributes, such as high functioning, as opposed to the negative attributes such as avoiding disease.

SELECTED BIBLIOGRAPHY

Allen, T. C., Cagle, P. T., & Popper, H. H. (2008). Basic concepts of molecular pathology. *Archives of Pathology and Laboratory Medicine*, 132, 1551–1556.

Copstead. L. C., & Banasik, J. L. (2010). *Pathophysiology* (4th ed.). St. Louis: Saunders Elsevier.

Davidson, M. R., London, M. L., & Ladewig, P. A. (2008). *Olds' maternal-newborn nursing and women's health across the lifespan.* Upper Saddle River, NJ: Pearson Prentice Hall.

Fessele, K. L. (2008). Genomics in cancer care. *ONS Connect*, October, 10–14.

Frye, D. K., Mahon, S. M., & Palmieri, F. M. (2009). New options for metastatic breast cancer. *Clinical Journal of Oncology Nursing*, 13(1), 11–18.

Gomez-Gallego, F., Santiago, C., Gonzalez-Freire, M., Muniesa, C. A., Fernandez Del Valle, M., Perez, M., et al. (2009). Endurance performance: Genes or gene combinations? *International Journal of Sports Medicine*, 30(1), 66–72.

Gulseth, M. P., Grice, G. R., & Dager, W. E. (2009). Pharmacogenomics of warfarin: Uncovering a piece of the warfarin mystery. *American Journal of Health-System Pharmacy*, 66, 123–133.

Haslam, R. H., & Valletutti, P. J. (Eds.) (2004). *Medical problems in the classroom: The teacher's role in diagnosis and management* (4th ed.). Austin: Pro-ed.

Hilderbrand, M. S., & Smith, R. J. (2008). Advances in understanding genetic hearing loss. *Hearing Health,* Summer, 28–32.

Hudson, K. (2008). The health benefits of genomics: Out with the old, in with the new. *Health Affairs*, 27(6), 1612–1615.

Huether, S. E., & McCance, K. L. (2008). *Understanding pathophysiology* (4th ed.). St. Louis: Mosby Elsevier.

Lavine, G. (2009). HHS panel examines effects of patents, licenses on genetic testing. *American Journal of Health-System Pharmacy*, 66, 114, 116.

Mahon, S. M., & Palmieri, F. M. (2009). Metastatic breast cancer: The individualization of therapy. *Clinical Journal of Oncology Nursing*, 13(1), 19–28.

Manolio, T. A. (2007). Study designs to enhance identification of genetic factors in healthy aging. *Nutrition Reviews*, 65(12), S228–S233.

Manolio, T. A., Brooks, L. D., & Collins, F. S. (2008). A Hapmap harvest of insights into the genetics of common disease. *Journal of Clinical Investigation*, 118(5), 1590–1605.

Maradiegue, A. (2008). A resource guide for learning about genetics. *Online Journal of Issues in Nursing*, 13(1), 10–10. Retrieved February 26, 2009, from CINAHL Plus with Full Text database.

McCarthy, M. I., Abecasis, G. R., Cardon, L. R., Goldstein, D. B., Little, J., Ioannidis, J. P., et al. (2008). Genome-wide association studies for complex traits: Consensus, uncertainty and challenges. *Nature Reviews Genetics*, 9, 356–369.

Meigs, J. B., Shrader, P., Sullivan, L. M., & Mcateer, J. B. (2008). Genotype score in addition to common risk factors for prediction of type 2 diabetes. *New England Journal of Medicine*, 359(21), 2208–2219.

Moore, A. (2008). Gene genie. *Nursing Standard*, 22(51), 18–19.

Olson, H., Jirikowic, T., Kartin, D., & Astley, S. (2007). Responding to the challenge of early intervention for fetal alcohol spectrum disorders. *Infants and Young Children*, 20(2), 172–189.

Patton, K. T., & Thibodeau, G. A. (2010). *Anatomy and physiology* (7th ed.). St. Louis: Mosby Elsevier.

Pedersen, A. (2008). Noninvasive prenatal diagnosis of monogenic disease backed. *Diagnostics and Imaging Week*, II(49), 1, 12–13.

Porth, C. M., & Matfin, G. (2009). *Pathophysiology: Concepts of altered health states* (8th ed.). Philadelphia: Lippincott Williams & Wilkins.

Poust, J. (2008). Targeting metastatic melanoma. *American Journal of Health-System Pharmacy*, 65, 509–515.

Schwartz, E. B., Postlethwaite, D. A., Hung, Y., & Armstrong, A. (2007). Documentation of contraception and pregnancy when prescribing potentially teratogenic medications for reproductive-age women. *Annals of Internal Medicine*, 147(6), 370–376.

Thibodeau, G. A., & Patton, K. T. (2010). *The human body in health and disease* (5th ed.). St. Louis: Mosby Elsevier.

Van Ness, B. (2008). Genomic research and incidental findings. *Journal of Law, Medicine and Ethics*, 36(2), 292–297.

Wattendorf, D. J., & Muenke, M. (2005). Fetal alcohol spectrum disorders. *American Family Physician*, 72(2), 279–285.

Webber, K. M., Perry, G., Smith, M. A., & Casadesus, G. (2007). The contribution of lutenizing hormone to Alzheimer disease pathogenesis. *Clinical Medicine and Research*, 5(3), 177–182.

Wolkoff, L., Kelly, A., & Passut, J. (2008). Gene therapy offers hope for hereditary blindness. *Ocular Surgery News*, 26(10), 1,5.

Zacho, J., Tybjaerg-Hansen, A., Jensen, J. S., Grande, P., Sillesen, H., & Nordestgaard, B. G. (2008). Genetically elevated C-reactive protein and ischemic vascular disease. *New England Journal of Medicine*, 18(359), 1897–1908.

3

Cancer

No doubt the mere mention of "cancer" elicits fear and anxiety. Cancer is the growth of abnormal cells that tend to invade neighboring tissue and spread to distant body sites. It is a condition of uncontrolled cellular proliferation that knows no limits and serves no purpose for the host. According to the American Cancer Society, approximately 1.4 new cancer cases were predicted to be diagnosed in 2008.

The term cancer refers to more than 100 forms of the disease. Although each cancer has unique features, all cancers develop by following a few shared processes that in turn depend upon crucial genetic alterations. For a cell to become cancerous, these genetic alterations must spur cell growth, inactivate genes that normally slow growth, allow cells to keep dividing, thereby immortalizing them, and allow cells to live on with abnormalities that otherwise would cause them to undergo apoptosis. In addition, genetic alterations must occur that allow cancer cells to recruit normal cells to support and nourish them, and to develop strategies that prevent the immune system from destroying them. These processes that cancer cells share and that differ substantially from those of normal cells are the focus of this chapter and of the ongoing, worldwide research effort to prevent and cure cancer.

● Physiologic Concepts

CELLULAR REPRODUCTION

Although all cells reproduce during embryogenesis, only certain cells continue to do so after birth. Cells that continue to reproduce, such as liver, skin, and gastrointestinal (GI) cells, duplicate their DNA exactly before splitting into two new daughter cells. Cells reproduce by going through a process called the **cell cycle**, described fully in Chapter 2. Advancement through the cell cycle is tightly controlled and can be stopped or started depending on the conditions of the cell and the signals it receives, some of which are described below.

Cell cycling is controlled by the contributions of a variety of genes that respond to cues on cell crowding, tissue injury, and growth needs. In general, cells go through the cell cycle when stimulated to do so by hormones and growth factors secreted by distant cells, by locally produced growth factors, and by chemical cues released from neighboring cells, including cytokines produced by immune and inflammatory cells. These external cues act by binding to specific receptors on the plasma membrane of the target cell. Once bound, the receptor complex activates a second messenger system, which delivers the growth signal to the nucleus. When the signal reaches the nucleus, certain proteins there, called transcription factors, turn on or off specific genes that in turn produce proteins that control cell proliferation. Activated genes also produce proteins that feed back on each of the steps of signaling and messenger stimulation to amplify or minimize the effects of the initial stimulus.

The following discussion describes the external cues controlling cell growth and provides an example of an important second messenger system. Finally, the two broad categories of genes whose end products ultimately control the cell cycle are presented: the tumor suppressor genes and the proto-oncogenes.

Hormones and Growth Factors that Control Cellular Reproduction

Various hormones and growth factors may stimulate cells to increase or decrease their rate of reproduction. Table 3-1 includes selected growth hormones and their significance. Some of these substances inhibit growth of other cells while stimulating cell division and growth in target cells.

Chemicals that Control Cellular Reproduction

Various chemicals may stimulate cells to increase or decrease their rate of reproduction. These chemicals may be released by injured or infected neighboring cells or by immune and inflammatory cells drawn to an area after tissue

TABLE 3-1 Growth Factors and Associated Significance

Growth Factor	Significance
Epidermal growth factor (EGF)	Regulates cell growth, proliferation, and differentiation of epidermal cells and other types of cells
Fibroblast growth factor (FGF)	Facilitates angiogenesis and wound healing; proliferation and differentiation of fibroblasts, endothelial cells, myoblasts
Hemopoietic cell growth factors	Proliferation and differentiation of blood cells
Insulin-like growth factors (IGFs)	Regulate response of other cells to other growth factors; regulate differentiation of some cells types; promote cartilage and bone growth
Interleukin-2 (IL-2)	Proliferation of T lymphocytes; discriminates between foreign and self; promotes natural response to microbial infection
Nerve growth factor (NCF)	Promotes axon growth; stimulation and differentiation of sympathetic and some sensory nerves
Platelet-derived growth factor (PDGF)	Regulates proliferation of connective-tissue cells and neurological cells; facilitates angiogenesis
Transforming growth factor β (TGBβ)	Regulates response of most other cells to other growth factors; regulates differentiation for some cell types; impacts immunity, cancer, heart disease, diabetes, Marfan syndrome; antiproliferative factor in epithelial cells
Vascular endothelial growth factor	Stimulates new blood vessel formation; regulates proliferation, migration, invasion, survival, and permeability of endothelial cell function

injury. Many cytokines, released by cells of the immune system, stimulate cellular proliferation and differentiation. Cells possess receptors on their plasma membranes for immune and inflammatory mediators. Binding by some of these substances causes cells to produce more receptors for other immune proteins, thereby amplifying the initial response.

Physical Cues that Control Cellular Reproduction

Neighboring cells appear to communicate with each other about tissue crowding and tissue type by releasing locally active chemicals, and by passing ions and other small molecules through channels called gap junctions. Normal cells respond to physical and chemical cues released by a large number of similar cells by slowing or stopping their rate of reproduction. This allows cellular growth and proliferation to be controlled based on tissue space requirements. These methods of communication allow cells to recognize other cells of the same type (e.g., kidney cells recognize other kidney cells).

Cytoplasmic Second Messenger System Controlling Cellular Reproduction

The cytoplasmic signal cascade begins after a protein hormone, growth factor, or other chemical binds to a cell membrane receptor and turns on a specific second messenger system. Activated second messenger proteins relay the growth-controlling signal to the nuclear transcription proteins. An example of an important cytoplasmic messenger is the *ras* protein. The normal *ras* protein transmits stimulatory signals from bound growth factor receptors on a cell's membrane to other proteins down the line that ultimately turn on cell cycling. Many cancer cells show a mutation in the gene that produces the *ras* protein, such that it is always produced, even when growth factor receptors are not stimulated. Mutation of the *ras* protein was discovered as the first human oncogene in bladder cancer cells. This mutation results in uncontrolled cellular proliferation even when growth factors are not present. Hyperactive *ras* proteins are found in approximately one-fourth of all human tumors.

Tumor Suppressor Genes

Several different genes, called **tumor suppressor genes**, control cell cycling by coding for proteins that inhibit cellular growth and reproduction. Tumor suppressor genes are vitally important in all normally functioning cells. As described later, although cancer results from many accumulated mutations, the first mutation that sets a cell on its way to becoming cancerous often occurs in one of the tumor suppressor genes. For cancer to occur, the tumor suppressor gene must be inactivated.

Tumor suppressor genes act by producing proteins that slow down or stop the second messenger brigade, including proteins that interfere with the functioning of the stimulatory *ras* protein. Tumor suppressor genes may also code for proteins that make up surface receptors that bind growth-inhibiting hormones or factors. Other tumor suppressor genes, when activated, stimulate a damaged cell to undergo apoptosis (programmed cell death). Finally, some tumor suppressor genes produce proteins that code for important brakes that act directly on cells about to commit to going through the cell cycle; these genes include the *Rb* gene and the *p53* gene.

The Rb Gene

The *Rb* gene codes for the pRb protein, the master brake of the cell cycle. Without this protein, the cell cycle is constantly in the "on mode," and cellular reproduction can occur nonstop. Mutations in this gene have been identified in a variety of human cancers including bone, bladder, pancreatic, small cell lung, and breast cancer, and the cancer after which the gene was named, retinoblastoma. Mutations in the Rb locus have been identified in up to 70% of individuals with osteosarcoma.

The p53 Gene

The *p53* gene codes for the p53 protein, which normally monitors the health of the cell and the integrity of cellular DNA. The p53 protein can act as a powerful brake to halt cell division before it is too late if errors in DNA transcription are present or if cellular conditions are not favorable. The p53 protein can cause the cell either to pause in the cycle indefinitely until a DNA error is corrected, or to undergo apoptosis. By controlling cellular replication, the *p53* gene ensures that a genetic error is not passed on and only healthy cells reproduce. Deletion or mutation of the gene occurs in approximately 75% of colorectal cancer cases. It has also been associated with breast cancer, small cell lung carcinoma, hepatocellular carcinoma, astrocytoma, and many other tumors. Mutations in the *p53* gene are shown to occur in at least 50% of all types of tumors making it the most common genetic change in human cancer.

Other Tumor Suppressor Genes

Although *Rb* and *p53* have been the most extensively studied tumor suppressor genes, Table 3-2 includes other genes and their associated pathologies when mutations occur.

Proto-oncogenes

Proto-oncogenes are genes found in all cells that, when activated, stimulate a cell to go through the cell cycle, resulting in cellular growth and proliferation. These genes may stimulate cell cycling at all levels, including (1) producing proteins that make up membrane receptors for growth-stimulating hormones and chemicals, (2) increasing the production of second messenger proteins, including the *ras* protein, that transfer growth signals to the nucleus, and (3) producing transcription factors that turn on vital genes to force cell growth forward (e.g., the family of *myc* genes).

The myc Genes

The *myc* genes are a family of proto-oncogenes that code for transcription factor proteins that drive cellular reproduction. In healthy cells, *myc* genes are

TABLE 3-2 Tumor Suppressor Genes and Associated Pathologies	
Tumor Suppressor Gene	**Pathology**
APC gene	Familial adenomatous polyposis coli; colorectal cancers; malignant melanoma; ovarian cancer
WT-1 gene	Wilms tumor; many breast cancers
NF-1 gene	Neurogenic sarcomas
VHL gene	Renal-cell carcinoma; hemangioblastoma of the brain, pheochromocytoma
FHIT gene	Cancers of the kidney, lungs, digestive tract
p15 and *p16* genes	Tumors of the breast, pancreas, and prostate
DPC4 gene	Pancreatic carcinoma
BRCA1 and *BRCA2* genes	Breast and ovarian cancer
PTEN gene	Prostate cancer; gliomas; thyroid cancer; Cowden syndrome

activated only in response to growth factors acting on the cell surface. In many types of cancer, however, the *myc* gene is turned on constantly, even in the absence of growth factors. Typically, low levels of proliferating lymphocytes stimulate the gene and mature lymphocytes stop the *myc*. Cellular proliferation can occur without control when this gene is damaged.

When normal proto-oncogenes become overactive and cause uncontrolled cell division, they are called **oncogenes**, or cancer-causing genes. Typically, after early embryonic life oncogenes are turned off or tightly controlled. Exposure to a carcinogen can damage the cell's DNA and cause overstimulation of the oncogene resulting in development of cancer cells. Overstimulated oncogenes produce excess cyclins that interfere with suppressor genes and thus interrupt the balance between cell growth initiation and suppression. Approximately 70 oncogenes have been identified and it is noteworthy that these are not abnormal genes. They are part of a normal cell and only become problematic when exposed to a carcinogen.

CELLULAR DIFFERENTIATION

Differentiation is the process of development in which cells acquire specialized characteristics including structure and function. Normal cells differentiate during development and aggregate with similar differentiated cells. For example, some embryonic cells are destined to become cells of the retina, whereas others are destined to become cells of the skin or heart. The more highly differentiated a cell, the less frequently it will go through the cell cycle to reproduce and divide. Neurons are highly specialized cells and do not retain the ability to reproduce after the nervous system is completely developed. Skin and mucosal cells continue to be proliferative. Cells that seldom or never go through the cell cycle are unlikely to become cancerous, whereas cells that go through the cell cycle frequently are more likely to become cancerous.

Differentiation is a sequential process and appears to occur from the selective suppression of certain genes in some cells, whereas in other cells those same genes are active. Differentiation of each cell and tissue appears to affect differentiation of neighboring cells and tissues. Cells release specific growth factors that initiate or guide differentiation of neighboring cells.

CELL RECOGNITION AND ADHESION TO LIKE CELLS

Normal cells adhere to others of the same type and group together. Although the mechanism by which cells recognize each other is not well understood, it appears to involve chemical cues secreted only by certain cells and bound by receptors present only on similar cells. Surface proteins present on one cell type that match up with proteins on similar cells, also appear to assist in similar cell recognition. These surface proteins are cell adhesion molecules that maintain contact between cells and the extracellular matrix. They provide signals that maintain cell survival and cell type differentiation. Cell-to-cell recognition is demonstrated by placing cells of many different types together in a Petri dish; after a certain period, the cells will have moved into clusters with only same-type cells in each cluster.

Other adhesion molecules exist between cells and the underlying tissue matrix. These connections anchor cells to one location. When normal cells become detached from each other or experience a loosening of their attachment to underlying tissue, they respond by initiating apoptosis, which prohibits cells from floating free of their tissue of origin.

THE CELL CLOCK

Normal human cells reproduce a predictable number of times, after which they stop and become senescent. This predictability implies that cells possess some counting system that tells them when to stop dividing. This system is important because if cells divided indefinitely we would have many more cells than is compatible with life. The mechanism by which cells tick off their own divisions involves a telomere-based counting system.

Telomeres, described in Chapter 2, are the end pieces of chromosomes that shorten with each division. When the telomere length becomes sufficiently short (indicating that it has divided a certain number of times) the cell stops dividing. Putting the brakes on cell division in response to telomere shortening requires that the cell has functioning Rb and p53 proteins. Occasionally, a cell continues to divide after the telomere reaches its threshold length; usually these cells soon self-destruct as their chromosomes begin to chaotically fuse and randomly break.

Cell crowding also results in neighboring cells releasing signals that inhibit the further replication of cells. This is called **contact inhibition**.

● Pathophysiologic Concepts

UNCONTROLLED CELLULAR REPRODUCTION

Cancer cells do not respond to the normal cues controlling cellular reproduction. Instead, they go through the cell cycle more often than normal, resulting in an overabundance of abnormal cells. Cancer cells spend little time in the gap stages of interphase and are frequently found in the M (mitosis) and S (DNA copying) stages. This information is vital when selecting treatment for different types of cancer.

Uncontrolled cellular reproduction occurs when cells become independent of normal growth control signals. This characteristic of cancer cells is called **autonomy**. Autonomy results when cells do not respond to the cues controlling contact inhibition—for example, growth inhibitors released by neighboring cells or inhibitory growth factors and hormones traveling in the circulation. Cancer cells may disregard these signals by not producing membrane receptors that bind the inhibitory growth signals or by not activating appropriate second messengers that transmit inhibitory information to the nucleus. Other cancer cells may overproduce membrane receptors that respond to growth stimulatory signals. Cancer cells may also produce their own growth factors that bind to their cell membranes, thereby promoting self-proliferation and allowing them to be independent of any outside control.

When placed in an in vitro experimental setting, cancer cells aggressively grow on top of each other and produce layers of disorderly cells, ignoring not only chemical signals but the tendency to respect neighboring borders. Autonomy is demonstrated in the tendency of cancer cells to detach from neighboring cells and spread to distant body sites. It has been suggested that the adhesion molecules that exist between cells of the same type and between normal cells and the extracellular matrix no longer exist for cancer cells. Cancer cell autonomy may result from the inactivation of tumor suppressor genes or the change from proto-oncogenes to oncogenes.

ANAPLASIA

A change in the structure of a cell with loss of differentiation is known as anaplasia. Cancer cells demonstrate various degrees of anaplasia. By undergoing anaplasia, a cancer cell loses its ability to perform its previous functions and bears little resemblance to its tissue of origin. Highly anaplastic cells may appear embryonic and begin to express functions of a different cellular type. Some cancer cells may become ectopic sites of hormone production. For instance, antidiuretic hormone (ADH) or adrenocorticotrophic hormone (ACTH), hormones that are normally synthesized by cells of the hypothalamus and anterior pituitary, respectively, may be secreted by ectopic sites of hormone production. Lung cancers frequently become ectopic sites of hormone production such as ADH or parathyroid hormone (PTH).

Because the immune system poorly responds to embryonic antigens, the presence of highly anaplastic cells may interfere with the host's immune response to the tumor and usually indicates a particularly aggressive cancer.

LOSS OF THE CELL CLOCK

Many cancer cells secrete an enzyme, telomerase, that acts to replace the telomere ends of chromosomes that shorten with each cell division. This leads to a destruction of the cell counting system and immortality of the cell. Not only does telomere replacement allow a cancer cell to continue to divide, increasing its number, but it also gives the cancer cell time to accumulate more mutations, some of which may improve the cell's ability to evade the immune system or produce newer, more potent growth-stimulatory factors.

NUCLEAR AND CYTOPLASMIC DERANGEMENT

Cancer cells often demonstrate multiple derangements of the nucleus, cytoplasmic organelles, and cytoskeleton. The nucleus is frequently enlarged and deformed, with obvious chromosomal breaks, deletions, additions, and translocations. The rate of mitosis is usually increased. In the cytoplasm, intracellular structures show disorganization and changes in size and shape. Changes in the microtubules that support the cell and are necessary for the control of virtually all intracellular functions are especially significant. The mitochondria become disorganized and misshapen.

TUMOR CELL MARKERS

Some cancer cells release tumor cell markers, which are specific substances secreted by a tumor into the blood, urine, or spinal fluid of an individual with a particular cancer. These markers are especially helpful in identifying the origin of a metastatic or poorly differentiated tumor. Tumor cell markers may be immunoglobulins, fetal proteins (oncofetal antigens), enzymes, hormones, genes, antigens, antibodies, or cystoskeletal and junctional proteins. Because fetal antigens often do not provoke an immune response, they may mask the tumor against the host's immune system. Tumor cell markers may even include fragments of DNA that are detectable, with increasingly sensitive measurement techniques, in the circulation when produced in excess by certain tumors.

Clinical Implications of Tumor Cell Markers

Tumor cell markers are clinically important because they offer a means of identifying those at high risk for cancer, identifying certain cancers, and monitoring cancer's progression before, during, and after treatment. For instance, if a specific tumor cell marker is identified in a patient, it suggests that cancer may exist in the person, and further diagnostic evaluation is necessary. Furthermore, in patients with a known malignancy, if after radiation or chemotherapy the tumor cell marker is not detectable, it suggests that the cancer is in remission. If, however, the tumor cell marker fails to decrease during therapy or reappears in high concentration after therapy, the tumor is unlikely to be in remission.

Examples of Tumor Cell Markers

Table 3-3 includes examples of tumor cell markers and associated cancers.

TABLE 3-3 Tumor Cell Markers	
Tumor Cell Marker	**Associated Cancer**
Acid phosphatase and prostate-specific antigen (PSA)	Prostate cancer
Adrenocorticotropic hormone (ACTH)	Pituitary adenoma
Alpha-fetoprotein (AFP)	Liver cancer
	Ovarian and testicular cancer
CA-125	Ovarian cancer
Carcinoembryonic antigen (CEA)	Colorectal, liver, pancreas, lung, breast cancer
Catecholamines	Pheochromocytoma
Estrogen and progesterone nuclear receptors	Breast cancer
Human chorionic gonadtropin (hCG)	Choriocarcinomas (usually uterine), teratoma, islet cell cancer
Leukocyte common antigen (LCA)	Malignant lymphoma
Lewis A antigen (CA 19-9)	Pancreatic and gastrointestinal cancer
Monoclonal immunoglobulin	Multiple myeloma
Neurofilament proteins	Neuroblastoma and ganglioneuroma
Thyroglobulin	Thyroid cancer
Urinary Bence–Jones protein	Multiple myeloma

Although the presence of a tumor cell marker may indicate the presence or recurrence of cancer, sole reliance on the presence or absence of a cell marker is not recommended. Interpretations must be made in the context of a thorough assessment. For example, PSA is detectable in all adult men; only an unexpected rise in PSA in a given individual, or an elevation above a certain age-dependent threshold, is suggestive of disease. Likewise, pregnant women have increased hCG, and CA-125 may be increased in women for reasons other than ovarian cancer. Failure to detect a tumor cell marker does not mean that an individual is cancer-free.

TUMOR GROWTH RATE

Each tumor grows at a certain rate dependent on characteristics of both the host and the tumor itself. Important characteristics of the host that affect a tumor's growth rate include the person's age, sex, and overall health and nutritional status. The status of the host's immune system is also important. An individual who is immunosuppressed may be unable to recognize a tumor as foreign, or may be unable to respond to a tumor that he or she recognizes. Certain hormonal states (e.g., pregnancy) may stimulate certain tumor growth rates, while stress may affect the host's ability to restrict the development or growth of a tumor.

Important characteristics of a tumor that affect its growth rate include its location in the body and its blood supply. The degree of cellular anaplasia and the presence or absence of tumor growth factors are also important characteristics. Many tumors depend on circulating or self-produced growth factors to stimulate their growth. Therefore, the tumors that grow most rapidly often populate their surface membranes with receptors for these factors. In addition, some tumor cells secrete chemicals that make the local environment more favorable to their growth. An example is secretion of tumor angiogenesis factors, described below.

TUMOR ANGIOGENESIS FACTORS

Tumor angiogenesis factors are substances secreted by tumor cells that stimulate the development of new blood vessel formation. To survive, all cells require an adequate blood supply for the delivery of oxygen and nutrients and the removal of waste products. Once a group of cancer cells has grown to a certain size (approximately 1–2 mm in diameter), it will outgrow its original blood vessel supply and must stimulate the development of new blood vessels to grow further.

Measuring tumor angiogenesis factors in the blood or urine may allow for early diagnosis of some cancers. Even more exciting are new treatments for cancer that involve blocking the production of tumor angiogenesis factors. Experiments demonstrate that without angiogenesis, tumors soon shrink and sometimes disappear. Interventions to block tumor angiogenesis factors in humans with cancer are a promising avenue of targeted drug therapy.

DESCRIPTIONS OF TUMOR GROWTH AND SPREAD

Growth and spread of a tumor is often described clinically; some of the different terms used are listed below. Tumor treatment often depends on the grade and stage of the cancer.

- Grading: Tumors are classified as grade I, II, III, or IV based on cellular or histologic characteristics. The more poorly differentiated (highly anaplastic) the cells, the higher the grade (Box 3-1).

B O X   3 - 1   Grading of Malignant Tumors

Gx Cannot be determined
G1 Well differentiated, low grade of malignance, slow growing
G2 Moderately differentiated
G3 Poorly differentiated, few normal cell characteristics
G4 Poorly differentiated, no normal cell characteristics, unable to determine tissue
    of origin

- Staging: A clinical decision concerning the size of a tumor, the degree of local invasion it has produced, and the degree to which it has spread to distant sites in a given individual. The tumor classification system, also known as the TNM Classification System, developed by the American Joint Committee on Cancer (AJCC) is included in Box 3-2.

B O X   3 - 2   TNM Classification System

T (tumor—size and spread of local primary tumor)

Tx Tumor cannot be adequately assessed
T0 No evidence of primary tumor
Tis Carcinoma in situ
T1-4 Progressive increase in tumor size or involvement

N (nodes)

Nx Regional lymph nodes cannot be assessed
N0 No evidence of regional node metastasis
N1-3 Increasing involvement of regional lymph nodes

M (metastasis)

Mx Not assessed
M0 No distant metastasis
M1 Distant metastasis present, specify site

- Ploidy defines the tumor chromosomes as normal or abnormal based on number and appearance. Normal ploidy (euploidy) has the typical 46 chromosomes. Cancer cells may gain or lose chromosomes and have an abnormal structure (aneuploidy). The degree of malignancy increases with the degree of aneuploidy.
- Doubling time: An estimate of the mean amount of time required for the division of the tumor cells. Tumor cells that rapidly divide have a short doubling time.

Tumors may grow only locally, or may spread to distant sites in the process called **metastasis**. It is the metastasis of tumors that may ultimately lead to death of the individual.

LOCAL GROWTH OF A TUMOR

The term cancer refers to the crablike projections put out by a growing tumor into the local tissue. Tumors spread locally when these crablike projections injure and kill neighboring cells. Growing tumors injure and kill neighboring cells both by compressing the cells and blocking off their blood supply. Tumor cells also appear to release chemicals or enzymes that destroy the integrity of a neighboring cell's membrane, causing the cell to lyse and die. When neighboring cells die, the tumor can easily grow to occupy that space. As described earlier, to grow beyond a certain size, tumors must stimulate the development of their own blood supply to meet high metabolic demands.

METASTASIS

Metastasis is the movement of cancer cells from one part of the body to another and is the leading cause of death from cancer. Metastasis usually occurs through the spread of cancer cells from the original (primary) site to a new, secondary site. Metastasis may occur by direct invasion or extension, seeding, or via blood or lymphatic pathways. The term malignancy refers to the ability of a tumor to metastasize. See page C1 for illustrations.

The process of direct invasion or extension can occur when cancer cells synthesize and secrete enzymes that break down proteins and allow their spreading into adjacent tissues. It is often difficult to determine the exact demarcation where cancer cells end and normal cells begin thus necessitating the removal of normal cells during surgical removal of cancer cells. Seeding is the result of shedding from the tumor cells. Seeding primarily occurs in the peritoneal cavity; however, the pleural cavity, pericardial cavity, and joints may be involved. Seeding is a risk during surgical removal of cancers. Metastasis via blood and lymphatic pathways is discussed below.

The Process of Metastasis

Steps involved in the metastasis of a primary tumor to a distant site include detachment, invasion, dissemination, and seeding (Fig. 3-1).

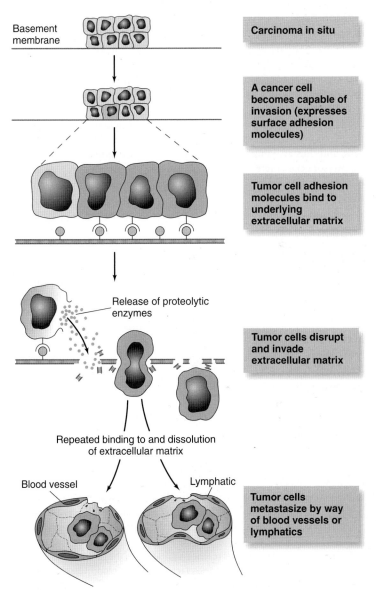

Basement membrane

Carcinoma in situ

A cancer cell becomes capable of invasion (expresses surface adhesion molecules)

Tumor cell adhesion molecules bind to underlying extracellular matrix

Release of proteolytic enzymes

Tumor cells disrupt and invade extracellular matrix

Repeated binding to and dissolution of extracellular matrix

Blood vessel   Lymphatic

Tumor cells metastasize by way of blood vessels or lymphatics

FIGURE 3-1 *Metastasis.* Cancer cells detach from like cells due to loss of adhesion. These cancer cells secrete an enzyme that destroys the basement membrane and allows entrance into blood or lymph vessels. Cancer cells are then disseminated downstream from the site of origin. (From Hall, J. [2006]. *Sauer's manual of skin diseases* [9th edition]. Philadelphia: Lippincott Williams & Wilkins).

Detachment

To metastasize, cancer cells must first detach from their primary cluster. Recall that normal cells are linked to neighboring cells and underlying matrix tissue, and thus detach with difficulty. In addition, if a normal cell senses that it has become detached from its neighbors, it undergoes apoptosis. Cancer cells, in contrast, lose adhesion with like cells and the extracellular matrix, allowing for relatively easy detachment. Likewise, a cancer cell may produce chemicals that mimic those secreted by neighboring cells, thereby fooling its internal checkpoints into thinking that it is still attached to other cells, and thus avoiding apoptosis. Cancer cells may also deactivate tumor suppressor genes, thereby eluding apoptosis by this means as well. As cancer cells detach, they begin to invade surrounding membrane barriers and enter the circulation.

Invasion

To spread to distant sites, detached tumor cells must gain entrance to a blood or lymph vessel. To do so, the tumor cells must (1) cross the basement membrane (a thin layer of tissue) separating its tissue of origin from the rest of the body, and (2) cross the basement membrane of a local blood or lymph vessel. To break down basement membrane walls and gain access to the circulation, tumor cells secrete specific enzymes that attack the integrity of the tissue. One such enzyme secreted preferentially by cancer cells to break down walls of a capillary is collagenase type IV. Collagenase type IV is effective in the spread of cancer cells because the new blood vessels formed in response to tumor angiogenesis factor are relatively thin and easily breached.

Dissemination and Seeding

Movement of tumor cells in the blood or lymph is called dissemination. Eventually, and especially if they are traveling in clumps, some tumor cells will get caught in a capillary or lymph network downstream from the primary site. Although many cells may die, a few tumor cells at this new site may survive and begin to seed the area. The more the cells detach from the primary tumor, the more likely it is that at least one will survive the journey and start a new tumor growth elsewhere.

When the secondary site has reached a critical size, the tumor cells will again begin to produce tumor angiogenesis factor and new blood vessel formation will be initiated to support the growth of this secondary site. Current research has focused on the role of the microenvironment in facilitating cancer cells to establish metastatic sites. Elements of the microenvironment include at a minimum the extracellular matrix, endothelial cells, myoepithelial cells, and macrophages.

Progress of a Metastasizing Tumor

Because cancer cells tend to be large, most lodge in the nearest lymph or capillary bed downstream from the primary tumor site. Because of this, the lungs, which receive systemic venous blood directly from most organs, are the most common sites of metastasis. Venous blood from the GI tract and pancreas travels first to the liver through the hepatic portal blood flow system, causing the liver to be the most common site of cancers from these organs. Metastasis is evaluated by observing for secondary sites in the lymph nodes nearest to the primary site, and then progressively further from this site. If exploration of the node closest to the primary site—called the **sentinel node**—is negative for tumor cells, it is likely that more distant nodes will not have been seeded either. Exceptions to this rule are tumor cells that show a striking preference to colonize certain tissues not necessarily downstream. The classic example of this preference is the tendency of prostate cancer to metastasize to bone. It has been suggested that in these cases, complementary adhesion molecules draw the tumor cells to the distant tissue. Finally, rough handling of a tumor during evaluation or surgery may cause cancer cells to break off from the primary site, thus increasing the likelihood of metastasis. Table 3-4 lists the most common sites of metastasis from primary tumor sites.

THE IMMUNE SYSTEM AND CANCER

The presence in the blood of antibodies, T cells, and natural killer (NK) cells produced against specific tumor antigens has been confirmed in individuals

TABLE 3-4 Common Sites of Metastasis	
Primary Tumor	**Common Site of Metastasis**
Brain	Central nervous system
Breast	Bone, lung, brain, liver
Colorectal	Liver, lymph nodes, adjacent structures
Head and Neck	Lymphatics, liver, bone
Liver	Lungs
Lung	Brain, bone, liver, lymph nodes, pancreas
Lymphomas	Spleen
Melanoma	Lymphatics, lung, liver, brain, gastrointestinal tract
Ovarian	Peritoneal surfaces, diaphragm, omentum, liver
Prostate	Bone (esp. lumbar spine), pelvic nodes, liver
Sarcoma (extremity)	Lungs
Testicular	Lungs, liver, brain

with cancer. In addition, individuals who are immunocompromised, including those with AIDS or those taking immunosuppressant drugs, have an increased chance of developing cancer. Potent anticancer cytokines, including tumor necrosis factor alpha (TNFα), have been identified that assist the immune system in identifying and destroying cancer cells. All of these findings demonstrate clearly that the immune and inflammatory systems have important roles in fighting and preventing cancer.

Cancer Cell Evasion of the Immune Response

Despite an apparent immune response to tumors, cancer cells are frequently able to evade the immune system. Highly anaplastic cells that primarily express oncofetal antigens are most likely to evade immune detection and are especially malignant. Other cancer cells may demonstrate changes in the expression of the major histocompatibility (MHC) antigens that normally stimulate a cell-mediated immune response, which may also allow cancer cells to evade the immune system. Cancer cells may also survive a host immune response by producing blocking antibodies that capture all host antibodies built against the tumor, allowing the tumor to continue to grow. These and other means by which tumor cells may escape immune recognition or destruction are being investigated. Experiments to boost the immune response to a tumor are also under way.

Cancer Cell Stimulation by the Immune Response

A too robust immune or inflammatory response also has been implicated in the development of cancer. For example, about 25% of cancers appear to be related to chronic infection. Liver cancer often develops after years of chronic infection by the hepatitis B or C virus, while stomach cancer is related to infection by *Helicobacter pylori*. Some research suggests that some of the cytokines released by white blood cells in response to infection, including TNFα, may block apoptosis of damaged or mutated cells, thus leading to abnormal cell proliferation and cancer. Other proinflammatory cytokines may stimulate the production of angiogenesis factors normally required for wound healing or reactive oxygen species that further damage the cell.

● Conditions of Disease

CANCER

There are several categories of cancer, and several theories as to how cancer develops. This section reviews the categories of cancer and presents the theory of carcinogenesis.

TABLE 3-5   Characteristics of Benign and Malignant Tumors

Benign Tumors	Malignant Tumors
Grow slowly	Grow rapidly
Grow by expansion	Spread by direct invasion, seeding or via blood or lymph pathways
Typically do not spread to other tissues	Spread to other tissues
Encapsulated	Not encapsulated
Cells adhere to each other	Lack adhesion
Rarely recur after removal	May recur
Usually regular in shape	Poorly defined shape
Well-differentiated	Poorly differentiated
Slightly vascular	Moderately to highly vascular
Not life-threatening	Potentially life-threatening

Categories of Cancer

Tumors are identified based on the tissue from which they develop. The suffix "oma" is usually added to the tissue term to identify it as a tumor, either benign or cancerous. Characteristics of benign and malignant tumors are included in Table 3-5. Several general categories of cancer are presented in Table 3-6. Individual cancers are discussed in chapters pertaining to specific organs or systems.

The Theory of Carcinogenesis

Cancer development, or carcinogenesis, is a multistep process that usually requires decades to occur. Factors that interact to influence cancer development include genetic predisposition, exposure to carcinogens, and immune function.

Initiation

The first step in carcinogenesis is most likely a mutation in the DNA of an individual cell during DNA replication (copying). Although mistakes in DNA copying are not unusual, most mistakes are identified by proofreading enzymes that travel down the DNA strands to check for errors, signaling the cell cycle to stop for repair when necessary. If a mistake cannot be repaired, the cell normally is instructed to self-destruct.

The theory of carcinogenesis suggests that in certain individuals, an error in DNA copying may not be noticed, the cell cycle may not stop in time for repair, or the defective cell may not self-destruct. If the DNA error is not identified and corrected, the genetic change becomes a permanent mutation and

TABLE 3-6 Cancer Classifications

Classification/Category	Tissue of Origin
Carcinoma	Epithelial cells including skin, testis, ovary, mucus-secreting glands, melanin-secreting cells, breast, cervix, colon, rectum, stomach, pancreas, esophagus
Carcinoma in situ	Abnormal epithelial cells that are confined; preinvasive lesions
Adenocarcinoma	Glandular tissues
Erythroleukemia	Erythrocytes
Glioma	Brain and spinal cord
Leukemia	Leukocytes
Lymphoma	Lymphatic tissue including lymph capillaries, lacteals, spleen, lymph nodes, and vessels
Melanoma	Pigment cells
Myeloma	Plasma cells
Sarcoma	Connective, muscle, bone

is passed on to all daughter cells. This step is irreversible and is called cellular initiation.

Agents capable of inducing cancer are referred to as carcinogens. Carcinogens can be categorized as complete or partial. Complete carcinogens are capable of initiating genetic damage and promoting cellular proliferation. Partial carcinogens stimulate growth but are not capable of initiating genetic mutations. Ultraviolet (UV) and ionizing radiation, viruses, chemicals, tobacco, and asbestos are examples of known carcinogens. Responses to carcinogens will vary with individuals and are influenced by the duration and extent of exposure as well as each person's unique genetic makeup.

Promotion

For a cancer to develop from this first, irreversible event, years of additional interactions with the cell by endogenous (internally produced) and exogenous (environmental) factors that cause additional genetic changes must occur, and all must lead to the production of a cell that proliferates aggressively and without quality control. If the cancer cell is unable to proliferate, it cannot form a tumor and therefore poses no threat.

Additive effects that enhance proliferation are called promoters. If the promoting events have significance related to a cell becoming autonomous, they may cause the cell to become cancerous. Factors that promote the acceleration of the cell cycle through stimulation of oncogenic genes and those that allow an abnormal cell to avoid detection by the immune system are most likely to result in a mutated cell becoming carcinogenic. Promotion may be reversed by the removal of the promoter although any cell that has been irreversibly initiated has the potential to be promoted for an indefinite period of time (Fig. 3-2).

A key point in this scenario is that the failure to detect or repair a DNA error is the first step of the cascade. This failure usually occurs in an individual who inherited a mutation in a tumor suppressor gene from one parent and developed a mutation in the other gene later in life, or in an

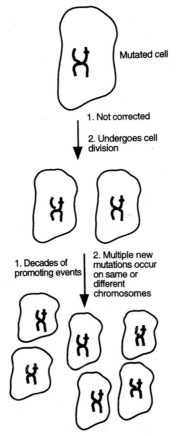

FIGURE 3-2 An uncorrected mutation passes to new daughter cells. If promoting events and new mutations occur, the cell may be released from normal growth controls to proliferate uncontrollably.

individual who developed, over the course of a lifetime, mutations in both of the genes coding for a particular tumor suppressor, neither of which were themselves caught and repaired. This description explains how tendencies to develop cancer can be present in families, how those with such tendencies tend to develop cancers earlier in life than those without, and how cancer incidence increases with age as more and more spontaneous mutations occur.

Progression

During the progression stage cancer cells become malignant. Before progression occurs, the tumor must develop and form its own blood supply by making tumor angiogenesis factor that triggers capillaries to develop branches into the tumor. The new blood vessel system nourishes the tumor and facilitates growth. As the cancer cells divide new characteristics appear and tumor cells acquire malignant changes that result in invasion and autonomous growth tendencies.

The multistep theory of carcinogenesis also allows for the acceptance of many causes of DNA mutation, many different variables that interact over the span of years, and roles for both heredity and environment.

Effect of Frequent Cell Cycling on Transcription Errors

The more number of times the DNA is copied and a cell replicates, the greater the chances of an error being made, a mistake being overlooked, and a mutation being passed on. Under some circumstances, these mutations may result in cancer. Cells that reproduce and divide frequently are at greatest risk of becoming cancerous.

Monoclonal Tumor Development

When a tumor develops, it appears to do so from a mistake passed on from a single cell. This results in a monoclonal tumor from one ancestral cell. This theory is consistent with there being one mutated cell that eventually develops into a cancer.

Promoters of DNA Replication Errors

Although some mistakes in DNA replication occur randomly, certain physical agents, chemicals, and microorganisms are known to cause DNA errors. Such agents, also referred to as carcinogens, include ionizing radiation, UV radiation, components of cigarette smoke, aromatic hydrocarbons, certain dyes, nitrosamines (present in preserved meats), aflatoxin (present on moldy peanuts), and asbestos. Some of these physical agents appear to damage the DNA directly by breaking DNA base pair bonds, or indirectly by producing free radicals or other intermediates that react with and damage the DNA. Aging increases the risk of cancer in part through increased production of free radicals.

Certain viruses have been identified that can cause DNA mutations. These viruses may damage the DNA directly by causing a transcription error, or may insert into the host DNA and turn on cellular proliferation. Cancers known to be caused *directly* by a virus include Burkitt lymphoma, caused by the Epstein–Barr virus; cervical cancer, caused by certain strains of the human papilloma virus (HPV); and liver cancer, caused by the hepatitis B virus. Kaposi sarcoma also may be caused by a virus and occurs especially in those suffering from acquired immunodeficiency syndrome (AIDS).

In addition to directly altering the DNA and causing cancer, viruses and other microorganisms may irritate the cell and cause chronic inflammation. Inflammation associated with the release of proinflammatory cytokines may stimulate cellular proliferation and angiogenesis. Inflammation also may stimulate the cell to divide more frequently, thus increasing the likelihood of DNA transcription errors.

Effect of any Mutating Agent

Any physical, chemical, or viral agent may cause mistakes in DNA replication or destroy proofreading enzymes. The worst-case scenario is that a mutating agent may deactivate a tumor suppressor gene that controls cell division. If this first mistake is followed by a mutation that transforms a proto-oncogene into an oncogene, cell proliferation may occur without control. Recall from the earlier discussion that a large proportion of human cancers result from mistakes in the *p53*, *ras*, or *myc* family of genes and that there are two copies of each gene. It is hypothesized that cancer results from many hits: damage to one gene that is followed by subsequent damage to others. This damage requires more than one genetic error to occur in a cell over many years. Even then, cancer will not develop unless promoting effects have turned the mutation deadly.

Promotion

A mutated cell is not a cancerous cell; many years of promoting events must occur before that cell becomes cancerous. It is suggested that various promoting agents may act to cause a mutated cell to become cancerous by accelerating the proliferation of the cell. Some promoters may stimulate cellular proliferation by stimulating oncogenes or increasing surface receptors for growth factors.

Other promoting agents may not cause an actual mutation in the DNA of a gene, but rather may cause a given tumor suppressor gene to be deactivated or "silenced." This type of change in the DNA is referred to as an **epigenetic** change in that it is separate from a change in the genome itself. Silencing of a gene usually occurs when the DNA in the area of the gene's promoter (activator) region is methylated (has a CH_3 group added to it); this process leads to the promoter region being unavailable to stimulation, and hence the gene is unable to be turned on. In the case of epigenetic changes, because the DNA itself has not been altered, the effects of the promoter may be reversible if exposure to it is stopped or if an antimethylating drug is administered.

Examples of promoters include endogenous hormones such as estrogen, certain food additives such as nitrates and salt, drugs, cigarette smoke, and alcohol; the latter two have a synergistic effect. Some substances, for example, tobacco, may act both as an initiator of a mutation and a promoter of cell proliferation.

Risk Factors

Some mistakes in DNA replication throughout a lifetime are inevitable. However, certain conditions or behaviors, known as risk factors, can increase or decrease the likelihood of a mutation arising and a mutated cell being promoted until it is cancerous.

Risk factors for cancer include exposure to any physical, chemical, or viral substance that is known to be mutagenic, and prolonged exposure to any promoter. Mutagens may be inhaled or eaten, or may act on the skin, such as in the case of UV radiation.

Behavioral Risk Factors

Certain behaviors increase the likelihood that an individual will be frequently exposed to cancer-causing stimuli. Behavioral risk factors may include cigarette smoking, other environmental toxins and diets rich in animal fat and preserved meats. Approximately 80% of cancer in North America has been linked to external factors. One third of all cancers in the United States can be attributed to cigarette smoking, and the American Cancer Society estimates that nearly 3000 nonsmokers die each year as a result of secondhand smoke.

The most common cancer associated with smoking is lung cancer, but it has also been linked to cancer of the bladder, kidney, pancreas, mouth, esophagus, and cervix. As a carcinogen, tobacco smoke has been classified as both an initiator and a promoter. It has been estimated that approximately 20% of cancer deaths in the United States have been associated with nutrition and physical activity factors. Research has indicated a link between high-fat diets and prostate, colon, and breast cancer. Food additives, preservatives, and preparation methods such as charbroiling, may also contribute to cancer development. Obesity also may be an independent risk factor for cancer because of the increased accumulation of fat-soluble toxins and potentially carcinogenic hormones in the fatty tissue.

Research has indicated a link between breast, esophageal, laryngeal and liver cancer and alcohol consumption. Alcohol has the potential to promote cancer growth in several ways including (1) liver impairment that interferes with metabolism of hormones and hazardous substances, (2) increased estrogen levels, and (3) effect on insulin secretion. Even a moderate level of alcohol consumption is linked to an increase in breast cancer, as is a sedentary lifestyle. Compared to smoking and diet, other environmental factors, including exposure to asbestos, radon, and coal tar, account for a small percentage each of cancer cases. Radiation exposure from sunlight, the primary cause of skin cancers, accounts for less than 2% of all cancers in the United States, although in other countries, including Australia, the incidence is higher.

Other behavioral risk factors include those associated with sexual behavior. A high number of sexual partners and an early onset of sexual activity increase the risk of becoming infected with the HPV, which is associated with genital neoplasms, and the AIDS virus, which is associated with Kaposi sarcoma. Some evidence suggests that infection with the sexually transmitted virus herpes simplex 2 may also increase cervical cancer risk. Hepatitis B virus can be passed sexually and increases the risk of liver cancer.

Hormonal Risk Factors

Although research has not found a direct carcinogenic effect from hormones, there is evidence that hormones do support carcinogenesis. Hormones tend to make target tissues more receptive to the carcinogen and facilitate cell division of malignant tissues. Estrogen may act as a promoter for certain cancers, such as breast and endometrial cancer. Because estrogen levels are high in menstruating women, the risk for developing breast cancer is increased in women who started menstruating early and reached menopause late. Delayed childbearing or choosing not to bear children increases the risk of breast cancer. This increased risk appears to be related to many years of uninterrupted exposure to estrogen. Estrogen replacement therapy in postmenopausal women appears to be associated with an increase in the risk of breast cancer.

Genetic Risk Factors

Five to ten percent of cancers are hereditary in nature. A family history of cancer, especially clustered as one type, is a risk factor for developing cancer. Genetic tendencies for carcinogenesis may involve fragile or mutated tumor suppressor genes, susceptibility to certain mutagens or promoters, faulty proofreading enzymes, or a poorly functioning immune system. Inherited defects in the *p53* gene and the *Rb* gene have been documented to be associated with a high risk of cancer. Certain cancers have a higher tendency to run in families than others. For example, although most cases of colon cancer arise spontaneously, some families carry mutations that increase the risk of this disease.

Likewise, although most cases of breast cancer arise without any clear genetic link, inheritable breast cancer accounts for approximately 5% to 19% of all breast cancers. Two genes have been identified that increase a woman's chance of developing of breast cancer: *BRCA1* and *BRCA2*. These genes are in the category of tumor suppressor genes, but their exact function in controlling cell proliferation is still unclear. Mistakes in one or both of these genes are present in increased frequency in women with breast cancer compared to women without breast cancer, and may account for approximately half of the heritable cases of breast cancer. The presence of a mutation in either of these genes does not guarantee the development of breast cancer; however, a woman carrying a mutation in the *BRCA1* gene has a 56% chance of developing breast cancer before the age of 70 and a 16.5% chance of developing ovarian cancer. Like other cancers with a genetic predisposition, familial cases of breast cancer tend to occur at a younger age.

Pediatric cancers likely have a genetic component. In children, the development of cancer is accelerated from several decades to only one or two decades. Acceleration may occur if a child inherits in the germ line (egg or sperm) one defective gene controlling a tumor suppressor or proto-oncogene product or develops such a mutation early in embryogenesis. Later, a second gene error would cause early cancer growth. Similarly, inheriting defective genes for proofreading enzymes would increase the risk of early cancer development.

It is likely that each of us has a certain genetic tendency toward developing cancer, which results in a small percentage of individuals developing cancer without exposure to known mutagens or promoters, whereas others with long-term exposures will remain cancer-free. In general, our genetic tendency toward cancer is overshadowed by risk factors we encounter in our environment and, most importantly, by the risks we take in our lifestyles and behaviors.

Viral Risk Factors

Some viruses have the potential to alter cells by infecting the host DNA. The result is cellular mutation and unregulated proliferation. The Epstein–Barr virus has been associated with Burkitt lymphoma, Hodgkin disease, and nasopharyngeal cancer. Cervical cancer has been linked to HPV, cytomegalovirus, and herpes simplex virus type 2 while other viruses have been linked to hepatocellular carcinoma and leukemia. The risk of cancer due to viruses is increased with age and in individuals with an altered immune system.

Immune Dysfunction

Malnutrition, advancing age, chronic disease, immunosuppressant medication, and stress have the potential to damage the immune system. A compromised immune system is unable to destroy cancer cells faster than they are proliferating.

Factors that are Protective against Cancer Development

Studies suggest that women who breastfeed for at least 6 consecutive months and women who have had multiple pregnancies have a reduced risk of developing breast cancer. These findings most likely relate to the decreased number of menstrual periods experienced by these women. Progesterone appears to be protective against breast cancer by inhibiting the stimulatory effects of estrogen. Progesterone level is high during pregnancy, which may explain why women who have had many pregnancies have a reduced risk of breast cancer. There is also a reduced risk of breast cancer in women who exercise even moderately. This finding may be related to reduced estrogen levels or to a decrease in fat consumption and obesity.

Dietary factors are important in reducing cancer risk. Diets rich in substances known to scavenge or remove dangerous free radicals, called free-radical scavengers or antioxidants, may reduce the risk of certain cancers. These substances include vitamins A, E, and C and folic acid, all of which are prevalent in green, leafy, and colorful vegetables and fruits. Vitamins C and D, selenium and beta-carotene have been beneficial in cellular repair resulting from free-radical damage. High-fiber diets have been found to indirectly serve a protective function. Fiber reduces fecal bile acid concentration, dilutes colon contents, and decreases colon transit time thus decreasing the contact time of potential carcinogens with the colon mucosa. Although research has been inconclusive, the current recommendation is to consume a diet low in fat, high in fiber, and high in natural antioxidants. Physical activity facilitates better weight control thus decreasing the risk of cancers related to being overweight.

Clinical Manifestations

Cancers may be diagnosed in routine examinations before any clinical manifestations appear. When clinical manifestations develop, they are usually specific to the tumor, its site, and the extent of metastasis. Some general clinical manifestations that most patients with cancer demonstrate include the following:

- Cachexia is a term used to describe the general wasting of fat and protein seen in many patients with cancer. Weight loss accompanies cachexia and is common in patients with cancer, many times being the presenting complaint. There appears to be a variety of causes of cachexia, including loss of appetite (anorexia), poor digestion, and the increased metabolic rate of the cancer cells as they continue to go through the cell cycle and reproduce excessively. Cancer cells have high-energy demands and steal nutrients needed by other cells for survival. Anorexia may be the result of toxins released from cancer and immune cells. Metabolism of foodstuffs may be altered, especially if the cancer involves the liver. Cachexia also appears to be caused, at least in part, by the presence of certain cytokines produced by the immune system to fight the cancer, including tumor necrosis factor (TNF). Cytokines and TNFs tend to contribute to the hypermetabolic state.

- Anemia occurs for many different reasons and in many different types of cancers. Most individuals with metastatic cancer eventually develop anemia. It occurs early in those with cancer of the blood-forming cells of the bone marrow. This is true whether the cancer specifically affects the red or white blood cells (leukemia). Cancers that result in chronic bleeding, such as colorectal or uterine cancer, cause anemia. Platelet abnormalities are common, contributing to blood loss. Some forms of chemotherapy and radiation may depress the bone marrow, causing anemia even in patients without previous bleeding or bone marrow disease.

- Fatigue frequently occurs as a result of poor nutrition, protein malnutrition, and poor oxygenation of tissues resulting from anemia. Certain cytokines produced to support the immune response against cancer are also known to cause fatigue. Growing tumors collapse the blood supply to healthy cells while stimulating their own blood supply. They take over the nutrient and oxygen supply of normal cells, causing widespread fatigue The fatigue is peripheral and central and is believed to be the result of a dysregulation of brain serotonin.

Diagnostic Tools

Methods to diagnose cancer vary with the location and type of suspected cancer. Methods include blood tests for tumor markers, tissue biopsy, cytologic studies, endoscopy, mammography, ultrasound, x-ray, computed tomography (CT), magnetic resonance imaging (MRI), and positron emission tomography (PET).

- Diagnosis of cancer involves a holistic assessment including the patient's clinical presentation, information on personal habits such as smoking, and investigation of the patient's genetic background for cancer.

- Screening tests, such as Pap smears to detect cervical cancer, mammograms to detect breast cancer, and digital examinations of the prostate coupled with a blood assay for prostate-specific antigen (PSA) to detect prostate cancer, can help to identify cancer early in its development. Testing for other cancer markers may be performed based on suspicion.

- Immunohistochemistry involves identification of tissue- or organ-specific antigens to help determine the primary tumor source.

- Microarray technology involves the use of gene chips to detect and count genes. Additional information gained from this process includes identification of tissue types, prognosis predictions, responses to therapy, and classification of hereditary tumors.

- Advanced methods to diagnose and localize cancer include radiographs, CT scans, and MRIs. Special bone scans may also be used.
- Noninvasive diagnostic tests for oral cancer are being developed that involve testing for the presence of salivary bacteria not normally present in healthy individuals.
- Cancer diagnosis is confirmed by surgically extracting a sample from a suspicious lesion, a procedure known as a biopsy, and performing a microscopic examination of the cells.

Complications

- Infections are common in those with cancer. Infections develop as a result of protein malnutrition, other dietary deficiencies, and immune suppression (especially bone marrow suppression), which often accompanies conventional therapies. Hormones released in response to the long-term stress of cancer can also cause immune suppression. When the immune response is suppressed, the body may perceive normal flora to be virulent and thus develop an opportunistic infection. Complications from surgery also may result in infections in patients with cancer. Infection is the major cause of complications and death in those with cancer.
- Pain may occur as a result of the invading tumor pressing on nerves or blood vessels in the area. Compression of the blood vessels can lead to tissue hypoxia, lactic acid accumulation, or cell death. Pain also occurs because the cancer cells release lytic enzymes that directly injure cells. Pain occurs as part of the immune and inflammatory reactions to the developing cancer. Fear and anxiety can worsen the pain for many patients with cancer. Most patients with advanced cancer experience pain. It is important for health care professionals to consider all treatments available to reduce pain severity and frequency in their patients.
- Pain caused by compression of nerves and blood vessels occurs especially in tissues that exist in space-limiting compartments, such as the bone or brain. For example, headaches are a common manifestation of advanced brain cancer, and bone pain is common with childhood hematologic cancers and bone cancer at any age. GI pain occurs when the smooth muscle of the gut is stretched.
- Paraneoplastic syndromes are systemic effects that accompany a malignancy and are most likely the result of excessive hormone or cytokine production by the tumor. Although the occurrence is between 10% and 15%, the syndrome may be the first indication of an unknown cancer, it can represent a life-threatening problem and it can interfere with appropriate treatment. Such syndromes may include Cushing syndrome, syndrome of inappropriate ADH, hypercalcemia, hypoglycemia, carcinoid syndrome, polycythemia, myasthenia, acanthrosis nigricans, dermatomyositis,

hypertrophic osteoarthropathy, clubbing of the fingers, venous thrombosis, endocarditis, anemia, and nephrotic syndrome.

- Leukopenia and thrombocytopenia may be the result of cancer invading the bone marrow and/or a side effect of treatment. The risk of infection and hemorrhage is greatly increased.

Treatment

Several treatments for cancer are available, as outlined below and shown in Table 3-7. All have the highest rate of success with early identification of the cancer.

- Surgery is useful in the diagnosis and treatment of cancer. For diagnostic purposes an incisional biopsy, excisional biopsy, needle biopsy, or endoscopy is performed to remove a tissue sample. Microscopic examination of the sample confirms a definitive diagnosis of cancer and facilitates staging of the tumor. Surgery has a better chance of curing a cancer if used on solid, well-circumscribed tumors. Tumors that have metastasized may be

TABLE 3-7 Cancer Therapy, Actions, and Effects		
Cancer Therapy	**Mode of Action**	**Adverse Effects**
Surgery	Reduce tumor size to alleviate pain; prevent metastasis if used early; diagnosis	Pain; deformity
Radiation	Damage dividing cells; stimulate apoptosis; halt cell cycle	Injures and leads to death of normal cells; bone marrow depression; skin desquamation
Chemotherapy	Multiple actions on cells to stop progression through cell cycle; may involve combination therapy and may act selectively or nonselectively	Injures and kills normal cells; anorexia; nausea; bone marrow depression
Immunotherapy/ biotherapy	Activate host immune system to better recognize and destroy tumor cells; specifically block enzymes and growth factors required for metastasis; allow evaluation of treatment	Some drugs may cause flulike symptoms

treated with surgery to give the patient relief from pain of the pressure of the growing tumor on surrounding nerves. Surgery is also used to debulk the tumor, which reduces tumor burden and improves the response to chemotherapy or radiotherapy. Reconstructive surgery may be done for the patient who has functional or cosmetic deficits with the major goal of improving function.

- Radiation therapy uses ionizing radiation to kill tumor cells and at least 50% of cancer patients are treated with radiation sometime during their illness. Radiation works on the principle that the cells most susceptible to the damaging effects of radiation are those in the S or M stages of the cell cycle. Tumor cells are most likely to be found in those stages. Unfortunately, many normal cells are also in those stages of the cell cycle at any given time, and may be killed by the therapy. It appears that radiation kills cells primarily by altering the DNA enough that brakes on the cell cycle, especially those put on by the p53 protein and the ras protein, are activated, leading to cell suicide. Unfortunately, many times cancer cells have deactivated normal braking genes, and therefore do not undergo apoptosis when DNA damage is present. This limits the usefulness of radiation therapy. Another limitation is the scarring of normal tissue that can occur, leading to fibrosis and reduced organ function. For some cancers—for example, Hodgkin lymphoma—radiation may be used alone for curative purposes. Often, radiation is used in addition to surgery and chemotherapy or to shrink the tumor, reducing tumor load. Three types of radiation therapy are now being used:

  - External radiation therapy involves several small doses over a designated period of time.

  - Photodynamic therapy uses light-sensitive molecules that form oxygen radicals that alter the DNA, cytoplasm, and the cell membrane causing the cells to die.

  - Internal radiation therapy or brachytherapy uses sealed radioactive implants placed into or on the tumor. High doses of radiation are delivered over a short period of time.

- Chemotherapy uses cytotoxic drugs to treat cancer and has been a standard of treatment since the 1970s. The goal of chemotherapy is a cure; however, it also may be used to interfere with tumor cell multiplication, control disease spread, and for palliatative purposes. Drugs of several different classes destroy cells in the S, M, or initial G stages of the cell cycle. Because different drugs work at different phases of the cell cycle a combination of chemotherapeutic agents may be used to increase the chances of killing more cancer cells. Tumors grow rapidly and therefore have the most number of replicating and dividing cells and are most susceptible to chemotherapy. However, healthy cells are also susceptible to the damaging effects of chemotherapy. Chemotherapy is frequently used in addition to surgery or radiation therapy, but may be used alone. Chemotherapy usually causes bone marrow suppression, which in turn causes fatigue, anemia, bleeding tendencies, and an increased risk of infection. Selected drug therapies will be discussed below.

One emerging type of adjuvant chemotherapy involves using reproductive hormone antagonists to fight reproductive cancers. The best example of this type of drug is tamoxifen, used clinically to fight estrogen-dependent breast cancers. Tamoxifen also appears to prevent the development of breast cancer in some women at high risk of the disease. Tamoxifen and similar drugs, collectively known as selective estrogen receptor modulators (SERMs), exert estrogenic effects on some tissues, for example, uterine endometrial tissue, bone, and the cardiovascular system, but exert antiestrogenic effects on the breast. This observation may allow different drugs to be tailored to the specific needs of each woman. Clinical trials to evaluate the use of tamoxifen to prevent the development of breast cancer are continuing.

- Drugs have been developed that block receptors for growth factors overexpressed on certain cancer cells. The best known of this type of drug is Herceptin (trastuzumab), which binds to and blocks HER2 receptors that are overexpressed in some women with breast cancer. HER2 receptors normally bind circulating epidermal growth factor (EGF); when overabundant, the proliferative effect of EGF is excessive. By binding to the HER2 receptors, Herceptin blocks the effect of EGF. Herceptin also may act to alert the immune system to the abnormal cancer cells, thereby targeting them for destruction. In an exciting development, when patients with metastatic breast cancer positive for overexpressed HER-2 receptors were treated with Herceptin combined with chemotherapy, they demonstrated a significant decrease in the risk for breast cancer recurrence compared with patients who received the same chemotherapy without Herceptin.

- Kinase inhibitors, also referred to as tyrosine kinase inhibitors, block transmission of signals inside the cancer cell thus blocking proliferation of the cells. By identifying kinases that actually facilitate cancer growth, inhibitors to treat various cancers can be developed.

- A mircrotubule inhibitor, ixabepilone, has been shown to be effective in treating metastatic and locally advanced breast cancer not responsive to other drugs. Microtubules facilitate chromosome separation during cell division. Microtubule inhibitors interfere with cell division in the mitotic phase, which ultimately results in cell death.

- Immunotherapy is a form of cancer treatment that takes advantage of the two cardinal features of the immune system: specificity and memory. Immunotherapy may be used to identify a tumor and any sites of hidden metastasis. Immunotherapy may stimulate the host's own immune system to respond more aggressively to a tumor, or tumor cells may be attacked by antibodies developed in the laboratory. Each of these options is described below.

- Fluorescence-labeled antibodies: To identify a tumor, antibodies can be produced in a culture against tumor-specific antigens taken from a patient. The antibodies can then be labeled with a fluorescent isotope and injected into the patient before, or at different times during or after treatment. If the antibodies encounter their specific type of tumor cells, the antibodies will bind to the tumor cells and the resulting fluorescence can be detected, located, and measured. This use of immunofluorescent antibodies allows clinicians to identify recurrent or metastasized tumors.

- Immune stimulants: Boosting the host's natural immune response to tumor cells involves activating B and T cells to notice the presence of a growing tumor. This approach has been used in skin tumors by injecting antigens capable of stimulating the immune system. Natural immunostimulants, such as interferon or some interleukins administered to patients with certain cancers, also appear to boost a cell-mediated response to these tumors.

- Attacking antibodies: Antibodies produced against specific tumor antigens are being used to attack and destroy tumor cells. For example, monoclonal antibodies have been developed against malignant B cells and used in patients with lymphoma. Various other attacking antibodies also are available for use in cancer therapy.

- Therapies based on the unique molecular biology of tumor cells compared to normal cells are being developed. These treatments take advantage of the recent discoveries of how cancers grow to invade local tissues and metastasize into the blood or lymph. Examples of biologic therapies being developed against tumors include drugs that specifically block tumor angiogenesis factors and enzymes such as collagenase type IV. Tumors make their own growth factors and populate their cell membranes with receptors for these factors and other substances that stimulate their growth. Drugs that block the production of tumor growth factors and the receptors for growth factors also are under development.

- Gene therapy is being developed to fight cancer. In gene therapy, pieces of DNA containing special messages are delivered to cancer cells with the hope that the cancer cell will take up the DNA and begin expressing the message for which the DNA codes. Although gene therapy is far from being available clinically, early studies have provided exciting leads. The most tantalizing developments to date have been attempts to incorporate genes that inhibit angiogenesis into mice suffering from various tumors. Other ideas include infecting cancer cells with genes that code for the production of toxic chemicals that destroy the cell when produced. Another idea involves providing cancer cells with instructions to produce a therapeutic protein that would correct a faulty tumor suppressor gene or compensate for a variety of genetic errors. Other pieces of DNA may cause the cancer cell to produce a surface receptor that would bind a specific chemotherapeutic drug. Finally, the idea that it may be possible to vaccinate against a certain cancer uses gene therapy as well. In this scenario, a cancer cell may be tagged with certain genes that make it more visible to the immune system. This could improve the host immune response and lead to destruction of all cells carrying that tag. At this time, the best option would be to tag the cancer cells with genes that express certain cytokines that, when produced, alert the immune system to the cancer. This approach combines immunotherapy with gene therapy.

- Genomic information has the potential to be used to individualize cancer treatment based on an individual's normal cells as well as the specific type of cancer cells. Matching specific mutations with the appropriate cytotoxic drug increases the possibility of a cure. Pharmacogenomics is useful in determining how an individual metabolizes a specific drug thus helping to identify the drug with the highest potential for cure and the least possibility of side effects and toxicity.

- DNA methyl transferase inhibitors that reverse epigenetic processes associated with the methylation of tumor suppressor genes are under investigation.

- The World Health Organization has outlined treatment strategies to reduce pain and has devised an analgesic ladder for pain that includes the use of nonopioid analgesia first, followed by a weak opioid and then a strong opioid. The opioid drug morphine is the drug of choice for moderate to severe cancer pain. Other drugs, including those derived from other plant sources and some animal sources, are useful as well.

- Administration of recombinant erythropoietin (EPO) to treat anemia and so reduce the debilitating fatigue experienced by many patients with cancer has proven highly successful. EPO is a hormone released by the kidney in response to hypoxia, and stimulates the production of red blood cells by bone marrow.

- Bone marrow transplantation involves the injection of hematopoietic cells into the bone marrow of the cancer patient. The cells may come from a compatible donor (allogeneic) or from the patient (autologous) if the individual has adequate stem cells. With an autologous transplant, the patient's bone marrow is harvested and frozen before chemotherapy or radiation and then reinfused after the other treatments are complete. Peripheral blood stem cell transplantation is also being used. Umbilical cord blood is rich in stem cells and offers new possibilities in cancer treatment. Research is still needed on the long-term effects and many ethical issues are still being discussed.

- Exercise has been shown to be effective in reducing symptoms and improving the physical and psychosocial functioning of patients with cancer.

Cancer Prevention

Cancer prevention is the ultimate goal. Although cancer will occur in some people regardless of lifestyle or personal behavior, certain types of lifestyles and behaviors increase cancer risk, while others decrease it. Cancer prevention involves primary and secondary prevention.

Primary Prevention

Primary prevention is focused on preventing the occurrence of cancer. This approach is most effective when the cause of a specific cancer type is known.

- Avoidance of known and potential carcinogens. Avoidance of cigarette smoking is the number one behavior that can reduce the risk of cancer, both for the individual who smokes and for family members and coworkers exposed to secondhand smoke. Children appear to be at increased risk of developing cancer after exposure to secondhand smoke even in utero. Chewable tobacco products also are associated with an increased risk of oral cancer and should be avoided. Chewing tobacco is a major health concern in adolescent medicine. Skin protection during sun exposure is extremely important in preventing the development of skin cancer.

- Modify associated factors. Although the exact cause of a cancer may not be known, conditions that increase the risk need to be avoided. For example, alcohol consumption, low-fiber high-fat diets, and multiple sexual partners have been shown to increase the risk of certain types of cancers. Limiting alcohol consumption to no more than 1 ounce per day and consuming a diet rich in fruits, vegetables, and fiber and low in animal fat are dietary modifications that may lower the risk of cancer development. Limiting sexual partners and practicing safe sex decreases the risk of sexually transmitted diseases, which reduces the risks of developing cancers related to infectious processes.

- Removal of tissues that have a high risk for developing into cancer. Skin lesions, colon polyps, and breast tissue that is highly suspicious may be removed prophylactically.

- Chemoprevention. The use of chemicals and nutrients in individuals with precancerous lesions, a history of cancer, and decreased immune system and even in healthy people with no specific cancer risk may be helpful. The purpose of chemoprevention is to reverse gene damage and stop the transformation process.

- Vaccination. The only approved vaccine at this time is Gardasil for the prevention of HPV, which is a strong risk factor for cervical cancer.

Secondary Prevention

The aim of secondary prevention is early detection that greatly increases the prognosis. Routine screening based on recommendations from the American Cancer Society does not decrease the incidence of cancer but does have the potential to decrease death through early intervention. Specific screening guidelines will be discussed with each specific type of cancer, but some examples of screening may include mammography, colonoscopy, PSA, and screening for gene mutations. Early cancer detection may be facilitated by teaching individuals self breast examination, self testicular examination, and regular skin examination.

Cancer Detection

Early detection of cancer, while not a preventive measure, can lead to containing or destroying a cancer before it has metastasized throughout the body. Early detection depends on identifying the risk factors for a specific patient and using appropriate physical examination techniques. Teaching individuals to report early warning signs included in Box 3-3 to the health care provider is imperative. Some screening tests, including Pap smears, tests for intestinal polyps, and biopsies of abnormal skin lesions, may allow for intervention even before dysplastic cells (cells showing early signs of abnormality) become cancerous.

B O X   3 - 3   Warning Signs of Cancer

Changes in bowel or bladder habits
A sore throat that does not heal
Unusual bleeding or discharge
Thickening or lump in the breast or elsewhere
Indigestion or difficulty swallowing
Obvious change in a wart or mole
Nagging cough or hoarseness

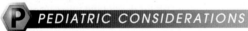

PEDIATRIC CONSIDERATIONS

- Cancer warning signs in children include:
  - Continued and unexplained weight loss
  - Headaches accompanied by vomiting in the morning
  - Increased swelling or continual pain in bones and joints
  - Lump or mass (abdomen, neck, other sites)
  - Development of whitish appearance in pupil
  - Recurrent fevers not caused by infections
  - Excessive bleeding or bruising
  - Noticeable paleness; persistent tiredness
- Childhood cancers are most likely the result of interaction between genetics and environment.
- Most common cancers involve soft tissue, bone, kidneys, hematopoietic system, and nervous system.
- Cancer incidence is highest in the early years and during puberty/adolescence.

GERIATRIC CONSIDERATIONS

- Older adults have the highest rate of most cancers, the lowest rate of early detection, and an increased risk of complications, disability, and death. Possible explanations for the increased incidence include decreased mitochondrial activity, altered immunity due to decreased T-cell activation, interleukin-2 levels, and mitogen response, and prolonged exposure to carcinogens.

- Cancer is the second leading cause of death in those 65 years of age and older.

- Early warning signs are often attributed to the aging process or comorbidities.

CULTURAL CONSIDERATION

- African Americans have a higher incidence of cancer and a higher death rate; most likely due to decreased access to care.

SELECTED BIBLIOGRAPHY

Alberts, B., Johnson, A., Lewis, J., Raff, M., Roberts, K., & Walter, P. (2008). *Molecular biology of the cell* (5th ed.). New York: Garland Sciences.

American Cancer Society (2007). *Cancer Facts and Figures 2007*. Retrieved from http://www.cancer.org/docroot/STT/content/STT_1x_Cancer_Facts_Figures_2007.asp.

American Cancer Society (2008). *Cancer Facts and Figures 2008*. Atlanta: The American Cancer Society.

Aschenbrenner, D. S. (2008). Advances in cancer therapy: Kinase and microtubule inhibition. *American Journal of Nursing*, 108(4), 50–51.

Banasik, J. L. (2010). Neoplasia. In L. C. Copstead, & J. L. Banasik (Eds.). *Pathophysiology* (4th ed.). St. Louis: Saunders Elsevier.

Beals, J. K. (2008, December 15). PTPRD a strong candidate for new human tumor suppressor gene. *Cancer Research*. Retrieved from http//www.medscape.com/viewarticle/585391.

Eliopoulos, C. (2010). *Gerontological nursing* (7th ed.). Philadelphia: Lippincott Williams & Wilkins.

Fessele, K. L. (2008, October). Genomics in cancer care. *ONS*, 23(10), 10–14.

Lambie, D. (2010). Caring for the patient with cancer. In K. S. Osborn, C. E. Wraa, & A. B. Watson (Eds.). *Medical-surgical nursing: Preparation for practice*. Upper Saddle River, NJ: Pearson.

Merkle, C. J. (2009). Neoplasia. In C. M. Porth, & G. Matfin (Eds.). *Pathophysiology: Concepts of altered health states* (5th ed.). Philadelphia: Lippincott Williams & Wilkins.

Min, Y., & Finn, O. J. (2006). DNA vaccines for cancer too. *Cancer Immunology and Immunotherapy*, 55, 119–130.

Mongha, A., Narayan, S., Das, R. K., & Kundu, A. K. (2008). Fever and leukemoid reaction: A rare paraneoplastic manifestation of bladder carcinoma. *Indian Journal of Cancer*, 45(3), 131–132.

Rubin, R., & Strayer, D. S. (Ed.). (2008). *Rubin's pathology: Clinicopathologic foundations of medicine* (5th ed.). Philadelphia: Lippincott Williams & Wilkins.

Santiago, C., Gonzalez-Freire, M., Muniesa, C. A., Fernandez del Valle, M., Perez, M., Foster, C., et al. (2009). Endurance performance: Genes or gene combinations? *International Journal of Sports Medicine*, 30(1), 66–72.

Virshup, D. M., & McCance, K. L. (2008). Biology of cancer and tumor spread. In *Understanding pathophysiology* (4th ed.). St. Louis: Mosby Elsevier.

Workman, M. L. (2010). Cancer development. In D. D. Ignatavicius, & M. L. Woodman (Eds.). *Medical-surgical nursing: Patient-centered collaborative care* (6th ed.). St. Louis: Saunders Elsevier.

Effective
and Ineffective
Health Protection

4

The Immune System

The immune system includes the bone marrow, lymph nodes, thymus gland, tonsils, and spleen. The immune system works to:

- protect the body from infection by microorganisms
- assist in healing
- remove or repair damaged cells if an infection or injury does occur
- identify self from nonself: the cells, tissues, and organs of the host versus the cells and tissues of foreign origin
- recognize and eliminate host cells that have been altered by intracellular viruses or cancer.

Abnormal responses by the immune system can cause an attack against the body's own cells, the development of cancer, or an inability to fight or heal from infection.

● Physiologic Concepts

CELLS OF THE IMMUNE RESPONSE SYSTEM

The immune response is under the control of specialized cells, the **white blood cells**. White blood cells protect the body from infection and cancer and assist in healing. White blood cells include the neutrophils, eosinophils, basophils, monocytes, and macrophages, and the B and T lymphocytes. Platelets are fragments of cells that also play a role in healing. All white blood cells and

TABLE 4-1 Normal Lab Values	
Blood Component	**Normal Range**
White blood cell count (WBC)	4,000–11,000 cells/mm³
Neutrophils	50–70% of total WBC
Basophils	0.1–1.0% of total WBC
Eosinophils	1–4% of total WBC
Monocytes	2–8% of total WBC
Lymphocytes	20–40% of total WBC
Platelets	150,000–400,000 mm³

platelets derive from a basic stem (originator) cell, called the pluripotent stem cell, in the bone marrow. From this cell, succeeding generations of stem cells differentiate and commit to producing one type of cell. Normal values for selected blood components are included in Table 4-1. Blood cells and their differentiation are discussed in Chapter 12.

Neutrophils, Eosinophils, and Basophils

Neutrophils, eosinophils, and basophils are called granulocytes because of the cytoplasmic granules that dominate their appearance under the microscope. The granulocytes remain in the bone marrow or circulation until they are drawn to an area of infection, inflammation, or trauma by substances released from damaged tissues, by microorganisms, or by the B or T lymphocytes. The cytoplasmic granules contain enzymes that break down and destroy microorganisms and digest cellular debris. Once granulocytes complete their function, they die. In a serious infection, granulocytes may only survive a few hours.

The neutrophils are the first white blood cells to arrive at an area of injury or infection and are key players in the processes of inflammation. Neutrophils arriving on the scene begin phagocytizing the cells and debris immediately. They also release chemicals that damage microorganisms and attract other white blood cells to the area, in a process called **chemotaxis**. Neutrophils initiate the inflammatory responses of vasodilation and increased capillary permeability. Clinically, neutrophils are often referred to as polymorphonuclear cells (PMNs) or segmented neutrophils ("segs") because of the segmented appearance of their multilobed nuclei. Eosinophils have several functions. First, they are involved in the allergic response (described later). Second, they are important in the defense against parasitic (helminthic) infections. They also protect the host by reducing the inflammatory response by destroying histamine. The eosinophils phagocytize cell debris, although to a lesser degree than do neutrophils. The level of eosinophils may increase during an allergic response or in response to helminthic infection.

Basophils circulate in the bloodstream and, when activated by injury or infection, release histamine, bradykinin, and serotonin. These substances increase capillary permeability and blood flow to the area, bringing to the area other mediators required to eliminate infection and promote healing. Basophils secrete the natural anticlotting substance heparin, which ensures that clotting and coagulation pathways do not continue unchecked. Basophils are also involved in producing allergic responses. They are similar in function to important initiators of tissue inflammation, the mast cells, but unlike mast cells, basophils circulate in the blood.

Monocytes and Macrophages

Monocytes circulate in the blood and enter injured tissue across capillary membranes that become permeable as part of the inflammatory reaction (described later). They arrive at the site of injury hours to days after neutrophils. Monocytes are not phagocytic, but after several hours in the tissue area, they mature into macrophages. Macrophages are large cells capable of withstanding an acidic environment and ingesting large quantities of cell debris and bacteria. Macrophages can phagocytize lysed red blood cells and other white blood cells. Some macrophage cells colonize tissues such as skin, lymph nodes, and lungs for months or years. These cells are readily available to scavenge microorganisms that may enter the body through those routes. The monocyte–macrophage cell system is called the reticuloendothelial system.

Lymphocytes

Lymphocytes include the B and T lymphocytes and a type of cell called the natural killer (NK) cell. Lymphocytes are produced in the bone marrow and mature there or in other lymphoid tissues.

B lymphocytes (B cells) mature in the bone marrow. After maturation, a B cell circulates in the blood in an inactive state and becomes active only after exposure to a specific molecule, usually a protein or large carbohydrate of foreign origin, to which it has been genetically programmed during fetal development to respond. When activated, the B cell becomes a **plasma cell**, a specialized cell that mounts an immune response against the molecule that activated it. B lymphocytes comprise the humoral immune system, meaning that they circulate in the blood (the humor).

T lymphocytes comprise the cellular immune system. T-cell maturation occurs during passage through the thymus gland. Like a B cell, the mature T cell stays inactive until it encounters the specific molecule to which it has been programmed during development to respond; once it does so, it becomes activated and may directly attack and destroy the cell expressing that molecule. The T cell may also release chemicals that alert B cells to the presence of the invader, thereby initiating a humoral response. T cells can stimulate or in some circumstances inhibit the inflammatory responses via the release of pro- or anti-inflammatory peptides known as **cytokines**. T cells are important for recognizing and destroying parasites and viruses that hide intracellularly, where the B cells are unable to encounter them.

NK cells are produced in the bone marrow and provide innate defense for the body. The NK cells react to foreign molecules, but do not demonstrate specificity, that is, they may respond to more than one foreign molecule. They recognize abnormal cells by one of two mechanisms: killer-activating receptors or killer-inhibiting receptors. The natural history of NK cell origin and maturation is unclear.

Platelets

Platelets are not cells, but cytoplasmic fragments that develop from specialized cells in the bone marrow called megakaryocytes. Like white blood cells, platelets are drawn to an area of inflammation. Once the platelets arrive at the site of injury, they adhere to the vessel wall, forming aggregates or plugs. Adhering to the vessel wall activates the platelets, causing them to release several biochemical mediators, including serotonin and histamine, which temporarily decrease blood flow and bleeding. This vasoconstriction is short lived, however, and soon blood flow increases to deliver other white blood cells to the area. If the injury is small, the platelet plug is usually sufficient to allow for healing. Platelets circulate in the blood for about 10 days before they become nonfunctioning and are phagocytized by neutrophils and monocytes. If a person has too few platelets, he or she is at increased risk of developing multiple small hemorrhages under the skin and throughout the body.

THE SPECIFIC AND INNATE IMMUNE RESPONSES

The immune system includes both specific and innate responses. *Specific* immune responses are those that involve activation of the B and T lymphocytes. B and T lymphocytes are capable of responding with specificity and precision to virtually any foreign molecule an individual may encounter in a lifetime. Once the original response is made, the B or T cell retains a memory of it. If a second encounter with that molecule occurs, the B- or T-cell response will be faster and more effective than before.

The *innate* immune response, in contrast, includes the inflammatory responses to infection or injury and the white blood cells that participate in those responses: the neutrophils, basophils, eosinophils, and monocytes and macrophages. Species resistance, mechanical barriers, chemical barriers, secretions, inflammation, interferon, and complement are all part of the innate immune system. The inflammatory response is stimulated after tissue injury or infection, with the goal of delivering white blood cells and platelets to the tissues to limit damage and promote healing. The inflammatory reactions are not characterized by specificity or memory, but they are fast and effective.

ANTIGENS

An **antigen** is any molecule that can stimulate a specific immune response against itself or the cell that carries it. Billions of B and T lymphocytes are produced during fetal development with the potential to bind to at least 100 million distinct antigens. Antigens that can bind to a T or B lymphocyte include those present on the cell wall of bacteria or mycoplasmas, the coat of a virus, or on certain pollens, dusts, or foods. Every cell of a person has surface proteins that would be recognized as foreign antigens by B or T lymphocytes from another person. If an antigen causes either the B or T lymphocyte to become activated and to multiply or differentiate further, it is an immunogenic antigen.

B-LYMPHOCYTE RESPONSE TO AN ANTIGEN

When a B lymphocyte encounters its specific antigen, it binds to it in a "lock and key" fashion, causing the B cell to differentiate into a **plasma cell**. The plasma cell in turn begins to secrete millions of molecules of **antibodies** made specifically against that antigen. Once produced, the antibodies, also called **immunoglobulins**, circulate throughout the bloodstream seeking to eliminate the antigen that stimulated their production. Antibody-mediated responses are important for defense against bacteria and circulating viruses and against toxins released from bacteria.

Immunoglobulins/Antibodies

There are five specific immunoglobulins produced in response to an antigen: IgG, IgM, IgA, IgE, and IgD. A description of each is included in Table 4-2.

Antibody Structure

All antibodies are similar in appearance. They consist of two long heavy chains called the Fc portion, and two small heads called the Fab portion. The Fc portion is identical for all antibodies of a single class (e.g., IgG or IgM). The Fab portion is specific for each antibody and contains the specific binding site for an antigen. Binding of antigen to the Fab portion of the antibody activates the Fc portion, leading to destruction of the microorganism or other antigen-bearing cell. An antibody is shown in Figure 4-1.

Antibody Destruction of a Microorganism

Antibodies cause the destruction of bound antigen by a variety of mechanisms. Usually, the antibody does not kill the cell, but instead coordinates the attack by turning on NK cells, activating complement, and enhancing phagocytosis. Under some circumstances, an antibody may directly inactivate an antigen.

NK cell activation occurs when binding of the antigen to the Fab (specific) portion of the antibody allows an NK cell to establish connections with the

Immunoglobulin/Antibody	Description
TABLE 4-2 Description of Immunoglobulins/Antibodies	
IgG	Most common immunoglobulin; makes up 75–80% of all circulating antibodies; crosses placental barrier from mother to baby during pregnancy; imparts natural passive immunity to the neonate; levels increase slowly during first exposure to an antigen, but with the second exposure they rise immediately and to a greater extent
IgM	Synthesized by immature B cells to become a part of their plasma membrane; produced first and in highest concentration during primary exposure to an antigen; largest antibody in size; protection from gram-negative bacteria
IgA	Present in mucus membranes and secretions such as saliva, tears, vaginal mucus, breast milk, gastrointestinal and lung secretions, and semen; provides protection against viral and respiratory pathogens
IgE	Responsible for hypersensitivity and allergic responses; cause mast cells to release histamine; protection against parasites
IgD	Facilitates maturation and differentiation of B lymphocytes; low concentrations in the plasma

Fc (nonspecific) portion, thus linking up the NK cell with the antigen (Fig. 4-2). The NK cell then releases toxic chemicals that directly kill the antigen target.

Complement activation will be described in more detail shortly. Complement is a series of molecules that, when activated, leads to the initiation of an inflammatory response and the killing of the antigen-bearing cell. Like NK cell activation, binding of the antigen to the Fab portion of the antibody allows the first molecule in the complement chain (C1) to bind nonspecifically to the Fc portion. Such binding hooks up the antigen-bearing cell with the complement, ultimately leading to the destruction of the antigen-bearing cell.

Phagocytic stimulation occurs similarly; when the antigen binds to the Fab portion of the antibody, this allows a phagocytic cell (usually a macrophage or neutrophil) to bind to the nonspecific Fc portion, stimulating phagocytosis of the linked antigen and the cell that bears it.

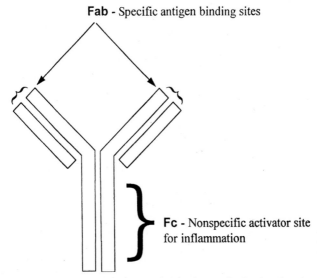

FIGURE 4-1 Diagrammatic representation of an antibody, showing sites for antigen binding and inflammatory activation.

Direct effects of an antibody may occur if, for example, an antibody binds to a virus at the same site that the virus uses to bind to and enter a susceptible cell. This would inactivate the virus. Similarly, the antibody may bind to a bacterial toxin at the same site that the toxin would use to interact with susceptible cells. This would eliminate the effect of the toxin.

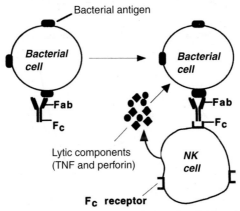

FIGURE 4-2 Activation of NK cell after binding of antibody to bacterial antigen. Activated NK cell secretes lytic components that lyse the bacterial cell. Similar patterns occur after the binding of complement or phagocyte.

Opsonization

Binding of an antibody to an antigen on a bacterium causes **opsonization**, a change in the bacterial cell wall that renders otherwise impenetrable bacteria susceptible to phagocytosis. The complement also serves as an opsonin (an agent that can cause opsonization).

The Role of the T Cell in B-Cell Response to an Antigen

To mount an antibody attack against a microorganism, T-cell support is almost always required. As described below, cytokines released by activated T lymphocytes trigger B-cell proliferation and differentiation into antibody-secreting plasma cells.

Memory Cells

Some B lymphocytes do not become antibody-secreting plasma cells after antigenic stimulation, but rather become **memory cells**. Memory cells circulate indefinitely in the blood and become active immediately upon repeated exposure to the antigen.

The first time a B lymphocyte is exposed to its antigen (the primary exposure), production of antibodies against the antigen can take 2 weeks to more than 1 year, although normally antibodies to an antigen are detectable in the blood within 3 to 6 months. Because of memory cells, the next time the antigen is encountered, the antibody response occurs almost immediately (see Fig. 4-3).

T-LYMPHOCYTE RESPONSE TO AN ANTIGEN

When a T lymphocyte binds to an immunogenic antigen, it is stimulated to mature and reproduce. This reproduction results in up to four subtypes of

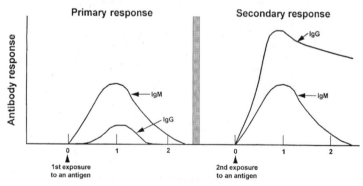

FIGURE 4-3 Primary and secondary antibody responses to an antigen.

T cells capable of acting in response to the antigen: cytotoxic T cells, helper T cells, regulatory T cells, and memory T cells. The T-cell response to antigen is called a cell-mediated response, because the T cells respond directly; they do not need to become plasma cells and secrete antibody to destroy the antigen.

Cytotoxic T cells directly destroy the antigen by releasing toxic chemicals. These chemicals punch holes in the membranes of the cells carrying the foreign antigen. Cytotoxic T cells are also called CD8 cells because of a specific protein present on their plasma membrane.

Helper T cells secrete peptides, called **cytokines**, which act as cell messengers to coordinate the response of cytotoxic T cells and B cells. There are two general categories of helper T (Th) cells: Th1 and Th2 cells. Th1 cells release cytokines that are proinflammatory, in that they draw neutrophils and monocytes to the area of injury or infection and stimulate macrophage phagocytosis. Th1 cytokines increase the production of prostaglandins, leading to increased blood flow and interstitial edema, and induce systemic symptoms of inflammation, including fever. Th1 cytokines favor the production of cytotoxic T cells and induce cell-mediated immune responses. Th2 cells generally secrete anti-inflammatory cytokines, which put the brakes on potentially dangerous inflammatory reactions. Th2 cells favor activation of humoral (B-cell driven) responses. Normally, Th1 and Th2 immune responses are in balance with each other.

Regulatory T cells act to suppress the host's immune response, a function that under some circumstances may increase the risk of infection, but under other circumstances may serve to protect the host against an overzealous immune system. Although their mechanism of action is still under investigation, regulatory T cells appear to suppress immune function via direct contact with B cells or other T cells, and/or by releasing anti-inflammatory cytokines. A deficiency in regulatory T cells has been suggested to play a role in the development of autoimmune disease, while overactive regulatory T cells may protect tumor cells from immune attack. Some evidence suggests that certain viruses, including the human immunodeficiency virus (HIV), exploit regulatory T cells' ability to dampen the body's antiviral response. Regulatory T cells are characterized by C25 receptors on their cell membranes.

Memory T cells circulate in the bloodstream until the specific antigen that stimulated their production is encountered again. Subsequent responses to that antigen occur rapidly.

RECOGNITION OF SELF VERSUS FOREIGN ANTIGENS

It is essential that the immune system recognizes self-antigens and only initiates attack against nonself or damaged cells. To ensure only appropriate immune responses, potential antigens are always presented to the immune system, and to the T cells in particular, in combination with self-antigens, called major histocompatibility complex (MHC) proteins. Because these antigens are expressed in such high concentrations on leukocytes, they are often referred to as human leukocyte antigens (HLA).

Self-Antigens

Each individual possesses cell surface antigens that are unique to that individual. These antigens, the MHC proteins or histocompatibility antigens, serve as a sort of cellular fingerprint. There are two groups of MHC proteins: **MHC I** and **MHC II**. The MHC I proteins are found on nearly all cells of the body except the red blood cells. The MHC II proteins are found only on the surface of macrophages and B cells. MHC proteins have two functions: (1) they present self-antigens to T cells and (2) they bind foreign antigens and present these to T cells. The MHC I molecules bind and present antigens only to cytotoxic T cells. The MHC II molecules bind and present antigens only to helper T cells (both Th1 and Th2 types).

The MHC Genes

The MHC proteins are inherited as four closely linked loci (groups of genes) on chromosome 6. These genes, called the MHC, are usually inherited together, with one set of loci received from each parent. There are many different possible alleles for each loci, resulting in more than one trillion possible antigen combinations. Therefore, it is virtually impossible for two unrelated individuals to have matching MHC proteins. Identical twins will have the same proteins, and an individual's siblings and offspring will likely have MHC proteins that are more similar than those of unrelated individuals.

The Role of the MHC Proteins in Controlling Immunity

After a foreign or unknown cell has been phagocytized by a macrophage or has become bound to a B cell, antigens from the cell are expressed on the macrophage or B cell adjacent to host MHC II antigens. The foreign antigens and the MHC II antigens are presented together to passing helper T (CD4) cells. Each passing helper T cell compares the foreign or unknown antigen to the host's MHC II antigens (Fig. 4-4). If in comparing the unknown antigen to the MHC II antigens, a helper T cell recognizes the antigen as foreign, the helper T cell will secrete cytokines that activate the B cell to become an antibody-secreting plasma cell. If the antigen presented is seen by helper T cells as too similar to the MHC II proteins on the B cell or macrophage, the helper T cells will not become activated, or perhaps may become T regulatory cells, and the antigen will not be attacked.

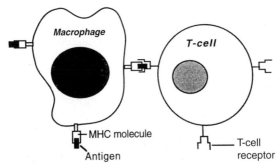

FIGURE 4-4 Antigen presentation to a T cell. The macrophage presents processed antigen along with the MHC self molecule to the T cell, which becomes activated against the antigen.

To activate cytotoxic (CD8) cells, MHC I proteins must be presented in association with the unknown or foreign antigen. All cells express MHC I proteins; therefore, any cell can present foreign antigens to CD8 cells for comparison. Cells infected with a virus make abnormal proteins, as do cancerous cells. These abnormal proteins are recognized as antigens and presented to CD8 cells along with host MHC I proteins. When cytotoxic T cells encounter abnormal proteins compared to the MHC I proteins, they are stimulated to initiate killing of the cells.

Graft Rejection and MHC Proteins

A poor match of MHC proteins is the major cause of graft rejection. Not all cellular antigens need to match; however, the closer the MHC profile match between donor and host, the greater the chance a graft will be accepted. Graft rejection is an example of cell-mediated immunity.

Development of Self-Tolerance

During gestation, hundreds of thousands of T and B cells are formed. Some of these T and B cells fit lock and key with host antigens and are therefore capable of reacting against them. To eliminate the potential of attack against host cells, T cells residing in the thymus and B cells in the bone marrow are exposed during a critical period of embryogenesis to a multitude of host antigens. If, during this time, a B or T cell encounters an antigen to which it matches, the B or T cell is programmed to undergo apoptosis and self-destruct. This leaves behind only cells tolerant to host antigens. This theory of tolerance is called the **clonal deletion theory** because it explains the elimination of clones of immune cells that react with self-antigens.

A second method also exists to ensure the elimination of cells with the potential to attack host antigens. This mechanism, called **clonal inactivation**, occurs outside the thymus during fetal development and throughout life. In this scenario, MHC II antigens are presented to helper T cells. If a helper T cell encounters the specific antigen to which it matches among the MHC proteins, the helper cell undergoes apoptosis.

Because helper T cells are essential in activating B cells to become plasma cells, clonal deletion and clonal inactivation of T cells can eliminate humoral and cellular immunity against self-antigens. In these processes, tolerance is recognized as an active process, essential for the survival of the host. Occasionally, tolerance to host cells may be lost, which leads to the development of an immune response against those cells and may cause autoimmune disease.

Exceptions to Clonal Elimination

Some tissues grow during fetal development without exposure to immature T cells. These tissues normally are kept sequestered from the immune system after birth. If they are later exposed to immune cells, however, an attack against them may occur. Cells that are normally kept sequestered from the immune system include certain cells of the testes and eye.

B- AND T-LYMPHOCYTE RESPONSES TO A FOREIGN ANTIGEN

In a **B-cell response**, B cells bind a foreign antigen. Helper T cells are presented pieces of the antigen, either by the B cell directly or by macrophages that have begun phagocytizing the antigen. If the antigen is different enough from the MHC II proteins expressed by the B cell or macrophage, the helper T cell releases cytokines that activate the B cell, causing it to become an antibody-secreting plasma cell. The antibody will bind the antigen throughout the body and orchestrate its destruction. The T cells also stimulate macrophages to increase phagocytosis of the organism and activate other white blood cells and complement to assist in the defense response.

In a **cell-mediated response**, cells of any type infected with an intracellular organism or cells that have become cancerous present foreign proteins to cytotoxic T cells along with their own MHC I proteins. This activates the cytotoxic cells to destroy the cells carrying the foreign protein.

RED BLOOD CELL ANTIGENS

There are at least 80 different antigens present on the red blood cells. The most important of these are the ABO antigens and the Rh antigens. Blood types are referred to as ABO and Rh.

ABO Antigens

The ABO blood group consists of A and B antigens. An individual receives from each parent an A antigen gene and a B antigen gene, or neither (called the O antigen). The A and B antigen genes are each dominant over the O antigen gene, but are codominant with each other. Thus, an individual who receives an A antigen gene from one parent and an A or an O from the other (AA or AO) will have type A blood. An individual who receives a B antigen gene from one parent and a B or an O from the other (BB or BO) will have type B blood. An individual who receives an A antigen gene from one parent and a B antigen gene from the other will have AB blood. Type O blood is possible only if an individual receives neither the A nor B antigen gene from either parent (OO).

Rh Antigens

The Rh antigens are a complex group of antigens present on the red blood cell. If a particular type of Rh antigen is present on the red blood cells, an individual is considered to be Rh positive. If this antigen is not present, an individual is considered Rh negative. Each individual receives one Rh gene from each parent. The Rh-positive gene dominates, such that an individual with one Rh-positive gene and one Rh-negative gene is Rh positive. Rh antigens, when mismatched between mother and fetus, can be responsible for a severe reaction in the fetus. This reaction is characterized by red blood cell lysis and anemia (hemolytic disease of the newborn and erythroblastosis fetalis), which occurs when an Rh-negative mother produces antibodies against the red cells of an Rh-positive fetus. Antibodies may cross the placenta and cause destruction of fetal red blood cells before or during birth.

Immune Reactions against Mismatched Blood

An individual with type A blood given a transfusion of type B blood may develop a severe immune reaction against the B blood, called a transfusion reaction. In a transfusion reaction, lysis and agglutination of the donated red blood cells occur. Inflammation, blood clotting, and death may result. A similar reaction would occur if an individual with type B blood were to receive a donation of type A blood. An individual with Rh-negative blood who receives an Rh-positive blood transfusion may also have an immunologic reaction, although typically the response is less intense.

Individuals with type A or type B blood can safely receive type O blood because type O blood will not stimulate an antibody reaction. Individuals with O-negative blood are called universal donors because they can supply blood to anyone. Individuals with AB-positive blood are universal recipients because they will not react against any type blood. O-negative is the blood of choice

TABLE 4-3   Blood Types and Transfusion Compatibility

Genotype	Blood Type	Red Cell Antigen	Serum Antibodies	Compatible Donor
OO	O	None	Anti-A, Anti-B	O
AO	A	A	Anti-B	A, O
AA	A	A	Anti-B	A, O
BO	B	B	Anti-A	B, O
BB	B	B	Anti-A	B, O
AB	AB	AB	None	A, B, AB, O

for an emergency trauma patient who has not been cross-matched (blood type determined). See Table 4-3 for a summary of blood types and transfusion compatibility.

IMMUNITY

Immunity is the state in which one is protected from disease development. Immunity may be innate, passive, or acquired after exposure to a microorganism or toxin.

Innate Immunity

Innate immunity is the immunity that exists due to an organism's natural resistance. Innate immunity includes barriers to infection provided by the skin, gastrointestinal (GI) juices, and tears, as well as the protection provided by the nonspecific mediators of inflammation discussed previously.

Passive Immunity

Passive immunity refers to the immunity provided to an individual by transfer of antibodies from someone else or by delivery of a prepared antitoxin. Antitoxins are antibodies produced specifically against a certain bacterial toxin (e.g., diphtheria antitoxin). An example of passive immunity is when antibodies produced in one individual against the hepatitis B virus are harvested and given to another individual who has been exposed to the virus, but whose cells have not yet been infected by it. Clinically, the transferred antibodies are referred to as hepatitis B immunoglobulin. Likewise, an individual bitten by a rattlesnake may be given antivenom. The antivenom consists of antibodies produced by a person who was bitten by a rattlesnake and survived the bite. The hope in this situation is that the passively provided antibodies will take out of circulation the poisonous venom before the person is killed or seriously affected. Passive immunity also occurs when maternal IgG antibodies cross the placenta and when IgA and other antibodies are provided to the infant in breast milk.

Passive immunity works by providing a person with preformed, specific antibodies when that person is incapable of forming antibodies (a fetus or infant) or when there is insufficient time for antibodies to be produced before infection or death occurs. Passive immunity offers immediate, but temporary protection, and does not provide a memory response.

Active Immunity

Active immunity is the cellular and humoral immune response developed by an individual who has been significantly exposed to a microorganism or toxin. Exposure may occur in a disease process or as a result of an immunization. Active immunity is characterized by memory in the B and T lymphocytes and the production of specific antibodies and T cells. An antibody titer (level) may be measured in a serum sample to document the development of immunity to a microorganism or toxin. Active immunity takes longer to develop but is natural and lasts for years. A positive titer (except in an infant) implies active immunity.

Immune Status of the Fetus and Newborn

Cell-mediated (T-cell) immunity begins in utero. A primary humoral immune response (IgM) to various microorganisms can be stimulated in the fetus in the last trimester of gestation. Other immune responses to an antigen (IgG and IgA), neutrophil and macrophage phagocytosis, and the production of inflammatory mediators, however, are not significantly present until 6 to 8 months after birth. This makes the fetus and newborn vulnerable to infection and disease. In utero, maternal IgG antibodies are actively transported across the cells of the placenta and can be detected in the newborn for at least 6 months after birth. These antibodies offer the fetus and infant passive immunity against various microorganisms. IgA and other immunoglobulins may pass to the newborn through breast milk.

A time of particular vulnerability for a newborn is at approximately 5 to 6 months after birth when maternal IgG levels are being cleared, although the infant's own immune system is not yet working at its peak. This vulnerability is especially true if the infant is not breastfeeding.

THE INFLAMMATORY RESPONSE

The inflammatory response occurs after tissue injury or infection to eliminate pathogenic injury and remove injured tissue so that healing can occur. Inflammation may precede a specific immune response or be initiated by one. There are two stages in an acute inflammatory reaction: vascular and cellular (see page C2 for illustrations).

Vascular Stage of Inflammation

The vascular stage of inflammation begins almost immediately after an injury or in response to infection or toxin exposure. Arterioles at or near the site briefly constrict and then undergo a prolonged vasodilation (relaxation). The brief constriction pulls the endothelial cells lining the arterioles apart, allowing for passage of early arriving white blood cells. The subsequent vasodilation occurs primarily as a result of mast cell degranulation and the release of chemical mediators (described later). Dilation of the arterioles causes increased fluid pressure in the downstream capillaries. At the same time, histamine and other chemicals cause an increase in the permeability of surrounding capillaries. Increased permeability combined with increased blood flow leads to increased movement of a plasma filtrate into the interstitial space. The result is swelling and edema of the interstitial space and increased viscosity of the blood left behind in the capillary. Occasionally, red blood cells may move into the area surrounding injured cells.

Cellular Stage of Inflammation

The cellular stage of inflammation begins with the movement of white cells in the blood to the area of injury or infection. These cells and platelets are drawn to the area by chemicals released from injured cells, from mast cells, by complement activation, and by cytokine production that occurs after antibody–antigen binding. Attraction of white blood cells to an area of injury is called chemotaxis. Once at the site of injury, the various stimulants cause the capillary endothelial cells and the white blood cells, especially neutrophils and later monocytes, to express complementary adhesion molecules. The endothelial cells become sticky for the white blood cells, causing the white blood cells to move to the periphery of the capillary, in a process called margination. This leads to the emigration of the white blood cells through the capillaries to surround and phagocytize the damaged cells. Platelets entering the area stimulate clotting to isolate the infection and control bleeding. Cells brought to the site will eventually be responsible for healing the injured area.

The Mast Cell

Mast cells are specialized cells filled with vasoactive chemicals. These cells are found throughout the loose connective tissue surrounding the blood vessels, especially in the lungs, GI tract, and skin. Inflammation begins when mast cells release their intracellular contents during tissue injury, exposure to toxins, activation of the proteins of the complement cascade, and antibody–antigen binding. Releasing the contents of the mast cell is called **mast cell degranulation**. Histamine, serotonin, and other substances are released with mast cell degranulation and contribute to vasodilation, increased capillary permeability, and the drawing of white blood cells and platelets to the area.

Chemical Mediators of Inflammation

The main chemical mediator of inflammation is **histamine**, which is released by basophils, platelets, and mast cells. Histamine participates in both steps of the vascular response to inflammation: relaxation of blood vessels leading to increased blood flow and increased capillary permeability. Histamine is also active in nonvascular tissues. In the respiratory passages, histamine causes constriction of bronchiolar smooth muscles. In the gut, histamine stimulates acid secretion. Histamine also causes itching. Histamine binds to H_1 receptors in the respiratory passages and the vascular system, and to H_2 receptors in the gut. Binding to the H_1 receptors causes a decrease in further release of histamine from the mast cells, an example of a negative feedback response.

Neutrophil and **eosinophil chemotactic** factors are chemicals released from white blood cells (neutrophils or eosinophils) that draw other cells to the area.

Prostaglandins, especially of the E series, are important mediators of inflammation. Prostaglandins are produced when a cell membrane is damaged, or a cell bursts, and arachidonic acid, a main constituent of the cell membrane, is metabolized by the cycloxygenase (COX) enzymes I and II. Prostaglandins (PGE_1 and PGE_2) increase blood flow and increase capillary permeability. They also augment the effects of histamine, cause fever in response to infection, and stimulate pain receptors. Other substances produced from arachidonic acid metabolism include vasoconstrictive prostaglandins and thromboxane A_2, a promoter of platelet aggregation and vasoconstriction. Prostaglandin synthesis is inhibited by nonsteroidal anti-inflammatory drugs (NSAIDs), such as aspirin and ibuprofen, which act by blocking the COX I and COX II enzymes.

Leukotrienes also are end products of arachidonic acid metabolism. These substances increase vascular permeability and increase the adhesion of white blood cells to the capillary during injury or infection. They also act as chemoattractant chemicals. One type of leukotriene, called slow-reacting substance of anaphylaxis, plays an important role in the bronchiolar constriction of asthma and in allergic reactions. Leukotriene production is not blocked by COX enzyme inhibitors.

Cytokines are a family of peptides produced by a variety of immune and inflammatory cells, including macrophages, monocytes, neutrophils, and B and T lymphocytes. They are also produced by noninflammatory cells, including fibroblasts and endothelial cells. Cytokines are often referred to by specific names related to their function or numbered following the general term "interleukin." Cytokines function as local hormones that affect the host defense response to injury or infection. Each cytokine may have multiple effects on a variety of interrelated processes. In general, cytokines serve as communication links between different arms of the immune and inflammatory responses. Cytokines are discussed further in Chapter 7.

There are two general categories of cytokines: proinflammatory and anti-inflammatory. *Proinflammatory* cytokines (e.g., interleukin-1, interleukin-2, interleukin-6, tumor necrosis factor, and interferon-gamma) promote the inflammatory responses and cause fever and malaise. These proinflammatory cytokines are released from macrophages and monocytes (interleukin-1) or activated Th1-type lymphocytes (interleukin-2, interleukin-6, tumor necrosis factor, and interferon-gamma). Interleukin-2 and tumor necrosis factor stimulate cytotoxic T cells to attack and kill cancer cells or cells infected with a virus. They also alert macrophages to increase phagocytosis. A variety of other cytokines are important for stimulating the bone marrow to increase white and red blood cell production (hematopoietic colony-stimulating factors). These cytokines cause the increase in white blood cells that typically accompanies infection. *Anti-inflammatory* cytokines (e.g., interleukin-4 and interleukin-10) decrease the secretion of the proinflammatory cytokines and stimulate activation of B cells.

Interferons are a type of cytokine specific for preventing intracellular infection by viruses or parasitic organisms. They are produced by T cells (interferon-gamma) or other white blood cells (interferon-alpha) or fibroblasts (interferon-beta) and function to alert neighboring cells to secrete chemicals that will prevent them from becoming infected. The interferons have been used clinically to stimulate the immune system of patients with cancer and other diseases.

Chemokines are a type of cytokine that act as chemotactic agents to regulate leukocyte movement. They may act to attract all types of white blood cells, or may be specific for certain white blood cells. Chemokines interact with target white cells by binding to receptors on the cell membrane. They work by a variety of mechanisms, one of which is to cause the cell to express adhesion molecules complementary to those expressed by capillary endothelial cells. These adhesion molecules make white blood cells sticky for the capillary, resulting in migration and emigration of the cells.

COMPLEMENT SYSTEM

The complement system consists of 20 or more plasma proteins that are activated one by one in a domino fashion when the first protein (C_1, the classical pathway) or the third protein (C_3, the alternative pathway) is activated. The C_1 protein is activated when the Fc portion of an IgG or IgM antibody is turned on after antigen binding to the Fab portion. The C_3 protein is usually activated by pieces of bacterial or fungal cell wall released during phagocytosis. Activation of complement is an effective mechanism for destroying extracellular microbes.

The first five complement proteins (C_1–C_5) stimulate mast cell degranulation, white blood cell chemotaxis, and opsonization of bacteria. Activation of complement proteins 6 through 10 (C_6–C_{10}) causes bacterial cell lysis by making the cell wall leaky to water.

COAGULATION PATHWAY

The coagulation pathway involves another series of at least 13 proteins that activate in a step-by-step cascade. The coagulation cascade functions like the platelets (but more powerfully) to stop bleeding. The result of the coagulation cascade is the formation of an insoluble clot and a meshwork of fibers that entrap microorganisms and prevent the spread of infection.

The coagulation cascade can be stimulated by many substances present with inflammation or injury. The intrinsic pathway is activated when one of the plasma proteins, factor XII (the Hageman factor), comes into contact with an injured blood vessel. The extrinsic pathway is stimulated when a different plasma protein, factor VII, comes into contact with a substance called tissue thromboplastin, which is released by injured cells. Both pathways result in the formation of a fibrin clot. The coagulation pathway requires calcium ion for most steps. Coagulation is kept in check by a series of natural anticoagulants that act with naturally occurring heparin (from platelets) to stop the coagulation cascade and prevent uncontrolled thrombus formation.

● Pathophysiologic Concepts

LOCAL SIGNS OF INFLAMMATION

The five cardinal local characteristics of inflammation are included in Table 4-4 along with the underlying pathology.

TABLE 4-4   Local Signs of Inflammation

Sign/Symptom	Physiology
Redness	Increased blood flow to the area
Heat	Increased blood flow to the area
Swelling	Increased capillary permeability allows plasma proteins and exudates to enter the interstitial space
Pain	Stretching of nerves caused by pressure from exudates and stimulation of nerve endings by mediators of inflammation
Loss of function	Caused by the pain and swelling

SYSTEMIC SIGNS OF INFLAMMATION

Signs of the inflammatory response may be local or systemic depending on the severity. Fever and leukocytosis are the classical systemic signs. The patient may also have vague complaints and general malaise.

Fever

Fever is the elevation of the temperature set point in the hypothalamus. With an increase in set point, the hypothalamus sends out signals to increase body temperature. The body responds by shivering and increasing the basal metabolic rate.

Fever occurs in response to production of certain cytokines, including interleukin-1, interleukin-6, and tumor necrosis factor. These cytokines are considered to be endogenous pyrogens (heat producers). The pyrogenic cytokines are released by several different cells, including monocytes, macrophages, T-helper cells, and fibroblasts, in response to tissue infection or injury. The endogenous pyrogens cause fever by producing a prostaglandin, probably PGE, that raises the hypothalamic thermoregulatory set point. When the source of the pyrogen is removed (e.g., after a successful response of the immune system against a microorganism), its level decreases, which returns the set point to normal. For a short time, body temperature will lag behind the return of the set point and the hypothalamus will perceive the body temperature as too high. In response, the hypothalamus will stimulate responses such as sweating to cool the body. Aspirin and other NSAIDs inhibit fever by blocking prostaglandin synthesis.

Although the function of endogenous pyrogens has been recognized for more than 30 years, it is still uncertain exactly how they transmit the message of infection from the periphery to the central nervous system (CNS). The primary hypothesis proposed to explain this occurrence is that locally produced interleukin-1 stimulates the firing of the vagus nerve, which then transmits the information to the CNS. Once the signal reaches the CNS, brain prostaglandin is produced and raises the hypothalamic thermoregulatory set point. An alternative hypothesis is that the interleukins may themselves cross the blood–brain barrier, and directly stimulate hypothalamic PGE production.

Fever has been shown to occur in every observed animal, suggesting an evolutionary role in species survival. Research suggests that fever helps an organism fight infection and thus is beneficial to the host. However, high fevers may damage cells, especially those of the CNS.

Leukocytosis

Leukocytosis is an increase in circulating white blood cells (leukocytes). An increase in neutrophils is responsible for the initial leukocytosis that accompanies an infection or inflammation. With infection, the number of immature cells (myeloid cells) in the blood increases as the mature neutrophils and other mature granulocytes are used up. As the inflammation continues, immature neutrophils (bands) are released from the bone marrow. This shift toward immature cells is called a **left shift**. With resolution of inflammation or infection, a **right shift** occurs as mature cells are released from the marrow and again dominate in the circulation.

CHRONIC INFLAMMATION

Chronic inflammation is an inflammatory reaction lasting longer than 2 weeks. Chronic inflammation may follow acute inflammation, for example, an unresolved infection or a poorly healed wound. Chronic inflammation may also occur without a preceding acute inflammation, for example, if the body encounters a microorganism it cannot kill, it often encloses the microorganism within a wall to isolate it. Examples of microorganisms that may lead to chronic inflammation include the mycobacteria responsible for tuberculosis and leprosy. These bacteria survive in macrophages, which group together to form a protective capsule of cells called a granuloma.

HYPERSENSITIVITY REACTIONS

Hypersensitivity reactions are abnormal immune and inflammatory responses. There are four types of hypersensitivity reactions.

Type I Hypersensitivity Reactions

Type I hypersensitivity reactions are allergic reactions mediated by the IgE antibody. In type I reactions, an antigen—called an **allergen**—to which the individual is sensitive is recognized by a B cell, which is then stimulated to make IgE antibodies against the antigen. IgE binds the antigen as well as a nearby basophil or mast cell via a high-affinity IgE receptor present on those cells. The inciting allergen is typically multivalent (has many IgE-binding sites), so the allergen actually links several IgE antibodies together. This linking triggers a cascade of signals that cause degranulation of the mast cells and basophils, and the release of histamine, cytokines, chemokines, and leukotrienes. These mediators, as well as activated complement and eosinophil chemotactic factor, cause peripheral vasodilation and increased capillary permeability, leading to localized swelling and edema. Symptoms are specific according to where the allergic response occurs. Binding of the antigen in the nasal passages causes allergic rhinitis with nasal congestion and inflammation of the tissues, while binding of an antigen in the gut may cause diarrhea or vomiting.

A severe type I hypersensitivity reaction is termed an **anaphylactic reaction**. Anaphylaxis involves a rapid IgE–mast cell response after exposure to an antigen to which the individual is highly sensitive. Histamine-induced dilation of the entire systemic vasculature can occur, leading to the collapse of the blood pressure. A severe decrease in systemic blood pressure during an anaphylactic reaction is called anaphylactic shock. Because histamine is a potent constrictor of bronchiolar smooth muscle, anaphylaxis involves closure of the respiratory passages. Anaphylaxis in response to some drugs such as penicillin, or in response to a bee sting, may be fatal in highly sensitized individuals, as a result of circulatory collapse or respiratory failure. Symptoms of an anaphylactic reaction include itching, abdominal cramps, flushing of the skin, GI upset, and breathing difficulties.

Type II Hypersensitivity Reactions

Type II hypersensitivity reactions occur when IgG or IgM antibodies attack tissue antigens. Type II reactions result from a loss of self-tolerance and are considered autoimmune reactions. The target cell is usually destroyed.

In a type II reaction, antibody–antigen binding causes complement activation, mast cell degranulation, interstitial edema, tissue destruction, and cell lysis. Type II hypersensitivity reactions lead to macrophage phagocytosis of the host cells. Examples of type II autoimmune diseases include Graves disease, which involves antibodies produced against the thyroid gland; autoimmune hemolytic anemia, which involves antibodies produced against red blood cells; transfusion reactions, which involve antibodies produced against donor blood cells; and autoimmune thrombocytopenic purpura, which involves antibodies produced against platelets. Systemic lupus erythematosus (SLE) also has aspects of type II reactions (described later).

Type III Hypersensitivity Reactions

Type III hypersensitivity reactions occur when circulating antibody–antigen complexes precipitate out in a blood vessel or in downstream tissue. Antibodies are not directed against those particular tissue sites, but are trapped in their capillary meshwork. In some cases, foreign antigens may adhere to tissues, causing formation of antibody–antigen complexes at those sites.

Type III reactions activate complement and mast cell degranulation, causing damage to the tissue or capillaries where they occur. Neutrophils are drawn to the area and begin to phagocytize the injured cells, causing release of cellular enzymes and the accumulation of cell debris. This continues the inflammation cycle.

Examples of type III hypersensitivity reactions include serum sickness, in which antibodies form against foreign blood, often in response to intravenous drug use. The antibody–antigen complexes deposit in the vascular system, joints, and kidneys. With glomerulonephritis, antibody–antigen complexes form in response to an infection, often by streptococcal bacteria, and deposit in the glomerular capillaries of the kidneys. With SLE, antibody–antigen complexes form against collagen and cellular DNA, and deposit in multiple sites of the body.

Type IV Hypersensitivity Reactions

Type IV hypersensitivity reactions are T cell–mediated reactions, in that cytotoxic (CD8) or helper (CD4) T cells are activated by an antigen, leading to destruction of the cells involved. Cytotoxic cell–mediated reactions are often against virally infected cells and can lead to extensive tissue damage. CD4 cell–mediated reactions are delayed, taking 24 to 72 hours to develop. They are characterized by the production of proinflammatory cytokines that stimulate macrophage phagocytosis and increase swelling and edema.

Examples of conditions caused by type IV reactions include autoimmune thyroiditis (Hashimoto disease), in which T cells are produced against thyroid tissue, graft and tumor rejection, and delayed allergic reactions, such as the reaction to poison ivy. The tuberculin skin test indicates the presence of delayed cell-mediated immunity against the tuberculin bacillus.

IMMUNE AND INFLAMMATORY DEFICIENCIES

Immune and inflammatory deficiencies inhibit the body's ability to respond to infection or injury, and may result from impaired function of any or all white blood cells. Complement or coagulation proteins may also be deficient. Immune and inflammatory deficiencies may be congenital (present at birth) or acquired after illness, infection, or prolonged stress. The deficiencies may be temporary or permanent.

Congenital Immunodeficiency

Congenital immunodeficiency occurs as a result of a genetic defect. Congenital immunodeficiency may involve one type of T or B cell, all the T cells (DiGeorge syndrome), or all the B cells (Bruton agammaglobulinemia). Most commonly, one immunoglobulin (usually IgA or IgG) is missing. Individuals with selective immunoglobulin deficiency may have an increased susceptibility to certain infections or may be asymptomatic. Severe cases of IgG deficiency may be treated with replacement injections. Typically, selective IgA deficiency is not treated because patients may develop IgG antibodies to administered IgA, which may cause anaphylaxis. With total B-cell deficiency, the missing immunoglobulins can be provided to the individual by intravenous administration. Infants with primary T-cell deficiency have severely impaired ability to fight infection because T cells are required not only for cellular immunity but humoral immune responses as well. If the pluripotential bone marrow stem cells are dysfunctional, T and B cells and all other white blood cells may be deficient. This condition is called severe combined immunodeficiency syndrome (SCIDS). SCIDS used to be fatal in early childhood, but treatment with harvested stem cells is yielding promising results.

Congenital immunodeficiency may also occur if an individual is born without certain MHC proteins. Without these proteins, dysfunctional self-antigen presentation to the T cells occurs, leading to a failure of T-cell immune function. This condition usually causes death in early childhood.

Acquired Immunodeficiency

Acquired immunodeficiency is reduced functioning of the immune system developing after birth. Acquired immunodeficiency may arise in response to infection, malnutrition, chronic stress, certain medications, or pregnancy. Systemic illnesses such as diabetes, renal failure, and cirrhosis of the liver can cause immunodeficiency. Individuals receiving corticosteroids to prevent transplant rejection or to reduce chronic inflammation are immunosuppressed, as are those receiving chemotherapeutic drugs and radiation therapy. Surgery and anesthesia may also depress the immune system.

Acquired immunodeficiencies can be of B- or T-cell function, or both. Because B cells require helper T-cell stimulation to successfully fight infection, T-cell deficiencies also cause dysfunction of the humoral immune system.

Consequences of Immunodeficiency

Immunodeficient individuals repeatedly develop frequent severe and unusual infections and are often unable to fight them. Individuals with T-cell deficiencies frequently develop viral and yeast infections; individuals with B-cell deficiencies are especially susceptible to infections by bacteria that normally require opsonization. HIV destroys the helper T (CD4) cells and infects other white blood cells. Live virus vaccines are contraindicated in individuals who are immunodeficient.

● Conditions of Disease or Injury

Autoimmune disorders affect approximately 5% of the U.S. population. During embryonic development, some lymphocytes may develop that are unable to differentiate between self and nonself. If these autoreactive lymphocytes are not suppressed or eliminated, immune tolerance will not develop. The lack of immune tolerance may be the result of (1) contact with a previously sequestered antigen, (2) neoantigen development, (3) complications from an infectious disease, (4) emergence of a forbidden clone (mutant cell), or (5) a suppressor T-cell alteration. The peak onset for autoimmune diseases is between 15 and 45 years of age. Most autoimmune conditions have periods of remissions and exacerbations. A brief overview of several autoimmune diseases is presented in Table 4-5. A more in-depth discussion is included in the chapter associated with the particular system involved. Allergy, SLE, and HIV/AIDS are discussed in this chapter.

TABLE 4-5 Autoimmune Diseases

Disease	Description
Addison disease	Hyposecretion of adrenal hormones; clinical manifestations may include decreased appetite, weight loss, chronic and severe fatigue, hypotension, skin hyperpigmentation, and hypoglycemia
Cardiomyopathy	One theory is that an abnormal gene damages the heart muscle and fibrous and fatty tissue attempt to repair the damage resulting in hypokinetic areas which eventually interferes with adequate pump function; clinical manifestations may include palpitations, light-headedness, syncope, fatigue, and cardiac dysrhythmias
Diabetes mellitus	Lymphocytes infiltrate and destroy insulin-producing cells in the pancreas resulting in insulin deficiency; affects carbohydrate, fat, and protein metabolism; clinical manifestations may include hyperglycemia, polyuria, polyphagia, polydipsia, weight loss, and fatigue
Glomerulonephritis	Antigens from immune complexes deposit in the kidney and alter filtration resulting in fluid and electrolyte imbalances and possibly kidney failure; may be triggered by a streptococcal infection; clinical manifestations may include mild edema, oliguria, azotemia, increased BUN, and hematuria
Goodpasture syndrome	Circulating antibodies attack antigens intrinsic to glomerular basement membrane resulting in glomerulonephritis; clinical manifestations include those associated with acute glomerulonephritis, and pulmonary symptoms such as shortness of breath, cough, and hemoptysis
Graves disease	Most common cause of hyperthyroidism; more common in women; thyroid stimulating immunoglobulins activate thyroid stimulating hormone receptors on thyroid follicular cells, which increases thyroid hormone production; clinical manifestations may include weight loss, increased appetite, exertional dyspnea, nervousness, goiter, palpitations, heat intolerance, and fatigue

table continues on page 136

TABLE 4-5 Autoimmune Diseases (continued)

Disease	Description
Hemolytic anemia	Noxious stimuli causes increased breakdown of RBCs; clinical manifestations may include fatigue, shortness of breath, and hypoxia
Hashimoto disease or chronic lymphocytic thyroiditis	Most common cause of hypothyroidism; immune system attacks thyroid tissue causing a decrease in thyroid hormone production which slows the metabolic rate; clinical manifestations may include weight gain, cold intolerance, constipation, mental lethargy, dry skin, thinning hair, and edema
Multiple sclerosis (MS)	Demyelination in the brain and spinal cord; activation of T cells specific for myelin basic protein; the T cells release cytokines in the CNS which initiates an immune response that causes damage to the myelin sheath and axons; clinical manifestations may include fatigue, vertigo, nystagmus, sensory loss, altered gait, weakness of the extremities, and optic neuritis
Myasthenia gravis	Destruction of acetylcholine receptors at the neuromuscular junction; it is speculated that the epithelial myoid cells from the thymus may become antigenic and initiates an autoimmune attack; clinical manifestations may include progressive muscle weakness, fatigue, ptosis, diplopia, difficulty chewing and swallowing, and difficulty talking
Pernicious anemia	DNA synthesis of the RBC is impaired resulting in large, immature blood cells; clinical manifestations may include gastrointestinal (smooth beefy red tongue, anorexia, and nausea), integumentary (hyperpigmentation), and/or neurological symptoms (peripheral neuropathy, ataxia, confusion, and memory loss)
Reproductive infertility	Destruction of gametes due to antigens on sperm or tissue surrounding ovum
Rheumatic fever	Abnormal autoimmune response to inappropriately treated group A beta-hemolytic Streptococcus leading to scarring and malformation of cardiac valves; clinical manifestations may include fever, malaise, headache, erythema marginatum, swollen tender joints, weakness, shortness of breath, chorea, and elevated WBC count

Disease	Description
Rheumatoid arthritis (RA)	Antiglobulin antibodies combine with immunoglobulin in the synovial fluid and complexes are formed; neutrophils migrate to the joint space and cause destruction; clinical manifestations may include fatigue, anorexia, joint pain, low-grade fever, joint deformity; synovial inflammation may spread to other tissues
Scleroderma	Immune system stimulates excess production of fibroblasts resulting in excess collagen; clinical manifestations may include hard, shiny and painful skin, immobile mask-like face, joint pain, and muscle weakness
Systemic lupus erythematosus (SLE)	Autoantibodies and antibody–antigen response causes damage to joints and soft organs; strong familial tendency; clinical manifestations may include fatigue, unexplained fever, swollen joints, red rash (butterfly rash on face), arthralgia, unexplained hair loss, and photosensitivity
Ulcerative colitis	Suspected that a defect in intestinal permeability allows antigen leakage through the mucosa resulting in inflammatory response; clinical manifestations may include low-grade fever, malaise, anorexia, weight loss, abdominal distention, blood and mucus in the stool, and tenesmus

ALLERGY

An allergy is an overstimulation of inflammatory reactions that occurs in response to a specific environmental antigen. An antigen that causes an allergy is called an allergen. Allergic reactions may be antibody mediated or T cell mediated. Type I hypersensitivity reactions are examples of antibody-mediated allergies, whereas Type IV hypersensitivity reactions are examples of T cell–mediated allergies.

An individual with a Type I hypersensitivity allergic response has developed sensitized IgE antibodies to an allergen. When the allergen is encountered by the antibody, the antibody is overexpressed, causing excessive mast cell degranulation and release of histamine and other inflammatory mediators (leukotrienes, chemokines, and cytokines). Type IV hypersensitivity reactions occur after transdermal (across the skin) transport of an allergen that is presented to T cells sensitized to that allergen. Manifestations of an allergic response depend on where the allergen is encountered—whether in food, in inhaled particles, or through the skin. The timing of an allergic reaction varies depending on whether the response is type I (immediate) or type IV (delayed). A type I reaction involving the skin is called atopic dermatitis; a type IV reaction is called **allergic contact dermatitis**. The skin response to poison ivy is a type of allergic contact dermatitis and is discussed in Chapter 5.

Cause of Allergies

The cause of allergies is unclear but the IgE-mediated antibody–antigen response is the hallmark of allergic reactions. An antigen stimulates overproduction of IgE antibodies that cleave to the mast cells. When these antibodies interact with an allergen, histamine and proinflammatory mediators are released from mast cells and cause the typical clinical manifestations associated with allergies. Excessive IgE binding, easily provoked mast cell degranulation, or excessive helper T cell response may also be involved. Recent work suggests that a deficiency in T regulatory cells may contribute to overresponsiveness of the immune system and allergy. Overexposure to certain allergens at any time, including during gestation, may cause an allergic response. Genetic predisposition is the most consistent factor. There is a 25% risk factor in the general population for developing an allergy. The risk increases to 50% if one parent has allergies and to 75% if both parents have allergies.

Clinical Manifestations

- Localized swelling, itching, and redness of the skin, with skin exposure to an allergen. Type IV reactions are often characterized by blistering and crusting over of the affected area.
- Diarrhea and abdominal cramps, with exposure to a GI allergen.
- Allergic rhinitis, characterized by itchy eyes and runny nose, with exposure to a respiratory allergen. Swelling and congestion occur. Breathing difficulties may occur because of histamine-mediated constriction of the bronchiolar smooth muscle of the airways.

Diagnostic Tools

- Skin tests help in diagnosing an allergy. A small amount of the suspected allergen is injected under the skin. Individuals allergic to that allergen will respond with marked erythema, swelling, and itching at the injection site.
- Serum immunoglobulin analysis may indicate increased basophil and eosinophil count.

Complications

- A severe allergic reaction may result in anaphylaxis, which is characterized by a decrease in blood pressure and closure of the airways. Itching, cramping, and diarrhea may occur. Without intervention, severe reactions can lead to cardiovascular shock, hypoxia, and death.

- Allergic contact dermatitis (e.g., with a poison ivy reaction) may lead to secondary infection from excessive scratching.

Treatment

- Antihistamines and drugs that block mast cell degranulation may reduce the symptoms of allergy.
- Corticosteroids, inhaled, administered nasally, or taken systemically, act as anti-inflammatory agents and can reduce the symptoms of an allergy. Inhaled or intranasal therapy needs to be used for extended periods of time before becoming effective. Inhaled corticosteroids exert their effects only on the respiratory passages and may have few systemic effects.
- Inhaled mast cell stabilizers reduce mast cell degranulation and may reduce type I allergic symptoms.
- Desensitization therapy, involving repeated injections of small amounts of an allergen to which an individual is sensitive, may cause the individual to build IgG antibodies, called "blocking antibodies," against the allergen. These blocking antibodies also bind the allergen and by doing so interfere with the ability of the allergen to covalently link multiple IgE molecules together; this prevents mast cell degranulation, so allergic symptoms are reduced. IgG antibodies are produced each time the allergen is encountered and eventually may stop the allergic response.

LATEX ALLERGY

Contact with natural latex can result in a type I allergic reaction or a type IV cell-mediated reaction. With type I, the release of IgE antibodies can cause redness, itching, urticaria, asthma, and conjunctivitis. The potential to progress to anaphylactic shock also exists. With type IV the reaction may be delayed for up to 48 hours after exposure and produce dryness, itching and cracking of the skin followed by redness and swelling.

Contact with latex may occur through direct contact or via inhalation. Increased glove use has significantly increased exposure to latex and resulted in more allergies. It is essential to identify those with latex allergies and provide latex-free products for use. Education about sources of the latex protein is imperative. Foods with a similar structure protein (kiwi, avocado, strawberries, bananas) have the potential to trigger an allergic response. Patients who require frequent procedures with latex products (urinary catherterization, surgeries) are also at risk for developing a latex allergy.

SYSTEMIC LUPUS ERYTHEMATOSUS

SLE is a chronic autoimmune disease in which antibodies against several different self-antigens are produced. The antibodies are usually IgG or IgM and may be produced against DNA and RNA, proteins of the coagulation cascade, skin, red blood cells, white blood cells, and platelets. Antibody–antigen complexes can precipitate in the capillary networks, causing type III hypersensitivity reactions. Chronic inflammation can follow.

Causes of SLE

The cause of SLE is unknown, although it often occurs in individuals with a genetic tendency for autoimmune disease. Additional evidence to support a genetic role is the high concurrence among identical twins, and an increased incidence in blacks compared to whites. The tendency to develop SLE may be related to alterations of specific MHC genes and how self-antigens are expressed and recognized. Women are more likely to develop SLE than men, suggesting a role for the sex hormones. Recent research has identified a gene (interleukin-1 receptor–associated kinase 1) on the X chromosome believed to influence two key genetic loci for the development of SLE. Continued studies will explore the impact of this gene, which appears to cause serological and cellular reactivity and pathological autoimmunity.

SLE can be brought on by stress, often related to pregnancy or childbearing. In some individuals, excessive exposure to ultraviolet radiation may initiate the disease. Infections and medications such as procainamide, anticonvulsants, hydralazine, hormones, and some antibiotics may aggravate or trigger an exacerbation. Typically affected are young women during their childbearing years. The disease may remain mild for years, or may progress and lead to death.

Clinical Manifestations

- Polyarthralgia (joint pain) and arthritis (inflammation of the joint). Fever from chronic inflammation.
- Facial rash, in a malar (butterfly) pattern across the nose and cheeks. The word lupus means wolf and refers to the wolflike appearance of the rash.
- Fingertip lesions and bluing caused by poor blood flow and chronic hypoxia. Sclerosis (tightening or hardening) of the skin of the fingers.
- Sores on the oral or pharyngeal mucous membranes.
- Scaling lesions on the head, neck, and back.
- Eye and feet edema may signify renal involvement and hypertension.
- Sensitivity to light, retinopathy, retinal detachment, or loss of vision.
- Anemia, chronic fatigue, weakness, frequent infections, and bleeding are common because of the attack against the red and white blood cells and the platelets.

Diagnostic Tools

- Antinuclear antibodies are present in at least 95% of individuals with SLE, but may occur in those without the disease.
- Antibodies against double-stranded DNA are diagnostic for SLE.

- Elevated lupus erythematosus (LE) prep and presence of anti-Sm antibody and complement proteins C3 and C4.
- Hematuria and proteinuria signal renal damage.
- Antineuronal antibodies may be present.

Complications

- Renal failure is the most common cause of death in individuals with SLE. Renal failure may develop as a result of the deposit of antibody–antigen complexes in the glomeruli with resultant complement activation leading to cellular injury, an example of a type III hypersensitivity reaction.
- Pericarditis (inflammation of the sac surrounding the heart) may develop.
- Inflammation of the pleural membrane surrounding the lungs can restrict respirations. Bronchitis is common.
- Vasculitis of all peripheral and cerebral vessels may occur.
- CNS complications include stroke and seizure. Alterations in personality, including psychosis and depression, may develop. Personality changes may be related to drug therapy or the disease.

Treatment

- Anti-inflammatory drugs including aspirin or other NSAIDs are used to treat fever and arthritis.
- Systemic corticosteroids are used to treat symptoms and reduce renal and CNS pathology.
- Immunosuppressive drugs, such as methotrexate, and cytotoxic drugs (azathioprine) are used if steroids are ineffective or symptoms severe.
- Antimalarial drugs such as hydroxychloroquine are used to treat skin rashes, arthritis, and other symptoms. Also helpful in reducing abnormal blood clots.
- Rituximab, an intravenous antibiotic to decrease B cells, has been found to facilitate remission.
- Mycophenolate mofetil helps reverse lupus kidney disease.
- Plasmapheresis for vasculitis, and severe brain and kidney involvement.
- Splenectomy in severe cases to minimize platelet destruction and minimize the risk for bleeding.
- Balance rest and exercise to minimize fatigue and maintain muscle tone and joint movement.

ACQUIRED IMMUNODEFICIENCY SYNDROME

Acquired immunodeficiency syndrome (AIDS) is a viral disease that causes the collapse of the immune system. Until recently, once diagnosed with AIDS, an individual had a high probability of dying within 10 years. However, advances in treatment of patients with AIDS have made long-term survival possible. Since AIDS was first described in the early 1980s, much has been learned about how this and other viruses work and about the important roles of all white blood cells in host defense.

AIDS is caused by infection with the HIV. There are at least two HIV viruses, HIV-1 and HIV-2. HIV-1 is common in the United States, whereas HIV-2 is found primarily in West Africa. HIV-1, first identified in the early 1980s, is a retrovirus, meaning that it carries in its core two single strands of RNA that, with infection of a host cell, are delivered to the nucleus and transcribed into the host DNA. Transcription of the virus into host DNA occurs by the actions of an enzyme called **reverse transcriptase** that also is carried as part of the virus into the host nucleus. Once integrated into host DNA, the virus replicates and mutates over the course of many years, slowly but steadily killing off cells of the immune system.

Cell Infection and Death

HIV only infects cells that carry certain membrane receptors to which it can bind, one of which is the CD4 antigen. On the virus is a complementary surface antigen, called group 120 antigen, which fits lock and key with the CD4 receptor. Cells that carry the CD4 antigen, and so can be infected by HIV, include macrophages, the skin immune cells called Langerhans cells, astrocytes of the CNS, and the helper T cells, already identified previously as CD4 cells. Most of the macrophages and helper T cells concentrate in the lymph nodes, spleen, and bone marrow, acting as a huge reservoir of virus-containing cells that continually pass the virus on to healthy cells traveling through those sites. Because of the high density of infected cells in secondary lymph organs, the number of *circulating* cells infected by the virus grossly underestimates the true number of infected cells. This means that even if the virus is undetectable in the blood, it is likely to still exist in noncirculating cells.

As previously mentioned, in order to infect a cell, it is required that the virus binds the CD4 antigen; however, this requirement is not in itself sufficient for infection to occur. Besides binding the CD4 receptor, HIV must also bind a second surface receptor before it can enter a host cell. Chemokine receptors on macrophages and helper T cells have been identified that provide the necessary second binding sites for HIV. On macrophages, this receptor is the chemokine receptor identified as CCR5; on the helper T cells, the second surface receptor is the chemokine receptor identified as CXCR4. A key point to understand is that naturally occurring HIV readily binds CCR5 receptors and so quickly infects macrophages, but ineffectively binds CXCR4 receptors. *This means that at first the virus infects primarily macrophages.* Once inside, HIV does not destroy the macrophage, but can survive inside the cell for years, replicating constantly, and mutating frequently. Eventually a mutated strain develops that is equally capable of binding the CXCR4 receptor, and so the virus then can infect helper T cells as well as macrophages. With this shift, the virus soon becomes deadly, because HIV kills the helper T cells it infects, eventually causing levels of helper T cells to fall to fewer than 200/μL of blood (normal levels are approximately 1000/μL). When helper T cells fall to this level, the development of opportunistic infections and other AIDS-defining illnesses is inevitable.

HIV destroys the helper T cells when it takes over the cell's genetic machinery and begins to make new viral components, using a second enzyme—**protease**—carried by the virus into the host cell. As the virus reproduces, it destroys the host cell membrane, perhaps by interfering with the cell's ability to protect itself from free radicals or by producing a superantigen that destroys the cell. Once HIV reproduces and kills the helper T cell, many more viruses are released into the circulation. These go on to infect other cells. Contributing to the death of the helper T cells is the immune response the host killer cells mount in an attempt to eliminate the virus and infected cells. As the number of helper T cells decreases, the cell-mediated immune system becomes progressively weaker. B cell and macrophage function also fail as T cells are lost. Loss of immune function allows microorganisms that would normally be kept in check to proliferate wildly, leading to disease and death from a variety of infections. Without immune surveillance, cancers develop as well, contributing to the high death rates seen in individuals infected with AIDS.

The Course of HIV Infection

An individual infected with HIV may remain asymptomatic for 8 or more years during the time the infection is mostly restricted to the macrophages. Once the virus begins destroying helper T cells, it will progress rapidly, usually over the course of 2 to 5 years, if untreated. An individual is diagnosed as having AIDS when the T-cell count decreases to fewer than 200 cells/μL, or when an opportunistic infection (i.e., toxoplasmosis, cytomegalovirus, pneumocystis carinii pneumonia, hepatitis B, hepatitis C), cancer, or AIDS dementia develops.

It should be emphasized that HIV infection is not AIDS, and occasionally an individual infected by the virus will survive more than 12 years with no signs of AIDS developing even without treatment. However, infection with the virus means the individual is contagious to others, whether symptoms of AIDS are present or not.

AIDS-Resistant Genes

Reports of HIV resistance have been described in the literature for many years. Approximately 10% to 20% of individuals repeatedly exposed to HIV will not become infected with the virus, and some people who become infected experience an atypically long time period without symptoms. Recently it has been shown that some of the resistance to HIV results from mutations present in certain genes, including the gene coding for the *CCR5* receptor. Specifically, it has been demonstrated that approximately 10% to 14% of Caucasians carry one mutant *CCR5* gene and approximately 1% of Caucasians carry two mutant genes (one from each parent). If an individual is homozygous for a mutation in the *CCR5* gene, he or she is usually resistant to HIV infection. If an individual is heterozygous for the mutant gene, he or she may become infected but will show a delay in the onset of overt AIDS by at least 2 to 3 years. Rates of resistance in populations other than Caucasians are lower; only 3% of African-Americans carry a single mutated gene offering resistance, and virtually no Native Americans, native Africans, or East Asian people carry even one copy of the mutant gene. Therefore, these populations have an increased susceptibility to infection compared to Caucasians.

Because of the presence of the mutant gene in Caucasians compared to other races, it has been hypothesized that the mutation in the *CCR5* gene developed relatively recently in evolutionary terms, after the major races split from each other. It has been suggested that a mutation in the *CCR5* gene survived in the Caucasian population because it conferred some sort of protection against a deadly disease experienced mostly by this group; this disease has been suggested to be the bubonic plague or a similar disease that ravaged Central Europe approximately 700 years ago. Research is under way to explore this hypothesis and to determine whether the *CCR5* protein can be disabled in those with two good copies, thereby offering AIDS resistance to others.

The astute reader will notice that it was mentioned earlier that an individual carrying two mutant copies of the *CCR5* gene is usually incapable of becoming infected with HIV. This caveat exists because even if an individual does not have the *CCR5* protein, that individual could still become infected with HIV if exposed to already mutated HIV. This situation occurs most frequently if an individual is infected with the virus from someone in the late stages of infection; if this happens, the virus can infect the T cells immediately without needing to infect the macrophages first.

Passage of HIV

HIV is passed between individuals during the exchange of body fluids, including blood, semen, vaginal fluid, and breast milk. Urine and GI contents are not believed to be a source of HIV transmission unless they visibly contain blood. Tears, saliva, and sweat may contain the virus, but in quantities thought to be too low to cause infection.

Individuals at Risk of Developing HIV

Whether an individual exposed to HIV becomes infected depends on several factors, including the individual's immune, nutritional, and general health status, and the amount of virus to which the individual is exposed. The age and sex of an individual also influence risk.

Individuals at high risk for becoming infected with HIV include those who exchange blood with infected persons in a blood transfusion or through contaminated needles. A contaminated needle-stick exposure may occur accidentally in the health care setting or through the sharing of needles during drug use. The risk of becoming infected after an accidental needle-stick injury with a contaminated syringe is low (0.32%). The risk of becoming infected after a single exposure to contaminated injection-drug equipment is higher (0.67%). Although the risk of becoming infected from a transfusion with infected blood is very high (almost 100%), the blood supply in industrialized countries is routinely tested for the presence of antibodies to HIV and contaminated blood is discarded. However, at certain times after infection with the virus, antibodies may not appear in infected blood, making a contaminated transfusion theoretically possible. These times include the period after infection before antibody response has developed and at the end stages of AIDS, when an individual's immune system may be so depressed that antibody levels are negligible.

Other individuals at risk of becoming infected with HIV are those exposed to semen or vaginal fluid during sexual intercourse with an infected individual. Most at risk of being infected via sexual intercourse are men who receive anal sex from other men, with the probability of HIV transmission after unprotected receptive anal intercourse estimated to be 0.8% to 3.2%. This higher risk is in part due to the breakdown and bleeding of rectal cells that occur during anal intercourse. Heterosexual transmission of the virus also occurs, however, and in fact is the primary mode of transmission in some countries, including sub-Saharan Africa and parts of the Caribbean. In general, heterosexual transmission more easily occurs from male to female, in which the probability of becoming infected from a single encounter with an infected partner is approximately 0.09% for a woman and 0.03% for a man. Although the incidence of infection in male homosexuals is still greater than in heterosexuals in the United States, the incidence of AIDS is increasing rapidly among heterosexual adults, especially women of color or Hispanic origin.

The likelihood of becoming infected with the virus during heterosexual or homosexual intercourse depends on many factors. Exposure to HIV from a partner experiencing a primary infection (i.e., before an antibody response has developed) appears to increase the risk of infection compared to exposure from a partner who has had the infection for a longer period and has already produced antibodies. Similarly, a partner nearing the end of an infection has a higher titer of virus than at other times and may show virtually no remaining immune resistance. The presence of a sexually transmitted disease in either partner also increases the risk of sexual transmission because of the presence of open wounds with some sexually transmitted diseases and the increased number of white blood cells in an area of infection. In women, cervical ectopy, a change in the structure of the cervix that causes it to be more fragile and likely to bleed, increases the likelihood of infection from a given exposure. Cervical ectopy is more common in teenagers, pregnant women, and women taking oral contraceptives, placing women from these categories at increased risk. Sex during menstruation may increase the risk of transmission from both sexes. And finally, the incidence of HIV in uncircumcised men is eight times as high as in men who are circumcised. This increased incidence may be related to the co-occurrence of sexually transmitted diseases in uncircumcised men or to an abundance of immune cells present in the foreskin that offer the virus a quick opportunity for infection. There is also a greater risk of infection in sex partners of uncircumcised men. This may explain why some African countries reporting a cultural preference against circumcision show especially high rates of heterosexual transmission.

Spread to Women and Children

In the United States, HIV infection is increasing among women, usually after sexual intercourse with infected intravenous drug users or bisexual men. Today, women make up over 50% of all HIV-infected individuals worldwide. Women are more susceptible than men to infection during heterosexual intercourse because of the normal microscopic vaginal tears and bleeds that occur with intercourse. In addition, infected semen remains in the woman's vagina up to 48 to 72 hours longer than the amount of time the penis is exposed to vaginal secretions. Women tend to be diagnosed later and have a higher morbidity and mortality because of not receiving treatment in a timely manner.

A woman infected with HIV may pass the infection on to her infant across the placenta, usually during the third trimester, or after exposure of the infant to contaminated blood and amniotic fluid during the birth process. An infant born to an untreated, infected mother has at least a 25% chance of becoming infected with the virus. The use of anti-HIV drugs administered to an infected mother during pregnancy, and to an infant of an infected mother soon after birth, significantly reduces the rate of infant infection, to less than 10% in some studies. Because of this documented protection to the infant, it is recommended that all pregnant women be tested for HIV infection as soon as pregnancy is confirmed. A woman may also acquire the virus after giving birth and pass it to her infant during breastfeeding.

Clinical Manifestations

- Flulike symptoms, including a low-grade fever, aches, and chills, may develop a few weeks to a few months after infection. Symptoms resolve after the initial immune response reduces the number of virus particles, although the virus survives in other infected cells.

- During the latent period, an individual infected with HIV may be asymptomatic, or in some cases may experience persistent lymphadenopathy (swollen lymph nodes).

- Two to 10 years after HIV infection, most individuals, if untreated, begin to experience opportunistic infections. These illnesses indicate the onset of AIDS and include vaginal and oral yeast infections and various viral infections such as varicella zoster (chickenpox and shingles), cytomegalovirus, or persistent herpes simplex virus infection. Women may develop chronic yeast infections or pelvic inflammatory disease.

- Once AIDS is established, respiratory infections, often with the opportunistic organism *Pneumocystis carinii*, become frequent. Multiple drug–resistant tuberculosis may develop because a patient with AIDS is unable to mount an effective immune response to fight the bacteria, even with the help of antibiotics. Patients with AIDS who develop tuberculosis typically experience a rapidly worsening course of the disease, leading to death within a few months. The disease frequently spreads to extrapulmonary sites, including the brain and bone.

- CNS manifestations include headaches, motor defects, seizures, personality changes, and dementia. Patients may become blind and eventually comatose. Many of these symptoms result from opportunistic viral and bacterial infections of the CNS, which cause inflammation of the brain. HIV also directly infects and injures brain cells.

- Diarrhea and wasting away of body fat are common in patients with AIDS. Diarrhea results from opportunistic viral and protozoal infections. Oral and esophageal yeast infections (thrush) cause pain when chewing and swallowing, and contribute to the loss of body fat and failure to thrive. Wasting syndrome is a hallmark manifestation of AIDS.

- Various cancers occur at an increased rate in patients with AIDS because of the lack of a cell-mediated immune response against neoplastic cells. The most common tumor in HIV-infected individuals is Kaposi sarcoma, a cancer of the vascular system characterized by red skin lesions. Most individuals who develop Kaposi sarcoma have been infected through homosexual intercourse. Recent evidence suggests that coinfection with a unique herpesvirus, human herpesvirus 8, may be required for the development of Kaposi sarcoma. Human herpesvirus 8 is uncommon in the general population, but common in the U.S. homosexual population.

Diagnostic Tools

- Immediately after infection, CD4 (helper T) cell counts may decrease, but soon return to near normal as the initial immune response contains the infection.

- Rapid HIV antibody tests give results in 10–60 minutes, but a Western blot must be done to confirm a positive diagnosis.

- Enzyme immunoassay (EIA) detects serum antibodies that bind to HIV antigens. Antibodies against HIV usually appear 4 to 6 weeks after infection, but may take 6 months or longer in some cases to develop. The time period between actual HIV infection and detection of the virus or antibodies in the blood is referred to as the *window period*. If a serum sample is identified as HIV positive (having a positive antibody titer), a Western blot test will be performed to confirm infection. Uninfected infants born to infected mothers may appear HIV positive for more than a year after birth because of the presence of maternal antibodies.

- CD4+ T-cell counts to monitor disease progression. Helper T-cell counts eventually begin to decrease. When levels reach fewer than 200 to 300 cells/µL of blood, opportunistic infections develop. The progress of the disease and the success of various treatments are followed by measuring a patient's helper T cells over time.

- Tests to measure the viral load (polymerase chain reaction [PCR], or bDNA) present at any given time in the blood of an infected individual have been shown to be highly accurate in predicting the occurrence of symptoms, the prognosis, and the general state of health of an individual. Those found to have high amounts of virus have an accelerated progression of the disease regardless of the number of helper T cells. The greater the number of virus particles present in an individual, the greater the infectivity during sexual intercourse and between mother and infant.

- Tests to measure HIV RNA also are predictive of host status. HIV RNA levels often are followed to evaluate the success of AIDS treatment.

Treatment

At this time, there is no cure for AIDS; thus, prevention of HIV infection is essential. Prevention means avoiding contact with HIV-contaminated body fluid. Because it is usually impossible to know in advance whether body fluid is contaminated with HIV, one should assume contamination unless proven otherwise. To avoid exposure to HIV one should:

- Practice sexual abstinence or mutually monogamous sexual intercourse with a noninfected partner.

- Be tested for the virus at least 6 months after the last unprotected sexual intercourse, because it may take at least 6 months after exposure to the virus to build antibodies. Oral sex may also pass the virus.

- Use a latex condom during sexual intercourse with a person whose HIV status is unknown.

- Refrain from sharing needles with anyone for any reason.

- Prevent infection to a fetus or newborn. A woman should know her own and her partner's HIV status before pregnancy. If a pregnant woman is positive for HIV, anti-HIV drugs or antibodies can be given to her during pregnancy and to the infant after birth. Treatment in utero may also be effective in preventing transmission of the virus to the fetus or newborn. An infected mother should not breastfeed her infant. Breast pumps should not be shared.

- Postexposure prophylactic treatment with a reverse transcriptase inhibitor after accidental needle-stick or sexual exposure decreases the odds of acquiring primary HIV infection.

If infection occurs, drug treatment regimens are available that can dramatically change the course of infection. The medications are costly and some side effects can be challenging for the patient. Support and information about available resources are vital.

- HIV/AIDS is treated by following the treatment regimen known as highly active antiretroviral therapy or HAART. HAART involves a combination of drugs that include one or more of the following:
  - A nucleoside reverse transcription inhibitor (NRTI). This type of drug (e.g., azidothymidine or AZT) interferes with viral transcription into host DNA by blocking the action of the viral enzyme reverse transcriptase by interfering with the availability of a nucleoside (thymidine).
  - A non-nucleoside reverse transcription inhibitor (NNRTI). This type of drug acts via noncompetitive binding to block the active site on the reverse transcriptase enzyme. These drugs are effective in combination with other medications such as the NRTIs.
  - A protease inhibitor, which blocks the action of the HIV protease enzyme necessary for the production of mature viral particles. While effective, protease inhibitor therapy is associated with a condition known as HIV-associated lipodystrophy, characterized by hyperlipidemia, insulin resistance, and a redistribution of body fat to the abdomen, breast, and back. The etiology of this syndrome is multifactorial, and includes an effect of the protease inhibitors on fat loss from adipose tissue and on preadipocyte differentiation.
  - A fusion inhibitor inhibits the fusion of the virus and cell membranes and thus interferes with the entry of HIV-1 into the host cells.
- The HAART regimen does not cure AIDS, but can dramatically prolong survival time and improve the quality of life for infected individuals. Questions exist regarding when to initiate therapy, with concerns over drug side effects and the potential for the virus to gain resistance to the medications. Recent data suggest that initiating therapy early in the course of infection may stave off most serious side effects and improve survival.
- HAART appears to be safe and effective in pregnant women, although questions regarding teratogenesis remain. Current recommendations are that, if possible, therapy be discontinued during the first trimester and then resumed.
- HAART is safe for use in infants born to mothers infected with HIV.
- Besides the side effect described for the protease inhibitors, side effects of the NRTI and the NNRTI medications include nausea, headaches, and bone marrow suppression, leading to anemia and fatigue. Adherence to HAART is difficult and may be impossible for some patients. Drugs must be taken frequently and at certain times of the day. The cost of long-term combination therapy is high and HIV disproportionately affects the poor; thus, therapy may be impossible in some countries and for uninsured individuals.

- A healthy diet and stress-free lifestyle are important. Treatment should include education to avoid alcohol, smoking, and illicit drugs. Stress, poor nutrition, alcohol, and other drugs are known to impair immune functioning.
- Patients should avoid other infections because they could lead to activation of T cells and may accelerate the replication of HIV. To prevent infection, available vaccines should be administered as long as live-viruses vaccines are not used.
- Treatment for specific infections and cancers should be administered as they arise.

PEDIATRIC CONSIDERATIONS

- Vaccines provide protection to the immunized individual and to other members of the community who have not been immunized (herd immunity). Childhood immunization is by far the most cost-effective public health program available today. Vaccines have significantly reduced the incidence of many illnesses previously common in childhood, including measles, rubella, chicken pox, and polio. Pediatric hepatitis B immunization has reduced the incidence of liver cancer worldwide.
- Before maternal antibodies are cleared from the infant's bloodstream, it is impossible to tell whether an infant showing IgG antibodies against a specific microorganism is reflecting maternal infection or whether the infant is himself or herself actively infected by the microorganism. Maternal antibodies begin to decrease after 6 months; therefore, the infant's antibody titer (level) after 6 months should be measured to identify true infection versus passive immunity. This is important to keep in mind when identifying which infants of mothers infected with HIV are infected and which only carry maternal antibodies to the virus. Infants who are infected with the virus may benefit from drug therapies that would be unnecessary and possibly dangerous to uninfected infants. Measuring the presence of HIV virus or viral antigens in an infant, rather than antibodies against HIV, allows for earlier diagnosis of infant HIV status.
- Infants and children exposed to cigarette smoke are at greater risk of developing asthma and other respiratory allergies.

GERIATRIC CONSIDERATIONS

- As an individual ages, the number and function of immune cells decrease, resulting in an increased prevalence of infection and malignancy in the elderly. Moderate exercise may improve immunocompetence in the elderly by increasing the number of NK and cytotoxic T cells.
- The elderly are often immunodeficient, in part because of the progressive decrease in function of the thymus with aging, but also because of poor blood flow and reduced delivery of the mediators of immunity and inflammation that many elderly experience as a result of atherosclerosis. Other systemic diseases such as diabetes mellitus,

which increases in incidence with age, contribute to a depressed immune response as well. Poor nutrition, caused by poverty, isolation, or bad dentition, contributes to poor immune function in the elderly.

- Approximately 10% of all HIV/AIDS cases occur in those 65 years of age and older. Considered a disease of the young, the older adult may not be diagnosed and treated in a timely manner.

- The older adult typically has a lower core temperature (95 to 97°F) so even a low-grade fever could be indicative of a major infection.

SELECTED BIBLIOGRAPHY

Beals, J. K. (2009). Gene on X chromosome plays critical role in systemic lupus erythematosus. *Proceedings of the National Academy of Science USA*. Retrieved April 6, 2009, from http://www.medscape.com?viewarticle/590699.

Copestead, L. C., & Banasik, J. L. (2010). *Pathophysiology* (4th ed.). St. Louis: Saunders Elsevier.

DeFranco, A. L., Locksley, R., & Roberston, M. (2007). *Immunity: The immune response in infectious and inflammatory disease*. Sunderland, MA: Sinauer Associates.

Deval, R., Ramesh, V., Prasad, G. B., & Jain, A. K. (2008). Natural rubber latex allergy. *Indian Journal of Dermatology, 74*(4), 304–310.

Ignatavicius, D. D., & Workman, M. L. (2010). *Medical-surgical nursing: Patient-centered collaborative care* (6th ed.). St. Louis: Saunders Elsevier.

Karunanayake, M., & Adair, C. (2009). HIV-associated lymphoma. *Baylor University Medical Center Proceedings, 22*(1), 74–76.

McGrogan, A., Seaman, H. E., Wright, J. W., & de Vries, C. S. (2008). The incidence of autoimmune thyroid disease: A systematic review of the literature. *Clinical Endocrinology, 69*(5), 687–696.

Osborne, K. S., Wraa, C. E., & Watson, A. B. (2010). *Medical-surgical nursing: Preparation for practice*. Upper Saddle River, NJ: Pearson.

Patton, K. T., & Thibodeau, G. A. (2010). *Anatomy & physiology* (7th ed.). St. Louis: Mosby Elsevier.

Peltola, V., Toikka, P., Irjala, K., Mertsola, J., & Ruuskanen, O. (2007). Discrepancy between total white blood cell counts and serum C-reactive protein levels in febrile children. *Scandinavian Journal of Infectious Disease, 39*, 560–565.

Porth, C. M., & Matfin, G. (2009). *Pathophysiology: Concepts of altered health states* (8th ed.). Philadelphia: Lippincott Williams & Wilkins

Rubin, R., & Strayer, D. S. (2008). *Rubin's pathology: Clinicopathologic foundations of medicine* (5th ed.). Philadelphia: Lippincott Williams & Wilkins.

Sato, T., Kobayashi, R., Toita, N., Kaneda, M., Hatano, N., Iguchi, A., et al. (2007). Stem cell transplantation in primary immunodeficiency disease patients. *Pediatrics International, 49*, 795–800.

Schonfeld, J. E., & Berger, W. E. (2008). Anaphylaxis: Commonsense ways to reduce risk. *Consultant, 48*(10), 786–792.

Seshan, S. V., & Jennette, J. C. (2009). Renal disease in systemic lupus erythematosus with emphasis on classification of lupus glomerulonephritis. *Archives of Pathology and Laboratory Medicine*, 133, 233–248.

Soysal, A., Millington, K. A., Bakir, M., Dosanjh, D., Aslan, Y., Deeks, J. J., et al. (2005). Effect of BCG vaccination on risk of *Mycobacterium tuberculosis* infection in children with household tuberculosis contact: A prospective community-based study. *Lancet*, 366, 1443–1451.

Storey, M., & Jordan, S. (2008). An overview of the immune system. *Nursing Standard*, 23(15–17), 47–56.

Thibodeau, G. A., & Patton, K. T. (2010). *The human body in health & disease* (5th ed.). St. Louis: Mosby Elsevier.

Touhy, T. A., & Jett, K. F. (2010). *Ebersole and Hess' gerontological nursing & healthy aging* (3rd ed.). St. Louis: Mosby Elsevier.

Washkewicz, T. (2009). Systemic scleroderma: The truth beneath a "skin disease." *Clinician Review*, 19(3), 9–11, 15–16.

Werneck-Silva, A. L., & Prado, I. B. (2009), Gastroduodenal opportunistic infections and dyspepsia in HIV-infected patients in the era of highly active antiretroviral therapy. *Journal of Gastroenterology and Hepatology*, 24(1), 135–139.

The Integument

The skin is the largest organ of the body and the first line of defense. Hair, nails, glands, and the skin make up the integumentary system. The skin functions to protect and insulate underlying structures, activate vitamin D, and assist with immune regulation, and it serves as a calorie reserve. The skin mirrors our emotions and stresses and impacts how others relate to and treat us. In a lifetime, the skin may be cut, bitten, irritated, burned, or infected. The skin has enormous resilience and capacity for recovery.

● Physiologic Concepts

STRUCTURE AND FUNCTION OF THE SKIN

The skin is composed of three layers, each consisting of different cell types and serving different functions. The three layers are the **epidermis, dermis,** and **subcutaneous** layer. A diagram of the skin is shown in Figure 5-1.

Epidermis

The outermost layer of the skin, the epidermis, is fairly thin all over the body except for the palms of the hands and soles of the feet. The cells of the epidermis continually undergo mitosis and are replaced approximately every 30 days. The epidermis contains sensory receptors for touch, temperature, vibration, and pain.

The main component of the epidermis is the protein keratin, produced by cells called **keratinocytes**. Keratin is an extremely durable, tough substance

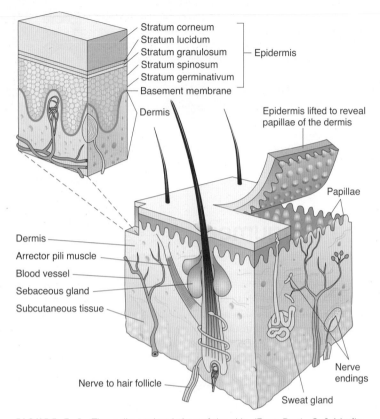

FIGURE 5-1 Three-dimensional view of the skin. (From Porth, C. & Matfin, G [2009]. *Pathophysiology, concepts of altered health states* [8th edition]. Philadelphia: Lippincott Williams & Wilkins.)

that is insoluble in water. Keratin prevents the loss of body water and protects the epidermis from irritants and infection-causing microorganisms. Keratin is the main component of the skin appendages: the nails and the hair.

Melanocyte cells are present at the base of the epidermis. Melanocytes synthesize and secrete melanin in response to stimulation by melanocyte-stimulating hormone, which is produced by the anterior pituitary. Melanin is a black pigment which disperses throughout the epidermis to give color pigmentation to the skin and protect cells from ultraviolet (UV) radiation.

Immune cells, called **Langerhans' cells,** or dendritic cells, are present throughout the epidermis. The cells originate in the bone marrow but are deposited in the deep layer of the epidermis early in life. Langerhans' cells recognize foreign particles or microorganisms that enter the skin and present them to T lymphocytes as the first step in initiating an immune attack. Langerhans' cells may be responsible for recognizing and eliminating dysplastic or neoplastic skin cells. Langerhans' cells are physically associated with sympathetic nerves, suggesting a relation between the nervous system and the ability of the skin to fight off infection or prevent skin cancer. Stress may affect the functioning of Langerhans' cells by increasing sympathetic stimulation. UV radiation may damage Langerhans' cells, reducing their ability to prevent cancer.

Merkel cells or tactile epithelial cells provide sensory information. They connect to sensory nerve endings and serve as light touch receptors.

Dermis

Lying immediately under the epidermis, the dermis is considered loose connective tissue and is composed of fibroblast cells that secrete the proteins collagen and elastin. The collagen and elastin fibers are arranged haphazardly, giving the dermis distensibility and resilience. A gel-like substance, hyaluronic acid, is secreted by the connective tissue cells. Hyaluronic acid surrounds the proteins and gives the skin elasticity and turgor (tension). In addition to the protective function, the dermis also serves as a reservoir for water and electrolytes. Throughout the dermis are blood vessels, sensory and sympathetic nerves, lymphatic vessels, hair follicles, and sweat and sebaceous glands. The somatic sensory receptors in the dermis process sensory information such as touch, pressure, pain, and temperature. Mast cells, which release histamine during injury or inflammation, and macrophages, which phagocytize dead cells and microorganisms, are also present.

Blood vessels in the dermis supply the dermis and epidermis with nutrients and oxygen and remove waste products. Dermal blood flow offers a means for the body to control its temperature. With a decrease in body temperature, sympathetic nerves to the blood vessels are activated and increase the release of norepinephrine, causing constriction of the vessels and a conservation of body heat. If body temperature is too high, sympathetic stimulation of the dermal blood vessels is reduced, dilating the vessels and allowing for the transfer of body heat to the environment. Arteriovenous (AV) connections, called anastomoses, are present on some blood vessels. AV anastomoses facilitate skin temperature regulation by allowing blood to bypass the upper layers of the dermis in times of severe cold. Sympathetic nerves to the dermis also innervate sweat glands, sebaceous (oil) glands, and hair follicles.

Subcutaneous Layer

Although not always considered a part of the skin, the subcutaneous layer or hypodermis lies beneath the dermis and connects skin with underlying body structures. The subcutaneous layer of the skin is composed of fat and connective tissue and acts both as a shock absorber and a heat insulator. The subcutaneous layer is a calorie reserve station as well: fat can be stored in this layer and, if needed, broken down to serve as an energy source.

HAIR AND NAILS

The nails are keratinized plates that extend from the fingers and the toes. The nails protect the fingertips and are most likely evolved with an original purpose of defense. A layer of epithelium underneath the nail is the nail bed. The nail bed is highly vascular and monitoring the color of the nail beds can offer valuable information about oxygenation of the blood.

The hair is hardened keratin that grows at variable rates on different parts of the body. The lanugo which covers the fetus in utero is replaced by vellus hair before or shortly after birth. This hair is strong, fine, and less pigmented. Terminal hair that appears around puberty in the pubic and axillary area is coarse. Hair grows as a follicle shaft in a canal, beginning deep in the dermis. In addition to a hair follicle, each canal contains a sebaceous gland and a smooth muscle fiber, called an arrector pili muscle. When this muscle cell is stimulated by the sympathetic nervous system, it causes the hair to stand on end. Hair on the head may protect against sunburn. Hair color is largely determined by the amount, type, and distribution of melanin. With aging, hair turns white because of the inability to continue melanin production.

SEBACEOUS GLANDS

The sebaceous glands accompany the hair follicles. They secrete an oily substance called sebum into the surrounding canal to prevent damage to the surrounding hair and skin. Sebaceous glands are present all over the body, especially on the face, chest, and back. Testosterone increases the size of the sebaceous glands and the production of sebum. Testosterone levels increase in males and females during puberty.

SWEAT GLANDS

There are two types of sweat glands: eccrine and apocrine. Eccrine sweat glands open directly onto the surface of the skin and are distributed over the entire body. Eccrine glands function mainly in cooling the body by means of evaporative heat loss. They are especially concentrated on the hands, feet, and forehead. Apocrine glands are mainly located in the axillae (armpits) and in the pubic and anal areas. These glands secrete sweat into the canals of the hair follicles. When acted upon by surface bacteria, the secretions of the apocrine glands cause the characteristic odor of perspiration.

VITAMIN D

The skin plays a vital role in the body's use of vitamin D. Vitamin D is a hormone obtained in the diet in an inactive form. It is required both for the absorption of calcium from the gut and in order to reduce the renal excretion of calcium. For vitamin D to function, however, it first must be activated by the body. The initial step in vitamin D activation occurs in the skin as a result of UV radiation, after which it is further acted upon by the kidney and the liver. Vitamin D activation is increased in response to a decrease in serum calcium. Because vitamin D acts as a hormone, the skin may be considered an endocrine gland.

● Pathophysiologic Concepts

Many different lesions occur on the skin. They are described on the basis of size, depth, color, and consistency. See pages C3, C4, C5, and C6 for illustrations of common skin lesions.

BULLA

Measuring more than 1.0 cm in diameter and filled with watery fluid, a bulla is a large, raised area on the skin. Bullae are large blisters that can occur after a burn.

CRUST

A crust is the accumulation of dried serous (serum-like) or seropurulent (pus) exudate on the skin (e.g., the crust seen on an impetigo or herpes lesion). It is usually golden in color.

CYST

An elevated, circumscribed encapsulated lesion in the dermis or subcutaneous layer is called a cyst. It may be filled with liquid or a semisolid substance.

EROSION

An erosion is an area on the body characterized by the loss of superficial epidermis. Typically the area is depressed, moist, and glistening but does not bleed (e.g., the skin after bursting of a blister or vesicle).

EXCORIATION

An excoriation is a scratch on the skin with loss of the epidermis (e.g., a skinned knee). It may be a hollowed-out, crusted area with slight bleeding.

FISSURE

A fissure is a linear crack in the skin from the epidermis to the dermis, for example, as seen with athlete's foot. The fissure may be pink or red, dry or moist, and usually there is no bleeding.

KELOID

A keloid is a scar formation on the skin, occurring after a trauma, injury, or piercing, that is out of proportion to the injury. Keloids are caused by excessive collagen formation during the healing process. They appear raised, red, and firm. There is a genetic tendency to develop keloids, and this type of scarring is especially common in African Americans. An individual prone to keloid formation should alert a health care provider when a skin injury occurs. Prevention of keloid formation is supported by careful surgical techniques, pressure dressings, good wound care, and adequate nutrition. There is no single best treatment for an existing keloid, although topical dressings, steroid injections, and laser therapy all have been used with some success. Immunotherapy is under investigation. Removal of a keloid may worsen scarring in some cases.

LICHENIFICATION

Thickened, roughened skin that may occur with constant irritation is known as lichenification. This condition is seen, for example, in skin with atopic dermatitis.

MACULE

A macule is a flattened area of the skin, characterized by a change in color. A macule (e.g., a freckle or a flat mole, also called a nevus) is typically smaller than 1.0 cm in diameter.

NODULE

A nodule is a solid, elevated mass measuring between 1.0 cm and 2.0 cm in diameter. It is firmer in consistency than a papule and occurs deeper in the dermis (e.g., a cyst).

PAPULE

A papule is a solid, elevated mass, smaller than 1.0 cm in diameter. Examples of papules include elevated moles and warts.

PATCH

A patch is a flat, nonpalpable irregularly shaped macule measuring greater than 1.0 cm in diameter. Examples include vitiligo, Mongolian spots, and port-wine stains.

PETECHIA

A deep red spot of pinpoint hemorrhage under the skin is called petechia. Petechiae may signify a bleeding disorder or fragility of the capillaries and may accompany a serious infection.

PLAQUE

A plaque is a raised surface with a flat top and measures larger than 1.0 cm. Examples of plaques are several papules grouped together or the lesions seen with psoriasis.

PRURITUS

Pruritus refers to itching of the skin. Pruritus may occur as a primary response to a surface irritant or inflammation, for example, after a mosquito bite, or with dry skin. Primary pruritus results from release of histamine during inflammation. Pruritus may occur secondarily to a systemic disease, such as liver or kidney failure. With systemic disease, metabolic toxins may accumulate in the interstitial fluid under the skin.

PURPURA

A purpuric lesion is a large patch of purple discoloration under the skin associated with hemorrhage. It may result from a variety of causes, including thrombocytopenia (decreased platelets), trauma (a "black and blue mark"), or an allergic response. A purpuric lesion occurring without trauma may be a red flag for bleeding elsewhere in the body, including the brain.

PUSTULE

A pustule is an elevated vesicle filled with pus. Examples of pustules are the lesions of impetigo or acne.

SCALE

An irregular collection of keratinized cells or a flake of epidermis is referred to as a scale. It may be thick or thin, dry or oily, and can vary in size. Examples of scaling are seen in dandruff or dried skin.

SCAR

A scar is an area of the body where the skin has been replaced by fibrous tissue (e.g., a burn scar). A scar may be thin or thick.

TELANGIECTASIA

Capillary dilation will manifest as fine, irregular lines such as seen with rosacea.

TUMOR

A tumor is a large, solid mass that is elevated and larger than 2.0 cm. Tumors may be neoplastic or benign, as, for example, a breast cancer versus a lipoma (a benign tumor made up mostly of adipose tissue).

ULCER

An ulcer is an area with loss of epidermal and deeper layers of the skin that may bleed and scar. Ulcers have a concave appearance and may vary in size. An example of an ulcer is a decubitus ulcer (pressure sore).

URTICARIA

Urticaria, also known as hives, consists of raised edematous plaques (wheals) associated with intense itching (pruritus). Urticaria results from the release of histamine during an inflammatory response to an allergen to which the individual has become sensitized. Chronic urticaria may accompany systemic disorders such as hepatitis, some cancers, or thyroid abnormality.

VESICLE

A vesicle is a small, raised circumscribed area on the skin with a measurement of less than 1.0 cm. It is formed by the presence of serous fluid within the skin layers (e.g., a chickenpox blister).

WHEAL

A wheal is a raised area of skin edema that exists only temporarily and itches (e.g., the area surrounding a mosquito bite or an area of the skin during an occurrence of urticaria [hives]). The center of a wheal is pink or red, with a surrounding circle of paler skin.

● Conditions of Disease or Injury

BENIGN SKIN DISORDERS

Cysts

A cyst is dome shaped, freely movable, pale, and ranges in size from 0.5 to 5 cm. It is filled with keratin and has a central opening which drains a pasty, malodorous substance. If it becomes infected, treatment may include antibiotics and surgical removal.

Keratoses

A horny overgrowth or abnormal growth of keratinocytes is referred to as keratosis. The most common premalignant skin lesions on sun-exposed areas are **actinic keratosis.** Beginning as hyperemic, poorly defined lesions, they develop into dry, brown, scaly macules with a reddish tinge and a rough surface. The lesions are typically less than 1 cm in diameter and the surrounding skin may have a weathered appearance. The lesions are more easily felt than visualized. Approximately 20% of actinic keratoses eventually convert to squamous cell carcinoma. Treatment may include cryosurgery, liquid nitrogen, or topical chemotherapeutic agents such as 5-fluorouracil or imiquimod creams. Aldara may be used to stimulate the immune system to remove the lesions.

Seborrheic keratosis is characterized by a sharply circumscribed round or oval wartlike lesion. It may be black, tan, brown, yellow, or pink in color and ranges in size up to several centimeters. Although benign, lesions need to be monitored for changes in color, size, or texture which may be indicative of malignant transformation.

Lipoma

A nodular collection of fat tissue under the skin is a lipoma. It is slow growing, freely movable, soft and may be up to several centimeters in diameter. Surgical removal is possible if desired for cosmetic reasons.

Nevi or Moles

Moles can be flat or raised, hairy or nonhairy and vary in color and size. Although harmless, moles should be monitored for changes in size, color, or texture which may be indicative of malignant transformation.

Skin Tags

Soft, brown, or flesh-colored papules seen in aging adults are skin tags. Ranging in size from pinpoint to pea sized, they most commonly develop on the neck, axilla, and intertriginous areas.

PIGMENTATION ALTERATIONS

Pigmentation alterations are the result of changes in normal skin color. **Café-au-Lait spots** and **liver spots (solar lentigo)** are two examples of hyper-pigmentation. Café-au-Lait spots are flat cutaneous pigmentations ranging from 0.5 to 20 cm in diameter. They are considered benign, but six spots or more may be indicative of neurofibromatosis. Liver spots or age spots are sharply demarcated dark areas on sun-exposed skin. They generally occur in Caucasians over 60 years of age with a familial tendency. Prevention through limited sun exposure and the use of sunscreen is recommended. Bleaching creams may lighten the areas and for cosmetic purposes, skin resurfacing with laser and liquid nitrogen is an option.

An acquired or hereditary decrease in melanin causes a hypopigmentation of the skin. **Vitiligo (leukoderma)** is a localized loss of melanocytes in the skin and hair. White patches of skin with definite borders may appear on the face, neck, axillae, or extremities. Possible causes include pernicious anemia, hyper-thyroidism, autoimmune disease, or inhibition of melanogenesis.

ALLERGIC AND HYPERSENSITIVITY DISORDERS

An inappropriate or exaggerated response of the immune system is referred to as hypersensitivity. Allergic responses are one type of immune hypersensitivity and may cause an immediate or a delayed response. Examples include atopic dermatitis, contact dermatitis, drug-induced skin eruptions, and urticaria.

Atopic Dermatitis

Atopic dermatitis (atopic eczema) is an inflammation of the skin involving overstimulation of T lymphocytes and mast cells. Histamine from the mast cells causes itching and erythema. Water loss from the epidermis and decreased skin lipid levels cause the skin to be dry. Scratching can cause skin breakdown. Atopic dermatitis is frequently seen in infants and children, but it may persist into adulthood. There appears to be a genetic tendency toward the disease and 75% to 85% have a personal or family history of allergic rhinitis or asthma.

Clinical Manifestations

- Severe pruritus.
- Periods of remissions and flare-ups.
- Irregular, red papular patches, weepy, shiny, thickened.
- Infantile characteristics include vesicle formation, oozing, crusting, excoriation, pale cheeks, extra creases under the eyes (Dennie–Mrogan folds), erythema.
- Adult characteristics include dry red patches, leathery skin, lichenification, scaling, excoriation.

- In infants, lesions often appear on the face, scalp, buttocks, extensor surfaces of the extremities. In older children and adults, the lesions appear more commonly on the hands, feet, neck, behind the knees, and in the bends of the elbows.

Diagnosis

- Diagnosis is usually accomplished with the help of a good history and physical examination.
- Increased serum IgE, elevated interleukin-4, elevated eosinophils.

Complications

- Infection of the skin with common surface bacteria, especially *Staphylococcus aureus*, or with viruses such as herpes simplex may develop. Individuals should avoid inoculation with live, attenuated viruses.
- Thinning of the skin with continued steroid use.

Treatment

- Avoidance of known irritants or allergens.
- Use of emollients for skin hydration (limit number of baths and use tepid water with mild, unscented soap).
- Antihistamines to help control itching.
- Soft, light cotton clothing made of natural fiber.
- Cool compresses to reduce inflammation.
- Topical low-dose steroids to reduce inflammation and allow healing.
- Minimize stress and temperature extremes to minimize vascular and sweat response.
- Antibiotics as needed to prevent or treat secondary infections.

Contact Dermatitis

Contact dermatitis is an acute or chronic inflammation of the skin caused by exposure to an irritant (irritant dermatitis) or allergen (allergic dermatitis). The location of the dermatitis on the skin corresponds to the site of exposure. Allergic contact dermatitis occurs when Langerhans' cells process and present an allergen to nearby T cells. The T cells respond with a type IV hypersensitivity response against the allergen. The response is delayed in that it takes hours to days to become evident. Several exposures may be incurred before a reaction occurs. The extent of the reaction is dependent on the duration and intensity of the exposure. Irritant dermatitis occurs when the skin is exposed to a substance that dries out or irritates it. Irritant dermatitis is only inflammatory and does not involve a specific immune response.

Common causes of allergic dermatitis include poison ivy or poison oak, latex, and chemicals found in jewelry. Common causes of irritant dermatitis include soaps, detergents, household cleaners, insecticides, and dusts. Some foods and spices may also cause contact dermatitis.

Clinical Manifestations

- Both types of dermatitis present acutely with localized papules, erythema (redness), and oozing vesicles in an area of contact. The vesicles burst and crust.
- Pruritus may be intense.
- Allergic dermatitis typically presents 1 to 2 days after exposure.

Diagnosis

- Dermatitis usually follows the pattern of exposure—for example, poison ivy typically travels vertically up the legs or may be present only on areas of the skin that were uncovered when exposed to the plant. A circle of lesions around the wrist may indicate an allergy to a bracelet or watch, whereas lesions below the umbilicus may indicate an allergy to the metal of a zipper. Reddened, irritated hands may indicate an inflammatory response to dishwashing. A good history accompanying the physical pattern is the key to diagnosis.
- Allergy skin testing may be indicated.

Complications

- Chronic conditions may cause lichenification, fissures, and scales.
- An infection of the skin may result from repeated scratching and skin breakdown.
- A severe response to poison ivy or another potent allergen may result in significant reddening and swelling of the face. The eyes may be closed because of edema.

Treatment

- Identifying the cause of the dermatitis and avoiding exposure prevents recurrence.
- Cool compresses reduce inflammation. Oatmeal soaks or baths in other soothing chemicals may provide relief. Antihistamines may be used to reduce itching.
- Short-term, topical, anti-inflammatory, steroidal therapy may be used to interrupt the inflammation. For severe attacks involving the eyes and face, a burst of systemic corticosteroids is often used.

Drug-Induced Skin Eruptions

Many drugs can cause a local or generalized skin eruption although it occurs more commonly in females. T cells recognize the medication as a foreign substance and react. Cutaneous reactions typically occur within 7 days of drug exposure. Ampicillin, penicillin, cephalosporins, and barbiturates are the most common drugs causing a reaction. Reactions can range from a mild rash to epidermal skin detachment and bullous skin lesions (erythema multiforme minor, Stevens–Johnson syndrome, and toxic epidermal necrolysis).

Clinical Manifestations

- Erythema, pruritus, urticaria
- Maculopapular lesions in symmetrical, generalized distribution (face is usually not involved)
- Fever and other systemic symptoms may also be present.

Diagnosis

- Thorough history with specific questioning about any new medication. Also determine if this type of rash has occurred before and if so, what medications was the patient taking.

Complications

- With extensive involvement, dehydration and hypothermia may occur.

Treatment

- Discontinue the medication.
- Antihistamines for itching.
- Systemic corticosteroids for widespread or severe reaction.

Urticaria

Also referred to as hives, urticaria involves fluid leakage from the skin's blood vessels. Histamine release from mast cells and basophils causes increased permeability of the microvessels in the skin and surrounding tissue. This permits fluid leakage into the tissues which results in edema and wheal formation. Acute urticaria is a result of an IgE-mediated response and chronic urticaria is associated with circulating IgG antibodies to IgE receptors. Common causes include food, medications, insect stings, viral infections, dust mites, and exposure to pollen. Some autoimmune conditions may also trigger urticaria.

Clinical Manifestations

- Erythematous wheals. Raised red or pink areas surrounded by a paler halo. Blanch with pressure. Size varies.
- Intense itching.
- Angioedema may be present.

Diagnosis

- History of exposure to a possible causative agent.

Complications

- Angioedema of the face can cause airway compromise and temporary disfigurement.

Treatment

- Avoid known triggers.
- Antihistamines.
- Leukotriene inhibitors.
- Cold compresses or cool colloid-type baths.
- Oral corticosteroids for refractory cases.
- Epinephrine for angioedema of larynx and pharynx.
- Tricyclic antidepressants with antihistamine actions may be used.

VIRAL INFECTIONS OF THE SKIN

A variety of viral infections may present with a skin rash. Many of these rashes are most common during childhood (Table 5-1) but may occur at any time. Herpes simplex virus (HSV) is the most common viral skin infection seen in adults.

Herpes Simplex 1 and 2

The herpesviruses include herpes simplex 1 and 2. Herpesviruses cause characteristic skin and mucous membrane lesions and are passed by viral shedding

TABLE 5-1	Common Childhood Rashes		
Infection	Causative Agent	Characteristic of the Rash	Complications
Rubeola (10-day measles)	Paramyxovirus	Erythematous macular papular rash, beginning on face, moving to trunk and extremities; Koplik spots (pinpoint white) in mouth 1–3 days before rash	Measles encephalitis; secondary bacterial infection, including otitis and pneumonia
Rubella (3-day measles)	Rubella virus	Diffuse, red-pink macular rash beginning on face and trunk, spreading to extremities	Congenital rubella syndrome, if contracted by mother during pregnancy

Infection	Causative Agent	Characteristic of the Rash	Complications
Roseola	Herpesvirus 6	High fever followed approximately 3 days later by an erythematous macular rash, especially on the trunk	Unusual
Chickenpox	Herpes varicella-zoster	Macules, vesicles, and scabbings present at the same time. Intense itching	Varicella pneumonia, secondary bacterial infection, joint pain. Mothers infected during first trimester of pregnancy may suffer loss or congenital deformity of the fetus. Newborns infected at birth may have serious morbidity or mortality. Adults infected may become severely ill
Scarlet fever	Group A beta-hemolytic streptococcus	Sandpaper-like erythematous macular–papular rash	Poststreptococcal glomerulomephritis, rheumatic fever

from the lesions. The incubation period for both viruses is approximately 2 to 24 days after infection. A prodromal period often precedes the appearance of lesions. During the prodromal period and the time of open lesions (a 2- to 6-week period), the virus is contagious. After an initial infection, the virus may lie dormant in the sensory nerve tract innervating the primary lesion. The dormant virus may become active again at any time, causing the reappearance of lesions. Reactivation of a latent herpes infection may occur with illness, stress, excessive sun exposure, or at certain times of the menstrual cycle. Severity worsens with age and is most severe in the immunocompromised individual.

Herpes simplex 2 is typically a genital or anal infection, whereas herpes simplex 1 is usually responsible for cold sores on the face. Either virus, however, is capable of infecting any site on the body. Herpes simplex 2 is considered a sexually transmitted disease.

Clinical Manifestations

- Symptoms during the prodromal stage may include low-grade fever, malaise, and a burning or itching on the mouth or genitals.
- With active infection, clusters of painful vesicles on a red base erupt on the lips, face, skin, nose, oral mucosa, genitalia, or anus. The vesicles may burn and itch. The vesicles rupture within 3 to 4 days and crust over. They usually disappear within the next week.

Diagnosis

- Diagnosis is made by history and physical examination, although cell culture may be used to confirm a suspected outbreak.

Complications

- Secondary bacterial infection of the vesicles may develop.
- Herpes simplex may infect the eye, causing blindness (keratoconjunctivitis). A primary herpes simplex 2 infection during pregnancy may cause damage to the fetal central nervous system, including blindness and mental retardation. Risk to the fetus is especially high if the pregnant woman is exposed to the virus for the first time late in her pregnancy.
- Neonatal infection by the virus may occur with an ascending vaginal or cervical infection during the pregnancy or during passage of the newborn through an infected birth canal.

Treatment

- There is no cure.
- Oral or topical treatment with an antiviral drug (acyclovir, famciclovir, valacyclovir), may reduce the frequency, duration, and intensity of the lesions. In some cases, these medications may be used as daily prophylaxis.
- Lidocaine, diphenhydramine, and aspirin may decrease pain.
- Cesarean section is performed if active genital herpes infection is present or if there is suspicion that the pregnant woman is in the prodromal stage.

Herpes Zoster

More commonly referred to as shingles, herpes zoster is a reactivation of the varicella-zoster virus in people who have previously had chickenpox. With reactivation, the virus that has been dormant in the dorsal root ganglia of the sensory cranial and spinal nerves travels from the ganglia to the skin corresponding to the dermatome. Factors that alter the body's immunologic functioning (stress, medication, radiation, illness, and aging) may cause a re-activation. The majority of the estimated 1 million Americans affected annually are over 60 years of age. It is highly recommended that individuals over 60 years of age take the vaccine for herpes zoster. It has been shown to decrease the incidence of shingles as well as postherpetic neuralgia.

Clinical Manifestations

- Varying levels of pain ranging from mild irritation to excruciating pain prior to eruption of the lesions.
- Grouped vesicles on an erythematous base. Occur in a segmental distribution along the infected nerve. Typically occur unilaterally on the face, thorax, and trunk.
- Vesicles dry and form crusts.

Diagnosis

- Thorough history and classical distribution of lesions.
- Polymerase chain reaction (PCR) directly identifies the virus and may be used.

Complications

- Postherpetic neuralgia (pain) may occur in a large percentage (10% to 70%) of individuals suffering from shingles. Postherpetic neuralgia refers to pain that persists for longer than 1 month after the acute onset of shingles. It is most common in elderly patients and is difficult to relieve once it becomes established.
- Secondary infection with necrosis in immunocompromised individuals.
- Eye involvement can result in blindness.

Treatment

- Antiviral agents such as acyclovir, famciclovir, or valacyclovir—preferably started within 72 hours of rash development.
- Cool compresses, lidocaine patches.
- Narcotic analgesics, tricyclic antidepressants, fabapentin, anticonvulsants, and nerve blocks for postherpetic neuralgia.
- Use of corticosteroids is controversial.

Chicken pox

Chickenpox is a common childhood communicable disease caused by the vari-cella zoster virus. It is highly contagious and is transmitted from person to person by way of respiratory droplets. Chickenpox is usually an illness of childhood, but adults exposed to the virus for the first time may develop the disease. The varicella virus has an incubation period of 7 to 21 days and is contagious during a brief prodromal period (approximately 24 hours before lesions appear) and until all lesions are crusted over. The disease is usually self-limiting and resolves within 7 to 14 days.

Clinical Manifestations

- Low-grade fever and malaise may be present 24 hours before vesicles appear.
- The rash of chickenpox begins as red macules, usually first appearing on the trunk and spreading to the face and extremities. Within a few hours, the macules become fluid-filled vesicles, with more macules developing in the mouth, axilla, labia, and vagina. These latter vesicles progress to become fluid-filled. The vesicles burst after a few days and crust over.
- Numerous macules, vesicles, and scabs at different stages may be present at any one time.
- Mild to extreme pruritus.
- Cough, coryza, and photosensitivity may accompany the lesions.

Diagnosis

- Diagnosis is made by history and physical examination.

Complications

- Secondary bacterial infection of the vesicles may develop.
- Pneumonia, encephalitis, or joint inflammation and pain may follow chickenpox infection.
- Reye syndrome may develop in children given aspirin during a chickenpox infection.
- Adults who acquire chickenpox may have a particularly severe disease course and are at higher risk of developing pneumonia or other complications.
- Chickenpox may spread internally in immunocompromised individuals, leading to increased morbidity and mortality.

Treatment

- Prevention of chickenpox is possible with the varicella vaccine. This vaccine can be given to children or adults, and is highly successful in preventing infection. Some individuals (approximately 10%) may develop a few vesicles 10 to 20 days after immunization and may be contagious to others at that time. It is hoped that by preventing varicella, the incidence of shingles will also decline, although this has not as yet been documented.
- Treatment of active chickenpox infection is mainly supportive and is geared at preventing the development of secondary skin infections. Oatmeal baths,

calamine lotion, and antihistamines may be used to reduce itching. In children, the nails may be cut, or mittens may be worn, to reduce scratching.

- Antiviral drugs (acyclovir, vidarabine, sorivudine) may be prescribed after exposure or at the earliest sign of chickenpox infection in adults or in immunocompromised children to limit the degree of infection. The use of antiviral drugs in healthy children who have chickenpox may also be considered to reduce lesion number and the length of infection.

Rubeola

Rubeola, also called measles or red measles, is an upper respiratory tract infection caused by the paramyxovirus. Rubeola is usually seen in children and is transmitted by way of inspired droplets. It has a 7- to 12-day asymptomatic incubation period before signs of the disease appear and is highly contagious. Active disease is characterized by early (prodromal) symptoms followed by a rash.

Clinical Manifestations

- Prodromal symptoms include high fever, barking cough, runny nose, conjunctivitis, and enlargement of lymph nodes. Active infection is characterized by Koplik spots over the buccal (cheek) mucosa. A Koplik spot is a pinpoint white spot surrounded by a red ring.
- A maculopapular rash with erythema, beginning on approximately day 3 or 4, is another manifestation. The rash starts on the face, spreads to the trunk, and finally the extremities. The rash lasts approximately 4 days.

Diagnosis

- Diagnosis is usually made by history and physical examination.
- Antibody titer.

Complications

- Measles encephalitis is a common complication of rubeola. It may be caused by the measles virus, or it may be a secondary bacterial infection. Recovery is usually complete, but lasting brain damage and death might occur.
- Pneumonia, otitis media, or encephalitis may occur after measles.

Treatment

- Primary treatment is the prevention by vaccination with a live attenuated virus at 15 months after birth. A booster is usually administered at 4 to 6 years, and sometimes in the teen years. Treatment of measles infection is supportive and may involve antibiotics if a secondary bacterial infection develops.
- Darkened room, rest, fluids, antipyretics are used to treat symptoms.

Rubella

Rubella, also called German measles or 3-day measles, is a viral infection of the respiratory tract caused by the rubella virus. There is a 14- to 21-day incubation period after infection, followed by prodromal symptoms lasting 1 to 4 days. A rash then develops. Rubella is very contagious during the prodromal stage, but may not be contagious once a rash develops.

Clinical Manifestations

- Prodromal stage is characterized by low-grade fever, malaise, lymph node enlargement (especially postauricular), sore throat, and headache.
- Active infection is characterized by a diffuse maculopapular rash, which begins on the trunk and spreads to the extremities. The rash lasts for approximately 2 to 3 days.

Diagnosis

- Diagnosis is made by history and physical examination.

Complications

- Infection in a pregnant woman, especially during the first trimester, may cause severe birth defects in her infant.

Treatment

- Primary treatment is the prevention by vaccination with a live, attenuated virus at 15 months, at 4 to 6 years, and in the teen years. The typically used vaccine, called an MMR vaccine, for measles (rubeola), mumps, and rubella, is a combination vaccine for these three diseases.
- All women of childbearing age should be tested for the presence of antibodies against rubella (a rubella titer test). A woman who is antibody negative (has never had rubella or been adequately vaccinated against it) should be immunized against the virus.
- Treatment of rubella infection is supportive, and is focused on keeping the individual well-hydrated and rested.

Roseola Infantum

Roseola is a common infection of infants between the ages of 6 months and 2 years, although children as old as 4 years may also develop the infection. Roseola appears to be viral in origin and is characterized by a sudden onset of high fever (38.9°C to 40.5°C; 100°F to 104°F) in an otherwise well child, lasting 3 to 5 days. After this time, a rash develops, especially over the trunk.

Clinical Manifestations
- Sudden, high fever in an apparently well child, followed 3 to 5 days later by a red, lacy, macular rash over the trunk and neck.

Diagnosis
- Diagnosis is made by history and physical examination. Typically, there is no lymph node enlargement (adenopathy).

Treatment
- Reassurance is usually the only treatment required. Fever medication may be used.

Smallpox

Routine smallpox vaccination was stopped in 1972 and in 1980 the World Health Organization declared that smallpox had been eradicated. Concerns that some of the stored virus may have fallen into the hands of bioterrorists have prompted the Centers for Disease Control and Prevention to propose immediate isolation of anyone infected. Vaccination of those at risk is also recommended. Smallpox is spread by droplet nuclei or aerosol. Symptoms develop abruptly after an incubation period of 7 to 19 days. Fever, headache, backache, rigor, and malaise are followed by a centrifugal distribution of macules that progress to papules and then pustular vesicles. Pustules form scabs that leave depressed depigmented scars.

Warts

In humans, warts (verrucae) are caused by infection with the human papillomavirus (HPV). Irregular thickening of the stratum spinosum and increased thickening of the stratum corneum results in nipple-like lesions. Warts can occur anywhere on the skin and although most warts are benign papules, some have the ability to transform and become malignant. There are many different strains of HPV. Some strains preferentially infect the genital or anal region, causing genital warts, whereas others colonize the fingers and hands, causing simple warts. Plantar warts are warts on the bottom of the feet that grow in rather than out from the skin. Warts are passed by skin-to-skin contact. Genital warts are considered a sexually transmitted disease.

Some studies suggest that over 40% of young women using university health care centers for their gynecologic care have genital warts. Certain strains of genital warts have been identified as causing cervical cancer; other strains are unlikely to progress to cancer. The risk of developing cervical cancer is especially high in women with genital warts who smoke. This increased risk most likely occurs because cervical mucus concentrates tobacco toxins, which may then act synergistically with HPV to produce cancer.

Clinical Manifestations

- Skin warts may be flat or round, large or small, grayish white to tan, convex papules with a rough, pebble-like surface.
- Warts on the soles of the feet or the palms of the hand may be rough and scaly.
- Genital warts have a cauliflower-type appearance. They may be seen on the head or shaft of the penis, on the labia, in the vagina, or surrounding the anus.

Diagnosis

- Diagnosis is made by history and physical examination.
- Occasionally, a biopsy of the lesion may be taken for histologic confirmation of HPV. Typing of the lesion may be performed at that time as well.

Complications

- Cervical cancer in women may be considered a complication of HPV infection in that it most commonly results from infection with certain strains of the virus.
- Infrequently, a newborn exposed to genital warts during the birth process may develop esophageal warts.
- With genital warts, low self-esteem and feelings of guilt and shame may occur. Individuals who have HPV may be reluctant to establish new relationships.

Treatment

- For genital warts, prevention with the vaccine Gardasil has been approved by the Food and Drug Administration for females aged 9 to 26. It protects against the four HPV types responsible for 90% of genital warts and 70% of cervical cancer.
- Warts go away on their own when the immune system is stimulated to recognize their presence. Such stimulation typically happens with vascularization or bleeding of the wart.
- Irritation of a skin or plantar wart by the application of salicylic acid, formaldehyde, podophyllum, or other skin irritants may stimulate an immune reaction against the wart. All types of warts frequently reappear after treatment.
- Liquid nitrogen, cryosurgery, or laser may be used to remove stubborn or unsightly warts, or warts on the genital or esophageal regions.
- Occluding warts with duct tape.

BACTERIAL INFECTIONS OF THE SKIN

Impetigo

A superficial skin infection, usually caused by *Staphylococcus* or group A beta-hemolytic streptococcal infection, is known as impetigo. There are two types of impetigo: vesicular and bullous.

Vesicular impetigo most commonly occurs in children, presenting as pustules on the skin filled with a honey-colored fluid. The pustules burst and crust over. Vesicular impetigo is highly contagious, and easily passes from one area of the body to another and from person to person with contact.

Neonates may develop bullous impetigo from cross-contamination in the nursery. This type of impetigo is caused by *S. aureus* and is highly contagious. Bullous impetigo is characterized by vesicles that burst and crust. Any area of the body may be infected.

Clinical Manifestations

- Localized pustules, which burst and crust, anywhere on the body. Crusts and fluid are honey-colored.
- Lesions often spread.
- Pruritus may result in excoriation from scratching.

Diagnosis

- Diagnosis is made by history and physical examination.
- Bacterial culture and drug sensitivity testing is recommended.

Complications

- Acute poststreptococcal glomerulonephritis (inflammation of the nephron) may occur from antibody–antigen complexes depositing in the kidney (type III hypersensitivity response). Widespread infection in an infant is possible.

Treatment

- Systemic antibiotics may be administered after culture and identification of the organism. Topical antibiotics such as mupirocin may be adequate if the lesion is small.
- Removal of crusts with warm water and gentle antibacterial soap.
- Sterilization of towels and frequent hand washing must be done to prevent spread on the body and to family members.

Cellulitis

Cellulitis is a bacterial infection of the dermis or subcutaneous layer of the skin. Cellulitis typically occurs after a surface wound, bite, or untreated carbuncle or furuncle. The most common causative organisms are group A beta-hemolytic streptococci or *S. aureus*. The most common areas affected are the legs, hands, ears, and buttocks. Erysipelas is a superficial form of cellulites characterized by bright red, warm, tender, and well-defined lesions. Lymphatic involvement manifests with a red streak from the primary site.

Clinical Manifestations

- The skin appears swollen and red and is tender and warm to the touch. The area feels taut with poorly defined borders. An exudate of serous or purulent fluid may be present.
- Fever may be present.

Diagnosis

- Diagnosis is made by history and physical examination.
- Mild leukocytosis with a shift to the left or increased neutrophils.
- Wound culture.

Complications

- Septicemia, nephritis, or death if not treated appropriately.

Treatment

- Elevate and rest the area
- Warm soaks in an antibacterial medium or Burrow's solution may be used.
- Systemic antibiotics are necessary.
- Pain medication as needed.

Folliculitis

Infection of a hair follicle, usually by the bacterium *S. aureus*, is known as folliculitis. Inflammation occurs in the follicle due to chemotatic factors and enzymes that are released from the bacteria. Risk factors include trauma to the skin and poor hygiene.

Clinical Manifestations

- Surface pustules surrounded by erythema with pain, and swelling.

Diagnosis

- Diagnosis is made by history and physical examination.

Complications

- A boil, also called a **furuncle**, may develop if the inflamed follicle bursts and spreads the bacteria into the dermis. Pain and inflammation worsen. Oozing of pus and cellulitis may develop.

Treatment

- Soap and water and topical antibiotics.
- Warm compresses and incision of the lesion may be required.
- Systemic antibiotics may be required.

Carbuncle and Furuncles

When folliculitis extends into the subcutaneous and dermal layers and involves more hair follicles a carbuncle or furuncle develops. Occlusion of a sebaceous gland causes an inflammatory response. A carbuncle is about 3 to 10 cm in diameter and drains pus leaving craterlike nodules. A furuncle, often referred to as a "boil" is about 1 to 5 cm in diameter and is filled with pus. Abscess may develop as immune cells encircle the infection.

Clinical Manifestations

- A deep, hard, firm mass under the skin that is painful and may drain purulent material.
- Systemic signs of infection, including chills, fever, and malaise.
- Regional lymphadenopathy.

Diagnosis

- Diagnosis is made by history and physical examination.
- Drainage may be cultured.

Treatment

- Warm compresses and topical or systemic antibiotics. An abscess may require lancing and drainage.

Scarlet Fever

Although not a bacterial infection, scarlet fever is a skin rash caused by toxins released during infection with group A beta-hemolytic streptococci. Scarlet fever, also called scarletina, is usually associated with a pharyngeal streptococcal infection.

Clinical Manifestations

- The rash of scarlet fever is usually pink, mainly over the neck, trunk, axillae, thighs, and groin, with a feeling similar to fine sandpaper.
- The rash is typically accompanied by other signs of a pharyngeal streptococcal infection: high fever, sore throat, fever, headache, and nausea.
- Strawberry or raspberry tongue, skin desquamation.
- Facial flushing with circumoral pallor.

Diagnostic Tools

- A throat culture is usually positive for group A beta-hemolytic streptococci. This coupled with a good history and physical examination usually confirms scarlet fever.

Complications

- Poststreptococcal glomerulonephritis, rheumatic fever, otitis media, chorea, and peritonsillar abscess may all follow a streptococcal infection.

Treatment

- Treatment is with penicillin or, if the individual is allergic to penicillin, erythromycin or another macrolide.

FUNGAL INFECTIONS OF THE SKIN AND NAILS

Fungal infections of the skin are considered superficial infections and are typically described based on the site of infection. The infections of the skin are called tinea (mistakenly referring to a worm). **Tinea pedis** is an infection of the foot (e.g., athlete's foot); **tinea corporis** (ringworm), an infection of the body; **tinea barbae**, an infection of the beard; and **tinea capitis**, an infection of the scalp. **Tinea versicolor** is a fungal infection of the body that may result in patches of discoloration that are worsened by exposure to sunlight. The most common nail infection is **onychomycosis** or **tinea unduium**.

Fungal infections of the mouth (thrush), gastrointestinal (GI) tract, and vagina usually are a result of the yeast-like fungus *Candida albicans* and are called **candidiasis**. *C. albicans* is part of the normal human flora that, under some conditions, may multiply excessively and cause symptoms.

Deep fungal infections of the respiratory tract or brain usually occur only in immunocompromised individuals and are considered opportunistic infections. Histoplasmosis is a fungal infection of the respiratory tract that may develop in normal individuals as well.

Causes of Fungal Infections

Fungal infections occur in individuals who are somehow predisposed to their development. Predisposition may exist for no obvious reason, but often individuals are predisposed as a result of their environment or behavior, for example, frequent participation in athletic events associated with perspiration and frequent showering where the fungus may be present (e.g., locker rooms). A predisposition is also present in individuals suffering from decreased immune function (e.g., diabetics, pregnant women, and young infants). Those who have severe immunodeficiency, including those suffering from acquired immunodeficiency syndrome (AIDS), are at special risk of chronic, debilitating fungal infections. In fact, vaginal or oral yeast infections are frequently the first opportunistic infections seen in individuals infected with the human immunodeficiency virus (HIV). Persons who have chronic fungal infections should be evaluated for diabetes mellitus and HIV/AIDS.

Treatment with antibiotics for a bacterial infection may kill normal vaginal bacteria that usually exist in balance with vaginal yeast. This decrease in normal vaginal bacteria may predispose women or girls to vaginal yeast infections. Vaginal douching can also result in loss of normal vaginal flora.

Clinical Manifestations

- Skin infections cause inflammation with erythema and itching.
- Ringworm may present as a ring of erythema with a pale interior. Scaling of the edges may be present.
- Yeast infections may appear as inflamed pustules that itch and are painful. Erythematous macules surrounded by isolated pustules or papules at the boarder constitute the classical satellite lesions associated with yeast infections.
- Vaginal infections are associated with a cheese-like white discharge.
- Oral infections present with multiple white ulcerations surrounded by erythema, which may be extremely painful.
- Nails initially are white or silvery and then turn yellow or brown. They may become deformed, cracked, and thickened.

Diagnosis

- Fungal infections may be diagnosed by history and physical examination.
- Microscopic examination of nail or skin scrapings prepared with potassium hydroxide allows for identification of hyphae (characteristic spores and filaments of fungi) under the microscope.
- Viewing the affected area with a special UV light (Wood lamp) may also allow for recognition of fungal infections, as the spores fluoresce blue-green under this lighting condition. If hyphae or spores cannot be seen, scrapings may be sent for culture to confirm or refute diagnosis. Sometimes, cultures are sent even if hyphae or spores are seen.

Complications

- Surface infections may become secondarily infected by bacteria.
- Deep fungal infections (internal) may cause significant morbidity and mortality.
- Scarring of the skin or, with tinea capitis, alopecia (hair loss) may occur.
- Painful oral lesions that interfere with eating may contribute to the wasting seen in individuals suffering from AIDS.

Treatment

- Skin infections are treated with type-specific antifungal medications applied topically or occasionally given systemically. Scalp and foot infections are often treated with systemic agents.

- Candidiasis is treated with antifungal cream or suppositories.
- Treatment may be given to partners of women with chronic vaginal yeast infection.
- Deep fungal infections may require extensive, specific antifungal therapy and hospitalization.

INFLAMMATORY DISORDERS OF THE SKIN

Acne

Acne is a common inflammatory disease of a sebaceous gland associated with a hair follicle, called the **pilosebaceous unit**. There are two types of acne: inflammatory and noninflammatory. Both types of acne are characterized by excessive sebum production. The excess sebum accumulates in the follicle, causing the follicle to swell.

In inflammatory acne, the follicle becomes blocked by the sebum and a type of acne-specific bacterium, *Propionibacterium acnes*, proliferates in the canal. Eventually, the follicle ruptures and the sebum and bacteria are released into the dermis, causing inflammation of the dermal tissue. In noninflammatory acne, the follicle does not burst but remains dilated. The sebum either moves to the skin surface (a blackhead) or the canal remains blocked (a whitehead).

Acne is commonly seen in teenagers and young adults, beginning with the onset of puberty. Although both boys and girls suffer from acne, it is especially severe and common in boys. Adults, especially women, may have a recurrence of acne.

Causes of Acne

Sebum production is stimulated by androgens, especially testosterone. The sharp increase in androgens seen in both girls and boys during puberty is largely responsible for the onset and severity of acne. There is little research-based support for traditional biases to prove that diet or lack of facial cleansing contributes to acne, although *P. acne* infection of the obstructed follicle may be worsened by poor nutrition. Instead, there is a strong genetic influence over the development of acne that may be related to oversensitivity of the sebaceous glands to androgen or the presence of an environment favorable to the proliferation of bacteria. Other contributors to acne may be important and vary for any given individual. Protective against acne is estrogen, which opposes the action of androgen on the sebaceous glands and reduces the development of acne. In adult women, the development of acne may be related to other systemic conditions or may occur as the level of testosterone relative to estrogen begins to rise in the early perimenopausal years.

Acne rosacea is a condition of the skin that develops in middle-aged adults of both sexes and is characterized by redness (erythema), papules, and pustules, especially on the forehead, nose, cheeks, and chin. Although no specific cause of acne rosacea has been identified, it is associated with heightened sensitivity to the sun. The condition may come and go and is typically exacerbated by hot drinks and alcohol. It may result in hypertrophy of the sebaceous glands, with thickening of the nose (rhinophyma), a permanent development. Eye irritation, including conjunctivitis, may be present. There is also a genetic tendency to develop rosacea, with light-skinned populations especially susceptible.

Clinical Manifestations

- Acne may present with a variety of lesions on one individual. Lesions can include blackheads, whiteheads, nodules, pustules, cysts, and scars. Lesions commonly occur over the face, back, and shoulders.
- In women, acne may increase before or during the menstrual period when estrogen levels are the lowest.
- With rosacea, the face may turn bright red with even limited sun or alcohol exposure, and papules and pustules may develop.

Complications

- Scarring may occur in severe cases of acne.
- Self-esteem may be affected even with less-severe conditions.
- Rhinophyma may occur with rosacea.

Treatment

- Topical agents such as benzoyl peroxide and retinoic acid (vitamin A, Retin-A) are used to dry and peel the skin. This effect increases cell turnover and opens the follicles and facilitates the movement of sebum to the skin. Benzoyl peroxide also works to eliminate *P. acnes*. Retin A may lead to excessive drying and redness of the skin, and individuals using Retin A must avoid unprotected sun exposure. Pregnant women are advised to avoid using Retin A.
- Antibacterial soap may reduce bacterial contamination of the skin.
- Lasers damage oil glands and photodynamic light therapy treats overactive oil glands using the *P. acnes* bacteria.
- Topically applied antibiotics, often in combination with benzoyl peroxide, may be prescribed for use once or twice a day. Topical antibiotics, usually tetracycline, erythromycin, or clindamycin, work to reduce *P. acnes* proliferation. Treatment with this regimen typically takes at least 4 weeks to induce notable improvement.
- Oral low-dose antibiotic therapy (e.g., tetracycline, doxycycline) may be administered to reduce bacterial proliferation in the follicle. Antibiotic therapy requires several weeks to be effective and may induce photosensitivity. Oral tetracycline damages developing teeth; therefore, it is contraindicated in pregnant women or women planning to get pregnant. Tetracycline is also a drug of choice for rosacea.

- Birth-control pills containing estrogen can reduce sebum production. They may be used to treat acne in girls and women.
- Systemic 13-*cis*-retinoic acid (isotretinoin) may be used for severe nodular cystic acne. This drug can cause severe birth defects and should not be used by young women who are or may get pregnant. Males likewise should avoid impregnating a partner while on isotretinoin.

Psoriasis

Psoriasis is a chronic, autoimmune, inflammatory skin disease that affects approximately 2.6 million Americans. Psoriasis is characterized by rapid turnover of epidermal cells, leading to abnormal proliferation of the epidermis and the dermis. The skin demonstrates red, raised scaly plaques that can cover any body surface. Psoriasis has a strong genetic component and its prevalence varies by ethnicity, with Caucasians more frequently affected than those of African descent. The quality of life reported by patients with moderate or severe psoriasis can be quite compromised, with studies reporting life quality levels reduced to those reported by patients with severe diseases such as emphysema and heart failure. Psoriasis typically occurs between 15 and 30 years of age, but can develop at any age.

Causes of Psoriasis

Although previously described as a disease of benign epithelial proliferation, it has become increasingly clear that psoriasis is in fact an autoimmune disorder. T lymphocytes are activated in response to an unknown stimulus, through an association with the skin's Langerhans' cells. Activation of localized T cells leads to the production of proinflammatory cytokines, including tumor necrosis factor alpha, and growth factors that stimulate abnormal cellular proliferation and turnover. Normal epidermal cell turnover is approximately 28 to 30 days; with psoriasis, the epidermis in affected areas may shed every 3 to 4 days. Rapid cell turnover results in increased metabolic rate and increased blood flow to the cells to support the high metabolism. Increased blood flow causes the erythema, and the rapid turnover and proliferation lead to poorly developed and immature cells. Small trauma to the skin results in exaggerated inflammation, causing epidermal thickening and plaque formation.

Risk Factors for Psoriasis

There is a genetic tendency for the development of psoriasis, with an increased incidence among family members. Over a thousand genes, primarily immune response and proliferation genes, have been identified that appear to play a role in the pathogenesis and maintenance of psoriasis. Environmental factors, including trauma to the skin, viral or bacterial infection, cigarette smoking, and stress, may worsen the condition. Certain drugs, including angiotensin-converting enzyme inhibitors and lithium, can precipitate or worsen an outbreak.

Clinical Manifestations

- Well-demarcated (clearly bordered) erythematous plaques covered with silvery white scales develop, especially over knees, elbows, scalp, and in skin folds.
- Lesions typically develop insidiously, with just one or two lesions later coalescing into many.
- Nail pitting or separation of the nail is common.
- Symptoms typically improve in summer and worsen in winter.

Diagnosis

- Diagnosis is made based on history and physical examination. A family history of the disease may be recalled.
- Skin biopsy.

Complications

- Severe infections of the lesions may develop.
- A deforming arthritis similar to rheumatoid arthritis, called psoriatic arthritis, occurs in approximately 30% of individuals. When severe, this can be a disabling disease.
- Because of the impact on patients' self-esteem, psychological stress, anxiety, depression, and anger may develop.
- Research has indicated an increased risk for cardiovascular disease, metabolic syndrome, and malignancy. Extensive research is continuing.

Treatment

- The severity of disease determines treatment.
- Mild disease is usually treated successfully with topical emollients to soften plaques, vitamin D analogs to reduce inflammation, or topical retinoids to peel the skin, the latter often in combination with topical steroids to reduce inflammation. Coal tar is an old and effective treatment that is applied to the skin for several weeks. Its exact mechanism of action is unknown.
- Phototherapy with UVB may be used.
- For more serious conditions, photochemotherapy is often used. This type of treatment employs a light-activated drug, methoxsalen (Psoralen), given orally to a patient 1 to 2 hours before he or she is exposed to UV radiation. Activated methoxsalen blocks DNA synthesis and therefore slows cellular replication and turnover. This treatment is identified by the acronym PUVA, referring to its combination of Psoralen (P) and long-wave ultraviolet radiation (UVA). Some concerns exist regarding its long-term effects, and individuals using PUVA should be screened regularly for skin cancer.

- Moderate disease and flare-ups are often treated systemically, using chemotherapeutic drugs to affect cell turnover, antimetabolites to prevent cell cycling, or oral immunosuppressive drugs, such as corticosteroids, to suppress inflammation.
- New treatment strategies for moderate or severe disease include immune-modulating drugs. These drugs work by decreasing the number or functioning of pathogenic T cells or by blocking the effects of the proinflammatory cytokines. Examples of immune-modulating drugs approved by the FDA for the treatment of moderate or severe psoriasis include alefacept, efalizumab, and etanercept. Others are under development.
- Severe disease may require hospitalization and systemic steroids.

PARASITIC SKIN CONDITIONS

Pediculosis

Infestation with lice is known as pediculosis. Lice are gray, gray-brown, or red-brown wingless parasites that survive by sucking blood. There are three types that infest the human body: pediculosis capitus (head lice), pediculosis corporis (body lice), and pediculosis pubis (pubic lice). The female louse lays eggs (nits) along the hair shaft. When the eggs hatch, the lice secrete a toxic saliva that causes trauma and itching. Lice are spread through personal contact and cannot survive beyond a few hours without a live host. It is estimated that 10 to 12 million Americans are affected by head lice annually.

Clinical Manifestations

- Pruritus.
- Appearance of nits or lice.
- Red and excoriated scalp.
- On the body, the bites may be macular, papular, or wheals with a hemorrhagic puncture site.

Diagnosis

- Firmly attached nit which is a white or yellow oval speck.
- Live adult lice on the hair shaft.
- Ova of lice fluoresce under UV or Wood's light.
- Culture.

Complications

- Intense scratching can cause excoriation and possible secondary infections.
- Excessive use of over-the-counter treatment may result in resistant strains.

Treatment

- Combing hair with a nit comb.
- Pyrethrin or permethrin shampoos block nerve impulse transmission which paralyzes and kills lice.
- Malathion or shampoos.
- Lice suffocation with olive oil, petroleum, or mayonnaise is an old remedy that may or may not be effective.
- Antihistamines for itching.
- All linens and hair accessories should be thoroughly cleaned.

Scabies

Scabies is caused by the mite *Sarcoptes scabiei* that burrows under the skin and lays eggs in the stratum corneum. The fecal material of the mite in the burrows tends to cause severe itching. The most common areas affected are the interdigital webs of the fingers, flexor surface of the wrist, belt line, penis, nipple, and gluteal crease. Transmission occurs by person-to-person contact and by contact with infested clothing. The mite can live up to 2 days without a living host.

Clinical Manifestations

- Linear red to reddish-brown burrows.
- Pruritus.

Diagnosis

- Skin scrapping for mite, ova, or feces.

Complications

- Intense scratching can cause excoriation and possible secondary infections.

Treatment

- After bathing, application of permethrin, malathion, or other mite-killing agent for 12 hours.
- Disinfect linens and clothing with detergent and hot water.

SCLERODERMA

Scleroderma, which means hardening of the skin, is an autoimmune connective tissue disease. The immune system stimulates an excess production of fibroblasts and may involve only the skin or may occur systematically and involve the kidneys, heart, lungs, and gut. Women are affected more commonly than men.

Scleroderma is characterized by massive deposits of collagen under the skin or in internal organs, resulting in inflammation and fibrosis. Skin deposits are in the dermal and subdermal tissue. The disease may include a group of symptoms represented by the acronym CREST: calcium deposits, Raynaud's phenomenon characterized by spasms of the arterioles of the fingers, esophageal dysfunction, sclerodactyly (scleroderma of the fingers and toes), and telangiectasis (vascular lesion due to dilation). Although the actual cause is unknown, exposure to toxins such as silicosis and epoxy resins may predispose a person to the disease.

Clinical Manifestations

- The skin appears tight, shiny, and often red from inflammation.
- Flat affect.
- Rigid body movements.
- Fingertips and nails may be narrow or missing.
- Hard, calcium nodules under the skin may be visible and palpable.
- Muscular atrophy, pain, and deformity may develop.

Diagnosis

- Often diagnosed by excluding other connective tissue diseases and from the history and physical examination.
- Positive LE prep, elevated gamma globulin level, and presence of antinuclear antigen

Complications

- A mortality rate of approximately 50% if the disease progresses to involve internal organs.

Treatment

- There is no specific treatment for scleroderma. It is recommended that patients avoid exposure to cold temperature and smoking, both of which cause vasoconstriction and worsen symptoms.
- Steroidal anti-inflammatory medication may be used to slow the autoimmune response.
- Emollients for dry, itchy skin.

TATTOOS AND BODY PIERCINGS

A tattoo is a permanent mark on the skin made by injecting ink or dye with a needle into the dermis. Tattooing may be done by amateurs, professionals, or medical personnel. Body piercing is typically performed for the purpose of jewelry insertion and may involve any part of the body. For tattooing and body piercing the use of sterile equipment is imperative.

Complications

- Infection.
- Allergic reaction.
- Transmission of blood-borne pathogens and other infections (hepatitis B, hepatitis C, tuberculosis, tetanus, and HIV).
- Scarring and keloid formation.
- Some dyes may cause a reaction during magnetic resonant imaging.

BURNS

Burns may result from exposure of the skin to high temperature, electrical shock, or chemicals. Burns are classified according to tissue depth of the burn and the extent of the body surface area that has been burned.

Depth of a Burn

A burn may be classified as superficial first-degree, superficial partial-thickness second-degree, deep partial-thickness second-degree, full thickness third-degree, or full-thickness fourth degree. Table 5-2 (Burn Wound Classification) includes characteristic of each type.

Extent of a Burn

The extent of a burn refers to the total body surface area (TBSA) of an individual's body that has received superficial or deep second-degree burns or full-thickness burns (it does not include first-degree burns). To determine the extent of a burn, the percentage of TBSA affected is estimated. One method for estimating the percentage of a burn is by using **the rule of nines** (Fig. 5-2). With this method, each arm is considered 9% of the body surface area, each leg 18%, the front and back torso each 18%, the head 9%, and the genital area 1%. The percentages of the body burned are added to give the TBSA burned. For children, the rule of nines is slightly altered to more accurately reflect surface area based on growth and development. The Lund and Browder chart (Fig. 5-2 Estimating the Extent of a Burn), is a more accurate determination of body surface area because calculations are based on the surface area for each body part according to the age of the patient. If burns are scattered over the body, the patient's hand, which is about 1% of body size, can be used to roughly estimate the extent of the burn.

TABLE 5-2 Burn Wound Classification

Degree of Burn	Depth of Burn	Wound Characteristics
First-degree	Epidermis	Erythema and pain
		Heals in 3–4 days
		Example: sunburn
Superficial partial-thickness second degree	Epidermis and the dermis	Extremely painful with blister formation in minutes
		Heals in about a month
		Secondary infections may occur
Deep partial-thickness second degree	Epidermis and entire dermis	Hair follicles remain intact and regrow
		Partially sensitive to pain due to sensory neuron destruction but surrounding area is usually painful
		Heals in several weeks
		Surgical debridement and grafting
Full-thickness third degree	Epidermis, dermis, subcutaneous layer	Capillary, vein, and nerve destruction
		Not painful but surrounding area is painful
		Heals in months
		Surgical debridement and grafting
		Scars are hard and leathery
Full-thickness fourth degree	Epidermis, dermis, subcutaneous layer, muscle, bone, internal tissues	Dry, charred; mottled; brown, white, or red; no sensation; altered or absent movement in involved extremities

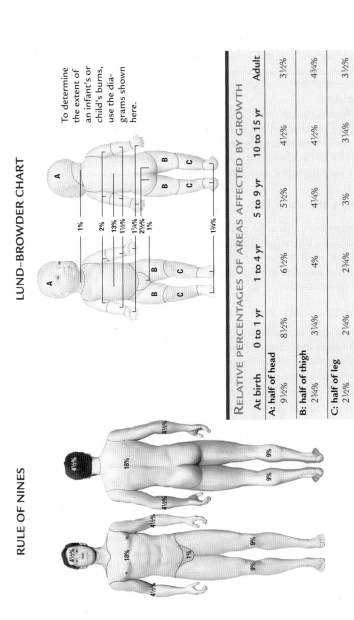

RULE OF NINES

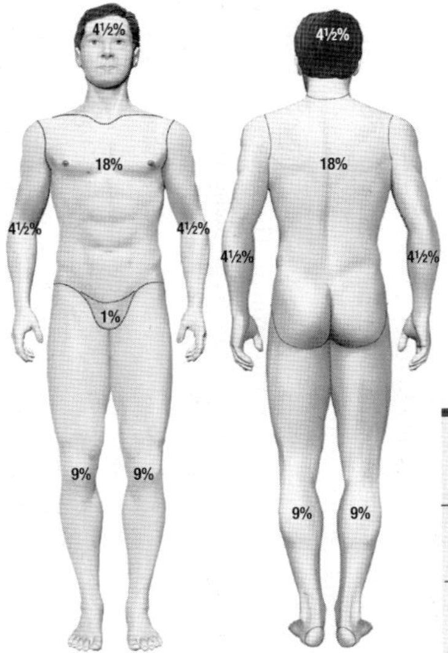

LUND–BROWDER CHART

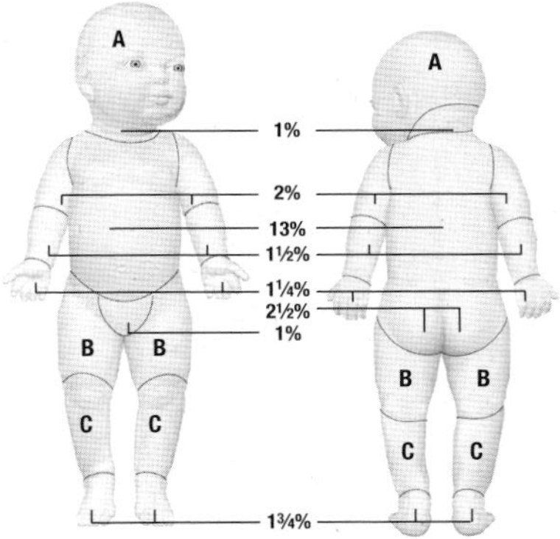

To determine the extent of an infant's or child's burns, use the diagrams shown here.

Relative percentages of areas affected by growth

At birth	0 to 1 yr	1 to 4 yr	5 to 9 yr	10 to 15 yr	Adult
A: half of head					
9½%	8½%	6½%	5½%	4½%	3½%
B: half of thigh					
2¾%	3¼%	4%	4¼%	4½%	4¾%
C: half of leg					
2½%	2¼%	2¾%	3%	3¼%	3½%

FIGURE 5-2 Estimating the extent of a burn. (From Anatomical Chart Company [year]. *Atlas of pathophysiology* [3rd edition]. Philadelphia: Lippincott Williams & Wilkins.)

The TBSA burned is especially important during the initial assessment when determining if a patient should be sent to a burn center and when calculating fluid and nutrient requirements. Based on TBSA burned, major burns are defined as those involving between 25% and 40% of the body surface area of an adult and between 15% and 25% of the surface area of a child. Burns of greater than 40% in adults or 25% in children are associated with significant mortality.

Besides considering TBSA burned and depth of burns, the overall health and age of the individual must be taken into consideration when predicting survival from any burn. Children and the elderly have increased mortality compared with middle-aged and young adults. An individual suffering from a severe burn should be transferred to a burn care facility as soon as possible.

Effects of a Major Burn

A major burn affects the metabolism and function of every cell in the body. All systems are compromised, especially the cardiovascular system. Given the dependence of every organ on adequate blood flow, alteration in cardiovascular function has wide-ranging implications for survival and recovery. Cellular changes also occur.

Cardiovascular Response to a Major Burn

Edema of the burned tissue and directly surrounding areas occurs immediately following a severe burn. Edema of the burned tissue results from a breakdown of the capillaries and from plasma fluid and protein leaking into the interstitial space. The edema leads to increased tissue pressure, exacerbation of tissue hypoxia, and worsening damage. Cytokines, prostaglandins, leukotrienes, and histamine all are released and further increase capillary permeability. White blood cells are attracted to the area, especially neutrophils, which produce free oxygen radicals and contribute to reperfusion injury.

After several more hours, edema spreads beyond the burned tissue, as the ability of distant capillaries to act as barriers to diffusion is lost as well. This later edema of nonburned tissue appears to result from a transient increase in capillary permeability to water and protein. The loss of capillary integrity is described as **a loss of capillary seal**. The accumulation of fluid in the interstitial space throughout the body results in a significant decrease in circulating blood volume, causing a fall in stroke volume and blood pressure. Pulse rate increases in compensation. Irreversible shock may develop.

During the period of capillary leakage, blood viscosity increases and blood flow is sluggish. Individuals are at increased risk of clot formation. With a weakly beating heart, blood accumulates in the lungs, causing pulmonary congestion and increasing the risk of embolus formation. Decreased blood flow to the kidneys causes renal hypoxia and a significant decrease in urine output. The renin–angiotensin system is stimulated, resulting in increased salt and water retention. Because the capillaries do not contain the increased volume, additional edema develops, further increasing the risk of pulmonary congestion and pneumonia. Hypoxia of the gut causes injury to the mucus-producing cells, leading to gastric and duodenal ulcers (called Curling ulcers). Within approximately 24 to 48 hours after a burn, the capillaries reseal and the fluid is slowly reabsorbed back into the circulation. However, the effects of the loss of seal remain, and the risk of morbidity and mortality continues to be high.

Cellular Response to a Burn

In response to a major burn, cells outside the burned area may become permeable to electrolytes, causing sodium and calcium to accumulate intracellularly, and magnesium and phosphate to leak out from cells. Water diffuses into the cell and the cell swells. Injured cells burst, releasing potassium into the extracellular fluid. These changes affect the membrane potential of all cells and can lead to cardiac dysrhythmias and alterations in central nervous system function.

Immune function is inhibited by a major burn. Loss of immune function, combined with loss of the barrier function of the skin, puts an individual at high risk for infection. Decreased immune function appears to result from the release of hormones, including but not limited to cortisol. Cortisol is released with stress and is an immunosuppressant at high concentrations.

Metabolic rate is significantly increased with a major burn. Hypermetabolism may result from activation of the sympathetic nervous system and the stress response, as well as from attempts to balance the heat loss that occurs when the insulatory function of the skin is lost. Healing of the burn also requires huge amounts of energy. The temperature control center in the hypothalamus is affected by the response to a major burn, leading to an increase in hypothalamic set point. This increase may result from cytokines and other peptides released during the widespread inflammatory response. The hypermetabolism, as well as the increase in cortisol and epinephrine (hormones of the postabsorptive state) and changes in insulin sensitivity, leads to tissue breakdown and protein and fat wasting. Protein breakdown contributes to severe muscle wasting.

Clinical Manifestations

- A superficial first-degree burn is characterized by redness and pain. Blisters may develop after 24 hours, and the skin may later peel.
- A superficial partial-thickness second-degree burn is characterized by rapid blister formation (within minutes) and intense pain.
- A deep partial-thickness second-degree burn is characterized by blisters or thin dry tissue that covers the wound and peels off. The wound may not be painful.

- A full-thickness third-degree burn appears flat, thin, and dry. Coagulated blood vessels may be seen. The skin may be white, red, or black and leathery.
- Electrical burns may appear similar to thermal burns, or may appear as silver, raised areas. Electrical burns usually occur at points of electrical contact. The internal damage caused by an electrical burn may be much more severe than is apparent from the external wound.

Diagnostic Tools

- Diagnosis may involve only an inspection of the burn site if the burn is small and uncomplicated. However, for significant burns, the American Burn Association recommends additional evaluation. With a burn of the face or neck, or when a burn covers a large percentage of TBSA, checking the airway is essential since such burns can lead to airway edema requiring intubation. Additionally, determining the mechanism of injury and a comprehensive physical examination to look for other sites of trauma are required.
- The rule of nines is used to evaluate the percentage of body surface burned in adults (over age 15). In children, the Lund and Browder chart is used to determine TBSA burned.
- Urine output is followed closely during the period of burn shock and after resealing of the capillaries. This is essential for evaluating the success of volume replacement during burn shock. When urine output returns to normal, the capillaries are said to have resealed.
- Depth of wound is evaluated to determine the local and surgical treatment of wounds.

Complications

- Any burn may become infected, causing further disability or death. Methicillin-resistant *S. aureus* is an especially frequent cause of hospital-acquired (nosocomial) infection in burn patients. Infections are the leading cause of morbidity and mortality in patients who initially survive a major burn.
- Sluggish blood flow may lead to the development of a blood clot, causing a cerebral vascular accident, a myocardial infarct, or a pulmonary embolus.
- Lung damage may occur from smoke inhalation or embolus formation. Pulmonary congestion may result from left-heart failure or a myocardial infarct. Adult respiratory distress syndrome may develop. The combination of smoke inhalation and a severe body burn increases mortality.
- Electrolyte disturbances may lead to a cardiac dysrhythmia and cardiac arrest.
- Burn shock may irreversibly damage the kidneys, leading to renal failure within the first week or two after the burn. Renal failure may also develop as a result of renal hypoxia or rhabdomyolysis (myoglobin obstruction of the kidney tubules secondary to widespread muscle necrosis).

- Decreased blood flow to the gut may result in hypoxia of the mucus-producing cells, leading to peptic ulcer disease.
- Disseminated intravascular coagulation (DIC) may occur with widespread tissue destruction.
- Fluid resuscitation may exacerbate some chronic conditions such as congestive heart failure or renal failure.
- With a major or disfiguring burn, psychological trauma may lead to depression, family breakup, and thoughts of suicide. Psychological symptoms may occur any time after a burn. Symptoms may come and go repeatedly over a lifetime as patients grieve and re-grieve over the losses encountered from the burn injuries.
- The financial burden to the family of an individual who has a severe burn is enormous. Not only are wages lost if the individual is an adult, but care is continuous and costly.

Treatment

- Individuals experiencing a burn should immediately be removed from the burning agent, and the burned area of the skin should be immediately immersed under cool water to stop further tissue destruction. The application of ice should be avoided because ice decreases blood flow to the area and may worsen the degree of the burn. Clothes should not be removed from a serious burn, because removing clothes may also remove skin.
- Edema associated with superficial or partial-thickness burns may be controlled by cold-water immersion. The intravenous administration of large macromolecules, such as albumin, dextran, and starch, may improve non-burn edema, but is unlikely to improve edema of the burned tissue. Heparin may maintain blood flow in burned injuries, but may also contribute to edema.
- Individuals who have a severe burn must receive medical treatment. Infants, young children, and the elderly who suffer anything other than a minor burn should be evaluated by a medical provider, as should those who have any chronic illness or condition. Burns to the hands, face, and genitals should be evaluated by medical personnel.
- First-degree burns usually require only prolonged exposure to large amounts of cool water or the application of cool compresses and anti-inflammatory medication.
- First-degree chemical burns should be flushed with cool water for several minutes.
- Burns deeper than first-degree require antimicrobial therapy and should be evaluated by medical personnel. Application of silver-based ointment is especially effective, as silver inhibits bacterial growth. Silver is toxic, however,

to keratinocytes and fibroblasts necessary for tissue healing, so risks and benefits should be weighed. Silver nitrate has the potential to cause severe electrolyte imbalances (hyponatremia and hypochloremia).

- Major burns require quick intravenous fluid replacement to combat the loss of capillary seal. To maintain blood pressure and prevent irreversible shock, infusions in an adult may reach the staggering amount of 30 L in 24 hours. The high rate of fluid replacement also flushes the kidney and reduces the risk of renal failure.

- Early and continued nutritional support is required for severely burned individuals. Because of the hypermetabolic response to a severe burn, calories and protein must be in adequate supply to prevent muscle catabolism and wasting. Enteral feeding is optimal for those who suffer severe burns, both because of its ability to provide adequate calories for healing and because it appears to protect the gut mucosa, reducing damage to the gut barrier.

- In second-degree partial-thickness burns, special dressings that support cell division and growth are applied.

- Second-degree, total-thickness, and third-degree burns require near immediate debridement (surgical excision of the wound) and grafting. If possible, grafting should be from nondamaged skin of the burn patient (autograft). Other grafting sources are human donors, alive or dead (allograft), or nonhuman donors, usually pigs (xenograft). Cultured autografts and artificial skin grafts have been developed as well.

- Tissue-expansion techniques have been used to improve the chances for successful skin grafting. These techniques stimulate a stretch-induced signal transduction pathway whereby stretch increases the growth of keratinocytes and stimulates protein synthesis in skin to be used for autografts.

- Pain relief and pain management are major goals of burn therapy. Burns themselves can be excruciatingly painful, as can the treatments used to help a burn to heal. Alleviating pain as much as possible reduces stress, which may improve immune function and healing. Adequate pain relief also may relieve the psychological trauma associated with burns, some of which continues long after the burn is physically healed.

DECUBITUS ULCER

Decubitus ulcers are of concern worldwide and incur costs in billions of dollars each year. Research has also indicated that pressure ulcers and their treatments negatively impact the patient physically, mentally, emotionally, and socially. Decubitus ulcers, also called pressure sores or bed sores, are lesions on the skin that occur after the breakdown of the epidermis, the dermis, and, occasionally, the subcutaneous tissue and underlying bone. Decubitus ulcers are usually seen in individuals who are bedridden or have significantly decreased mobility, especially if these conditions are accompanied by poor nutritional status. Even if mobility is normal, those suffering a reduced sensitivity to pain (e.g., individuals who have diabetes mellitus, spinal cord injuries, or stroke) may develop an ulcer. The severity of an ulcer is based on the depth of erosion into the tissue. Even ulcers that look small on the surface of the skin may be associated with significant injury under the skin. Clinically, the designation "decubitus ulcer" includes any skin area with blanching erythema, nonblanching erythema, decubitus dermatitis, an ulcer at any stage of healing, or gangrene. See page C7 for illustrations and staging of decubitus ulcers.

There are four forces that together produce a decubitus ulcer: pressure, shearing, friction, and moisture. A decubitus ulcer usually forms on an area of the skin overlying a bony process. It develops when the **pressure** in that area goes unrelieved for a long period, causing collapse of the supplying blood vessels. This collapse leads to tissue hypoxia and cellular death. Decubitus ulcers are common on skin areas exposed to sliding or **shear** forces, where there is a high degree of **friction** between the skin and the surface, and on skin exposed for prolonged periods to the **moisture** of **urine** or **feces**, which further breaks down the skin and makes it susceptible to infection.

Clinical Manifestations

- A sign of early injury is an area of redness that does not disappear with fingertip pressure (nonblanching). An ulcer (erosion) on the skin is seen with more severe injury. A visible skin lesion may be partial or full thickness, extending through the dermis or even through the subcutaneous tissue. A full-thickness injury may damage the bone.
- Pain and systemic signs of inflammation, including fever and increased white blood cell count, may develop.

Diagnosis

- Decubitus ulcers are diagnosed with the help of a good history and physical examination. Individuals at high risk should be checked frequently for an early stage of ulcer development. Early stage is suggested by skin that remains blanched with pressure for more than a brief period.
- The Centers for Medicare and Medicaid Services (CMS) are now differentiating between community-acquired and hospital-acquired pressure ulcers and will no longer reimburse for hospital-acquired pressure ulcers.

Complications

- Infection leading to prolonged disability and hospitalization may occur with even small ulcers.

Treatment

- Prevention is essential! Risk assessment tools such as the Braden Scale for Predicting Pressure Sore Risk are helpful in the early identification and subsequent modification of risk factors.
- Prevention of a decubitus ulcer is essential and involves turning bedridden individuals frequently (at least every 2 hours), maintaining a dry surface free of debris, and ensuring adequate nutrition.
- Careful and frequent observations to recognize the earliest signs of skin breakdown.
- Caloric intake should be kept high to assist in immune function and to maintain overall general good health.
- Adequate hydration.
- If a pressure sore does develop, relief of the pressure on the skin and the placement of a clean, flat, nonbulky dressing are required.
- Wound care is based on the stage of the ulcer and may include semipermeable or occlusive dressings, debridement surgically or with proteolytic enzymes, and skin grafts.

SKIN CANCER

Skin cancer is the most common form of cancer in the United States, with over a million cases diagnosed each year. The incidence of skin cancer varies geographically, peaking at high altitude and in sunny regions of the country. Skin cancer is more common in light-skinned individuals than it is in dark-skinned individuals, although individuals from all races are at risk. There are three types of skin cancer: basal cell, squamous cell, and malignant melanoma (Table 5-3). All types of skin cancer are increasing in incidence and developing in individuals at younger ages. These increases are most likely because of the increase in recreational sun exposure over the last several decades.

Basal Cell Carcinoma

Basal cell carcinoma is a superficial cancer of immature epithelial cells. The tumors typically are slow growing and seldom metastasize, although they can cause localized tissue destruction. Basal cell carcinoma is the most common skin cancer in light-skinned people. The two most common types are nodular ulcerative basal cell and superficial basal cell. Basal cell carcinoma is caused by cumulative exposure to UV radiation from sunlight and genetic factors are involved as well. With early diagnosis and treatment it is highly curable although it may reoccur.

Squamous Cell Carcinoma

Squamous cell carcinoma is a cancer of the epidermal cells that may spread horizontally over the skin or vertically into the dermis. Spread may be slow or

TABLE 5-3 Skin Cancer		
Type	**Characteristics**	**Treatment**
Basal cell	*Nodular ulcerative*: Flesh-colored or pink nodule, often depressed in the center, enlarges over time. Shiny/waxy, most frequently seen on sun-exposed areas, often the ear, face, or hand *Superficial*: Flat, nonpalpable, erythematous plaque. Red, scaly areas enlarge with nodular borders and telangiectatic bases. Occurs most often on chest or back	Excision
Squamous cell	Scaly, red, keratotic, slightly elevated lesion, with central area of ulceration. Irregular borders may be crusted in later stages. Most frequently seen on sun-exposed areas, often the face, helix of the ear, nose, lower lip, or on scarred areas	Excision. May require radiation therapy
Malignant melanoma	Rapidly growing lesion arising de novo or from a pre-existing mole. Usually raised, black or brown, or sometimes varied in color. The borders are irregular and asymmetrical; they may bleed. Most frequently seen on sun-exposed areas, but may develop anywhere. Related to burning sun exposures	Excision, surgical removal of surrounding tissue, lymph node biopsy. Radiation, chemotherapy, or immune therapy may be used

aggressive. Squamous cell carcinoma may metastasize to other sites of the body. Squamous cell cancer is most common in the elderly and develops after prolonged exposure to the sun. It frequently develops on areas of the skin demonstrating precancerous lesions or irregularities, such as keratosis (a horny growth), actinic dermatitis, or areas of previous discoloration. Squamous cell carcinoma may also develop at the site of a previous scar (e.g., a burn scar). The use of immunosuppressive drugs predisposes transplant patients to squamous cell carcinoma due to drug-induced sensitivity to UVA and UVB radiation. The risk for squamous cell carcinoma is highest in sunny climates, with Australia having the highest rates of squamous cell carcinoma in the world.

Malignant Melanoma

Malignant melanoma is an aggressive tumor of the melanin-producing cells at the base of the epidermis. Malignant melanoma may develop at the site of a pre-existing nevus (mole) or may develop spontaneously on the skin. This type of skin cancer often develops during middle age or older, and appears to result from intense burns with blistering at any time in life. Other risk factors include light skin, freckles, and fair-colored hair. Malignant melanoma represents 4% of skin cancers but 79% of cancer deaths.

Research suggests melanoma occurs from a radiation-induced decrease in the functioning of the skin's immune cells, the Langerhans' cells. This makes the cells of the skin less able to identify and repair DNA damage, thus increasing the risk of carcinogenesis. A genetic predisposition for melanoma is likely with gene studies underway. Metastasis is common and the incidence of melanoma is increasing, especially among the young.

Risk Factors

- Fair or light skin color.
- Family or personal history of skin cancer.
- Chronic sun exposure.
- Intermittent, yet intense sun exposure.
- Sunburns early in life.
- Large number of moles or freckles.

Clinical Manifestations

- Basal cell carcinoma usually appears on sun-exposed areas of the body, including the face, arms, and chest. Lesions may appear as dome-shaped papules or nodules, well circumscribed, with a pearly white color, as in the case of classic nodular basal cell carcinoma, or as scaly reddened patches or plaques (superficial basal cell carcinoma). The lesions are painless.
- Squamous cell carcinoma usually occurs on sun-exposed areas of the body or on scarred tissue. The lesions appear as scaly red plaques or raised nodules with central necrosis.
- Malignant melanoma may appear as a multicolored nodule growing vertically or as a circular spread of pigmentation larger than 1 cm. Borders of either lesion are irregular and often asymmetric, and bleeding may occur. Melanoma may develop on sun-exposed areas, or on the palms of the hands, the soles of the feet, or the oral or vaginal mucosa.

Diagnosis

- Skin cancer diagnosis is made as a result of a physical examination followed by the excision and biopsy of a suspicious lesion. Any lesion should be considered suspicious if it demonstrates one of the ABCDs of skin cancer: **A**symmetry, irregular **B**order, a change in **C**olor, or an increasing **D**iameter such that the lesion is greater than 0.5 cm (approximately the size of a pencil eraser).

Complications

- Local invasion and destruction of tissue may occur with any type of skin cancer.
- Metastasis to regional lymph nodes and throughout the body may occur, especially with malignant melanoma. Basal cell carcinoma has very low risk for metastasis, while squamous cell carcinoma demonstrates intermediate risk.

Treatment

- Prevention of basal and squamous cell carcinoma is possible with rigorous protection from the sun, including avoidance of the sun at peak hours and the use of hats, protective clothing, and broad-spectrum sunscreen.
- Individuals can reduce the incidence of malignant melanoma by avoiding sun exposure and by wearing protective clothing. Individuals should avoid or limit the use of indoor tanning beds, as research suggests a strong association between indoor tanning and melanoma. Sunscreen may not protect against the development of malignant melanoma.
- Basal cell carcinoma usually is surgically excised. Prognosis is good.
- Squamous cell carcinoma is surgically excised and radiation therapy may be required. Prognosis is good, especially if metastasis has not occurred.
- Malignant melanoma is surgically excised, along with a margin of surrounding tissue. Lymph node biopsy is performed to determine if metastasis has occurred. Sentinel lymph node biopsy, i.e., biopsy of the node closest to the malignancy, has been shown to be an effective predictor of metastasis and a means of directing therapy. Prognosis depends on the size of the lesion and the outcome of the lymph node biopsy. Nodular growth has a worse prognosis.
- Removal of cancerous cells may include curettage with electrodesiccation, surgical excision, laser, irradiation, chemosurgery, or cryosurgery.
- Chemotherapy and immunotherapy both may be required in addition to surgery for malignant melanoma and sometimes squamous cell carcinoma.
- Tumor vaccines active against specific antigens in malignant melanoma are being used in selected patients. Gene therapy for malignant melanoma is also being studied.

PEDIATRIC CONSIDERATIONS

- Rubella is a strong teratogenic agent (one that causes birth defects) and is most highly contagious before an individual develops obvious signs of infection. To protect pregnant women from infection and subsequent injury to a developing fetus, it is imperative that all children be vaccinated against the virus during early childhood. Vaccinating young children protects any pregnant woman with whom the child may come in contact.

- Impetigo is a common childhood skin infection. It is highly contagious in crowded environments, such as schools and day care centers, especially if sanitary practices are poor.

- Infants who have oral thrush may be asymptomatic or may nurse poorly. If a breast-feeding infant is diagnosed with thrush, both infant and mother should be treated because infection can pass back and forth between the mouth and the nipple.

- Burns are a major cause of morbidity and mortality in children. Most burns to children are preventable. Frequent sources of burns include scalds from kitchen stove spills, or hot water exposure. Because children have skin that is much thinner than that of adults, even brief exposure (less than a second) to hot water can scald a child. Fire injury from being unable to escape a burning home or car and electrical burn injuries from electrical sockets or cords also account for a substantial number of childhood burns. Children may be burned purposefully in situations of abuse. Signs of this type of burn include delays in seeking medical attention, contact burns to parts of the body such as the back of hands or the genitals, and burns on the buttocks and legs indicative of forced immersion in hot water. Any burn is a frightening, painful experience for a child, and all possible steps should be taken to prevent a burn from occurring.

 GERIATRIC CONSIDERATIONS

- As an individual ages, all three layers of the skin change. The epidermis loses its elasticity and turgor and has a reduced capacity to produce and distribute melanin. Age spots (concentrated deposits of melanin) appear. The hair and nails become thin and brittle. The hair grays as melanocytes are lost. The number of Langerhans' cells decreases, increasing the skin's susceptibility to solar damage. Both poor blood flow and decreased Langerhans' cell function increase the risk of infection. Sensory receptors are reduced in number, contributing to an increased risk of injury. Poor blood flow and reduced immune function delay wound healing. Decreased sebaceous and sweat gland functioning cause drying and wrinkling of the skin. The ability of the body to cool itself by sweating and vasodilatation, or to conserve heat by vasoconstriction, is reduced, most likely due to a decreased responsiveness of the vasculature to sympathetic stimulation. A reduced ability to cool or warm the body by changing the skin's blood flow increases the risk of hyperthermia in elderly adults exposed to prolonged heat and the risk of hypothermia in elderly adults exposed to severe cold.

- The elderly frequently present with purpura and petechia, especially on the legs. Petechia and purpura in the elderly usually indicate fragility of the blood vessels or a platelet disorder. However, in some cases, these lesions may be caused by a fall or may result from abuse. Idiopathic purpura may occur in young women.

- The prevalence of psoriasis increases with age, making it a common disorder of the elderly. Because of changes in renal and hepatic clearance rates in the elderly, there is an increased risk of adverse drug side effects and drug interactions with several of the treatment options.

 CULTURAL CONSIDERATIONS

- Pomade acne may be seen in African Americans and Hispanics as a result of some grooming products that contain lanolins isopropyl myristate.
- Capsaicin-induced dermatitis that includes erythema, irritation, and burning pain occurs in Hispanics from handling hot chili peppers.
- Ecchymotic streaks may result from the Asian practice of coin rubbing in the skin.
- Cupping practices may result in circular, ecchymotic, painful burns.

SELECTED BIBLIOGRAPHY

Abernathy, H., Cho, C., DeLanoy, A., Khan, O., Kerns, J. W., & Knight, K. (2006). What nonpharmacological treatments are effective against common nongenital warts? *Journal of Family Practice*, 55(9), 801–802.

Aldredge, L. M. (2009). Beneath the surface: Psoriasis is more than skin deep. *Advance for Nurse Practitioners*, 17(4), 27–30.

Bickley, L. S. (2007). *Bate's guide to physical examination and history taking* (9th ed.). Philadelphia: Lippincott Williams & Wilkins.

Byrd, T. (2008). A rapidly spreading rash on a child: Strep infections, gastroenteritis precede symptoms. *Advance for Nurse Practitioners*, 16(11), 24–25.

Cobb, C. (2009). Saving face: Strategies to fight father time. *Advance for Nurse Practitioners*, 17(4), 39–45.

Demling, R. H. (2005). The burn edema process: Current concepts. *Journal of Burn Care Rehabilitation*, 26, 207–227.

Eckman, M., Labus, D., & Thompson, G. (eds.). *Atlas of pathophysiology* (3rd ed.). Philadelphia: Lippincott Williams & Wilkins.

Eliopoulos, C. (2010). *Gerontological nursing* (7th ed.). Philadelphia: Lippincott Williams & Wilkins.

Ford, J. (2008). Pesticide-resistant head lice: A super bug spawns concern—and a cottage industry. *Advance for Nurse Practitioners*, 16(8), 53–55.

Guyton, A. C., & Hall, J. (2006). *Textbook of medical physiology* (11th ed.). Philadelphia: W.B. Saunders.

Hemmelgarn, M. H. (2009). Shedding light on vitamin D. *American Journal of Nursing*, 109(4), 19–20.

Ignatavicius, D. D., & Workman, M. L. (2010). *Medical-surgical nursing: Patient-centered collaborative care*. St. Louis: Saunders Elsevier.

Javier, J. (2009). The treatment and prevention of head lice infestation. *Advance for Nurse Practitioners,* Winter, 17(2), 1–8.

Ledezma, B. (2009). Ipilimumab for advanced melanoma: A nursing perspective. *Oncology Nursing Forum*, 36(1), 97–104.

Madariaga, M. G., Naldi, L., Chatenoud, L., Khan, S., Schon, M. P., & Boehncke, W. H. (2005). Psoriasis. *New England Journal of Medicine*, 353, 848–850.

Magin, P., Pond, D., Smith, W., & Watson, A. (2005). A systematic review of the evidence for "myths and misconceptions" in acne management: Diet, face washing and sunlight. *Family Practice*, 22, 62–70.

Murase, J. E., Lee, E. E., & Koo, J. (2005). Effect of ethnicity on the risk of developing nonmelanoma skin cancer following long-term PUVA therapy. *International Journal of Dermatology*, 44, 1016–1021.

Parrish, J. A. (2005). Immunosuppression, skin cancer, and ultraviolet A radiation. *New England Journal of Medicine*, 353, 2712–2713.

Patton, K. T., & Thibodeau, G. A. (2010). *Anatomy and physiology* (7th ed.). St. Louis: Mosby Elsevier.

Porth, C. M., & Matfin, G. (2009). *Pathophysiology: Concepts of altered health states* (8th ed.). Philadelphia: Lippincott Williams & Wilkins.

Poust, J. (2008). Targeting metastatic melanoma. *American Journal of Health-System Pharmacy*, 65, 509–515.

Rollet, J. (2008). Oil crisis: Today's treatment for adolescent acne. *Advance for Nurse Practitioners*, 16(8), 45–48.

Sherman, C. (2008). How to reduce the pain of herpes zoster. *The Clinical Advisor*, September, 11(9), 51–54.

Simandl, G. (2009). Disorders of skin integrity and function. In C. Porth, & G. Matfin, (Eds.). *Pathophysiology: Concepts of altered states* (pp. 1557–1602). Philadelphia: Lippincott Williams & Wilkins.

Stanger, C. B. (2009). Actinic keratosis: Do the numbers add up? *The Nurse Practitioner*, 34(2), 37–39.

Stotts, N. A., & Gunningberg, L. (2007). Predicting pressure ulcer risk: Using the Braden scale with hospitalized older adults: The evidence supports it. *Am J Nursing*, 107(11), 40–47.

Tanghetti, E. A. (2008, September). Managing acne vulgaris: Two important issues. *The Clinical Advisor*, 33–36, 40–43.

Thibodeau, G. A., & Patton, K. T. (2010). *The human body in health and disease* (5th ed.). St. Louis: Mosby Elsevier.

Tielsch-Goddard, A. (2008). Clinical issues of tattooing. *Clinician Reviews*, 18(12), 34–40.

Tofte, S. J. (2008). Atopic dermatitis: Stop the march to allergy and beyond. *Advance for Nurse Practitioners*, 16(9), 41–43, 70.

Homeostasis and the Stress Response

Stress is one of the most cited concepts in biomedical literature. Whether physical, mental, or emotional, stress has the potential to be positive or negative depending on the individual and the situation. From a positive aspect, stress can preserve life, but if left unresolved, maladaption, and even death can occur. The result of stress is dependent on many factors such as type, duration, adaptation, intensity, and coping abilities. The physiologic pathways and pathophysiologic effects of stress can be evaluated objectively and are described in this chapter.

● Physiologic Concepts

DEFINITION OF STRESS

Stress has been defined in many different ways for over 100 years. The modern concept of stress assumes that humans live in a world that has multiple threats (e.g., terrorism) and challenges (e.g., living in a 24-7 world) and that the ever-changing demands of daily life require constant psychological, behavioral, and physiologic adjustment. Thus, stress can be defined as anything that disrupts equilibrium, or any demand that exceeds the body's ability to cope. Stress is a subjective experience that can have negative health consequences.

TYPES OF STRESSORS

Stressors include a wide variety of factors ranging from psychological (e.g., speech anxiety, worry, and mental anguish) and environmental (e.g., natural disasters, socioeconomic status) to physical (e.g., exercise, trauma, and illness) and immunologic (e.g., infection, physical disease). Stressors can be pleasant ("eustress"), as in the case of a wedding or graduation, or unpleasant ("distress"), such as losing a job. They also vary in duration (i.e., acute vs. chronic) and frequency (e.g., daily vs. monthly). Acute stressors are temporary and identifiable. Chronic stressors are long term and may not be as easily identified. Constant exposure to a stressor tends to synthesize the individual to the situation so that the source of the stress may not be as obvious. The low level of stress may become a way of life and negatively impact the health of the individual.

A stressor does not always need to be physically present for a person to experience its negative consequences, as in the case of posttraumatic stress disorder (PTSD). Although they occurred in the past, remembered stressors, such as the events of September 11, 2001 or the death of a spouse, can be traumatic enough to provoke a stress response just from being recalled. While occasional stress exposure can provide stimulation and intellectual challenge, prolonged stress challenges the body's ability to maintain physical and emotional homeostasis and is associated with negative bodily responses.

HOMEOSTASIS

Homeostasis was defined by Walter B. Cannon, a noted American physiologist of the early 20th century, as the maintenance of the physiologic internal environment. Stressors threaten the body's ability to maintain physiologic homeostasis. The body responds to any change in internal conditions with reflexes designed to return itself to the previous state. Homeostasis is usually accomplished by activation of a negative feedback cycle. An initiating stimulus (i.e., the stressor) causes activation of a response, which then directly or indirectly leads to a lessening of the initiating stimulus. This feedback loop allows the body to remain in a dynamic steady state, whereby it continually adjusts to maintain its internal composition and function. Figure 6-1 shows a negative feedback cycle for a physical or mental stressor.

Cannon also noted the role that homeostasis plays in species survival. The fight-or-flight response, proposed in the early 1900s, is a prototypical mammalian stress response in which an organism (such as a human) either fights or flees when faced with a threat (such as a tiger) in order to survive. Thus, stressors trigger a coordinated cascade of biological and behavioral responses that are designed to ensure the safety and well-being of the organism. Under acute conditions, this biobehavioral cascade can be incredibly adaptive in preventing harm. In contrast, continued exposure to stressors and their consequent physiologic end products can result in damage to the body. These biobehavioral cascades are discussed in the following section.

NERVOUS SYSTEM AND HORMONAL RESPONSES TO STRESS

The response to stress involves activation of the sympathetic nervous system (SNS) and the release of various hormones and peptides, including those of

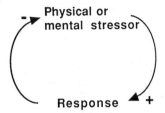

FIGURE 6-1 A stressor causes a response that acts in a negative feed-back manner to reduce the impact of the original stressor.

the hypothalamic–pituitary–adrenal (HPA) axis, the endogenous opioid system, arginine vasopressin (AVP), and oxytocin. The stress response also affects the release of growth and reproductive hormones. These responses prepare the body to cope with or overcome the stressor and are important for the survival and well-being of the organism.

The Sympathetic Nervous System

The fight-or-flight response begins with the activation of the SNS, a branch of the autonomic nervous system (ANS) (Fig. 6-2). Immediately following stressor exposure, the SNS responds with the release of the catecholamines epinephrine and norepinephrine from sympathetic neurons and the adrenal medulla, located in the center of the adrenal glands.

The responses to catecholamines are similar whether they are released from nerves or from the adrenal medulla. However, catecholamines released from the adrenal gland are rapidly metabolized and thus show more limited effects. Effects of the catecholamines include the following:

- Circulating and neurally released norepinephrine binds to receptors identified as alpha1 and alpha2. Binding to alpha1 receptors present on most vascular smooth muscle cells causes the muscle to contract resulting in decreased blood flow to organs supplied by those vascular beds. As a result, sympathetic activation causes a decrease in blood flow to the organs of the gastrointestinal (GI) tract, the skin, and the kidneys. This ensures maximum blood flow to the brain, heart, and skeletal muscles in times of stress. Norepinephrine also binds to receptors on the smooth muscle of the GI tract causing relaxation of the muscle and thereby slowing digestion and GI motility.
- Norepinephrine release causes an increase in plasma glucose levels by increasing the breakdown and release of glucose storage forms in the liver and skeletal muscles, thereby providing the body with a ready supply of energy.
- Norepinephrine released by sympathetic nerves innervating the eye causes dilation of the pupil, preparing the body for any type of attack or surprise.
- Circulating and neurally released epinephrine acts by binding to alpha-receptors and beta-receptors, identified as β_1 and β_2. By binding to β_1 receptors

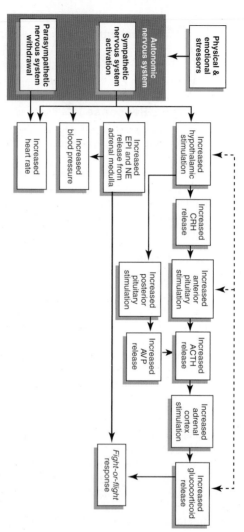

FIGURE 6-2 A simplified representation of the components of the autonomic nervous system (ANS) and hypothalamic–pituitary–adrenal (HPA) axis stress system. CRH, corticotropin-releasing hormone; ACTH, adrenocorticotropic hormone; EPI, epinephrine; NE, norepinephrine; AVP, arginine vasopressin. *Solid lines* represent direct or indirect stimulatory pathways. *Dashed lines* represent direct or indirect inhibitory pathways. (Adapted from Klein, L. C., & Corwin, E. J. (2002). Seeing the unexpected: How sex differences in stress responses may provide a new perspective on the manifestation of psychiatric disorders. *Current Psychiatry Reports*, 4, 441–448.)

on the heart, epinephrine causes an increase in the heart rate and an increase in cardiac contractility, both of which serve to increase the cardiac output during stress.

- Epinephrine binding to β_2 receptors in the liver and skeletal muscle causes an increase in glucose release, resulting in increased glucose available for all cells to use if fight or flight is necessary.

- Epinephrine binding to β_2 receptors present on bronchiolar smooth muscle increases airflow to the lungs by relaxing the muscle, thereby opening up the air passages and facilitating oxygenation of blood for tissues that may be called on during a stressful situation.

The Hypothalamic–Pituitary Hormones

The hypothalamus is the primary structure in the brain responsible for maintaining physiologic homeostasis. It is affected by both physical and psychological stressors. Considered the master endocrine (hormonal) gland of the body, the hypothalamus controls the secretion of several important hormones. The hypothalamus is also connected through a wide neural network to other structures throughout the cerebral cortex and the limbic system. The hypothalamus is the part of the brain that is important in controlling water balance, body temperature, body growth, and hunger (Chapter 9). It is involved in monitoring and responding to feelings of rage, passion, and fear. The hypothalamus also integrates the responses of the sympathetic and parasympathetic systems. Stress affects the hypothalamus and therefore the release of several important hormones and neurotransmitters.

Overview of HPA Axis Activation

SNS activation by stress stimulates the HPA axis (see Fig. 6-2). HPA axis activation begins with the secretion of corticotropin-releasing hormone (CRH) from the paraventricular nucleus of the hypothalamus into the hypothalamic–pituitary portal blood flow system, which in turn stimulates the secretion of adrenocorticotropic hormone (ACTH) from the anterior pituitary, as well as AVP from the posterior pituitary gland. While AVP acts centrally to support the fight-or-flight response, ACTH circulates to the cortex of the adrenal glands to stimulate glucocorticoid release, including release of the corticosteroids (e.g., cortisol, corticosterone). Corticosteroids themselves regulate continued HPA axis function through a negative feedback loop by dampening further CRH release from the hypothalamus and ACTH release from the anterior pituitary gland. Ultimately, these stress hormones mobilize energy stores so that an organism can adapt to the stressor.

Cortisol

Cortisol is the primary corticosteroid associated with stress. It can be measured in blood, urine, feces, and saliva, and has multiple effects on the body, many of which allow an individual to cope with and survive a stressor. The effects of cortisol include the following:

- Stimulates new formation of glucose (gluconeogenesis), which increases the availability of glucose as an energy source in times of immediate need.
- Stimulates the breakdown of stored energy molecules such as fat, protein, and carbohydrate to allow mobilization of energy if immediate fight or flight is required.
- Primes the body to respond to all stressors by promoting sympathetic responses, including those geared toward enhancing cardiac output and maintaining blood pressure.
- Appears to affect the central nervous system. When confronted by a stressor, arousal is initiated and maintained, and the individual becomes cognitively and emotionally equipped to respond.
- Regulates further HPA axis activation through a negative feedback loop by returning CRH release from the hypothalamus and ACTH release from the anterior pituitary gland toward baseline levels (see Fig. 6-2).
- Stimulates gastric acid secretion, which may lead to a breakdown of the gastric mucosa.
- Affects the release of other hypothalamic-releasing factors and hormones. It inhibits the gonadotropin-releasing factors that control ovulation in women and sperm production and testosterone synthesis in men.
- Appears to also stimulate the release of the hypothalamic hormone somatostatin, an inhibitor of growth hormone (GH) release. It is possible that these effects of cortisol contribute to the reproductive dysfunction and growth deficiencies seen in some individuals with long-term stress.
- A high level of cortisol has many effects on the immune and inflammatory reactions, all of which are geared toward reducing inflammation and immune function. For instance, cortisol inhibits the production and release of all white blood cells, blocks B-cell and T-cell functions, and blocks the production of interleukins, which allow for communication among white blood cells. Cortisol reduces white blood cell accumulation at sites of injury or infection, causing a reduction in the usual inflammatory reactions. As a result of its effects on the immune system, elevated levels of cortisol can cause an increased susceptibility to infection and may delay or block healing. Because of these negative effects, it is often wondered why cortisol release is stimulated during states of infection or tissue injury. It may be that a short-term release of cortisol helps to limit damage to tissues caused by inflammation, and it is only with chronic stress that harmful effects of prolonged immunosuppression become obvious.
- Chronic elevations in cortisol levels are associated with destruction of hippocampal neurons, thereby leading to problems in learning, memory, and

attention, as well as the development of psychiatric disorders such as episodes of repeated and severe depression.

The Endogenous Opioid Peptides

Endogenous opioid peptides (EOPs; also called β-endorphins) are derived from proopiomelanocortin (POMC), which is also the precursor for ACTH. Both ACTH and EOPs are released from the anterior pituitary. EOPs may be released directly in response to stress or following stimulation by CRH from the hypothalamus.

EOPs have several physiologic functions, including effects on pain, appetite regulation, and modulation of the stress response through the HPA axis. The functions of EOPs are believed to include the following:

- Reduce the perception and experience of pain (EOPs often have been called the body's "natural morphine"). Prolonged exposure to pain or other stressors, however, can deplete the store of EOPs, leading to increased pain perception and despair.
- May inhibit calcium channels and thus inhibit synaptic transmission of pain impulses.
- Improve mood and increase feelings of well-being.
- May play a role in the rewarding aspects of some drugs of abuse. For example, the U.S. Food and Drug Administration (FDA) has approved the use of naltrexone, a long-acting opioid antagonist (i.e., it blocks the effects of EOPs on the brain), in the treatment of alcoholism to curb alcohol cravings and decrease alcohol intake.
- May play a role in regulating social interactions such that elevations in EOPs seem to be associated with increased social affiliation, at least for women. EOPs also may be involved in psychopathologies of social functioning such as autism.

Arginine Vasopressin (Antidiuretic Hormone)

AVP, also known as antidiuretic hormone (ADH), is a hormone synthesized in separate magnocellular neurons of the supraoptic nuclei, paraventricular nuclei, and accessory nuclei of the hypothalamus. AVP is released from the posterior pituitary gland in response to stress and acts to support the fight-or-flight response by stimulating ACTH release (see Fig. 6-2). AVP is also an important hormone that controls salt and water handling by the kidney, stimulates the sensation of thirst, and is involved in the control of arterial blood pressure (see Chapters 13 and 18). AVP may also play a role in enhancing cognitive functioning, increasing affiliative behavior and motor behavior, and mood disorders such as depression.

Oxytocin

Structurally similar to AVP, oxytocin is also synthesized in the supraoptic nuclei, paraventricular nuclei, and accessory nuclei of the hypothalamus and is released from the posterior pituitary gland in response to stress (Fig. 6-3). Here is where the similarities between AVP and oxytocin appear to end. However, whereas AVP plays a stimulatory role in the HPA axis response to stress, oxytocin appears to dampen the HPA axis response to stress by inhibiting ACTH and, perhaps, CRH release. This stress-dampening effect of oxytocin on the HPA axis has been termed the "tend-and-befriend" response to stress, because elevated oxytocin levels are associated with increased affiliative (friendship-oriented) behavior, which can be particularly adaptive for females in fighting stress. More specifically, the tend-and-befriend response to stress suggests that for females, a more adaptive response to some stressors may not be either fight or flight, but rather the use of social interactions to provide physical and perhaps psychological protection against a stressor. Designed to increase the likelihood of survival when faced with a threat, the tend-and-befriend response promotes safety and diminishes distress through nurturing activities that protect the female and her offspring (i.e., "tending") and creating and maintaining social networks (i.e., "befriending"). Because oxytocin levels are higher in females than in males and the biobehavioral effects of oxytocin are enhanced in the presence of estrogen, oxytocin's stress-reducing effects appear to be more prominent in females. These stress-reducing effects include lowering of blood pressure, perceived stress levels, anxiety, aggression, and depression, and perhaps improved attention and memory.

Growth and Reproductive Hormones

Growth Hormone

GH is released from the anterior pituitary in response to a balance of stimulatory and inhibitory hormones from the hypothalamus. GH release is initially stimulated by stress and results in metabolic responses aimed at conserving energy. With prolonged stressor exposure, the release of GH is inhibited. Inhibition of GH with prolonged stress supports the clinical finding of failure to thrive in children exposed to physical or psychological abuse or neglect.

Reproductive Hormones

The reproductive hormones—estrogen, progesterone, and testosterone—are released primarily from the ovaries or testes in response to stimulation by gonadotropic hormones from the anterior pituitary. The gonadotropic hormones, in turn, are controlled by hormones from the hypothalamus. With prolonged stress, circulating levels of reproductive hormones may decrease,

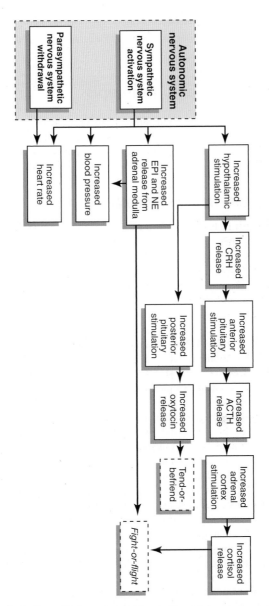

FIGURE 6-3 The role that oxytocin plays in the autonomic nervous system (ANS) and hypothalamic–pituitary–adrenal (HPA) axis stress system. CRH, corticotropin-releasing hormone; ACTH, adrenocorticotropic hormone; EPI, epinephrine; NE, norepinephrine.

leading to reductions in fertility and libido. Similarly, the pituitary hormones prolactin and oxytocin, which are essential for breastfeeding, may be reduced during prolonged stress.

● Pathophysiologic Concepts

The body's response to stress is adaptive in that it helps the organism meet the changing demands of the environment. A stress response that persists beyond the scope and timing of the challenge, however, can become maladaptive and lead to a multitude of negative health consequences.

GENERAL ADAPTATION SYNDROME

Endocrinologist Hans Selye's stress research, spanning a 40-year period, did much to popularize the notion of stress and to bring it to the attention of scientists in many disciplines. In doing so, he stimulated an extensive amount of research on the negative health consequences of stress. In the 1940s, Selye developed the concept of the **general adaptation syndrome (GAS),** a triad of stress responses that were nonspecific, he argued, because they appeared to result from any noxious or aversive event. In other words, Selye believed that all stressors, regardless of type, produced essentially the same pattern of pathophysiologic responding. Whereas Cannon's stress theory of fight or flight emphasized catecholamine secretion, Selye's theory emphasized adrenocortical responses to stress. The three stages of the GAS are alarm, resistance, and exhaustion. Table 6-1 includes a summary of the three stages and associated clinical manifestations.

The **alarm stage** begins with the activation of the reticular activating system, a part of the brain spread diffusely throughout the cerebral hemispheres that controls arousal. During this stage, the body becomes alerted to the presence of the stressor, and the body's defenses are mobilized to fight or flee the stressor (the fight-or-flight response; Fig. 6-2). The fight-or-flight response depends on the release of hormones and the activation of the SNS.

The **resistance stage** includes physical and psychological defenses focused on overcoming the stressor. From the hormonal and neural defenses mobilized during the alarm stage, certain responses are selected that can best cope with that particular stressor. During this phase, **allostasis** may occur. Allostasis achieves stability through change, which is in contrast to homeostasis which achieves stability by opposing change.

The **exhaustion stage** is the final stage of the GAS. This stage develops only if the stressor was not adequately defeated or avoided during the resistance stage. In stage 3, the body's defenses fail and homeostasis cannot be maintained. It is during stage 3 that an individual may show the onset of certain disease states.

TABLE 6-1 Three Stages of the GAS	
Stage	**Description and Clinical Manifestations**
Alarm stage	Exposure to a stressor results in fight-or-flight response
	Resistance is decreased
	Short-term response: from 1 minute up to 24 hours
	Increased secretion of glucocorticoids
	Increased norepinephrine secretion from adrenal medulla
	Increased activity of sympathetic nervous system
	Increased myocardial contractility
	Tachycardia
	Increased blood pressure
	Increased respiratory rate
	Bronchial dilation
	Decreased gastrointestinal motility
	Pupil dilation
	Increased perspiration
	Increased blood clotting
	Increased metabolism
	Decreased renal blood flow
	Increased renin
	Elevated glucose
	Anorexia, nausea, vomiting
	Anxiety
Resistance stage	Adaptation begins to occur
	Glucocorticoid and norepinephrine secretion returns to normal
	Sympathetic activity returns to normal
	Increased resistance
	Resolution of responses that occurred during the alarm phase
Exhaustion stage	Stress is extremely high or long lasting
	Glucocorticoid secretion increases and then decreases drastically
	Stress triad (adrenals hypertrophy, thymus and lymph nodes atrophy, bleeding gastric and duodenal ulcers)
	Loss of resistance and possibly death

Seyle's GAS model has received much criticism for several reasons, including the fact that it does not take into account that one's psychological *appraisal* of events is an important moderator of stress reactivity (e.g., that the event is challenging rather than threatening) and that individual differences exist in one's ability to cope with stress, including personality, perceptions, and biological constitutions. Despite these criticisms, Selye's model is a key theory in the stress field.

● Conditions of Disease

STRESS-RELATED ILLNESSES

Stress may influence the function of several systems and processes of the body, including the immune, cardiovascular, and reproductive systems, and the digestion and metabolism of foodstuffs. The skin may also exhibit signs of stress, and the central nervous system is an integral link in recognizing and responding to all stressors.

Because all parts of the body are affected by exposure to stressors, it is apparent why prolonged or intense physical or psychological stress can lead to changes in every organ or system. Examples of diseases or conditions that have been suggested to be stress related are shown in Box 6-1. How and if any

B O X 6 - 1 **Examples of Stress-Related Disorders**

Heart Disease/Coronary Artery Disease

Irregular heart rate and palpitations
Angina pectoris
Myocardial infarct
Elevated blood markers of coronary artery disease (e.g., elevated LDL and C-reactive protein)

Peripheral or Central Vascular Disorders

Hypertension
Stroke

Respiratory Disorders

Asthma
Hyperventilation
Hay fever

Gastrointestinal Disorders

Anorexia or obesity
Constipation or diarrhea
Gastric ulcer
Inflammatory bowel disease

box continues on page 215

B O X   6 - 1   **Examples of Stress-Related Disorders** (continued)

Endocrine Disorders

Type 2 diabetes mellitus
Amenorrhea

Musculoskeletal Disorders

Headache
Backache
Reduced growth/failure to thrive

Skin Disorders

Psoriasis
Acne
Neurodermatitis

Immune System Disorders

Frequent infections
Thyroid dysfunction
Autoimmune disease exacerbation
Rheumatoid arthritis
Cancer

Reproductive Disorders

Amenorrhea
Impotence
Sterility
Miscarriage

Behavioral Disorders

Dysregulated eating
Drug use (e.g., tobacco smoking, alcohol)
Aggression
Sleeplessness

Psychological Disorders

Fatigue
Anxiety
Depression
Difficulty concentrating/memory problems

one individual is affected by a particular stressor depends on a unique combination of genetics, personality, coping skills, current state of health and nutrition, family and social support systems, and previous experiences. Those in clinical practice see patients whose stress presents in a variety of ways, including GI upsets, headaches, skin outbreaks, hypertension, anxiety, and depression.

Clinical Manifestations

Specific clinical manifestations of the conditions mentioned in Box 6-1 are presented in chapters pertinent to the organ systems involved. Only the general clinical manifestations seen in response to a stressful situation are presented here. Clinical manifestations present during acute stress are different from the clinical manifestations present in response to chronic stress.

Acute stress is associated with:

- Increased heart rate and respiratory rate
- Sweating
- Dilated pupils
- Dry mouth
- A heightened state of awareness

Chronic stress may not be associated with any changes in cardiovascular or respiratory patterns, if local reflexes compensate adequately, although at other times changes may occur, including:

- Blood pressure may increase due to sympathetic stimulation of the cardiovascular system and increased arteriolar resistance.
- The person often appears distracted and distressed, is unable to sleep, and shows difficulty coping with the intense demands of the stressor.
- Family and professional relationships may suffer.

Complications

All the conditions described in Box 6-1 can be complications of stress. In regard to the immune system, high levels of acute stress, and even moderately intense chronic stress, have been associated with an increased susceptibility to viral infections and other illnesses. Besides the direct effects of cortisol on the immune system, studies have found SNS innervation of immune cells in the skin, the Langerhans' cells. This finding offers a mechanism by which neural excitation may alter immune function.

Treatment

Treatment is aimed at reducing the various symptoms of each disease or condition mentioned in Box 6-1. These types of treatments are provided in each pertinent chapter. Perhaps a better therapy is to help the individual with a stress-related condition avoid or remove the stressor or to develop more adaptive coping skills. If the stressor cannot be eliminated, the individual may be advised on how to deal more effectively with it. Therapies to reduce the impact of stressors include:

- If the stressor has a psychological component, the individual is encouraged to talk about his or her concern with family, friends, or a therapist. Studies have shown that having even one person to count on and talk to can reduce the health effects of acute or prolonged stress.

- If the stressor is physical, interventions to reduce pain and prevent infection are essential. Pain and infection are themselves stressors; without interruption or relief, they compound the effects of the original stimulus.

- For physical or psychological stressors, relaxation techniques, biofeedback, and visualization therapy may help the individual reduce the impact the stressor is having on his or her life. Regular exercise is known to increase endorphin release, which may relieve the impact of stressors.

 PEDIATRIC CONSIDERATION

- Intrauterine stress has the potential to result in fetal programming (relationship between events during fetal development and certain disease states later in life). Evidence supports a link between high levels of cortisol in utero and the development of elevated cholesterol, hypertension, and diabetes in adulthood. Examples of common stressors in the pregnant female include maternal malnutrition, smoking, and alcohol ingestion.

 GERIATRIC CONSIDERATIONS

- Possible sources of stress in the older adult may include decreased economic resources, loss of a spouse or close friend, relocation, poor health, or loss of independence.

- Personality, values, and past experiences will impact the older adult's response to stressful situations.

- Symptoms that indicate an older adult is experiencing negative effects of stress may include chronic high anxiety level, chemical use or abuse (alcohol, medications, etc.), jumpiness, chronic complaints, depression, sleep problems, and/or fatigue.

- Complementary and alternative approaches to stress management have been effective in older adults. These may include biofeedback, massage therapy, progressive muscle relaxation, breathing exercises, reading, music, or exercise such as yoga or walking.

SELECTED BIBLIOGRAPHY

Cannon, W. B. (1914). The interrelations of emotions as suggested by recent physiologic researchers. *American Journal of Psychology*, 25, 256–282.

Cannon, W. B. (1932). *The wisdom of the body*. New York: Norton.

Cannon, W. B., Britton, S. W., Lewis, J. T., & Groeneveld, A. (1927). The influence of motion and emotion in medulloadrenal secretion. *American Journal of Physiology*, 79, 433–465.

Cass, H., Gringras, P., March, J., McKendrick, I., O'Hare, A., Owen, L., et al. (2008). Absence of urinary opioid peptides in children with autism. *Archives of Disease in Childhood,* 93(9), 745–750.

Copstead, L. C., & Banasik, J. L. (2010). *Pathophysiology*. St. Louis, MO: Saunders Elsevier.

Corwin, E. J., & Pajer, K. (2008). The psychoneuroimmunology of postpartum depression. *Journal of Women's Health*, 17(9), 1529–1534.

Grillon, C., Duncko, R., Covington, M., Kopperman, L., & Kling, M. (2007). Acute stress potentiates anxiety in humans. *Biological Psychiatry*, 62(10), 1183–1186.

Guyton, A. C., & Hall, J. A. (2006). *Textbook of medical physiology* (11th ed.). Philadelphia, PA: W.B. Saunders.

Klein, L. C., & Corwin, E. J. (2002). Seeing the unexpected: How sex differences in stress responses may provide a new perspective on the manifestation of psychiatric disorders. *Current Psychiatry Reports*, 4, 441–448.

LeMoal, M. (2007). Historical approach and evolution of the stress concept: A personal account. *Psychoneuroendocrinology*, 32, S3–S9.

Mason, J. W. (1975). Emotion as reflected in patterns of endocrine integration. In L. Levi (Ed.). *Emotions: Their parameters and measurement* (pp. 143–181). New York: Raven Press.

Miller, G. E., Chen, E., & Zhou, E. S. (2007). If it goes up, must it come down? Chronic stress and the hypothalamic–pituitary–adrenocortical axis in humans. *Psychological Bulletin*, 133(1), 25–45.

Patton, K. T., & Thibodeau, G. T. (2010). *Anatomy and physiology* (7th ed.). St. Louis, MO: Mosby Elsevier.

Porth, C. M. (2009). *Pathophysiology: Concepts of altered health states* (8th ed.). Philadelphia, PA: Lippincott Williams & Wilkins.

Selye, H. (1946). The general adaptation syndrome and the diseases of adaptation. *Journal of Clinical Endocrinology*, 6, 117–230.

Selye, H. (1955). Stress and disease. *Science*, 122, 625–631.

Selye, H. (1976). *The stress of life*. New York: McGraw-Hill.

Steptoe, A., Hamer, M., & Chida, Y. (2007). The effects of acute psychological stress on circulating inflammatory factors in humans: A review and meta-analysis. *Brain, Behavior and Immunity*, 21(7), 901–912.

Storch, M., Gaab, J., Küttel, Y., Stüssi, A., & Fend, H. (2007). Psychoneuroendocrine effects of resource-activating stress management training. *Health Psychology*, 26(4), 456–463.

Tabloski, P. A. (2010). *Gerontological nursing* (2nd ed.). Upper Saddle River, NJ: Pearson.

Taylor, S. E. (2009). *Health psychology* (7th ed.). New York: McGraw-Hill.

Taylor, S. E., Klein, L. C., Lewis, B. P., Gruenewald, T. L., Gurung, R. A. R., & Updegraff, J. A. (2000). Female responses to stress: Tend-and-befriend, not fight-or-flight. *Psychological Review*, 107, 411–429.

Vincent, H. K., & Taylor, A. G. (2006). Biomarkers and potential mechanisms of obesity-induced oxidant stress in humans. *International Journal of Obesity*, 30, 400–418.

Watson, A. (2010). Stress and adaptation. In K. Osborne, C. Wraa, & A. Watson (Eds.). *Medical-surgical nursing: Preparation for practice* (pp. 214–250). Upper Saddle River, NJ: Pearson.

Wolf, G., Reinhard, M., Cozolino, L., Caldwell, A., & Asamen, J. (2009). Neuropsychiatric symptoms of complex posttraumatic stress disorder: A preliminary Minnesota multiphasic personality inventory scale to identify adult survivors of childhood abuse. *Psychological Trauma: Theory, Research, Practice, and Policy*, 1(1), 49–64.

Neuroendocrine–Immune Interaction

I t is not uncommon to experience health problems after an extremely stressful situation. Recognizing the harmful effects of stress, caregivers intuitively strive to provide a supportive, stress-free environment for patients. The mechanistic explanations for these real-life empirical observations can be found in the anatomic and functional connections between the central nervous system, the endocrine system, and the immune system. This interdisciplinary field of research is referred to as psychoneuroimmunology.

The exact biologic mechanisms that tie the central nervous, endocrine, and immune systems together continue to be clarified. One common stimulus that appears to integrate these systems is stress; the more intransigent aspect of this research may be understanding stress itself. The difficulty in reaching an understanding of stress is related to its subjective and inconsistent nature. For example, common experience has shown that conditions perceived as oppressive by some have no effect on others. Providing the means for a patient to avoid or to escape stress may represent the potential for therapy and for improved care giving.

● Physiologic Concepts

NEUROENDOCRINE CONTROL OF THE IMMUNE SYSTEM

Controlled experiments have shown that conditioned (Pavlovian) immune responses could be induced in animals by pairing the administration of an immunosuppressive drug (cyclophosphamide) with a neutral conditioning stimulus (saccharine in the drinking water). After sufficient paired conditioning, rats given the saccharine alone developed significantly reduced antibody titers when exposed to antigen, compared with unconditioned animals. This indicated a psychological influence on immune function unrelated to an infectious or inflammatory condition, thereby suggesting a neural or an endocrine effect.

An effect on the immune system by neural or endocrine activation has also been shown in controlled human studies. Psychological stress has been associated with the suppression of certain immune parameters. For example, the ability of lymphocytes to respond to mitogens (substances that initiate cell division) was depressed in blood samples taken from students just before oral fellowship exams. Lymphocyte responsiveness returned to normal several weeks after the examinations. Another study focused on the transient immunosuppression associated with chemotherapy. Re-exposure to similar sights and smells associated with chemotherapy administration revealed an immunosuppressive effect in patients even before receiving the next treatment. This further supports the association between the psychological and the physical.

Neuronal Connections to the Immune System

As early as the 1970s, a bidirectional relationship between the neuroendocrine system or the brain and the immune system was being investigated. If immune function is controlled by the brain, then interrupting (lesioning; i.e., cutting or damaging) neuronal pathways should disrupt normal immune function. Experiments have proved this. For example, lesioning the preoptic anterior hypothalamus (the structure that controls body temperature, eating, sleeping, and other vegetative functions) reduces the number of leukocytes in the spleen and thymus, reduces natural killer-cell function, and suppresses antibody production. Lesions to the limbic system (which is involved in emotion and motivation) have the opposite effect on the spleen and thymus. Interestingly, lesions to the cerebral cortex exhibit *lateralized* influences: lesions on one side of the cortex increase T-cell number and function in the spleen and thymus, and lesions on the other side have the opposite effect.

Electron microscopy studies have confirmed that the secondary lymphoid tissues (thymus, spleen, and lymph nodes) are innervated by the autonomic nervous system. In addition, all the elements necessary for synaptic signal transmission have been identified at the interface between nerve terminals and leukocytes in these tissues. Several neurotransmitters have been identified in the neurons innervating lymphoid tissue. Corresponding receptors for these neurotransmitters have been found on leukocytes, and leukocyte function is altered in vitro in response to these substances. As with any synapse, a mechanism needs to be in place to break down the neurotransmitters and thus terminate the individual signal; leukocytes possess appropriate enzymes to

TABLE 7-1	Effects of Neurotransmitters
Neurotransmitter	**Effects**
Substance P	Increased T-cell proliferation
	Increased B-cell antibody synthesis
	Increased cytokine production (including interleukin-1 and tumor necrosis factor)
	Increased reactive oxygen species by monocytes and macrophages
	Increased neutrophil chemotaxis
	Increased phagocytosis
	Increased release of histamine from mast cells
Somatostatin	Inhibited lymphocyte proliferation
	Inhibited antibody production
Norepinephrine	Enhanced lymphocyte proliferation via alpha-adrenergic receptors in low concentrations
	Diminished lymphocyte proliferation via beta-adrenergic receptors in high concentrations
Circulating epinephrine	Mobilization of preformed neutrophils and lymphocytes
	Low-dose simulates monocyte function
	High-dose inhibits monocyte function
Acetylcholine	Inhibited macrophage function

accomplish this. In addition, neurons have cytokine receptors (chemicals released by leukocytes) that make them susceptible to feedback control by leukocytes. And finally, leukocytes themselves make neuropeptides that can presynaptically influence neuronal function and signaling, further emphasizing the feedback loop. Examples of neurotransmitters that bind to immune tissue and their effects are included in Table 7-1.

Cytokine Connections

Another critical linkage between the neuroendocrine and the immune systems involves cytokines, the chemical mediators of inflammation described in Chapter 4. Cytokines may also function as neurotransmitters. They have the capability of stimulating sensory neurons in the viscera or crossing the blood–brain barrier to impact brain and nervous system function. Neuroendocrine signals can influence cytokine synthesis; conversely, cytokines can alter neuronal function and endocrine secretion. Since cytokines control the proliferative, cytotoxic, and synthetic activities of all the different leukocyte populations, neuroendocrine modification of cytokine synthesis or cytokine receptor expression can influence immune function more profoundly than can direct neuroendocrine action on individual leukocytes. Cytokines, in turn, modify neuroendocrine function (such as the hypothalamic–pituitary–adrenal axis) during times of infection or stress.

HYPOTHALAMIC–PITUITARY–ADRENAL AXIS

The effector mechanisms that fight infection (proteolytic enzymes, reactive oxygen species, and membrane-disrupting factors) are very destructive, and if these mechanisms are not controlled, they cause damage to a host's own cells. Cortisol, a hormone released from the adrenal gland, has pervasive immunomodulatory influences that provide this essential control at many levels. Cortisol is released both with stress and as part of the normal feedback control of immunologic and inflammatory processes. High physiologic and pharmacologic concentrations of cortisol keep the immune system under control by:

- Directly inhibiting macrophage phagocytosis, reactive oxygen species generation, and proteolytic enzyme release.
- Indirectly inhibiting reactive oxygen species production, proteolytic enzyme release, and other cytotoxic mechanisms by suppressing the production of the proinflammatory cytokines interleukin-1 and tumor necrosis factor.
- Inhibiting antibody synthesis and lymphocyte proliferation.
- Downregulating expression of substance P receptors.
- Stimulating expression of enzymes that break down substance P and other neuropeptides.
- Stimulating beta-adrenergic receptor expression.

Because of its ability to control so many aspects of inflammation, synthetic preparations of cortisol often are given clinically to reduce inflammation. The connection between infection and stress and the release of cortisol involves a feedback loop between the hypothalamus, the pituitary gland, and the adrenal gland. This cycle is shown in Figure 7-1. Infectious microorganisms or antigens stimulate secretion of interleukin-1 and other cytokines from macrophages. These cytokines travel to the hypothalamus and stimulate the release of corticotropin-releasing hormone (CRH). From here, the normal endocrine circuit begins with successive release of adrenocorticotropic hormone (ACTH) from the pituitary and cortisol secretion by the adrenal cortex. Cortisol then feeds back on the macrophages and inhibits further cytokine release, completing the loop.

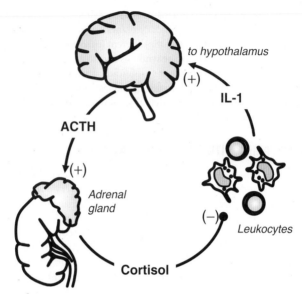

FIGURE 7-1 Hormonal feedback loop involving the hypothalamic–pituitary–adrenal axis.

As such, cortisol is an integral part of a normally functioning immune system. If this cytokine–cortisol loop is disrupted by adrenal cortical insufficiency or the actions of drugs, then exaggerated and damaging inflammatory responses can occur. This endocrine loop is vitally important but relatively slow (taking hours to develop). In contrast, a neural control loop also exists which acts within seconds or minutes.

HYPOTHALAMIC–PITUITARY–GONADAL AXIS

Women have a more responsive immune system than men. Thus, women are more resistant to infections, but they are also more susceptible to autoimmune diseases. Androgens, estrogen, and progesterone all have profound influences on immune function, but only estrogen receptors have actually been found on lymphocyte subpopulations. There is evidence that receptors for the other steroid hormones are located on the thymic epithelium and the bone marrow stromal cells that nurture leukocyte development from stem cell precursors. In addition, progesterone may influence mature leukocytes through glucocorticoid (cortisol) receptors that are expressed on all leukocytes (Fig. 7-2).

Estrogen and progesterone have complicated, concentration-dependent influences on cytokine production. Low concentrations of estrogen stimulate

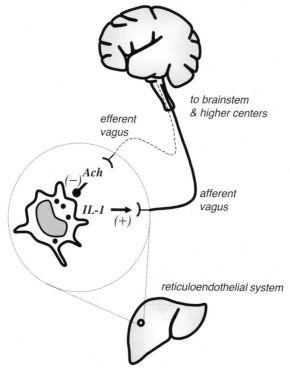

FIGURE 7-2 Reproductive–immune communication.

interleukin-1 production (compared with no estrogen at all). But the increase of concentrations through the normal range—experienced during a menstrual cycle—leads to dose-related inhibition of interleukin-1 secretion. Interleukin-1 synthesis is stimulated in a dose-related manner through the normal menstrual range of progesterone concentrations. However, high concentrations of progesterone, such as those reached during pregnancy, are inhibitory. This inhibitory influence of progesterone on the immune system is considered vital to the development of the immune tolerance that prevents the foreign tissue of the fetus from being rejected.

Although steroid hormones have received the most attention, the pituitary hormones involved in reproduction also have significant influences on immune function. Prolactin appears to have a supportive role in lymphocyte proliferation and can counteract cortisol-mediated inhibition. Stress can decrease circulating prolactin concentrations. Follicle-stimulating hormone may also stimulate interleukin-1 production.

VAGAL INFLAMMATORY REFLEX

The vagus is a cranial nerve containing a combination of afferent sensory fibers and efferent parasympathetic fibers. Its name comes from the Latin word for "wandering," which is appropriate because its branches reach out to the heart, lungs, gastrointestinal tract, liver, spleen, and kidneys. With the exception of the heart, these organs constitute major elements of the reticuloendothelial system; that is, contain particularly high concentrations of phagocytic, macrophage-like cells. The sensory fibers of the vagus can detect interleukin-1 and tumor necrosis factor released locally by the reticuloendothelial cells at the site of infection. This neural information is transmitted to the brainstem, where it stimulates the centers controlling the parasympathetic nervous system (Fig. 7-3). The efferent parasympathetic postganglionic fibers (including the vagus) release acetylcholine (as described in Chapter 8), which binds to nicotinic receptors on macrophages distributed throughout

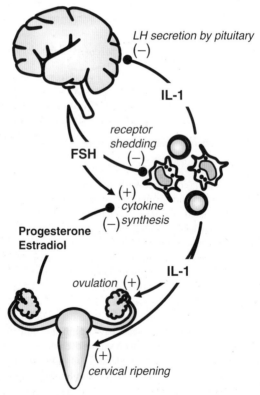

FIGURE 7-3 Neuronal feedback loop involving the vagus nerve.

the reticuloendothelial system. Binding of acetylcholine to the macrophages inhibits the secretion of proinflammatory cytokines, such as interleukin-1 and tumor necrosis factor, but has no influence on anti-inflammatory cytokines, such as interleukin-10. Studies with animals have shown that exaggerated and damaging inflammatory responses can occur if the vagus nerve is severed.

● Pathophysiologic Concepts

HYPORESPONSIVE AND HYPERRESPONSIVE IMMUNE REACTIVITY

A *hyporesponsive* immune system can lead to pathologic conditions because the host is unprotected from infectious microorganisms or tumors. A *hyperresponsive* immune system can be pathologic owing to nonspecific damage to host tissues caused by the overproduction of proteolytic enzymes and reactive oxygen species, or to specific damage to host cells triggered by autoantibodies.

STRESS-RELATED IMMUNOSUPPRESSION

Physiologically and emotionally stressful situations stimulate autonomic, limbic, and, possibly, cerebral cortical inputs to the hypothalamus which lead to the release of CRH and, subsequently, of cortisol. During prolonged or particularly severe stress, chronic elevations of cortisol are suspected of mediating immune dysfunction or, in some cases, immunosuppression. However, this is not at all a straightforward relationship. For example, plasma cortisol concentrations increase during exercise, but exercise also *decreases* the sensitivity of leukocytes to cortisol. Thus, leukocyte inhibition is not an automatic consequence of increases in cortisol concentration. Stress-related immunosuppression is more likely caused by a combination of factors (including, e.g., decreased prolactin concentrations) than strictly by increased cortisol concentrations. It is also noteworthy that the status of the immune system at the time of the stress has an influence as well. In an effort to cope with the stress, the body will upregulate or downregulate in an effort to achieve homeostasis.

AGE-RELATED IMMUNOSUPPRESSION

Aging is associated with an increased risk of cancer and reduced resistance to infectious disease. The critical lymphoid organ for T-cell development—the thymus—involutes (shrinks) with advancing age. This involution is characterized by reduction of the overall size of the thymus and, more importantly, by a proportionally greater loss of functional cells, with the mass replaced by inert fatty tissue. T-cell proliferation, T-killer-cell function, and T-cell enhancement of antibody synthesis all decline as well. These changes parallel age-associated declines in growth hormone. In animals, thymus involution can be reversed by growth hormone treatment (possibly in concert with other pituitary factors). These results raise hopes that hormone replacement therapy for senescent human immune systems can be devised which will improve immune surveillance against tumors and bolster resistance to infectious microorganisms.

IMMUNE ACTIVATION AND REPRODUCTIVE DYSFUNCTION

Increased concentrations of interleukin-1 in the brain can inhibit the luteinizing hormone (LH) surge, and therefore prevent ovulation. This may be an important protective mechanism that prevents conception during periods of infection or illness. On the other hand, recurrent spontaneous abortions have been associated with abnormally high uterine concentrations of cytotoxicity-promoting cytokines such as tumor necrosis factor and interferon-gamma. These cytokines are thought to help drive an inappropriately robust immunologic response that leads to the rejection of the fetus as a foreign intruder.

● Conditions of Disease

AUTOIMMUNE AND HYPERIMMUNE DISEASE

Neuroendocrine influences on the immune system are most drastically represented by diseases that have a strong gender bias or that wax and wane with stressful events. All of the disease conditions identified below are discussed in detail elsewhere in this book. A brief enumeration of them is as follows:

- Asthma (Chapter 14) is a condition of airway hyperresponsiveness characterized by bronchoconstriction (wheezing) caused by mast cell release of histamine into the pulmonary tissues and by a subsequent inflammatory reaction. Although many factors are probably involved in an asthmatic response, inappropriate or exaggerated neuronal release of substance P, which stimulates mast cell degranulation, has been implicated, possibly in conjunction with insufficient production or release of another peptide, vasoactive intestinal peptide (VIP), which inhibits histamine release.

- Crohn disease and ulcerative colitis are inflammatory bowel diseases (Chapter 15). Intestinal biopsies from patients indicate a possible neurogenic component in the inflammatory process such that abnormally high substance P and substance-P receptor concentrations exist and VIP concentrations seem lower than normal. Exacerbations are stress-related.

- Systemic lupus erythematosis (SLE) is an autoimmune inflammatory disease of connective tissue that can include skin rashes, joint pain, and fatigue (Chapter 4). The disease is more common in women than in men by a factor of 10:1. Androgens alleviate symptoms of SLE, and estrogen exacerbates the condition. Symptoms worsen during the luteal phase of the menstrual cycle but are not influenced to any great degree by pregnancy.

- Rheumatoid arthritis (RA) is an autoimmune disorder that results in the destruction of the synovial lining of the joints (Chapter 10). RA is more common in women than in men by a factor of 3:1, but it is relieved during the luteal phase of the menstrual cycle and during pregnancy—the high concentrations of progesterone at these times are thought to inhibit several of the inflammatory processes involved. Many cell types and inflammatory mediators have been implicated in this disease, but some possible neural–cytokine interactions deserve special note. Interleukin-1 and tumor necrosis factor concentrations are high in the synovial fluid of patients who have RA. These cytokines stimulate release of substance P, which in turn stimulates several proinflammatory processes, including increased production of interleukin-1 and tumor necrosis factor. Thus, a destructive positive feedback cycle is established.

Clinical Manifestations

Clinical manifestations of the above disease states are described in the chapters identified. A characteristic finding associated with all of the diseases mentioned above involves periods of remission and exacerbation.

Diagnostic Tools

Mechanisms for diagnosis of the above disease states are described in the chapters identified.

Treatment

A better understanding of the relation between neuroendocrine factors and immune or inflammatory effectors should lead to improved therapies for these and other pathologic conditions.

- Steroid hormone activity can be modulated by receptor antagonists and other drugs.
- Neuropeptide release can be influenced pharmacologically as well as behaviorally by avoidance of exposure to stressors or, when exposure is unavoidable, by adoption of relaxation techniques and coping strategies. For example, people are able to use biofeedback to lower their heart rate (through increased efferent vagal signals to the heart). Perhaps biofeedback can also be used to increase vagal anti-inflammatory signaling to the reticuloendothelial system.
- Antibodies and soluble receptors against tumor necrosis factor and receptor antagonists against interleukin-1 have been used clinically to reduce the rate of tissue destruction and relieve signs and symptoms of RA, but these treatments can also increase risks for serious infection. It can be difficult

to determine an optimal anticytokine dose that diminishes inappropriate destruction without seriously compromising host defense. Careful screening of patients for concurrent infection or use of immunosuppressive drugs including glucocorticoids seems necessary.

- Alternative therapies such as a back massage and hand holding have been shown to enhance contentment and increase relaxation, which may increase the protective function of the immune system and enhance healing.

SELECTED BIBLIOGRAPHY

Ader, R., Felton, D. L., & Cohen, N. (Eds.). (1991). *Psychoneuroimmunology* (2nd ed.). San Diego: Academic Press.

Briones, T. L. (2007). Psychoneuroimmunology and related mechanisms in understanding health disparities in vulnerable populations. *Annual Review of Nursing Research*, 25, 219–256.

Dantzer, R. (2005). Somatization: A psychoneuroimmune perspective. *Psychoneuroendocrinology*, 30, 947–952.

Dimitrov, S., Lange, T., Fehm, H. L., & Born, J. (2004). A regulatory role of prolactin, growth hormone, and corticosteroids for human T-cell production of cytokines. *Brain, Behavior, and Immunity*, 18, 368–374.

Huether, S., & McCance, K. (2008). *Understanding pathophysiology* (4th ed.). St. Louis: Mosby Elsevier.

Jordan, S. (2008). An overview of the immune system. *Nursing Standard*, 23(15–17), 47–56.

Langley, P., Fonseca, J., & Iphofen, R. (2006). Psychoneuroimmunology and health from a nursing perspective. *British Journal of Nursing*, 15(20), 1126–1129.

McCain, N., Gray, D., Walter, J., & Robins, J. (2005). Implementing a comprehensive approach to the study of health dynamics using the psychoneuroimmunology paradigm. *Advances in Nursing Science*, 28(4), 320–332.

Tsigos, C., & Chrousos, G. P. (2002). Hypothalamic-pituitary-adrenal axis, neuroendocrine factors and stress. *Journal of Psychosomatic Research*, 53, 865–871.

Integrated Control and Dysfunction

The Nervous System

The nervous and endocrine systems are the means by which different parts of the body communicate. The nervous system can be separated into the central nervous system (CNS), consisting of the nerve pathways of the brain and spinal cord, and the peripheral nervous system, consisting of nerves that innervate the rest of the body. The nervous system is the body's communication network and it functions to organize and coordinate all of the other body systems.

● Physiologic Concepts

THE NEURON

The neuron, also called a *nerve cell,* is the functional unit of the nervous system and is a highly specialized cell. Neural maturation occurs before or soon after birth. Although it was once believed that neurons did not undergo cellular reproduction and could not be replaced, new evidence is indicating that new neurons may be produced, but the functional significance is still unknown. Neurons generate and conduct electrical impulses and receive incoming stimuli from, and send outgoing stimuli to, other nerves, muscles, or glands. Neurons pass and receive signals through changes in the flow of electrically charged ions back and forth across the cell membrane.

Parts of the Neuron

Most neurons have four parts: the dendrite, an afferent end that receives incoming signals; the cell body, a central area containing the nucleus; the axon, a long efferent extension on which the signal passes; and the axon terminals, which branch off of the axon and deliver the signal to other cells. The axon and dendrite are referred to as nerve fibers. A typical neuron is shown in Figure 8-1.

Dendrite

A dendrite is a neural threadlike extension from the cell body that carries impulses to the cell body. The dendrite is the part of the neuron that receives stimulation from other nerves and is the main source of information. Each neuron may have many dendritic branches. Excitation of a neuron typically begins at the dendrite. The dendrite passes its excitation on to the adjacent segment, the cell body.

Cell Body

The cell body is responsible for high levels of metabolic activity because it must synthesize the cytoplasmic and membrane components necessary to maintain function of the axon and its numerous terminals. The cell body contains the typical organelles of a human cell. The nucleus, which contains the genetic information of the neuron, orchestrates the production of the proteins, enzymes, and neurotransmitters required by the nerve for its proper function. The cell body delivers these substances as needed to the rest of the neuron. Although neural excitation typically begins with the excitation of the dendrites, a cell body sometimes may be stimulated directly by incoming stimuli from other neurons and by chemical and electrical stimuli. The cell body delivers the electrical signal to the next segment, the axon.

Axon

Projecting from the cell body is the axon, the beginning of which is called the *initial segment* or trigger zone. The axon is a long fiber on which passes the electrical signal initiated in the dendrites and cell body. The axon transmits the original signal to another neuron or to a muscle or gland. Branching off the main stem of the axon may be multiple collateral fibers. Collateral fibers convey information to many other interconnected nerve cells, increasing the influence of the neuron throughout the nervous system. Down the length of the axon, contractile proteins and microtubules transport substances produced in the cell body.

In some nerves, the axons are covered by an insulating, protective, lipid sheath, called **myelin**. Myelin is produced when support cells wrap their plasma membranes around an axon. In the peripheral nervous system, the support cells are the *Schwann cells*. In the CNS, myelin is produced by a specialized type of cell, the *oligodendrocytes*. Myelin increases the velocity with which an

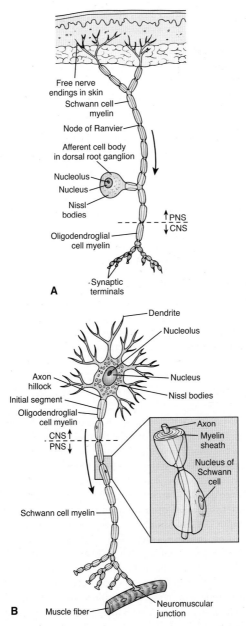

Free nerve
endings in skin

Schwann cell
myelin

Node of Ranvier

Afferent cell body
in dorsal root ganglion

Nucleolus

Nucleus

Nissl
bodies

Oligodendroglial
cell myelin

PNS
CNS

Synaptic
terminals

A

Dendrite

Nucleolus

Axon
hillock

Initial segment

Oligodendroglial
cell myelin

CNS
PNS

Axon

Myelin
sheath

Nucleus of
Schwann
cell

Schwann cell myelin

B   Muscle fiber

Neuromuscular
junction

Nucleus

Nissl bodies

FIGURE 8-1 The neuron. (From Porth, C. [2007]. *Essentials of Pathophysiology* [2nd ed.]. Philadelphia: Lippincott Williams & Wilkins.)

electrical signal is transmitted down an axon, as described later. Gaps in the myelinated axons, referred to as nodes of Ranvier, play a vital role in impulse conduction.

Axon Terminals

At the end of each main axon stem and collateral, the branching becomes extensive. These final divisions of the axon are called axon terminals. The synaptic knob or terminal knob is the enlarged distal end of each axon. The manufacturing, storage, and release of transmitter substances occur in the knob. It is through axon terminals that an electrical signal is passed to the dendrites or the cell body of a second neuron. In the peripheral nervous system, the signal may also pass to a muscle or glandular cell.

Categories of Neurons

Neurons that carry information from the periphery to the CNS are called sensory or **afferent neurons**. These neurons are the only type of nerve cell that do not have dendrites, but possess receptors on their distal ends that sense physical or chemical stimuli. Neurons that carry information out of the CNS to various target organs (muscle cells, other nerves, or glands) are called motor or **efferent neurons**. A third group of neurons passes messages between afferent and efferent neurons. These neurons are called **interneurons.** Almost 99% of all neurons in the body are interneurons, and all interneurons are in the CNS.

The Synapse

A synapse is the point of junction between two neurons. The synapse is made up of the knob, the synaptic cleft, and the portion of the cell receiving the impulse. Neurons communicate with each other by releasing chemicals into the small cleft (synaptic cleft) separating one from the other. The chemical released from a particular neuron is called a neurotransmitter. Transmitters have the ability to enhance or inhibit an impulse, but are unable to do both. Usually, a neurotransmitter is released from the axon terminal of one neuron, diffuses across the synaptic cleft, and binds to a receptor on the dendrite or cell body of the other neuron. However, a synapse can occur between two dendrites, between dendrites and a different cell body, or between an axon and an axon terminal. The cell that releases the neurotransmitter is called the **presynaptic neuron**. The neuron that completes the synapse is called the **postsynaptic neuron**. One postsynaptic neuron may receive input from thousands of presynaptic neurons. The postsynaptic neuron integrates and responds to the many signals influencing it. A synapse with two presynaptic neurons is shown diagrammatically in Figure 8-2.

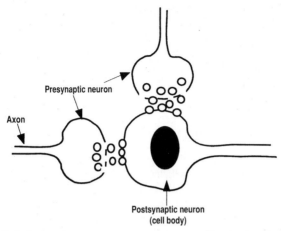

FIGURE 8-2 At a synapse, a presynaptic neuron releases chemicals that diffuse across the synaptic cleft and bind to a postsynaptic cell.

Neurotransmitters and Neuromodulators

Many neurotransmitters are used in the nervous system. Most neurotransmitters are synthesized in the cell body and transported down the axon to the axon terminal. Because neurotransmitters are released from presynaptic neurons, synaptic transmission usually occurs in one direction: from the presynaptic to the postsynaptic neuron. Neurotransmitters act rapidly to affect the postsynaptic neuron. To respond to a particular neurotransmitter, the postsynaptic cell must have specific receptors for it on its cell membrane.

Most neurons release one neurotransmitter, although some neurons may also release a cotransmitter. Frequently, cotransmitters, called neuromodulators, are a slightly different type of chemical than the neurotransmitter. Neuromodulators typically take longer to act than neurotransmitters, and may function to increase or decrease DNA transcription and protein synthesis. Neuromodulators often affect the response of a postsynaptic cell to a neurotransmitter, and are associated with long-term functions such as learning, mood, and development.

Examples of neurotransmitters and neuromodulators include the following: monoamines—norepinephrine, serotonin, dopamine, and histamine; amino acids—gamma-aminobutyric acid (GABA), glycine, glutamate, and aspartate; acetylcholine; and the neuropeptides, including the endorphins, enkephalins, substance P, vasoactive intestinal peptide (VIP), and adenosine triphosphate (ATP). Even some gases may serve as neurotransmitters, including nitric oxide and carbon dioxide (CO_2). Gases do not bind to postsynaptic receptors, but diffuse into the postsynaptic cell to exert an action.

A few neurotransmitters (e.g., acetylcholine and norepinephrine) can either excite or inhibit a postsynaptic cell. Often, however, a neurotransmitter has the same effect (excitatory or inhibitory) on all cells to which it binds. Examples of inhibitory neurotransmitters include GABA, glycine, nitric oxide, and usually dopamine. Glutamine is an example of an excitatory neurotransmitter. The neurotransmitters mentioned earlier may function in the CNS or the peripheral nervous system.

THE MEMBRANE POTENTIAL

The separation of the electrical charge across any structure sets up an electrical potential. Nerve cells, like all cells, have a separation of electrical charge across their cell membranes. The inside of the cell is negatively polarized (charged) compared to the outside, which is positively polarized. The difference in the electrical charge across the plasma membrane is called the membrane potential.

The membrane potential results from a balance between the concentration and electrical gradients that exist across the cell membrane and drive the movement of ions. These gradients unequally distribute electrically charged ions inside and outside the cell, setting up a membrane potential.

The Concentration Gradient Across the Cell Membrane

A concentration gradient exists across all cell membranes because the sodium–potassium pump transports three positively charged sodium ions out of the cell for every two positively charged potassium ions it pumps in. The separation of ions is shown in Figure 8-3. This sets up a concentration gradient with potassium in higher concentration inside the cell than outside, while sodium is in higher concentration outside the cell than inside (Chapter 1). Because potassium and sodium can readily move across the membrane, both tend to diffuse down their concentration gradients—potassium diffuses out of the cell,

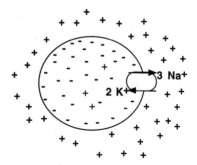

FIGURE 8-3 Excess positive charge on the outside of the membrane compared to the inside contributes to the membrane potential.

and sodium diffuses into the cell. The cell membrane is over 50 times more permeable to potassium than to sodium. Therefore, more positive charge moves out of the cell than comes in, making the inside of the cell negative.

The Electrical Gradient Across the Cell Membrane

Opposing the concentration gradient is an electrical gradient set up by potassium and sodium diffusion, and by the accumulation of negatively charged proteins inside the cell. Because the inside of the cell is negatively charged, potassium, sodium, and other positively charged ions are drawn inside the cell, whereas negatively charged ions such as chloride tend to leave the cell. This sets up an electrical gradient across each cell.

Net Result of Concentration and Electrical Gradients

The final balance reached between the electrical gradient and the concentration gradient across a resting cell is called the **resting membrane potential**. For any given cell, the resting membrane potential may range from 5 to 100 millivolts (mV), with the inside negative relative to the outside.

Changes in the Membrane Potential of Nerve and Muscle Cells

Cell membranes of neurons and muscles are unique because their permeability to sodium, potassium, chloride, and sometimes calcium can be changed by electrical or chemical stimulation. This allows the membrane potential of neurons and muscle cells to vary from the resting potential.

For neurons at rest, the membrane potential is approximately −70 mV (inside negative). If the inside of the cell becomes less negative, the cell is said to have become **depolarized**. If the cell becomes more negative inside, the cell is said to have become **hyperpolarized**. When the cell returns to its resting membrane potential, it is said to be **repolarized**. Changes in the cell membrane potential of a nerve cell may cause a local change in electrical current, called a graded potential, or may cause a large, propagated change in electrical current, called an action potential. It is through graded potentials and action potentials that the nervous system sends and receives signals.

GRADED POTENTIALS

A graded potential is an electrical potential that can vary in amplitude and duration. There are many examples of graded potentials in neurophysiology, including the synaptic potential, the receptor potential, and the muscle end-plate potential (EPP) (discussed in Chapter 10). Graded potentials are usually produced at a small site on the neuron (synapse, receptor, muscle end-plate) and die out as their charge spreads. Graded potentials are produced by chemical or electrical stimuli, and may be excitatory (depolarizing) or inhibitory (hyperpolarizing). If they are highly excitatory, they may cause an adjacent area of the neuron to depolarize and fire an action potential.

Synaptic Potentials

When a neurotransmitter is released from a presynaptic neuron and binds to a postsynaptic neuron, it will electrically excite (depolarize) or inhibit (hyperpolarize) the postsynaptic cell. If the neurotransmitter depolarizes the postsynaptic cell (makes it more positive inside), the synaptic signal is called an **excitatory presynaptic potential** (EPSP). EPSPs occur if the neurotransmitter opens channels that allow the passage of positive ions, such as sodium or potassium, into the postsynaptic cell. If the binding of the neurotransmitter to the postsynaptic neuron hyperpolarizes the postsynaptic cell (makes it more negative inside), the synaptic signal is called an **inhibitory postsynaptic potential** (IPSP). IPSPs occur if the transmitter opens channels that allow the passage of negative ions, usually chloride, inside the postsynaptic cell. Of the thousands of incoming signals on a postsynaptic neuron, some will be excitatory and others will be inhibitory. The electrical potential generated in the postsynaptic membrane varies in size, depending on the summation between the IPSPs and EPSPs received, and the amount of neurotransmitter released from each presynaptic cell.

If at the postsynaptic cell, the summation of all EPSPs and IPSPs results in significant excitation of the postsynaptic dendrite or cell body, the electrical excitation will be passed on to the postsynaptic cell through the activation of an action potential. If the summation of EPSPs and IPSPs is inhibitory, the postsynaptic cell will not create an action potential.

Muscle End-Plate Potential

The resting membrane potential of a muscle cell is approximately -90 mV. Stimulation by a motor neuron always causes depolarization at the site where the motor neuron synapses on the muscle cell, called the motor end plate. This depolarization is called an EPP. The EPP is a graded potential that spreads locally through the muscle fiber and usually causes contraction of the muscle. One motor neuron typically innervates many muscle fibers. One motor neuron and the fibers it innervates are called a **motor unit**.

Receptor Potential

A receptor potential is the electrical potential produced at the distal end of an afferent neuron after electrical or chemical stimulation.

Specialized cells in sensory organs produce receptor potentials that activate neurons in response to touch, sight, sound, smell, or taste.

A receptor potential is a graded potential; it varies in amplitude and duration and spreads through local current flow. When the receptor potential reaches the cell body, if it is large enough to cause the cell body to depolarize to threshold, the neuron will reach threshold and fire an action potential.

THE ACTION POTENTIAL

An action potential is a rapid ch
or muscle cell. An action potential
to cause the cell's voltage-sensitive
brane, to burst open. Once the gat
The incoming rush of sodium ions
become more positive, reaching appr
cell becomes more positive, the sodiu
the potassium gates, also affected by the
allowing potassium ions to rush out o
causes the cell to again become negative
cells, the action potential also opens calci

The action potential is an active, trans _____atic cell depolarization. Action potentials are different from _____u potentials in that they do
not vary in amplitude or duration. Instead, action potentials are considered
"all or none": if the electrical or chemical stimulus, or the EPSP, is great enough
to open enough voltage-dependent sodium channels to sufficiently depolarize
the membrane, the action potential will occur. If the stimulus is insufficient to
cause a certain level of depolarization, the action potential will not occur. The
level of depolarization at which a neuron fires an action potential is called the
threshold potential. In muscles, it takes one EPP to cause the muscle cell to
reach a threshold and contract. In nerves, it may take many EPSPs to cause the
nerve to reach threshold.

Spread of an Action Potential

When a nerve fiber reaches threshold and fires an action potential, the action
potential is propagated at an equal velocity and voltage along the entire length
of the axon, to the axon terminals. Propagation of the action potential occurs
because neighboring sites on the axon are affected by the change in current
generated by the original action potential. The change in current produced by
an action potential will be great enough to cause depolarization at a neighboring site on the neuron, and the action potential will be repeated. As the action
potential passes down the axon, the part of the axon that has just fired will be
refractory for a period of time until the membrane potential returns to the
resting level. Propagation of an action potential compared to the local spread
of a graded potential is shown in Figure 8-4.

The speed at which an action potential passes along a nerve fiber depends
on the diameter of the fiber and whether the fiber is covered by myelin. Because
large fibers present less resistance to the flow of current than small fibers, large
fibers transmit action potentials faster than small fibers. Fibers coated with
myelin pass action potentials faster than uncoated fibers because the myelin
acts as insulation to prevent the current from leaking out across the membrane.

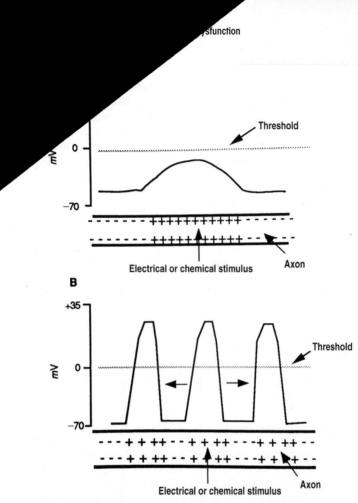

FIGURE 8-4 A graded potential **(A)** does not reach threshold and passes only a short distance on the membrane and dies out. An action potential **(B)** fires when depolarization reaches threshold and is repeated along the entire length of the axon. A neuron is capable of propagating an action potential in both directions, although in vivo an action potential starts at one end and travels in one direction.

This allows the action potential to spread by jumps down the axon in a process called **saltatory conduction**, rather than step by step. As shown in Figure 8-5, the areas where myelin is absent on the axon, called the nodes of Ranvier, contain a large density of sodium channels that open in response to the spread of current and quickly depolarize to threshold, propagating the signal with great speed. Without myelin covering, the current must depolarize each adjacent area of the axon, a process that slows neural transmission considerably.

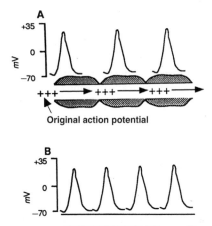

FIGURE 8-5 Propagation in myelinated fiber **(A)** compared to an unmyelinated fiber **(B)**. Action potentials pass by rapid saltatory conduction in myelinated fibers.

Synaptic Transmission of an Action Potential

Once an action potential reaches the axon terminal, it causes the opening of voltage-gated calcium channels. Although what happens next is not completely understood, it appears that when calcium ions enter into the presynaptic terminal, the ions bind to sites, called "release sites," on the inside of the surface of the presynaptic membrane. Binding at the release sites causes them to open, allowing that nerve's neurotransmitter to be discharged into the synaptic cleft. The neurotransmitter is packaged inside vesicles in the presynaptic terminal, each containing a few to several thousand molecules of neurotransmitter. The more calcium that enters the presynaptic terminal, the greater the number of vesicles that open to release their neurotransmitter. Discharge of a single presynaptic terminal is not generally enough to depolarize to threshold a postsynaptic cell—multiple EPSPs from multiple presynaptic neurons are usually required. If there are enough EPSPs, the postsynaptic neuron will depolarize and fire its own action potential. If there are not enough EPSPs, the summation of incoming signals on the postsynaptic neuron will not be enough to cause depolarization to threshold, and the signal will not pass on to the next neuron in the chain.

Summary of Synaptic Transmission

When an action potential reaches the synaptic knob, calcium channels are opened, causing the release of neurotransmitters across the synaptic cleft.

Neurotransmitters bind to receptors in the postsynaptic membrane causing certain ion channels to open.

When sodium and potassium channels open, sodium moves into the cell faster than potassium moves out causing the inside of the postsynaptic membrane to be more positively charged. This depolarization is the EPSP. An action potential is initiated if the EPSP reaches the threshold potential.

When potassium and chloride channels open, the outward flow of potassium and/or the inward flow of chloride result in a more negative postsynaptic membrane. This hyperpolarization is the IPSP. Initiation of the action potential is inhibited because the postsynaptic membrane is less likely to reach the threshold potential.

THE CENTRAL NERVOUS SYSTEM

The brain is a large mass of neural tissue located in the cranium (skull). It is one of the largest organs in the body and weighs about 1.4 kg. Neurons of the brain grow in size, but not in number after the first few months of postnatal life. The brain is composed of neurons and the supporting neuroglial cells. The brain is where reflexes are integrated to maintain the internal environment. It is also the source of several hormones and the site of integration of all sensory information. The brain receives approximately 15% of the cardiac output. Brain cells require glucose for energy metabolism and production of ATP. Figure 8-6 shows the CNS divided into the forebrain, midbrain, hindbrain, and spinal cord. The midbrain and hindbrain make up the brainstem. The cerebellum is described separately.

The Forebrain

The forebrain includes the diencephalon, which is located in the core of the brain, and the telencephalon, which forms the left and right cerebral hemispheres. The outer shell of the cerebral hemispheres is called the cerebral cortex. The cerebral hemispheres are connected together across a longitudinal fissure by axon bundles, one of which is the corpus callosum. The diencephalon includes the epithalamus, thalamus, subthalamus, and hypothalamus.

The Cerebral Cortex

The cerebral cortex is organized horizontally by function and divided vertically into layers. The vertical layers are clearly delineated and repeated throughout the cortex. The cerebral cortex is the most advanced part of the brain and is responsible for making sense of the environment and initiating thought and goal-oriented behavior. The cortex is called the gray matter because of the preponderance of neural cell bodies as opposed to neuronal axons, which tend to appear white. Different sections of the cerebral cortex, called lobes, perform different functions. Some parts of the cerebral cortex function as primary

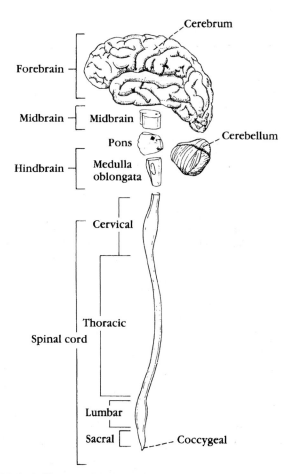

FIGURE 8-6 The central nervous system.

sensory areas and directly receive incoming sensory stimuli. These areas are bordered by secondary sensory areas that help interpret sensory stimuli. Other association areas receive information from primary and secondary sensory areas, and from other sites in the cortical and subcortical brain. Association areas allow for complex movements, interpretation and production of language, and appropriate response to friends, enemies, and strangers. The lobes of the cortex are shown in Figure 8-7.

The Frontal Lobe.
The frontal lobe includes the part of the cerebral cortex forward from the central sulcus (fissure or furrow) and above the lateral sulcus. It contains the motor

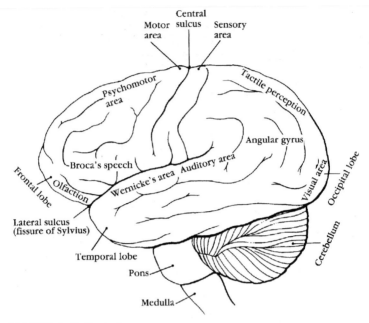

FIGURE 8-7 The brain.

and premotor areas. Broca's area is in the left frontal lobe and controls the production (or articulation) of speech. Many association areas in the frontal lobe receive information from throughout the brain and incorporate that information into thoughts, plans, and behavior. The frontal lobe is responsible for goal-oriented behavior, moral decision making, and complex thought such as reasoning, concentration, and abstraction. The frontal lobe also modifies (limits) emotional surges produced in the limbic system and the vegetative reflexes of the brainstem. Other functions include voluntary eye movement, recall of past experiences, and access to current sensory data.

Cell bodies in the primary motor area of the frontal lobe send axon projections to the spinal cord, most of which travel in pathways belonging to what is described as the corticospinal tract. In the corticospinal tract, motor neurons switch sides: motor information from the left side of the cerebral cortex passes down the right side of the spinal cord and controls motor movements of the right side of the body, and vice versa. Other axons from the motor area travel in extrapyramidal pathways. These fibers control fine motor movement and run outside the corticospinal tract to the spinal cord.

The Parietal Lobe.
The parietal lobe is the area of the cortex located behind the central sulcus, above the lateral fissure, and extending back to the parieto-occipital fissure.

The parietal lobe receives sensory input for touch and pain. Cells of the parietal lobe act as secondary association areas to interpret incoming stimuli. The parietal lobe passes sensory information such as taste and texture to many other areas of the brain, including the neighboring motor and visual association areas. The parietal lobe is responsible for understanding spatial relationships and perceptions, processing nonverbal stimuli, and plays a role in musical ability. Another vital function of the parietal lobe is filtering of extraneous noise and sensations.

The Occipital Lobe.
The occipital lobe is the posterior lobe of the cerebral cortex. It lies posterior to the parietal lobe and above the parieto-occipital fissure, separating it from the cerebellum. This lobe contains the visual cortex and the visual association areas. The occipital lobe receives information that originated as signals in the retina of the eye.

The Temporal Lobe.
The temporal lobe includes the part of the cerebral cortex extending down from the lateral fissure and back to the parieto-occipital fissure. The temporal lobe is the primary association area for auditory information and includes Wernicke's area, where language is interpreted. It is also involved in the interpretation of smell and is important for the formation and storage of memory. The temporal lobe is also responsible for integrating and interpreting information to garner socially appropriate responses. The hippocampus is part of the temporal lobe and is discussed later in the chapter.

The Diencephalon

The diencephalon structures lie deep between the cerebral hemispheres. The diencephalon includes the thalamus, the hypothalamus, and the basal ganglia.

The Thalamus.
The thalamus lies on either side of the third ventricle and receives all incoming sensory information (except smell) and in turn relays the information through numerous afferent tracts to the rest of the cerebral cortex. Descending fibers from the cerebral cortex also travel down to the thalamus. Function of the cerebral cortex depends on thalamic relay. The thalamus is part of the reticular activating system (RAS), an extensive group of neurons essential in arousal of the individual. The thalamus receives pain information and relays it to the cerebral cortex.

The Hypothalamus.
The hypothalamus makes up the base of the diencephalons and lies inferior to the thalamus. It is an important endocrine and neural organ responsible for maintaining homeostasis. The hypothalamus integrates and directs information concerning temperature, hunger, blood gas concentration, autonomic nervous system activity, and emotional status. It also regulates the levels of several hormones, including the pituitary hormones (Chapter 9).

The Basal Ganglia.

The basal ganglia are islands of gray matter lying deep in the diencephalon on either side of the thalamus and upper midbrain that process and influence information in the extrapyramidal nerve tracts. The basal ganglia are important for controlling highly skilled movements that require patterns and quickness of response without intentional thought. The precision of a baseball player and the grace of a ballerina require significant basal ganglia control.

The basal ganglia are composed of several structures that can be anatomically or physiologically separated, including the caudate nucleus, the putamen, and the globus pallidus. The basal ganglia are intimately associated with the substantia nigra and the subthalamic and red nuclei. Virtually all projections to and from the basal ganglia go through the thalamus. Lesions of the basal ganglia cause repetitive movements, grimaces, and tremors, as seen with Huntington disease (chorea) and Parkinson disease.

The Limbic System

The limbic system is a diffuse grouping of neurons from different areas of the brain. Neurons in the limbic system include fibers from all lobes of the forebrain and extensive connections from the hypothalamus and thalamus. Midbrain and hindbrain areas also send projections that contribute to the limbic system.

The hippocampus is considered part of the limbic system and plays an important role in coding and consolidating memories. Sensory information stimulates the hippocampus, which then sends information to other areas of the limbic system. The hippocampus organizes input in preparation for memory storage and plays a vital role in the transfer of information from short-term memory to long-term memory. Atrophy of the hippocampus has been associated with memory problems such as Alzheimer disease.

The amygdala, also considered part of the limbic system, is involved in the production of emotions, aggression, and sexual behavior. It helps with the interpretation of the surrounding environment to produce appropriate behavior. Learning and behavior are also influenced by several limbic system structures and connections.

The Brainstem

The brainstem, or stalk of the brain, performs sensory, motor, and reflex functions and is made up of the medulla oblongata, pons, and mesencephalon (midbrain). Many reflex centers are located in the medulla including the cardiac, vasomotor, and respiratory centers. The vomiting, coughing, sneezing, hiccupping, and swallowing centers are also located in the medulla. The pons contains the pneumotaxic centers that facilitate respiratory regulation. It is the reflex center for cranial nerves (CNs) six through eight and mediates mastication, saliva secretion, equilibrium, and hearing. The medulla has the cardiac-slowing center and the pons has the cardiac acceleration and vasoconstriction centers. The midbrain is responsible for pupillary reflexes and eye movements. It also contains the periaqueductal gray that may abolish pain when stimulated.

Neurons pass through the brainstem and carry motor information to and from the cerebral cortex, controlling equilibrium. Ten of the twelve CNs, controlling motor and sensory function of the eyes, face, tongue, and neck, leave from the brainstem. The secretory and motor functions of the gastrointestinal tract and the sensory functions of hearing and taste also are controlled by the CNs.

Cranial Nerves

Twelve CNs emerge from the undersurface of the brain and are identified by name and number. The name is associated with their area of distribution and the number indicates brain connection from anterior to posterior. Table 8-1 includes the name, number, innervation, and function of each CN.

TABLE 8-1 Cranial Nerves

Number and Name	Impulse Conduction	Function
CN I Olfactory	Nose to brain	Sensory: smell
CN II Optic	Eye to brain	Sensory: vision
CN III Oculomotor	Brain to eye muscles	Motor: eye movements, blink reflex, pupillary constriction, accommodation, eye and lid movement, somesthesia
CN IV Trochlear	Brain to external eye muscles	Motor: downward and inward eye movement
CN V Trigeminal	Teeth, skin, and mucus membranes of head to brain; brain to chewing muscles	Sensory and motor: Face, scalp and teeth sensation; Mastication
CN VI Abducens	Brain to external eye muscles	Motor: lateral eye deviation
CN VII Facial	Taste buds of tongue to brain; brain to face muscles	Sensory and motor: gustation, contraction of facial expression muscles
CN VIII Vestibulocochlear	Ear to brain	Sensory: hearing, sense of balance
CN IX Glossopharyngeal	Throat and tongue taste buds to brain; brain to throat muscles and salivary glands	Sensory and motor: throat sensations, taste, swallowing, salivary secretion

table continues on page 250

TABLE 8-1 Cranial Nerves (*continued*)

Number and Name	Impulse Conduction	Function
CN X Vagus	Throat, larynx, thoracic organs, and abdominal cavity organs to brain; brain to throat muscles, thoracic and abdominal cavity organs	Sensory and motor: throat, larynx, thoracic and abdominal cavity organs; swallowing, voice production, slowing of heart rate, acceleration of peristalsis in the gut
CN XI Accessory	Brain to certain shoulder and neck muscles	Motor: shoulder movements; head turning
CN XII Hypoglossal	Brain to tongue muscles	Motor: tongue movements

Reticular Formation

Running through the brainstem is a network of many small, branched neurons, called the reticular formation. These neurons include ascending and descending tracts, some of which cluster to form centers that control swallowing, vomiting, and respiratory and cardiovascular reflexes. The reticular formation is also essential for wakefulness and is necessary to focus attention. Functioning of the reticular formation is essential for life.

Wakefulness.
Various neurons in the reticular formation send information to higher brain areas to maintain wakefulness and arousal. These neurons and their projections are part of a functional rather than anatomic group of cells, called the RAS. The RAS maintains wakefulness, attention, and concentration. The RAS is stimulated by all sensory input, including painful stimuli.

Sleep.
The process of sleep is also under the control of the reticular formation. Like wakefulness, sleep is an active process. It occurs when certain centers in the brainstem send inhibitory signals to neurons throughout the RAS. These inhibitory signals appear to result from the release of the neurotransmitter serotonin by the reticular formation cells. Serotonin inhibits RAS firing, temporarily ending conscious behavior. Serotonin levels in the brain eventually decrease, and the person wakes up. Sleep and wakefulness normally follow a cyclic pattern unless that pattern is blocked, changed, or interrupted.

The Cerebellum

The cerebellum sits in the hindbrain posterior to the brainstem. The cerebellum helps maintain balance and is responsible for the smooth skeletal muscle responses that give grace and direction to voluntary movements. It controls fast, repetitive movements required for activities such as typing, piano playing, and bike riding. The cerebellum is also able to dampen muscle movement. As muscle movement begins, momentum is gained. Without a functioning cerebellum, motion would continue beyond the intended target.

THE SPINAL CANAL

The longitudinal axis of the skeleton is formed by the spinal canal or vertebral column. It is a long, thin column extending from the base of the skull to the sacrum (tailbone) with the spinal cord running down the middle. The spinal canal is filled with cerebrospinal fluid (CSF) and is surrounded by the bony vertebral column, which extends beyond the terminus of the spinal tract and offers protection to the delicate nerves inside. The spinal cord consists of interneurons whose axons travel up and down in organized tracts. Incoming to the ascending tracts are axon terminals that carry sensory information from peripheral afferent neurons. Many axon terminals synapse in the cord on an interneuron. If the summation of the various incoming IPSPs and EPSPs results in the interneuron reaching threshold, the interneuron will fire an action potential and pass the information further into the CNS. The sensory neuron may also stimulate a spinal reflex. This is accomplished when a sensory neuron synapses in the spinal canal directly on the dendrites or cell body of a motor neuron (monosynaptic reflex), or when it synapses on an interneuron that secondarily activates a motor neuron (polysynaptic reflex).

Also present in the spinal cord are descending interneurons that innervate dendrites and cell bodies of efferent nerves. Efferent nerves leave the spine in tracts and innervate muscle or endocrine cells.

Dorsal and Ventral Roots

Groups of afferent nerves entering at each level of the cord on the dorsal (toward the back) side are called dorsal roots. Efferent nerves leave each level of the cord in groups on the ventral (toward the front) side. These are called ventral roots. Dorsal and ventral roots at a given level of the spinal cord join together outside the cord to form 1 of 31 pairs of spinal nerves.

Gray and White Matter

The spinal cord can be separated into gray and white matter. Gray matter occupies the center of the tract and is filled with interneurons, cell bodies, dendrites of efferent neurons, axons of afferent neurons, and various support cells.

The white matter, consisting mostly of myelinated ascending and descending tracts, surrounds the gray matter.

THE MENINGES

The meninges are thin membranes surrounding the brain and spinal cord. There are three meninges: the dura mater (thick mother) on the outside, the arachnoid (spiderlike) as a middle layer, and the pia mater (little mother) lying immediately above the brain.

The space above the dura mater is called the epidural, and the space below the dura mater but above the arachnoid is called the subdural. The epidural and subdural spaces contain many small blood vessels. Damage to these vessels leads to blood accumulating in the epidural or subdural spaces. CSF circulates in the subarachnoid space (beneath the arachnoid, above the pia mater).

CEREBROSPINAL FLUID AND THE VENTRICLES

CSF is a clear fluid surrounding the brain and spinal cord. The CSF circulates in the subarachnoid space, and offers the brain protection against physical jarring. There is some exchange of nutrients and waste products between the CSF and the neural tissue. The CSF also plays a vital role in triggering homeostasis responses. For example, as CO_2 levels in the CSF change, a message is sent to the respiratory center in the brainstem to regulate the pH and CO_2 levels throughout the body. Although CSF is formed from plasma that flows through the brain, its concentration of electrolytes and glucose differs from that of plasma. Glucose and potassium levels are slightly lower in the CSF while chloride levels are higher.

CSF is formed as a result of filtration, diffusion, and active transport across special capillaries into the ventricles (cavities) of the brain, especially the lateral ventricle. The capillary network responsible for CSF formation is called the choroid plexus. Once in the ventricles, CSF flows toward the brainstem. Through small holes in the brainstem, CSF circulates to the surface of the brain and spinal cord. At the surface of the brain, CSF enters the venous system and returns to the heart. Thus, CSF is continually recirculated through and over the CNS. If the ventricle conduction pathways for CSF become blocked, fluid can accumulate, which results in a buildup of pressure inside and on the surface of the brain.

THE BLOOD–BRAIN BARRIER

The blood–brain barrier refers to the unique structure of the brain vascular system that prevents the passage of materials from the blood to the CSF in the brain. The blood–brain barrier is formed from tightly fused endothelial cells present in the brain capillaries and from cells (astrocytes) lining the ventricles that limit diffusion and filtration. Special transport functions regulate the fluid that crosses out of the general circulation to bathe brain cells. The blood–brain barrier protects delicate brain cells from exposure to potentially harmful substances. Many drugs and chemicals cannot cross the blood–brain barrier.

BRAIN BLOOD FLOW AND BRAIN METABOLISM

The brain receives 15% to 20% of the cardiac output. This high rate of blood flow is required to meet the brain's continually high demands for glucose and oxygen. The arterial blood supply is from the internal carotid arteries and the vertebral arteries. The circle of Willis serves as an alternate route for blood flow if one of the arteries is blocked. As a potent vasodilator, CO_2 regulates blood flow to ensure an adequate blood supply to the brain.

The brain is unique in that it normally uses only glucose as a source for oxidative phosphorylation and the production of ATP. Unlike other cells, brain cells do not store glucose as glycogen; therefore, the brain must continually receive oxygen and glucose through brain blood flow. Oxygen deprivation for as little as 5 minutes, or glucose deprivation for 15 minutes, can cause significant brain damage. Brain function depends so much on blood flow that it is possible to identify which parts of the brain are performing which tasks by measuring brain blood flow during specific brain activities.

Studies have shown that when performing a burst of mental work, the brain initially produces ATP by anaerobic glycolysis, rather than oxidative phosphorylation. Anaerobic glycolysis depends on glucose but does not require oxygen. The brain does this even if oxygen is readily available. The result is a rapid utilization and depletion of glucose, with a corresponding increase in oxygen levels. Within a short period, the brain begins oxidative phosphorylation.

INTRACRANIAL PRESSURE

The pressure inside the cranium is called the intracranial pressure (ICP). ICP is determined by the volume of blood in the brain, the volume of CSF, and the volume of brain tissue. Normally, ICP ranges from 5 to 15 millimeters of mercury (mm Hg). The Monro–Kellie hypothesis explains the compensatory response to a change in blood, CSF, or brain tissue. As one component increases, the other two decrease. Although the rigid skull poses some limitations, vasoconstriction reduces blood flow and CSF can be shunted to decrease pressure.

THE PERIPHERAL NERVOUS SYSTEM

The peripheral nervous system consists of nerves traveling between the brain or spinal cord and the rest of the body. There are 12 nerve pairs traveling to and from the brain and 31 pairs traveling to and from the spinal cord. The peripheral nervous system can be separated into afferent and efferent divisions. In all spinal nerves and most CNs, afferent and efferent fibers travel together in opposite directions. Some CNs carry only afferent information. Afferent neurons convey information to the CNS from all sensory organs, pressure and volume receptors, temperature receptors, stretch receptors, and pain receptors. Efferent neurons deliver neural stimulation to muscles and glands. Efferent neurons belong to either the autonomic or the somatic nervous system.

The Autonomic Nervous System

Autonomic nerve fibers leave the spinal cord and innervate smooth and cardiac muscle and the endocrine and exocrine glands. Autonomic nerve fibers are considered involuntary because there is little conscious control over their function. The two divisions of the autonomic nervous system, the sympathetic and parasympathetic divisions, are shown in Figure 8-8. Sympathetic and parasympathetic nerves innervate many of the same organs but typically cause opposite responses. The cell bodies of these neurons lie in the brain or spinal cord. In both divisions of the autonomic system, two nerve fibers participate in the efferent pathway.

The Sympathetic Nervous System

The first fibers of the sympathetic nerves, called the *preganglionic fibers*, leave from the thoracic or lumbar regions of the spine. Soon after leaving the spine, a preganglionic fiber joins other preganglionic fibers to form an autonomic ganglion. At this point, the preganglionic fiber synapses on the second nerve fiber of the system, the *postganglionic fiber*, and releases acetylcholine, which causes the postganglionic fiber to fire an action potential. From the autonomic ganglia, the postganglionic fiber travels to its target organ, the muscle or gland. The sympathetic postganglionic fiber usually releases the neurotransmitter norepinephrine. Target organ receptors for norepinephrine are called **adrenergic receptors**.

The Parasympathetic Nervous System

The fibers of the parasympathetic nervous system leave the brain in the CNs or leave the spinal cord from the sacral area. The preganglionic fiber of the parasympathetic system is typically long and travels to an autonomic ganglion located near the target organ. Preganglionic parasympathetic nerves release acetylcholine that then stimulates the postganglionic fiber. The parasympathetic postganglionic fiber then travels a short distance to its target tissue, a muscle or a gland. This nerve also releases acetylcholine. Preganglionic acetylcholine receptors (AChRs) for sympathetic and parasympathetic fibers are called **nicotinic receptors**. Cholinergic nicotinic receptors are stimulated in

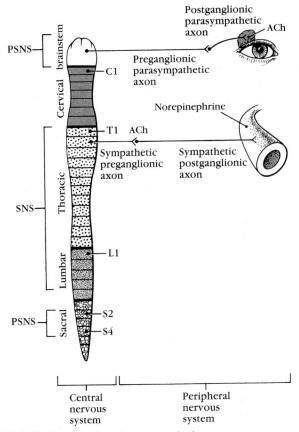

FIGURE 8-8 Sympathetic and parasympathetic systems.

the ganglia by presynaptic neurons. Postganglionic AChRs are called **muscarinic receptors**. These names relate to the experimental stimulation of the receptors by nicotine and muscarine (a mushroom poison).

Functions of the Sympathetic and Parasympathetic Nerves

Functions of the sympathetic and parasympathetic nervous system are included in Table 8-2.

The Somatic Nervous System

Somatic nerves of the peripheral nervous system consist of somatic motor neurons that leave the brain or spinal cord and synapse directly on skeletal muscle cells. Motor neurons are large myelinated nerves that release acetylcholine at

TABLE 8-2 Functions of the Autonomic Nervous System	
Sympathetic Nervous System	**Parasympathetic Nervous System**
Increased heart rate	Decreased heart rate
Increased strength of cardiac contraction	Conserves and restores energy
Increased cardiac output	
Pupil dilation	Pupil constriction
Inhibits accommodation for far vision	Stimulates accommodation for near vision
Stimulates pilomotor muscles resulting in "goose pimples"	
Vasoconstriction of all vessels except those supplying skeletal muscles	
Dilation of skeletal muscle vessels leading to increased blood flow to muscles	
Bronchial relaxation leading to increased oxygenation	
Decreased bronchial secretions	
Decreased gastrointestinal peristalsis; inhibition of defecation	Increased gastrointestinal peristalsis
Decreased digestive juice secretion	Stimulates digestive gland secretions
Closure of anal sphincter	Opens sphincter for defecation
Bladder relaxation which delays emptying	Bladder contraction that stimulates emptying
Increased epinephrine secretion	Airway constriction
Sweat gland stimulation	
Increased blood sugar	
Ejaculation	Erectile function
Increased lactic acid and release of free fatty acids	

the neuromuscular junction. Acetylcholine binds to receptors on a specialized area of the muscle cell, called the end plate. Binding of acetylcholine causes the muscle cell to reach threshold, resulting in an action potential and the opening of calcium channels (gates) in the membrane. This leads to an increase in intracellular calcium and contraction of the skeletal muscle fiber. Cholinergic nicotinic receptors are stimulated by acetylcholine from the somatic motor neuron. There are no inhibitory motor neurons.

SUPPORT CELLS

Cells in the central and peripheral nervous systems function to support nerve cells by providing nutrients, forming myelin, and clearing away cell debris and other material from the neuronal area. In the CNS, these cells are called neuroglia and are more numerous than nerve cells. Examples of neuroglia include the oligodendroglia cells, which make myelin; microglia cells, which support immune function in the CNS; and astrocytes, which carry nutrients from capillaries to nerve cells and remove excess neurotransmitters and ions that accumulate around neurons, thus ensuring optimal osmotic and ionic concentrations. Recently, neuroglial cells have received increased attention, with a gathering body of research indicating that they, especially the astrocytes, actually communicate with neighboring neurons. Through these interactions, neuroglial cells appear to influence the formation of synapses and help determine which neural connections become stronger and which become weaker over time. This function has important implications for learning and memory. In the peripheral nervous system, Schwann cells provide a source of nutrients for the neurons and produce myelin.

HOW THE BRAIN WORKS

Advances in technology, especially positron emission tomography (PET) and magnetic resonance imaging (MRI), have offered insights into how the brain allows us to think, remember, interpret stimuli, and understand and use language.

It appears that the mind breaks down complex functions into discrete components of a specific job, and delegates these components to specific neuronal networks. The outcomes from the different networks are then reassembled in a pattern that allows the brain to perform the activity or give meaning to a stimulus.

Communication Pathways

Perhaps best studied are the many steps involved in participating in a conversation. To begin with, spoken sounds are carried from auditory receptors in the ears through the thalamus to the primary auditory area of the cortex. At the same time, nonverbal visual clues are sent from the retina through the thalamus to the primary visual area. From the auditory cortex, signals travel to an area in the left temporal lobe, called Wernicke's area, where meaning is assigned to the words; and to associative areas where the impact of the words is perceived by the listener. To respond verbally, an area of the frontal lobe, called Broca's area, is activated, and an appropriate response is formulated. The reply is then spoken by activating the primary motor area of the brain, then passing the motor signals through the thalamus and down the spinal cord, resulting in activation of motor neurons to the face and throat.

The processing of various tasks by the brain is adaptable; as one becomes proficient at a task, the patterns of processing can change, becoming faster and often more efficient. One can learn to speak before thinking and listen without paying attention.

Memory

Memory is the internal recording of a prior event. Memory is a function of the cerebral cortex, specifically involving the temporal, parietal, and occipital lobes. The formation of memory is a multistep process that involves (1) focusing attention on a selected event, name, or number, to the exclusion of background events, (2) rehearsing the information, and (3) consolidating the information into chemical storage in the brain.

Focusing attention on one event or piece of information allows that information to enter short-term memory storage. This is an active state wherein the new event is compared with previous experiences. Short-term memory is considered to be the working memory and stores information for a few seconds or minutes. It is of limited capacity and if the information is not continually **rehearsed** or attended to, it will be lost when a new input arrives to distract attention. However, if the information is rehearsed, it will stay in short-term storage until it can be **consolidated** into long-term memory storage. Long-term memory is theoretically unlimited and permanent. Long-term memory depends on several excitatory neurotransmitters, including acetylcholine, dopamine, norepinephrine, and glutamate, and on hormones released during stressful events, including adrenocorticotropic hormone (ACTH), vasopressin, and epinephrine. Inhibitory transmitters, including GABA, can reduce the likelihood of consolidating memory from short-term storage to long-term.

Short-term memory involves temporary presynaptic inhibition or facilitation while long-term memory requires longer activation of presynaptic facilitation ultimately resulting in structural changes in the synapses of the cerebral cortex. It is believed that the neurotransmitter serotonin is released at the axoaxonal synapse, triggering the axon terminal of a presynaptic neuron to block the potassium channel. Because sufficient potassium is not available to rapidly depolarize the membrane, that action potential arriving at the presynaptic neuron lasts longer. As a result of the prolonged action potential, presynaptic calcium channels are open longer and trigger the release of more neurotransmitter, which facilitates synaptic transmission resulting in structural changes. These changes may involve one or a combination of the following: increased number of postsynaptic terminals, increased number of vesicles stored, increased number of sites for release of transmitters, and/or dendrite changes that allow post-synaptic facilitation.

When a short-term memory is consolidated into a long-term memory, it is done so by breaking the information to be remembered into separate units that are then processed in specific areas of the brain. For example, a visual experience is broken down into discrete attributes of color, shape, and size, and these attributes are stored separately.

There are two general types of long-term memory. **Declarative** memory is conscious memory for facts and events. This type of memory requires a well-functioning medial temporal lobe, which includes the hippocampus, and structures in the diencephalon. How these various parts of the brain interact during memory coding and retrieval is not known. The declarative memory is stored in the cerebral cortex, but again, how this occurs is not understood. **Nondeclarative** memory is involved with skill learning, repetition, and classical conditioning. Nondeclarative memory involves unconscious recollection and requires an intact cerebral cortex, basal ganglia, and cerebellum. With most types of dementia, declarative memory is lost before nondeclarative memory. Strokes (brain attacks) may interfere with nondeclarative and declarative memory.

● Pathophysiologic Concepts

ALTERATIONS IN CONSCIOUSNESS

Consciousness is the full awareness of self, location, and time in any environment. To be fully conscious, an intact RAS is required, as is the functioning of higher brain centers in the cerebral cortex. Connections through the thalamus must also be intact.

Alterations in consciousness typically begin with disruption in diencephalon functioning, characterized by dullness, confusion, lethargy, and finally stupor as the person becomes difficult to arouse. Continued decreases in consciousness appear with midbrain dysfunction and are characterized by deepening of the stupor state. Finally, dysfunction of the medulla and pons may occur, resulting in coma. This progressive decrease in consciousness is described as rostral–caudal progression.

Assessment Tools

One of the most widely used assessment tools for level of consciousness is the Glasgow Coma Scale (GCS) (Table 8-3). Areas of evaluation include eye opening, verbal response, and motor response. Possible scores range from 3 to 15 with a higher score indicating a higher level of consciousness. A score of 8 and below indicates a coma. When using the tool for serial assessments, it should be noted that it is not sensitive for altered sensorium.

The FOUR Score Consciousness Scale is a valid assessment tool that evaluates eye response, motor response, brainstem reflexes, and respiration. Each area is evaluated on a scale of 0 to 4 and can be used with the intubated patient. The scale is described in Table 8-4.

TABLE 8-3	The Glasgow Coma Scale	
Eye Opening (E)	**Verbal Response (V)**	**Motor Response (M) Upper Extremities**
4 = spontaneous	5 = normal conversation	6 = normal
3 = to voice	4 = disoriented conversation	5 = localizes to pain
2 = to pain	3 = words, but not coherent	4 = withdraws to pain
1 = none	2 = no words; only sounds	3 = decorticate posture
	1 = none	2 = decerebrate posture
		1 = none
		Total = E + V + M

ALTERATIONS IN PUPIL RESPONSES

The ability of our eyes to dilate or constrict, rapidly and equally, depends on an intact brainstem. Cerebral hypoxia and many drugs change pupil size and reactivity. Therefore, pupil size and reactivity offer valuable information concerning brain integrity and function.

Important pupil changes seen with brain damage are pinpoint pupils seen with opiate (heroin) overdose and bilaterally fixed and dilated pupils

TABLE 8-4	The FOUR Score Consciousness Scale		
Eye Response	**Motor Response**	**Brainstem Response**	**Respiration**
4 = eyelids open, tracking or blinking on command	4 = thumbs up or fist to command	4 = pupil and corneal reflex present	4 = not incubated, regular breathing
3 = eyelids open, not tracking	3 = localizing to pain	3 = one pupil wide and fixed	3 = not intubated, Cheyne–Stokes pattern
2 = eyelids closed; open to loud noise	2 = flexion to pain	2 = pupil or corneal reflex absent	2 = not intubated, irregular pattern
1 = eyelids closed; open to pain	1 = extensor posturing	1 = pupil and corneal reflex absent	1 = breathes above ventilator rate
0 = eyelids closed with pain	0 = no response to pain or myoclonus status epilepticus	0 = absent pupil, corneal and cough reflex	0 = breathes at ventilator rate or apnea

usually seen with severe hypoxia. Fixed pupils are typically seen with barbiturate overdose. Brainstem injury presents with pupils fixed bilaterally in the midposition.

ALTERATIONS IN EYE MOVEMENTS

In a fully conscious person, the steady gaze of the eyes at rest results from an intact cerebral cortex exerting control over the brainstem. With brain injury that involves loss of cortical function, the eyes typically rove and move together toward or away from the side of the brain injured, depending on the type of injury. Loss of higher brain centers results in reflexive eye movements, called doll's head movements. A doll's head movement is that which occurs when the eyes stare forward, always following the position of the head. Normally, when an individual's head is passively turned to one side, the eyes move to face the previous, forward direction.

With injury to the brainstem, loss of ocular movement occurs, and the eyes become fixed in a direct forward position. A skewed deviation, with one eye looking up and one down, suggests a compressive injury to the brainstem. Normal involuntary cyclic movements of the eyeball (nystagmus responses) in response to ice water delivered into the ear are lost with cortical and brainstem dysfunction.

ALTERATIONS IN BREATHING PATTERN

Brainstem Damage

The respiratory center in the lower brainstem controls respiration based on hydrogen ion concentration in the surrounding CSF. Damage to the brainstem causes irregular and unpredictable patterns of breathing. Opiate overdose damages the respiratory center and results in a gradual decline in the breathing rate until respiration ceases.

Cerebral Damage

A higher brain center normally maintains the rhythmic, regular breathing patterns seen in healthy individuals. This control center is lost with cerebral damage, and the individual begins to breathe in a pattern dependent on brainstem CO_2 and the hydrogen ion it produces. This type of CO_2–dependent breathing is called posthyperventilation apnea. In this pattern, respirations cease (apnea) until CO_2 builds up to a certain threshold, which causes the individual to hyperventilate (increase his or her respiratory rate) until the CO_2 is removed. At this point respirations cease again.

Cheyne–Stokes respiration also involves breathing based on CO_2 levels. In this case the respiratory center is over-responsive to CO_2, which results in a breathing pattern of smooth increases in rate and depth (crescendo breathing) that progresses until a certain CO_2 level is reached. The rate and depth of respirations then decrease smoothly until apnea occurs (decrescendo breathing). Cheyne–Stokes respiration is, like postventilation apnea, seen with damage to the cerebral hemispheres, and is often associated with metabolically induced coma.

ALTERATIONS IN MOTOR RESPONSES AND MOVEMENT

Abnormal motor responses include inappropriate or absent movements in response to painful stimuli. Brainstem reflexes such as sucking and grasping responses will occur if higher brain centers have been damaged. Flexion and rigidity of limbs also are motor responses indicative of brain damage. Muscle conditions that indicate abnormal brain function include hyperkinesia (excessive muscle movements), hypokinesia (decreased muscle movements), paresis (muscle weakness), and paralysis (loss of motor function). Specific loss of cerebral cortex functioning, but no loss of brainstem function, results in *decorticate posturing*. Decortication is characterized by flexion of the upper extremities at the elbows and internal rotation and extension of the lower extremities. This posture may be unilateral or bilateral. *Decerebrate posturing* occurs with severe injury to higher brain centers and the brainstem and is characterized by rigid extension of the limbs with pronation of the arms, plantar flexion, and backward arching of the head (opisthotonos).

DYSPHASIA

Dysphasia is impairment of language comprehension or production. Aphasia is total loss of language comprehension or production. Dysphasia usually results from cerebral hypoxia, which is often associated with a stroke but can result from trauma or infection. Brain damage leading to dysphasia usually involves the left cerebral hemisphere.

Broca Dysphasia

Broca dysphasia results from damage to Broca's area in the frontal lobe. Persons with Broca dysphasia will understand language, but their ability to meaningfully express words in speech or writing will be impaired. This is called expressive dysphasia.

Wernicke Dysphasia

Wernicke dysphasia results from damage to Wernicke's area in the left temporal lobe. With Wernicke dysphasia, verbal expression of language is intact, but meaningful understanding of spoken or written words is impaired. This is called receptive dysphasia.

AGNOSIA

Agnosia is the failure to recognize an object because of the inability to make sense of incoming sensory stimuli. Agnosia may be visual, auditory, tactile, or related to taste or smell. Agnosia develops from damage to a particular primary or associative sensory area in the cerebral cortex.

PERSISTENT VEGETATIVE STATE

A persistent vegetative state results from the loss of functioning of the cerebral hemisphere. It is a state in which a person is without cognitive function, is unaware of self, place, and time, and is unresponsive to the external environment. This state can occur after several different types of brain injuries and, as its title suggests, can persist for years. Although consciousness is lost, brainstem and cerebellum function remain intact; therefore, respiration, cardiovascular control, maintenance of body temperature, and certain brainstem reflexes such as yawning, grasping, and sucking will continue. Eyes may be open or shut, and a sleep–wake cycle will be followed, but there is no conscious perception of events or deliberate action. This diagnosis requires that the condition exists for at least one month. Criteria for the diagnosis include:

- Absence of awareness of self and environment
- Inability to interact with others
- Absence of sustained or reproducible voluntary behavioral responses
- Lack of language comprehension
- Adequate hypothalamic and brainstem function to maintain life
- Bladder and bowel incontinence
- Variably preserved CNs
- Spinal cord reflexes.

A coma is somewhat similar, except there is no opening of the eyes, and no sleep–wake cycle. Comas and persistent vegetative states have legal and ethical implications for the families of those affected and for society.

BRAIN DEATH

Brain death is the irreversible loss of cerebral hemisphere, brainstem, and cerebellum function. Consciousness is lost, as is the maintenance of respiration, cardiovascular, and temperature control function. There is no sleep–wake cycle, no pain response, and no reflexes. The electroencephalogram (EEG) is flat in an individual who is brain dead. Brain death is based on the criteria listed below.

- GCS < 3
- Apnea

- No pupillary response
- No gag or cough reflex
- No oculovestibular reflex
- No corneal reflex
- No oculocephalic reflex.

Establishing brain death has ethical and legal implications. A patient cannot be legally discontinued from life support without prior living will instructions unless brain death is established. Organ donation is allowed only when brain death is established. Unfortunately, a donated organ is more likely to be healthy when taken from an individual before brain death occurs.

DEMENTIA

Dementia is a loss of intellectual functioning without a loss of arousal or vegetative functioning. Memory, general knowledge, abstract thought, judgment, and interpretation of written and oral communication may be affected. Dementia may be caused by infection, drugs, trauma, or tumors. Biochemical disturbances and metabolic imbalance may also cause dementia. It is generally considered to be chronic and progressive, but some dementia is reversible if the initiating insult can be relieved. Other types of dementia, such as that caused by Alzheimer disease, are progressive and irreversible.

INCREASED INTRACRANIAL PRESSURE

ICP may increase with increases in cranial blood, CSF, or tissue. Cushing triad of a widening pulse pressure, bradycardia, and irregular respiratory pattern are classical, yet late signs of increased ICP. A significant increase in ICP is called intracranial hypertension. Intracranial hypertension causes delicate neurons and capillaries in the brain to become compressed, leading to hypoxia, neuronal injury and death, inflammation and swelling, and ultimately progressive deterioration of brain function. If ICP reaches systemic mean arterial pressure, blood flow to the brain will stop and the individual will die.

Causes of Increased Intracranial Pressure

Shifts in ICP are common, and occur with stimuli such as straining at stool, coughing, sneezing, or head-dependent positions. More significant increases in ICP can occur with conditions that increase blood flow to the brain, or that block blood flow out of the brain. Anything that significantly increases CSF production or blocks CSF outflow can increase ICP. Any increase in tissue mass (e.g., that associated with a growing brain tumor) can increase ICP. Stroke, trauma, and tumors are among the most common causes of increased ICP.

Edema and Swelling of the Interstitial Space

Important sources of increased ICP are any stimuli that lead to edema and swelling of the interstitial fluid compartment. Infection and inflammation are associated with interstitial swelling and edema resulting from the release of vasoactive mediators of inflammation that stimulate increased capillary blood flow and increased capillary permeability (Chapter 4). Bacterial toxins also cause significant cellular destruction and initiate capillary destruction, again causing interstitial swelling. Therefore, infection and inflammation significantly increase ICP.

Severe hypertension may increase ICP by causing filtration of plasma into the interstitial space, leading to edema and swelling. Severe trauma to the head, a burst aneurysm, or a hemorrhagic stroke cause bleeding in the brain, which increases ICP by acting as a source of expanding tissue (blood) and by causing inflammation with swelling and edema.

The Stages of Intracranial Hypertension

As volume in the brain increases, the brain directs response mechanisms designed to minimize increases in pressure and reduce the extent of brain damage. The response of the brain to increased ICP is called compensation. However, if the volume in the brain continues to increase, compensation will eventually lose its effectiveness. The brain goes through four stages in response to increased ICP.

Stage 1

An increase in one of the three volumes in the brain (blood, CSF, or tissue) is normally compensated for by a decrease in one or both of the other volumes. If successful, compensation will allow ICP to remain within the normal range even with a significant increase in one of the brain volumes. If there is increased volume in one compartment, but normal ICP because of compensation, the brain is said to be in stage 1 of intracranial hypertension. Usually, this stage involves decreased CSF production or increased CSF reabsorption, followed by increased arterial constriction to decrease blood flow into the brain. Persons in stage 1 may demonstrate only subtle behavioral changes, primarily drowsiness and slight confusion.

Stage 2

If the volume continues to increase despite early compensatory mechanisms, ICP begins to increase significantly and the individual is said to be in stage 2. This stage would occur with the progression of a tumor or continual bleeding from a severed artery or vein. During stage 2, the brain responds by constricting cerebral arteries in an attempt to reduce pressure by reducing blood flow. Reducing blood flow, however, leads to cerebral hypoxia and hypercapnia (increased CO_2 levels) and deterioration of brain function. Clinical signs include decreased level of consciousness, alterations in breathing pattern, and pupillary changes.

Stage 3

In response to worsening hypoxia and hypercapnia, the cerebral arteries undergo reflex dilation, with the goal of increasing brain oxygen delivery. As blood volume increases, however, ICP increases further, thereby worsening the situation. This cycle of increasing hypoxia leading to increasing pressure, thereby worsening the hypoxia, is called decompensation. With the onset of decompensation, the individual is said to enter stage 3 of intracranial hypertension.

In stage 3, the volume–pressure curve develops so that additional small changes in intracranial volume produce large changes in pressure. Fast-rising pressure compresses the arterioles and capillaries, worsening the hypoxia and the hypercapnia, and damaging the neural cells. The result is a pronounced decrease in consciousness, altered respiratory pattern, and loss of pupillary reflexes. As the brain senses worsening hypoxia and hypercapnia, it responds with reflexes geared toward increasing systemic mean arterial pressure in an attempt to increase its own oxygenation. A dramatic increase in systemic blood pressure only serves to further increase ICP, accelerating the destruction of the brain cells. Cerebral blood flow slows, and consciousness and reflexes are usually lost.

Stage 4

As the swelling and pressure in one compartment of the brain become very high, herniation (bulging) into another compartment occurs. Herniation increases pressure in the other compartment, and eventually the whole brain becomes involved. When ICP reaches mean systolic pressure, cerebral perfusion stops. The volume–pressure curve demonstrating the stages of increased ICP is shown in Figure 8-9.

Treatment of Intracranial Hypertension

Treatment of intracranial hypertension begins with the identification of the cause and effective monitoring of ICP. Osmotic diuretics (mannitol) to reduce blood volume, steroids to decrease inflammation and surgical removal of tumors or hematomas may also be used. In some cases, shunting devices may be necessary. In the past, a lot of emphasis was placed on measuring cerebral perfusion pressure. It is now believed that measures of oxygen utilization by the brain are a better assessment of brain ischemia. These measures are obtained by comparing the oxygen level of jugular venous blood and arterial oxygen levels. Significant differences in these values indicate inadequate brain perfusion. Hyperventilation is contraindicated under most conditions because it worsens cerebral ischemia. Research continues to identify best practices for the management of increased ICP.

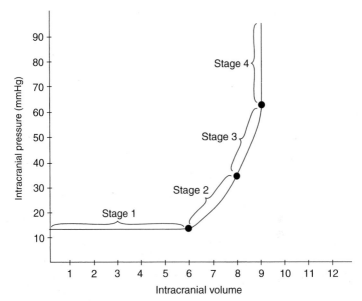

FIGURE 8-9 Intracranial volume versus pressure.

TESTS OF NEUROLOGIC FUNCTIONING

There are several methods to measure neuronal and brain electrical activity and observe for malformations, injuries, or tumors. Some of these techniques are presented briefly.

Electromyography

Electromyography (EMG) measures peripheral nerve function by recording the electrical activity of a motor nerve–muscle cell unit. A needle electrode is inserted through the skin into skeletal muscles to detect electrical activity. EMG is used to diagnose, describe, and monitor neuromuscular pathology in patients who are suspected of suffering a disorder in neural transmission or muscle cell function.

Electroencephalography

Electroencephalography measures electrical activity occurring in the brain through electrodes placed on the scalp. This technique offers a fast, real-time picture of brain activity. Electroencephalography is capable of picking up unusual brain wave signals indicative of brain damage or seizure activity. It is limited by an inability to accurately identify which area of the brain is generating the electrical signal, especially when the areas of desired evaluation are located deep in the brain.

Magnetoencephalography

Magnetoencephalography (MEG) is similar to electroencephalography, but is more accurate and allows more specific localization of brain function. It measures the magnetic fields from electrical activity in the brain via use of a superconducting quantum interference device which is extremely sensitive. This allows the brain to be visualized "in action" but the machines are cost prohibitive in many settings.

Magnetic Resonance Imaging

MRI captures what is happening in the brain physiologically before, during, and after an individual performs a task. MRI relies on the principle that each atom in the body will act like a little compass needle and line up in a predictable direction when exposed to a magnetic field. Signals unique to each atom are emitted and images can be formed from this information using specific computer programs. Organs are reproduced in more anatomic detail than by radiograph alone.

MRI has made a dramatic impact on the study of brain function and pathophysiology. It allows an investigator to noninvasively study oxygen concentration in the brain as an individual performs a task. Because the brain quickly shifts to anaerobic glycolysis with an activity spurt, oxygen levels increase in venous blood leaving an area performing a task. By looking for areas with high oxygen levels, researchers can identify blood flow patterns and active areas of the brain. Tissue structure and integrity can be imaged clearly with MRI. Automated software programs exist that allow clinicians and researchers to associate MRI data with specific anatomical regions, and to compare data originating from one region of the brain with data from other regions, including regions both participating and not participating in the activity.

Advantages of MRI include the absence of ionizing radiation and the high sensitivity the technique offers. It is the imaging technique of choice for most neurologic conditions. A limitation of MRI is the length of time required to scan the brain. Although ultrafast MRI is available, the ultrafast techniques are not as sensitive.

Magnetic Resonance Spectroscopy

Magnetic resonance spectroscopy (MRS) is an advanced type of MRI that offers information about the metabolite/biochemical aspects of tissue. This noninvasive approach provides chemical information about tissues using the frequency of the magnetic resonance.

Computed Tomography

Computed tomography (CT) scanning involves computer analysis of multiple radiologic images. In a CT scan, an x-ray beam is rotated around the patient, and passes successively through tissue from multiple directions. The pictures are then recreated by the computer to give a realistic three-dimensional representation of brain structure. Contrast media may be injected before the x-rays to improve fine detail of structures. CT scanning is readily available in most emergency rooms, and is used for rapid evaluation of neurologic emergencies. It is excellent for the visualization of bone and is able to detect acute hemorrhage. It is also the technique of choice when patients cannot undergo MRI due to the presence of foreign objects in the eye, pacemakers, or metal prostheses. Limitations of a CT scan involve multiple x-ray exposure and less detailed pictures than MRI.

Positron Emission Tomography

PET involves intravenous injection or inhalation of a positron-emitting iso-tope, followed by sequential radiographs of the skull that monitor the decay of the isotope in tissues that take up the label. This procedure allows the in-vestigator to study the distribution of a particular substance in the brain. It also allows the investigator to anatomically map the brain and determine blood flow patterns. By observing the flow of blood or the uptake of the isotope in different areas of the brain as an individual performs a task, one can identify which areas of the brain are most responsible for that task. Radiolabeled water is often injected when determining cerebral blood flow. Radiolabeled fluorodeoxyglucose is used to measure cerebral glucose metabolism, and carbon-11 is used to identify biochemical changes in the brain indicative of multiple sclerosis and Parkinson disease.

Single-photon emission computed tomography (SPECT) also involves the in-jection of a radionuclide to provide information on metabolic processes and blood flow, but involves decay to only a single photon. SPECT is typically less expensive than PET but offers poorer resolution of structure and metabolic activity.

Both PET and SPECT have been used to detect changes in neuropharmaco-logic parameters such as receptor numbers and neurotransmitter levels. These techniques allow researchers to determine the effects of substance abuse in the brain. For example, an acute increase in dopamine release, a decrease in sero-tonin transporter number, and increased occupancy of opiate receptors all have been documented to occur in response to various mood-altering substances.

Typically, blood flow patterns are determined at rest and during a specific task. Limitations to PET and SPECT involve the invasiveness inherent in in-jecting a radionuclide, although the ones chosen typically emit low levels of radiation and decay rapidly. Another limitation of these techniques is that neu-rons typically react faster than blood flow pattern can change, so some brain activity will be missed.

Ultrasonography

Ultrasound techniques use reflected sound to measure blood flow velocity, which is important for the assessment of cerebral blood flow when evaluating ischemic cerebrovascular disease. Ultrasound is used during surgical procedures on the brain to study the development of vascular spasm or blockage in real time. It is limited by the high degree of user proficiency required for its performance.

Myelogram

A myelogram involves the injection of air or contrast medium into the spinal subarachnoid space to visualize abnormalities of the vertebrae or spinal cord. Use of myelograms is gradually being replaced with MRIs, which offer much of the same information with less risk to the patient. Myelograms are typically reserved for conditions that involve weight-bearing flexion and extension which cannot be accomplished with an MRI or CT.

Cerebral Arteriogram

A cerebral arteriogram allows the visualization of the cerebral arteries following injection of dye. Flow of the dye is followed by radiographs to detect interruptions to circulation or changes in the vessel walls.

Evoked Potentials

This test is used to detect sensory nerve problems by measuring electrical signals to the brain due to hearing, touch, or sight. One set of electrodes is applied to the scalp and a second set is applied to the part of the body being tested. A stimulus is applied to the body part and the time it takes for the impulse to generate a response in the brain is recorded. The transmission should be instantaneous.

Cerebral Blood Flow Evaluation

A radioactive substance is inhaled or injected and is monitored via an external scintillation counter as it travels through the vessels in the brain. This test is being replaced by the SPECT, which is faster and of higher quality.

Lumbar Puncture

Lumbar puncture (LP) or spinal tap involves the insertion of a spinal needle into the subarachnoid space in the vicinity of the third and fourth vertebrae. LP can be used for several reasons such as to withdraw CSF for analysis, to inject medication or anesthesia, or to inject contrast medium or air for diagnostic studies. LP is rarely used when symptoms of increased ICP are present.

● Conditions of Disease or Injury

SEIZURE DISORDER

A seizure is the sudden, uncontrolled discharge of brain neurons, which produces changes in brain function. Many theories as to the cause of seizures are under investigation including altered membrane permeability, decreased inhibition of thalamic or cortical activity, and neurotransmitter imbalances resulting in excess acetylcholine and deficient gamma aminobutyric acid (GABA), which is an inhibitory neurotransmitter. Seizures result when certain cerebral neurons exist in a hyperexcitable or easily depolarized state. These neurons appear to have a less-negative-than-normal membrane potential at rest, or are missing important inhibitory connections. As a result, this group of neurons, called an epileptogenic focus, is always close to the threshold potential required for firing an action potential. Neurons of the epileptogenic focus respond to levels of stimuli that do not produce disorderly discharge in other neurons.

Once an epileptogenic focus begins to fire action potentials, the resulting current can spread to neighboring cells, causing them to discharge as well. It may spread to both sides of the brain and throughout cortical, subcortical, and brainstem areas. If the seizure begins diffusely throughout the cerebral cortex and includes both sides of the cortex, it is called a generalized seizure, and consciousness is always lost. If the seizure arises from a discrete focus and is limited to one side of the brain, it is called a partial seizure, and consciousness is usually not lost. Partial seizures may progress and become generalized. The time of unconsciousness after any generalized seizure is called the postictal phase.

As a seizure continues, inhibitory neurons in the brain fire and cause the neuronal discharge to slow, then stop. If one seizure is followed by a second or third seizure before the individual regains consciousness, or if a seizure continues for at least five minutes, status epilepticus is said to occur.

Seizure Syndromes

Generalized seizures affect the entire brain surface and include *tonic–clonic* seizures, characterized by sudden onset of rigid, intense contractions of arm and leg muscles (tonic seizure), followed by rhythmic contraction and relaxation of the muscles (clonic seizure). This is the most common type of generalized seizure and has been formally termed a grand mal seizure. Other generalized seizures may be purely *tonic*, purely *clonic*, or *atonic*. *Absence* seizures, frequently seen in children, are characterized by staring and sudden cessation of activity. With *atypical absence* seizures, staring is accompanied by myoclonic jerking and automatisms such as lip-smacking or other repetitive movements. Generalized seizures may occur idiopathically (for no known reason) or after brain trauma, infection, tumor, or bleeding.

Partial or focal seizures include *simple partial* seizures, during which consciousness is not impaired, and *complex partial* seizures, in which consciousness is impaired. A third type of partial seizure, secondary generalization, begins as a simple partial and progresses to impairment of consciousness. Partial seizures may occur idiopathically or after brain damage.

Consequences of a Seizure

During a seizure, cerebral oxygen demand increases more than 200%. If this oxygen demand cannot be met, brain hypoxia and brain damage may occur. Seizures that continue for extended periods, or the occurrence of status epilepticus, greatly increase the chance of brain damage.

Other consequences of a seizure, and especially of repeated seizures, include social isolation and reduced employment. Even the mildest forms of childhood epilepsy may be associated with lifelong social effects, including a reduced likelihood of marriage, childbearing, and academic achievement, even with normal intellectual functioning.

Causes of Seizure Disorders

Seizures can occur in anyone who experiences severe hypoxemia (decreased oxygen in the blood), hypoglycemia (decreased glucose in the blood), electrolyte imbalance, acidemia (increased acid in the blood), alkalemia (decreased acid in the blood), dehydration, water intoxication, or high fever. Drug withdrawal, drug abuse, and toxemia in pregnancy may also cause seizures. Some people seem to have a lower seizure threshold and therefore are more prone to seizures than others, suggesting a genetic tendency toward seizures. Seizures caused by metabolic disturbances are reversible if the initiating stimulus is removed. Syncope (fainting) is often misdiagnosed as a seizure because some muscle movements may be similar. Unconsciousness and muscle jerking related to fainting rarely last longer than 5 to 10 seconds, and fainting is not associated with postictal symptoms such as fatigue.

Epilepsy

Epilepsy refers to a seizure that occurs without a reversible, metabolic cause. According to the National Institute of Neurological Disorders and Stroke, epilepsy comprises two or more seizures. Epilepsy may be a primary or secondary condition. Primary epilepsy develops spontaneously, usually in childhood, and has a genetic predisposition. Mapping of several genes associated with primary epilepsy is under way. Secondary epilepsy occurs as a result of hypoxemia, head injury, infection, stroke, or CNS tumor. Adult-onset epilepsy is usually caused by one of these incidents.

Clinical Manifestations

Partial seizures may be associated with:

- Facial movements or grimaces
- Jerking beginning in one part of the body, which may spread

- Sensory experiences of sights, smells, or sounds
- Tingling
- An alteration in level of consciousness
- Complex partial seizures have impaired consciousness in addition to the characteristics above

Generalized seizures may be associated with:

- Unconsciousness, usually accompanied by a fall, except with childhood absence seizures
- Stiffening of the body with uncontrolled jerking of arms and legs
- A short period of apnea (breathing cessation) with possible cyanosis
- Pupillary changes and deviated gaze
- Salivation and frothing at the mouth
- Tongue biting
- Loss of ability to communicate
- Incontinence
- A postictal stage of stupor or coma, followed by confusion, headache, and fatigue; no memory of the seizure activity
- A prodroma may occur with any seizure type. A prodroma is a certain feeling or symptom that may precede a seizure by hours or days.
- An aura may occur with any seizure type. An aura is a certain sensory sensation that frequently or always immediately precedes a seizure.

Diagnostic Tools

- A detailed medical history is required for an accurate diagnosis of a seizure (specifically include details of the event and all medications).
- Thorough physical assessment with particular emphasis on the neurologic system.
- Basic laboratory evaluation must be performed to rule out metabolic causes or drug-induced seizures.
- LP is performed to rule out meningitis or encephalitis if suspected.
- MRI is the imaging modality of choice to identify brain lesions such as tumor, abscess, or vascular malformation as the cause of the seizure.
- A CT scan may be used for patients with emerging neurologic symptoms who need immediate diagnostic information.
- An electroencephalography may allow diagnosis of the type and location of the occurring seizure. Multiple electroencephalography recordings increase the diagnostic potential.
- PET scan.

Complications

- Hypoxic brain damage and mental retardation may follow repeated seizures.
- Depression and anxiety may develop. As described earlier, long-term social isolation may occur.

Treatment

- Identification of the type of seizure is essential for optimal treatment.
- Reverse the cause of the seizure disorder if possible.
- Maintain the airway and avoid injury during the seizure. Record all seizure activity including precipitating events, prodrome, aura, time, duration, actual activity, and postical state.
- Medications are available that may decrease the number of seizures an individual experiences. The goal of seizure treatment is zero seizure occurrence with a minimum of treatment-induced side effects. This can be extremely difficult in older patients. The medication selected must be appropriate for the seizure type.
- Resective surgery to excise the epileptogenic focus is becoming more common and is indicated in patients for whom antiepileptic drugs do not completely control seizures. Surgery may also be used to remove connections between the cerebral hemispheres, limiting seizure occurrence (called corpus callostomy).
- Vagus nerve stimulation involves an electrical device implanted in the infraclavicular area that provides a certain pattern of vagal stimulation to patients with seizures refractory to treatment. This treatment is a relatively new alternative to drug therapy. Vagal nerve stimulators have been shown to be effective in reducing the frequency of seizures in some patients.

HEAD INJURY

Head injuries may be open (penetrating through the dura mater) or closed (blunt trauma, without penetration through the dura). Open-head injuries allow environmental pathogens direct access to the brain. Damage will occur in either type of injury if blood vessels, glial cells, and neurons are destroyed or torn. Brain damage may develop after severe injury if bleeding and inflammation cause increased ICP.

Causes of Head Injuries

Causes of head injuries include automobile accidents, fights, falls, sporting injuries, and most recently military combat. Open-head injuries are often caused by bullet or knife wounds. While the incidence of open-head injuries in battle has decreased, the incidence of traumatic brain injury (TBI) from closed-head injuries has increased. It has been estimated that at least 8% and possibly up to 22% of wounded soldiers in the Afghanistan and Iraq wars have experienced a TBI due to explosions.

Types of Head Injuries

Several different types of head injuries are possible. Some involve an immediate loss of consciousness; others show delayed effects. Some head injuries result in obvious bleeding into the brain; others show no obvious signs of structural damage, but symptoms may develop.

Concussion

A concussion is a closed-head injury usually characterized by loss of consciousness. Concussion results in a brief period of apnea. A concussion can be mild, moderate, or severe, depending on the length of time the person is unconscious. A longer period of unconsciousness is predictive of a worse outcome. However, even mild concussions may be associated with subtle behavioral or cognitive changes, even if no obvious brain pathology exists. The condition, called postconcussive syndrome, may last for more than a year.

Epidural Hematoma

An epidural hematoma is the accumulation of blood above the dura mater. An epidural hematoma occurs acutely and is usually caused by a life-threatening arterial bleed.

Subdural Hematoma

A subdural hematoma is the accumulation of blood under the dura mater, but above the arachnoid membrane. Subdural hematomas are usually caused by a venous tear, although occasionally a subdural arterial bleed may occur. A subdural hematoma may develop rapidly, in which case it is called an acute subdural hematoma, or may result from a slow bleed, in which case it is called a subacute subdural hematoma. Chronic alcohol abusers and the elderly may experience a slowly developing hematoma over a period of months after a mild head injury, and may not show any obvious symptoms from the hematoma until it is large. This is called a chronic subdural hematoma. A chronic subdural hematoma is possible because the elderly and chronic alcohol abusers have reduced brain tissue, which allows the cranium to accommodate an expanding hematoma without a significant increase in pressure.

Subarachnoid Hemorrhage

A subarachnoid hemorrhage is the accumulation of blood under the arachnoid membrane, but above the pia mater. This space normally contains only CSF.

A subarachnoid hemorrhage usually results from a burst intracranial aneurysm, severe hypertension, an arteriovenous malformation, or a head injury. Blood accumulating on top of or under the meninges causes increased pressure on the underlying brain tissue.

Clinical Manifestations

- With a concussion, consciousness is often lost.
- Respiratory patterns may become progressively abnormal.
- Pupillary responses may be absent or progressively deteriorate.
- Headache may occur immediately or develop with increasing ICP.
- Vomiting may occur as a result of increased ICP.
- Behavioral, cognitive, and physical changes in speech and motor movements may occur immediately or develop slowly.
- Amnesia related to the event is common.
- Seizure.
- Restlessness or irritability.
- Disorientation or confusion.
- Diplopia.
- Gait changes.
- Personality changes.
- Bruising and tenderness of the scalp.
- Pupil changes, bradycardia, papilledema, elevated blood pressure, widening pulse pressure, and nuchal rigidity are associated with severe head injury.

Diagnostic Tools

- A skull radiograph may locate fractures or a developing bleed or blood clot.
- A CT scan or an MRI may pinpoint the site and extent of injury. A CT scan is usually the diagnostic tool of choice in the emergency room, although results of CT may be misleadingly normal.
- MRI is a more sensitive and accurate tool, capable of diagnosing diffuse axonal injury, but is costly and less accessible at most facilities.

Complications

- Bleeding inside the brain, called an **intracerebral hematoma**, may accompany a severe closed-head injury or, more commonly, an open-head injury. With bleeding in the brain, ICP increases, and neuronal and vascular cells are compressed. This is a type of secondary brain injury. With a hematoma, consciousness may be lost immediately, or may decrease later as the hematoma expands and the interstitial edema worsens.

- Subtle behavioral changes and cognitive deficits may exist and linger.

Treatment

Maintaining an open airway is the top priority. Treatment is focused on prevention and detection of increased ICP, maintenance of electrolyte balance, and monitoring of treatment and drug therapy.

- Mild and moderate concussions are usually treated with observation and bed rest.
- Surgical ligation of a bleeding vessel and evacuation of a hematoma may be required.
- Surgical debridement (removal of foreign material and dead cells) may be required, especially for an open-head injury.
- Decompression through the drilling of holes into the brain, called burr holes, may be required.
- Mechanical ventilation may be required.
- Antibiotics are required for open-head injury to prevent infection.
- Methods to decrease ICP may include the administration of diuretics and anti-inflammatory drugs.
- Antiepileptic agents may be given prophylactically.
- Barbiturate-induced coma is controversial although it has been used to treat intracranial hypertension not controlled by other methods. Barbiturates decrease metabolic demands, slow cerebral blood flow, stabilize cell membranes, and decrease vasogenic edema, which results in a more uniform blood supply to the brain.

SPINAL INJURY

Spinal injury usually involves a fracture or other injury to the vertebral bones. The spinal cord, running through the vertebral column, may be sliced, pulled, twisted, or compressed. Damage to the vertebral column or cord may occur at any level. Damage to the cord may involve the entire cord or be restricted to one half. Damage to the spine may result in temporary dysfunction or permanent damage if the cord is transected (cut).

Causes of Spinal Injury

Spinal cord injuries occur three to four times more often in males than in females. The most common causes of spinal injury are automobile and motorcycle accidents, falls, sports injuries, and wounds from guns and knives. Other causes include birth trauma, disc herniation, or bone spurs secondary to degenerative changes or osteoporosis.

Results of Spinal Injury

Microscopic Hemorrhages

Small hemorrhages develop with all vertebral or spinal cord injuries. These small bleeds, accompanied by inflammatory reactions that lead to swelling and edema, cause increased pressure in and surrounding the cord. Increased pressure compresses the nerves and decreases the vascular supply, which causes hypoxia and dramatically increases the extent of cord injury. Scar tissue can develop, causing the nerves in the area to become blocked or tangled irreversibly. Nerve growth factors are produced that may cause tangling of neurons and a worsening prognosis.

Loss of Sensation, Motor Control, and Reflexes

With severe spinal injury, sensation, motor control, and reflexes at and below the level of cord injury are lost. The loss of all reflexes is called **spinal shock**. Swelling and edema surrounding the cord may extend two vertebral segments above the site of injury. Therefore, sensory and motor loss and spinal shock may develop starting from two segments above the injury. Spinal shock typically goes away, but the permanent loss of sensation and motor control will continue if the cord has been transected or if severe swelling and hypoxia have occurred.

Spinal Shock

Spinal shock involves immediate loss of all reflexes from two segments above and below the site of cord injury. Lost reflexes include those controlling posture, bladder and bowel function, blood pressure, and maintenance of body temperature. Spinal shock appears to occur from the sudden loss of all of the tonic discharge normally carried in neurons descending from the brain, which acts to maintain the function of the reflexes. Spinal shock typically lasts 7 to 21 days, but may last longer. As spinal shock regresses, hyperreflexia may occur, characterized by muscle spasticity and reflex bladder and bowel emptying.

Autonomic Hyperreflexia

Autonomic hyperreflexia, also known as autonomic dysreflexia, is characterized by the reflex activation of sympathetic nerves below the level of the cord lesion, which leads to a dangerous increase in blood pressure. This condition can occur anytime after the cessation of spinal shock. Autonomic hyperreflexia occurs when a noxious sensory stimulus is relayed to the spinal cord and initiates a spinal reflex involving the activation of the sympathetic nervous system. With sympathetic activation, constriction of the blood vessels occurs and systemic blood pressure increases.

In individuals with an intact cord, such an increase in blood pressure would immediately be sensed by baroreceptors that monitor blood pressure (Chapter 13). In response to normal baroreceptor activation, the cardiovascular center in the brain would increase parasympathetic stimulation to the heart, thereby slowing the heart rate. In addition, the sympathetic nervous response would be blocked and dilation of the blood vessels would occur. The parasympathetic and sympathetic changes would serve to rapidly return blood pressure to normal. In an individual with a cord lesion, although the baroreceptors are activated and cause parasympathetic activation to slow heart rate and induce vasodilation above the site of injury, sympathetic reflex vasoconstriction below that level will continue.

With an occurrence of autonomic hyperreflexia, blood pressure can increase more than 200 mm Hg systolic, leading to a stroke or myocardial infarct. Other characteristics include severe headache, nasal stuffiness, flushing, and bradycardia. Stimuli that typically cause autonomic hyperreflexia include a distended bladder or bowel and the stimulation of surface pain receptors. Autonomic hyperreflexia is more likely to happen when the lesion is high (above T6) on the spinal cord.

Paralysis

Paralysis is the loss of sensory and voluntary motor function. With spinal cord transection, paralysis is permanent. Paralysis of the upper and lower extremities occurs with transection of the cord at level C6 or higher and is called quadriplegia. Paralysis of the lower half of the body occurs with transection of the cord below C6 and is called paraplegia. If only one half of the cord is transected, hemiparalysis may occur. Permanent paralysis may occur even when the cord is not transected, as a result of the destruction of the nerves following cord hemorrhage and swelling. In addition, demyelination of the axons in the cord can lead to clinically complete lesions, even though the spinal cord may not be transected. Demyelination of the axons most likely occurs as part of the inflammatory response to cord injury.

Clinical Manifestations

- Loss of sensation, motor control, and reflexes below the level of injury, and up to two levels above, will occur.
- Body temperature will reflect ambient temperature, and blood pressure will be reduced.
- The pulse rate is often normal, with low blood pressure.

Diagnostic Tools

- Physical examination
- CT and MRI to document vertebral and spinal injury and edema.

Complications

- If damage and swelling around the cord is in the cervical spine (down to approximately C5), respirations may cease because of compression of the phrenic nerve, which exits between C3 and C5 and controls the movement of the diaphragm.
- Autonomic hyperreflexia is characterized by high blood pressure with brady-cardia (low heart rate), and sweating and flushing of the skin on the face and upper torso.
- In the past, individuals suffering from a C2 or higher transection invariably died as a result of respiratory arrest. Although this is still true for many, recent advances in treatment modalities and better emergency rescue service responses have resulted in the survival of many individuals with high cord transection.
- Ascending spinal cord damage secondary to excessive edema.
- A severe spinal cord injury affects virtually all systems of the body to some degree. Commonly, urinary tract and kidney infections, skin breakdown and the development of pressure ulcers, and muscle atrophy occur.
- Depression, marital and family stress, loss of income, and large medical expenses are some of the psychosocial complications.
- Diabetes and stress ulcer development may occur with the use of high-dose corticosteroids.

Treatment

- Maintenance of a patent airway.
- Immobilization to prevent cord severing or additional damage after any head or neck injury is essential, even if a cord injury is not obvious.
- Early surgical intervention to relieve pressure on the cord caused by broken vertebrae or collapsed disks may reduce long-term disability.
- Immediate (within the first hour) large-dose administration of steroids has been shown to reduce cord swelling and inflammation and limit the extent of permanent damage. Strategies to stimulate axon regeneration, or to return impulse conduction along preserved but demyelinated axons, will likely lead to improved outcomes of patients with spinal cord injuries.
- Surgical fixation of the vertebral column hastens and supports healing.
- Physical therapy, including speech therapy if the lesion interferes with speech and respiratory movements, is begun soon after the patient's condition stabilizes.
- Education on avoidance and recognition of autonomic hyperreflexia can reduce the risk of stroke or myocardial infarct.
- Treatment of autonomic hyperreflexia includes antihypertensive medications and the removal of the initiating stimulus.

- For patients with permanent damage, education and counseling about long-term expectations and complications of skin, reproductive, and urinary systems are essential. Including family members in education and counseling sessions is essential.

CEREBRAL VASCULAR ACCIDENT

A cerebral vascular accident (CVA), often called a stroke or a brain attack, is an acute neurologic deficit related to an obstruction in brain blood flow. The term "brain attack" is being used more widely to raise awareness of the importance of early emergency intervention to minimize brain tissue damage. Especially at risk of suffering a CVA are elderly individuals with hypertension, diabetes, hypercholesterolemia, or heart disease. Other risk factors include smoking, coagulation disorders, obesity, excessive alcohol intake, and cocaine use. With a CVA, cerebral hypoxia leading to neuronal cell death and injury occurs. Inflammation, characterized by proinflammatory cytokine release, the production of oxygen free radicals, and swelling and edema of the interstitial space, occurs with cell damage and contributes to the worsening situation. Likewise, acidosis develops subsequent to hypoxia and further injures the brain via activation of acid-sensing neuronal ion channels. Ultimately, brain damage occurs after a CVA, typically peaking 24 to 72 hours after neuronal cell death.

There are two general classifications of CVAs: ischemic and hemorrhagic. Ischemic CVAs develop from a prolonged blockage in arterial blood flow to a part of the brain. Hemorrhagic CVAs occur as a result of bleeding into the brain. See page C8 for illustrations.

Ischemic Stroke

The arterial blockage causing an ischemic stroke may occur as a result of a thrombus (a blood clot in the cerebral artery) or an embolus (a blood clot that has traveled to the brain from elsewhere in the body).

Thrombotic Stroke

A thrombotic stroke occurs from occlusion of blood flow, usually resulting from severe atherosclerosis. Frequently, an individual will experience one or more transient ischemic attacks (TIAs) before a true thrombotic stroke occurs. A TIA is a brief, reversible disruption in brain function resulting from cerebral hypoxia. It is likely that a TIA occurs when an atherosclerotic vessel undergoes a spasm, or when the oxygen demand of the brain increases and this demand cannot be met because of advanced atherosclerosis. By definition, a TIA lasts fewer than 24 hours. Frequent TIAs suggest the likelihood of a true thrombotic stroke.

A thrombotic stroke typically develops over a period of 24 hours. During the period in which a stroke is progressing, the individual is said to be suffering from a stroke in evolution. At the end of that period, the individual is said to have suffered a completed stroke.

Embolic Stroke

An embolic stroke develops after arterial occlusion by an embolus formed outside the brain. Common sources of emboli leading to stroke include the heart after a myocardial infarct or atrial fibrillation, and emboli breaking off the common carotid arteries or the aorta.

Hemorrhagic Stroke

A hemorrhagic stroke occurs when a blood vessel in the brain is broken, leading to ischemia (reduced flow) and hypoxia downstream. Causes of hemorrhagic stroke include hypertension, a burst aneurysm, or an arteriovenous malformation (abnormal connection). Hemorrhage in the brain significantly increases ICP, worsening the resulting brain injury.

Clinical Manifestations

Specific clinical manifestations are dependent on the cerebral artery that is involved and the area of the brain being perfused by that vessel. General manifestations are listed below.

- Symptoms of a TIA may include temporary numbness of the face or limbs, slurring of words, confusion, dizziness, and changes or blackouts in vision. If any of these occurs, an individual should immediately seek medical assistance.
- With a CVA, the area of the brain that becomes ischemic determines the presenting clinical manifestations. Mentation, emotions, speech, vision, or movement can be affected. Many changes are irreversible, but some are reversible.
- Weakness of the arm and face.
- Ataxia.
- A hemorrhagic stroke is frequently accompanied by a severe headache and loss of consciousness.

Diagnostic Tools

A thorough history and complete physical with an in-depth neurologic assessment is vital. Specific diagnostic tools are listed below.

- Rapid diagnosis of a CVA is essential to minimize damage. CT scan is the method of choice for assessment of an acute presentation of a CVA. CT is highly sensitive to hemorrhage, an important consideration because there are vital differences in the treatment of ischemic versus hemorrhagic strokes. CT scans are also readily accessible, even in small or rural hospitals.

- Most MRI devices, although even more sensitive than CT at identifying early brain damage from a CVA, are slower than CT and thus are used less often in this emergency situation. However, after the initial CT scan, MRI is recommended to determine the exact location of damage and to monitor the lesion.
- More advanced MRI techniques such as perfusion- and diffusion-weighted imaging (DWI) reveal ischemia immediately and are vital for early diagnosis.
- CT angiography or magnetic resonance angiography (MRA) for vascular imaging.

Complications

- An individual suffering a major CVA to the part of the brain controlling respiration or cardiovascular response may die.
- Hypoxic destruction of expressive or receptive areas of the brain may lead to communication difficulties. Hypoxia of motor areas in the brain may lead to paresis.
- Emotional changes may occur with damage to the cortex, including the limbic system.
- An intracerebral hematoma may result from a burst aneurysm or a hemorrhagic stroke, causing secondary brain injury as ICP increases.

Treatment

The initial goal of emergency treatment is to reverse the evolution of ischemic brain injury. Subsequent goals include reperfusion and improved cerebral perfusion pressure. Treatments are listed below.

- In patients in whom the CVA can be identified as ischemic in nature, thrombolytic agents, such as tissue plasminogen activator (TPA), can be administered. TPA should be given as early as possible (at least within the first 3 hours of the attack) to be most effective in preventing long-term damage. However, it would be dangerous to treat a hemorrhagic stroke with a thrombolytic because this would increase bleeding and worsen outcome.
- A hemorrhagic stroke is treated with emphasis on stopping the bleeding and preventing another occurrence. Surgery may be required.
- Drug therapies that inhibit acid-sensing ion channels are being developed to limit stroke-induced damage.
- All stroke patients are treated with bed rest and a reduction of external stimuli to reduce cerebral oxygen demands. Measures to reduce intracranial edema and pressure may be instituted.
- Clinical trials to determine if the benefits outweigh the risks for procedures such as catheter-based recanalization, drug therapy to limit the calcium cascade, and hypothermia to decrease metabolic demands of the brain are in progress.
- Physical, speech, and occupational therapy are often required.

CENTRAL NERVOUS SYSTEM INFECTION

A CNS infection may involve the brain tissue (encephalitis), or the meninges (meningitis). Pathogens enter the CNS by crossing the blood–brain barrier or by direct invasion through an opening in the skull. With encephalitis and meningitis, inflammatory and immune responses cause increased swelling and edema in or around the brain, increasing ICP. Encephalitis also is associated with neuron death caused by the infecting microorganism.

Encephalitis

Encephalitis is usually a viral infection of the parenchyma of the brain. It is often carried by a mosquito vector (West Nile virus) or related to infection with herpes simplex 1 or cytomegalovirus. Nerve cell degeneration is widespread and edema and swelling are severe.

Meningitis

Meningitis is the most common serious infection of the CNS. It is usually caused by bacteria or a virus, although fungi, protozoa, and toxins are also causes. Meningitis frequently occurs from the spread of an infection elsewhere in the body, for example, the sinuses, ears, or upper respiratory tract. A posterior basilar skull fracture with a ruptured eardrum may also cause meningitis. With bacterial meningitis, released toxins destroy meningeal cells and stimulate immune and inflammatory reactions. Secondary encephalitis may occur. Even when treated, up to 40% of meningitis cases are fatal and up to 30% of survivors have neurologic complications.

In the past, most cases of meningitis were in children younger than the age of 5, and most often the causative agent was *Haemophilus influenzae*. Since 1990, a vaccine against *H. influenzae* has become available and is administered to most children in the United States and other countries as a series of injections, beginning in the second month of life. As a result of this important intervention, the incidence of meningitis in children aged 1 month to 2 years has decreased by 87%. Because of the dramatic decline in *H. influenzae*-type meningitis in this population, cases of bacterial meningitis overall in the United States have dropped by 55%.

Meningitis now occurs most commonly in adults aged 19 to 59. In this age group, the most common cause of bacterial meningitis is *Streptococcus pneumoniae* (pneumococcal meningitis). The next greatest incidence is in children aged 2 to 18, and the causal organism is most often *Neisseria meningitidis* (meningococcal meningitis). In the neonate, the causal organism is most often group B streptococcus; in infants aged 1 to 23 months the causal organism are split almost equally between *S. pneumoniae* and *N. meningitidis*.

While college students in general are no more likely to develop meningitis than other young adults of that age group, subgroups of college students are at increased risk. In particular, college freshmen living in dormitories have a sixfold greater risk of developing meningococcal meningitis than those not living in a dormitory. While most colleges now require vaccination against meningococcal meningitis, the vaccination is not effective against all strains.

Brain Abscess

A localized collection of pus in the brain parenchyma is known as a brain abscess. Streptococci, staphylococci, and anaerobes are the most common pathogens.

Clinical Manifestations

- Symptoms of increased ICP may develop with meningitis and encephalitis, including headache, decreased consciousness, and vomiting. Papilledema (swelling of the area around the optic nerve) may occur in severe cases. Typically, the symptoms are worse with encephalitis.
- Fever from infection is common in meningitis and encephalitis.
- Photophobia (painful response to light) from irritation of the CNs frequently accompanies meningitis and encephalitis.
- Inability to flex the chin to the chest without pain (nuchal rigidity) occurs in meningitis and encephalitis as a result of irritation of the spinal nerves.
- Encephalitis typically presents with dramatic signs of delirium and a progressive decrease in consciousness. Seizures, focal paralysis, muscle pain, a rash, and abnormal movements may occur.
- A brain abscess is seen as a space-occupying lesion with a focal infected core. As the infection progresses, it appears on a CT scan as a low-density core surrounded by an outer ring.

Diagnostic Tools

- In patients with suspected acute bacterial meningitis for whom there is no clinical contraindication, the CSF is collected through LP and examined for white blood cells and microorganism sensitivity. Elevated protein, elevated neutrophils, and low glucose in the CSF indicate meningitis.
- Laboratory studies for viral meningitis are not indicated (e.g., normal glucose, elevated lymphocytes).
- Rapid diagnosis of CNS infection is essential; this is especially true of meningitis. CT scan and MRI may be used to evaluate the degree of swelling and sites of necrosis. CT is very rapid and is most useful in emergency situations.
- Corticosteroid (dexamethasone) therapy to reduce inflammation appears to be beneficial for the adjuvant treatment of most adults with suspected pneumococcal meningitis.
- A diagnosis of encephalitis may be a diagnosis of exclusion.

Complications

- Individuals may suffer permanent disability, brain damage, or death from encephalitis or, less commonly, meningitis.
- Optic neuritis, visual impairment, deafness, personality changes, hydrocephalus, pneumonia, and endocarditis may result from meningitis.
- Seizures may develop.

Treatment

- A broad-spectrum antibiotic is administered after CSF collection and is changed if necessary after culture results.
- Antibiotic treatment may be accompanied by corticosteroids to prevent immune-mediated injury from bacterial cell wall lysis.
- An antiviral drug will be administered for encephalitis.
- Measures to reduce ICP will be initiated, especially for encephalitis.
- Some types of meningitis will require the patient to be isolated in the hospital.
- Antibiotics with excision or drainage are used to treat abscesses.

ALZHEIMER DISEASE

Alzheimer disease is a progressive dementia characterized by the widespread death of brain neurons, especially in an area of the brain called the nucleus basalis. Nerves from here normally project throughout the cerebral hemispheres to areas of the brain responsible for memory and cognition. These nerves release acetylcholine, which has been shown to be essential in building short-term memory at the biochemical level. The enzyme responsible for the production of acetylcholine, choline acetyltransferase, is reduced up to 90% in the brains of individuals who have died of Alzheimer disease compared to those who have died of other causes. Therefore, lack of acetylcholine can account for at least some of the forgetfulness and loss of cognitive function seen in individuals with Alzheimer disease. Other neurotransmitters also appear to be absent in individuals with the disease.

Alzheimer disease typically develops after the age of 65, causing senile dementia. However, it may occur earlier and result in presenile dementia. There is a genetic tendency to develop the disease, especially early onset disease. In fact, family history is second only to age as a risk factor for developing Alzheimer disease. The disease is the most common cause of dementia today.

Pathology

The pronounced autopsy findings of patients with Alzheimer disease include widespread development of neurofibrillary tangles, the axons of which coalesce into plaques, called amyloid-rich senile or neuritic plaques. The senile plaques include remnants of the dying nerve terminals, aluminum deposits, and abnormal protein fragments. The protein fragments always include pieces of a protein known as the amyloid beta peptide (Abeta). Abeta is a peptide fragment from a larger, membrane-spanning protein called amyloid precursor protein (APP). In addition, major morphologic changes include pronounced atrophy of the cerebral cortex with narrowing of the gyri, widening of the sulci and fissures, enlargement of the ventricles, loss of neurons, and significant vascular degeneration. These features are most pronounced in the frontal and temporal lobes. Similar tangles and chemical changes have been found in individuals with Down syndrome.

Development Theories

One theory concerning the development of Alzheimer disease involves the accumulation of Abeta in certain areas of the brain. Typically, the degradation of APP involves cleavage of the Abeta fragment as well, with the result that Abeta is lost from the area. In patients with Alzheimer disease, APP appears to be incorrectly cleaved, such that the Abeta fragment remains intact and accumulates in the surrounding plaques. It has been suggested that the abnormal processing of the larger APP allows pieces of Abeta to protrude out of nerve cell membranes, somehow initiating the tangles and killing the cells. Support for this theory comes from the finding that the gene coding for APP lies on chromosome 21, which when present in triplicate (rather than as a pair) causes Down syndrome. Virtually all individuals with Down syndrome who live into their 40s will develop Alzheimer disease. However, at least two other chromosomes have also been linked to Alzheimer disease in different groups of patients, suggesting that there may be more than one genetic cause of the disease.

A second theory as to the cause of Alzheimer disease involves the discovery that the risk of developing the disease increases with the inheritance of a certain gene coding for a specific type of cholesterol-shuttling protein, called apolipoprotein E (APO-E4). Inheritance of the gene for APO-E4, as opposed to one of the other varieties of this protein, APO-E2 or APO-E3, may somehow destabilize the nerve cell membrane, leading to tangling and neuronal cell death. Homozygotes for APO-E4 are at increased risk of developing the disease compared to heterozygotes.

Another area of research concerning Alzheimer disease involves glutamate, an excitatory neurotransmitter present throughout the brain. Glutamate plays an important role in learning and memory; however, some studies suggest that excess glutamate or abnormal cell sensitivity to glutamate may result in too much calcium entering nerve cells, causing neuronal cell death. The hippocampus, an area of the brain involved in memory, has been found to be especially sensitive to glutamate.

Research is indicating a link with gonadotropin luteinizing hormone (LH). LH has high receptor areas in the hippocampus, a vital area for cognitive functioning, which is diminished in those with Alzheimer disease. Elevated levels of LH have been found in those with Alzheimer suggesting that it may be an early indicator of disease progression. There is also data to support that LH regulates amyloid-B protein precursor processing.

Clinical Manifestations

The diagnosis of Alzheimer disease is usually a clinical one, based on history, physical, and biochemical and radiologic examinations. A clinical diagnosis of Alzheimer is typically highly sensitive in diagnosing positive cases, but may misdiagnose falsely, especially among the very old. Clinical manifestations include the following:

- Insidious, slowly progressing forgetfulness, decreased judgment, behavioral and personality changes developing over a period of up to 10 years.
- Progressive cognitive decline.
- Loss of visuospatial perception.
- Short-term memory loss and problems with math concepts are common.

Diagnostic Tools

- During a comprehensive physical examination, clinicians and attending family members often will recognize that patients suspected of dementia cannot provide reliable information on medical history. While not diagnostic, this is an important red flag.
- There is no definitive means of diagnosing Alzheimer disease during an individual's lifetime other than eliminating metabolic or vascular causes of the mental deterioration. However, increasingly sensitive MRI, PET, and SPECT scans can provide clinical support for the diagnosis. Newer techniques are likely to become available for more accurate identification of neuronal tangles and senile plaques.
- Although Alzheimer disease is the most common cause of dementia, approximately one-third of suspected dementia cases are caused by reversible disorders, including metabolic imbalance, drug effects, CVA, vitamin deficiencies, and depression. These causes must be ruled out using CT or MRI, a complete blood count, and metabolic studies.

Treatment

- Patient and family education regarding memory aids, diet, routines, simplifying tasks, using distraction, and safety issues may slow the progression of symptoms and help with the management of behavioral symptoms.
- Medications (Cognex) for the slowing or reversal of early Alzheimer symptoms are available and may delay the progression of symptoms in some patients.

- Cholinesterase inhibitors (donepezil, rivastigmine, and galantamine) that prolong the effective half-life of acetylcholine are the recommended drug therapy for mild to moderate dementia.
- Memantine, an *N*-methyl-D-aspartate (NMDA)-receptor antagonist, is approved for treatment of moderate to severe Alzheimer disease. Memantine works by moderately blocking glutamine receptors in the brain, allowing for some but not excessive glutamate stimulation.
- Some studies suggest that vitamin E and vitamin C supplementation may slow the progression of death, institutionalization, and severe dementia in some patients.
- Long-term benefits of all medications are undetermined.
- Research is currently under way related to the use of statins, anti-inflammatory agents, folate, and estrogen. Because cholesterol has been shown to cause ApoE, amyloid, and vascular damage, statins may be of benefit from a preventative perspective. Folate deficiency has been associated with increased homocysteine which is a possible risk factor for the disease and it has been suggested that estrogen may aid in prevention.

PARKINSON DISEASE

Parkinson disease is a progressive brain disorder characterized by the loss of neurons in an area of the *midbrain* known as the substantia nigra. These neurons use dopamine as a neurotransmitter and project their axons to the thalamus and the caudate and putamen areas of the basal ganglia. Parkinson disease results when about 80% of the cells that make up the substantia nigra are lost; there is also a reduction in dopamine receptors in the basal ganglia. Onset of the disease typically occurs in the sixth or seventh decade of life. It is the second most common neurodegenerative disease in adults. Although there may be a small genetic influence on the development of Parkinson disease, it seems mostly limited to early onset disease (before the age of 50).

Dopamine acts as an inhibitory neurotransmitter; thus, reduced dopamine stimulation in the substantia nigra and the basal ganglia leads to an imbalance between this inhibitory neurotransmitter and the excitatory neurotransmitter acetylcholine. Without dopamine, neurons are overstimulated by acetylcholine, resulting in excess muscle tone characterized by tremor and rigidity. A fixed facial tone projects a lack of emotional responsiveness, although there is often no emotional or cognitive deficit in patients with Parkinson disease.

Cause

The cause of Parkinson disease is unknown. As noted previously, recent evidence suggests that there is at least some genetic tendency toward developing the disease and some environmental issues that may be risk factors. Viruses, toxins such as pesticides, and ingestion of well water have been implicated in some studies.

Other Conditions Whose Symptoms Resemble Parkinson

Symptoms of Parkinson disease can develop in persons without the disease who suffer from certain types of brain trauma, infection, or tumors. Likewise, individuals who suffer from schizophrenia and require therapy with certain psychotropic drugs such as the phenothiazines may develop symptoms of Parkinson disease. Some symptoms of secondary Parkinson can be relieved by treatment of the injury or infection or by removal of the tumor or drug, but others may remain.

Clinical Manifestations

- Cardinal manifestations include bradykinesia, rigidity, tremor at rest, and postural instability due to loss of postural reflexes.
- "Pill-rolling" movement with hands.
- Micrographia or cramped, small handwriting.
- Drooling and dysphagia (difficulty swallowing).
- A shuffling gait, muscle rigidity, and stiffness.
- Akinesia, which is described as a lack of movement, including that involved with facial expressions and other voluntary movement, characterizes the disease.
- Secondary autonomic symptoms such as orthostatic hypotension, constipation, urinary incontinence, excessive sweating, and sexual dysfunction.
- Depression.

Diagnostic Tools

- In patients with Parkinson-like symptoms, diagnosis is often made based on history and physical examination. Other possible causes are ruled out.
- Diagnostic criteria includes a positive response to levodopa (strongly indicative), bradykinesia, and resting tremor or rigidity. Definitive diagnosis is confirmed by autopsy.

Complications

- Many patients with Parkinson disease develop dementia.

Treatment

- Dopaminergic (L-dopa) or anticholinergic drugs may be administered to reduce symptoms.

- Transplanting cells from the basal ganglia or adrenal medulla (where dopamine is also produced) of fetuses into the brains of patients with Parkinson disease to replace lost substantia nigra cells. This is experimental with ongoing research and many ethical concerns.
- Catechol-*O*-methyltransferase (COMT) inhibitors decrease levodopa metabolism making more available to cross the blood–brain barrier.
- The antiviral drug amantadine helps to minimize dyskinesias.
- The monoamine oxidase type B inhibitor, selegiline, decreases dopamine metabolism.
- Deep brain stimulation (DBS) is a procedure that places electrodes in areas of the brain which then receive high-frequency stimulation from an external pacemaker-like device.

HUNTINGTON DISEASE

Huntington disease (chorea) is a rare, degenerative disease of the basal ganglia and cerebral cortex. It is passed genetically as an autosomal-dominant disorder, apparently caused by expansion of a repeating codon located on chromosome 4. Onset of the disease typically occurs in the fourth or fifth decade of life.

With degeneration of the basal ganglia and cerebral cortex, several different neurotransmitters are lost. Many complications of the disease result from the loss of the inhibitory neurotransmitter GABA. There also appear to be gross abnormalities in energy production by the neuronal cell mitochondria.

Characteristic movements seen in patients with Huntington disease include extreme involuntary jerking, called chorea. These abnormal movements can occur all over the body and lead to physical exhaustion. Persons with Huntington disease undergo progressive loss of mental functioning, leading to dementia. The hallmark triad of the disease includes dominant inheritance, choreoarthetosis, and dementia. Death usually results within 10 to 15 years.

Clinical Manifestations

- Choreic (jerking) movements.
- Poor balance, dysphagia, hesitant or explosive speech, altered respirations, bowel and bladder incontinence.
- Poor judgment, memory lapses, and shortened attention span.
- Personality changes, depression, and slowly progressing dementia.

Diagnostic Tools

- Identification of the gene responsible for Huntington disease allows the diagnosis of the trait prenatally or before the onset of symptoms in an adult.

- Occasionally, MRI is used to image the brain. Atrophy is apparent in late disease. PET scan may be used to demonstrate hypometabolism of specific areas of the brain.

Treatment

- There is no treatment for Huntington disease. Because genetic identification of asymptomatic individuals who will likely develop the disease is possible, counseling is essential for those who choose to know their status and those who do not choose.

MULTIPLE SCLEROSIS

Multiple sclerosis is an autoimmune disease characterized by both a cell-mediated immune response and a humoral immune response with activated T cells and antibodies, both produced against self-antigens. These autoimmune activities lead to the destruction of neurons in the CNS. The peripheral nervous system is unaffected. It is unclear whether the immune attack is aimed at the myelin sheath directly, resulting in slowing of neural transmission down the axon, or is against the axon itself, causing severing of the axon and subsequent destruction of the myelin. In either case, the transmission of neural impulses in the brain and spinal cord is slowed, leading to dramatic alterations in movements and reflexes and, in some cases, changes in mental status such as deficits in memory, sustained attention, and rate of processing information. Mental status changes have been suggested to develop due to cholinergic deficits that may accompany increased cerebral glucose utilization. Continued inflammatory responses contribute to the disease by producing swelling and edema, which further injure the neurons and cause the development of scar tissue plaques on the myelin.

Categories of Multiple Sclerosis

There are four categories of multiple sclerosis, called syndromes, based on the original nerve tracts affected. These syndromes are the corticospinal syndrome, the brainstem syndrome, the cerebellar syndrome, and the cerebral syndrome. Initial symptoms usually fit into one of these syndromes. As the disease progresses, different tracts are affected and the symptoms become more widespread.

Besides separate neural tracts involved, multiple sclerosis can also take different forms based on the rate of progression of the disease. In the first type, **relapsing-remitting form**, the course of the disease is characterized by exacerbations of symptoms, followed by partial or full remission back to the preceding state. The second type, called **primary progressive form**, is characterized by a quick downhill course, without remission, from the beginning of the disease.

The third type, **secondary progressive form**, begins as the relapsing-remitting type, and then changes to a fast progression without remission.

Causes of Multiple Sclerosis

The cause of multiple sclerosis is unknown, but there appears to be a genetic tendency toward developing this and other autoimmune diseases. Some evidence suggests that a childhood viral infection, perhaps measles or a type of herpes infection, may initiate the immune response. It has been suggested that a breakdown in the blood–brain barrier during the time of the viral infection may have allowed a B-cell lymphocyte, developed against the virus, to gain entrance to and colonize the brain. An IgG clone (IgG from one B-cell line) is often present in the CSF of an individual with multiple sclerosis. These clones increase in number with the many exacerbations of the disease.

In support of this theory are observations that viral infections and multiple sclerosis occur more frequently in individuals who live at northern latitudes. An individual's risk of developing multiple sclerosis appears to be related to the latitude in which the individual lived for approximately the first 15 years of life, with those from northern latitudes most at risk.

Clinical Manifestations

- Early symptoms include fatigue, gait disturbance, vertigo, sensory loss, nystagmus, weakness in the lower extremities, spasticity, bladder problems, and optic neuritis.
- Episodes of motor, visual, or sensory disturbances that partially resolve and then recur.
- Bladder dysfunction may occur with some types of multiple sclerosis.
- Some individuals may develop cognitive or emotional disorders.
- Symptoms are frequently precipitated by stress. Stressors may include the birth of an infant, illness, fever, fatigue, or high temperatures.

Diagnostic Tools

- Clonal IgG bands in the CSF are found using electrophoresis techniques in approximately 90% of patients.
- Elevations in other types of CSF and plasma IgG are frequently present.
- MRI, and to a lesser degree CT scans, may allow for visualization of CNS plaques. MRI may identify disease activity even in the absence of acute clinical findings, and is capable of differentiating between old and new lesions.
- Techniques to measure muscle cell discharge will demonstrate delayed muscle excitation in some types of the disease.
- Visual evoked potential (VEP) to measure impulse transmission across nerve fibers (slowed in demyelinated areas).

Complications

- Severe neurologic deficits including loss of sight, increasing fatigue, and intellectual deterioration may develop over the course of the disease.
- Depression, loss of social support, family and spousal stress, and financial problems are common.

Treatment

- Aggressive immunosuppressant therapy at the start of the disease and with any exacerbation may limit the autoimmune destruction of the neuron or myelin.
- Antiviral drugs may slow the progress of the disease.
- Disease-modifying drugs such as interferon beta-1b and glatiramer acetate to slow progression.
- Antineoplastic drug, mitoxantrone, to suppress T-cell, B-cell, and macrophage activity.
- Natalizumab, a lab produced monoclonal agent, is available in limited and restricted distribution programs. It inhibits movement of damaged immune cells across the blood–brain barrier.
- Education on bladder training, sexual functioning, and avoidance of complications associated with reduced mobility may increase lifestyle satisfaction and overall health.
- Education regarding the need to avoid chronic fatigue and high temperatures may reduce symptoms.
- Innovative drug therapies are being tried that aim to foster antigenic self-tolerance by providing myelin protein for ingestion. These therapies are based on the hypothesis that an individual may tolerate (not attack in an immune response) a substance that enters the body through the GI tract.

AMYOTROPHIC LATERAL SCLEROSIS

Amyotrophic lateral sclerosis (ALS) is a rapidly progressing degenerative disease of the upper and lower motor neurons resulting in near total paralysis. The loss of motor neurons does not include CNs III, IV, and VI. Therefore, some facial movements, including blinking, are maintained. ALS is also known as Lou Gehrig disease and usually occurs in the fourth or fifth decade of life. The disease is usually fatal within 3 to 5 years, although some individuals may live longer. Degeneration of the motor neurons occurs without any obvious inflammation. Although the myelin is not a primary site of degeneration, loss of the nerve axon causes the subsequent loss of myelin, and scarring occurs. No known cause of ALS has been identified, although viral infection, metabolic disturbances, and trauma have been suggested. In addition, there is a familial form of ALS, which affects approximately 10% of ALS patients. Recent evidence suggests that a genetic link may be present in substantially more cases as well.

Clinical Manifestations

- Subtle onset and slowly progressive.
- Initial painless weakness develops in one muscle group, which progresses to weakness and paralysis in all skeletal muscles except the extraocular muscles.
- Spasticity, cramping, fatigue, fasciculations, dysarthria, dysphagia, and dyspnea.
- Intellectual and sensory functioning remains normal until death.

Complications

- ALS may be difficult to diagnose. Once confirmed, depression may occur. In many cases, severe family hardship develops as the disease progresses quickly.
- Aspiration, pneumonia, and respiratory problems as the muscles grow weaker.

Diagnostic Tools

Diagnosis is based on test findings and clinical presentations after other possible causes have been excluded. There is no specific tool for diagnosis but the following findings are consistent with a diagnosis.

- Muscle biopsy demonstrates lower neuron degeneration and small angulated atrophic fibers which confirms a strong clinical diagnosis.
- Creatine kinase (CK) is elevated.
- EMG findings include muscle fibrillations and fasciculations.
- Serial muscle testing reveals motor strength deficits.

Treatment

- Riluzole may extend survival time.
- Psychological support is essential for the individual and family, as is education on maintaining eye communication.
- Respiratory support.
- End-of-life care.

MYASTHENIA GRAVIS

Myasthenia gravis is a peripheral nervous system disorder characterized by autoantibody production against the receptors for acetylcholine present on the motor end-plate region of skeletal muscles. The IgG autoantibodies competitively bind to the AChRs, prevent acetylcholine from binding to the receptors, and therefore prevent muscle contraction. Eventually, receptors at the neuromuscular junction are destroyed.

Myasthenia gravis may first cause weakness of the muscles controlling eye movements (ocular myasthenia gravis) or may affect the entire body (generalized myasthenia gravis). Progression of the disease is variable and may be slowly progressing, with or without remissions, or rapidly progressing, leading to death by respiratory paralysis and failure.

The cause of myasthenia gravis is unknown but appears to be associated with a familial tendency toward developing autoimmune disease. The thymus gland is frequently hyperplastic and appears to function as it did in early childhood, suggesting it may be initiating or perpetuating the immune response.

Clinical Manifestations

- Weakness of the muscles of the eyes, causing ptosis (drooping of the eyelids), diplopia, ocular palsies.
- Poor posture.
- Respiratory compromise.
- Loss of bowel and bladder control.
- Muscle achiness, paresthesias, decreased smell and taste.
- Weakness of face, neck, and throat muscles, causing difficulty eating and swallowing.
- Continued spread of muscle weakness. Initially there is easy fatigue with recovery of strength after rest. Eventually there is no recovery of strength after rest.

Diagnostic Tools

- Normally acetylcholine is broken down at the neuromuscular junction by the enzyme acetylcholinesterase. A clinical diagnosis of myasthenia gravis can be confirmed on the basis of the return of muscle strength after intravenous administration of a medication that prevents the activity of acetylcholinesterase, thereby prolonging the half-life of acetylcholine. This medication, edrophonium chloride (Tensilon), allows acetylcholine to have a better chance of binding to its receptors, allowing voluntary muscle contraction. The effect of Tensilon lasts several minutes, after which muscle weakness reappears.
- Testing for AChR antibodies are elevated with myasthenia. A positive finding confirms the diagnosis, but a negative result does not rule out myasthenia.
- CT scan to determine if a thymoma is present.

- EMG measurements of skeletal muscle action potentials show reduced amplitude on motor neuron stimulation.

Complications

- Myasthenic crisis, characterized by severe worsening of skeletal muscle function culminating in respiratory distress and death as the diaphragm and intercostal muscles become paralyzed, may occur after a stressful experience such as an illness, emotional upset, surgery, or during pregnancy.
- Cholinergic crisis is a toxic response occasionally seen with the use of too much anticholinesterase drug. A hypercholinergic state characterized by increased intestinal motility, pupillary constriction, and bradycardia can develop. The individual may develop nausea, vomiting, sweating, and diarrhea. Respiratory distress may occur.

Treatment

- Frequent rest periods during the day conserve strength.
- Anticholinesterase medications are provided to prolong the half-life of acetylcholine at the neuromuscular junction. The medications must be taken on schedule each day to prevent muscle fatigue and collapse.
- Anti-inflammatory medications are used to limit the autoimmune attack.
- Immunosuppressants or chemotherapeutic agents to control symptoms.
- A myasthenic crisis may be treated with additional medication, and respiratory support if necessary.
- A cholinergic crisis is treated with atropine (acetylcholine blocker) and respiratory support, until symptoms resolve. Anticholinesterase therapy is withheld until toxic levels of the drug are reversed.
- Myasthenia crisis and cholinergic crisis present similarly but are treated differently. Tensilon administration is used to differentiate between the two disorders.
- Plasmapheresis (blood dialysis with the removal of IgG antibodies) and thymectomy (surgical removal of the thymus) are sometimes performed, with variable long-term results.
- Thymectomy may facilitate remission although it may not be immediately effective.

GUILLAIN-BARRÉ SYNDROME

Guillain-Barré (GB) syndrome is a peripheral nervous system disease characterized by the sudden onset of muscle paralysis or paresis. GB results from an autoimmune attack against the myelin surrounding the peripheral nerves. With destruction of the myelin, the axons can be damaged. Symptoms of GB disappear as the autoimmune attack ceases and the axons regenerate. If destruction of the cell body occurred during the attack, some degree of disability may remain. Although the cause of GB is unknown, the disease usually occurs 1 to 4 weeks after a viral infection or immunization. Possible explanations for the link between a viral illness and GB are: (1) viral illnesses cause an autoimmune response that may interfere with T-suppressor cell circuits, (2) if the viral causative agent has surface cell markers similar to myelin the body may accidentally attack itself, or (3) the virus may actually invade the cranial and spinal nerves.

The muscles of the lower extremities are usually affected first, with paralysis advancing up the body. Respiratory muscles may be affected, leading to respiratory collapse. Cardiovascular function may be impaired because of the interruption of autonomic nerve function.

Clinical Manifestations

- Ascending muscle weakness or paralysis.
- "Crawling-skin" sensation.
- Decreased or absent deep tendon reflexes.
- Ataxia.
- Respiratory compromise.
- Autonomic manifestations such as labile blood pressure, cardiac dysrhythmias.

Diagnostic Tools

- Nerve conduction tests will demonstrate neuronal dysfunction.
- Peripheral blood tests reveal leukocytosis early in the illness.
- Electrophysiologic studies (EPSs) reveal demyelinating neuropathy.
- Elevated protein in the CSF is common.
- CT and/or MRI may be done to rule out other causes.

Complications

- Respiratory or cardiovascular collapse may cause death.
- Weakness of some muscles may persist.

Treatment

- Plasmapheresis or immunoglobulin therapy.
- Ventilator support may be required if the respiratory muscles are affected.
- Anti-inflammatory medications may limit the autoimmune attack.

SPINA BIFIDA

Spina bifida is a congenital neural tube defect characterized by a failure of the vertebral arches to close. This results in a cystlike protrusion of the meninges alone (meningocele) or of the meninges and the spinal cord (myelomeningocele) out of the vertebral column. In the case of a meningocele, neural tissue is unexposed, and thus neural deficits are absent or minor. With a myelomeningocele, the spinal cord, in a cystlike protrusion with its nerves, suffers injury, inflammation, and scarring. The result is some loss of neural function, often including paralysis. Another type of spina bifida is one in which minor irregularities in the vertebral arches exist that are not obvious at birth. This is called spina bifida occulta (hidden).

A meningocele can occur in any area of the spine; cranial or upper cervical meningoceles are frequently associated with hydrocephalus. A myelomeningocele typically occurs in the lumbar or lumbosacral area.

Causes of Spina Bifida

Although the cause of spina bifida is unknown, a genetic predisposition may exist. Increased risk of the disorder occurs with maternal folic acid deficiency. Folic acid deficiency is common in women; therefore, it is strongly recommended that all women anticipating pregnancy begin taking folic acid vitamin supplements at least 3 months before conception.

Clinical Manifestations

Spina bifida occulta may be asymptomatic or associated with:

- Hair growth along the spine
- Midline dimple, usually in the lumbosacral area
- Gait or foot abnormalities
- Poor bladder control

A meningocele may be asymptomatic or associated with:

- A saclike protrusion of meninges and CSF from the back
- Clubbed foot
- Gait disturbance
- Bladder incontinence

A myelomeningocele is associated with:

- Protrusion of meninges, CSF, and spinal cord
- Neurologic deficits at and below the site of exposure

Diagnostic Tools

- Elevated levels of a fetal protein, called alpha-fetoprotein, in maternal serum may indicate fetal spina bifida.
- Ultrasound may diagnose the condition in utero.

Complications

- Hydrocephalus may occur with a meningocele or myelomeningocele.

Treatment

- No treatment may be required for spina bifida occulta or meningocele.
- Surgical repair of the myelomeningocele, and sometimes the meningocele, is required.
- If surgical repair is performed, placement of a shunt to allow for CSF drainage is necessary to prevent hydrocephalus and a subsequent increase in ICP.
- Planned cesarean section before the initiation of labor can be important in reducing the neurologic damage seen in an infant with a spinal cord defect.

HYDROCEPHALUS

Hydrocephalus (water on the brain) is characterized by an accumulation of CSF anywhere in the ventricles of the brain. Hydrocephalus may result from overproduction of CSF, obstruction of the flow of CSF within the ventricular system, or a decrease in the absorption of CSF out of the ventricles. Hydrocephalus can be apparent with a sonogram before birth, or it may develop in adulthood. In adults, hydrocephalus may develop suddenly after a head injury or slowly in response to a growing tumor.

Types of Hydrocephalus

There are two types of hydrocephalus: noncommunicating and communicating.

Noncommunicating Hydrocephalus

Noncommunicating hydrocephalus occurs as a result of obstruction of CSF flow within the ventricular system. This type of hydrocephalus may occur with a tumor or as a result of a congenital irregularity in the ventricular pathways.

Communicating Hydrocephalus

Communicating hydrocephalus occurs as a result of a blockage in the absorption of CSF. Causes of this type of hydrocephalus include a buildup of tissue (usually a neoplasm) or blood in the subarachnoid space. Head injuries may cause communicating hydrocephalus.

Effect of Hydrocephalus

ICP increases with hydrocephalus; this can directly injure underlying nervous tissue and compromise cerebral blood flow and the neuronal supply of oxygen and glucose. Compensation for increased ICP may occur with slowly developing hydrocephalus. With an acute brain injury, rapidly developing hydrocephalus dramatically increases ICP and compensation is usually ineffective.

Clinical Manifestations

- Newborns with hydrocephalus may have an enlarged head and a high-pitched cry.
- Acutely developing hydrocephalus causes a rapid increase in ICP and may present with a severe headache, decreased consciousness, papilledema, and vomiting.
- Slowly progressing hydrocephalus may present with irritability and changes in cognition and behavior.

Diagnostic Tools

- Ultrasound may allow diagnosis in utero.
- After birth, diagnosis is made by clinical inspection, measurements of head circumference, and observation of cranial suture lines.

Complications

- Mental retardation may result.

Treatment

- Placement of a shunt to drain CSF in utero or after birth may be performed.
- Treatment of the underlying cause is required.

CEREBRAL PALSY

Cerebral palsy (CP) is brain damage that occurs in an infant before, during, or soon after birth. It results in some degree of motor dysfunction. CP is non-progressive and is caused by cerebral hypoxia or increased ICP after physical trauma to the brain. Increased ICP may directly damage neuronal cells or may cause hypoxia by compressing the blood vessels. Frequently, hemorrhage is the cause of increased ICP.

There are several different types of CP. The most common, spastic CP, involves motor neurons and cerebral cortex injury. Dyskinetic CP involves injury to the basal ganglia or extrapyramidal tracts and ataxic CP involves the truncal muscles. There is a small percentage of individuals who have a mixed-variety disorder.

Clinical Manifestations

- CP may result in a motor deficiency in any or all limbs and usually involves muscle spasticity.
- Vision disturbances, mental impairment, and seizures may occur.
- Spastic CP: rigid extremities, clonus, exaggerated deep tendon reflexes, increased muscle tone, contractures, scoliosis.
- Dyskinetic CP: poor fine motor coordination, jerky movements that are rigid and uncontrolled.
- Ataxic CP: gait disturbances, instability, hypotonia at birth progressing to stiffness of truncal muscles.

Diagnostic Tools

- Typically, the infant is diagnosed based on clinical signs at birth or in early infancy.

Complications

- Developmental and social delays are common and may lead to family and marital stress.

Treatment

- Treatment depends on the extent of the physical impairment, mental status, and the occurrence of seizures. Surgery may be required to relieve contractions.
- All treatment regimens must include physical therapy.
- Counseling is important for the family and the child.

P PEDIATRIC CONSIDERATIONS

- Seizures in infants and young children brought on by a rapid increase in body temperature, also known as febrile convulsions, are common. Children who have febrile seizures do not appear to experience any long-term intellectual, academic, or behavioral effects.
- Falls are a major cause of head injuries in children. Head injuries in toddlers often are related to falls down the stairs or in playgrounds. An infant or young child who receives a head injury should be evaluated for nonaccidental head injury, often referred to as shaken-baby syndrome. This type of injury occurs from violently shaking an

infant or small child, and usually involves striking the head of the child against a hard surface. This type of injury is characterized by subdural or subarachnoid hemorrhage.

 GERIATIC CONSIDERATIONS

• Delirium is often confused with dementia. Delirium has a more abrupt onset, is secondary to a temporary source, and is usually reversed after the cause is removed.

• The prevalence of epilepsy increases with age. After age 70, it occurs two times more often than in the pediatric population and after 80 years of age it occurs three times more often.

• Falls are also a major cause of head injuries in the elderly. Falls may be related to poor vision, slippery rugs or tubs, and poor muscle strength in the elderly population. An elderly person who receives a head injury also may be the victim of elder abuse.

SELECTED BIBLIOGRAPHY

Alverzo, J. P. (2007). Improving stroke outcomes: Rehabilitation strategies that work. *American Journal of Nursing*, 107(11), 72B–72D, 72F.

Amato, M. P. (2005). Donepezil for memory impairment in multiple sclerosis. *Lancet Neurology*, 4, 72–73.

American Academy of Neurology. (2006). Practice parameters: Parkinson disease diagnosis and treatment. *Journal Watch*, 66, 968–975.

Arbelaez, J. J., Ariyo, A. A., Crum, R. M., Fried, L. P., & Ford, D. E. (2007). Depressive symptoms, inflammation, and ischemic stroke in older adults: A prospective analysis in the cardiovascular health study. *Journal of American Geriatrics Society*, 55(11), 1825–1830.

Atkinson, S. B., Carr, R., Maybee, P., & Haynes, D. (2006). The challenges of managing and treating: Guillain-Barre syndrome during the acute phase. *Dimensions of Critical Care Nursing*, 25(6), 256–263.

Berg, A., Bellander, B., Wanecek, M., Norberg, A., Ungerstedt, U., Rooyackers, O. et al. (2008). The pattern of amino acid exchange across the brain is unaffected by intravenous glutamine supplementation in head trauma patients. *Clinical Nutrition*, 27, 816–821.

Birks, J., Grimley Evans, J., Iakovidou, V., Tsolaki, M., & Holt, F. E. (2009). Rivastigmine for Alzheimer's disease. *Cochran Database of Systemic Reviews* 2009, Issue 2. Art. No.: CD001191. DOI: 10.1002/14651858. CO001191.pub2.

Boling, W., Aghakhani, Y., Andermann, F., Sziklas, V., & Olivier, A. (2009). Surgical treatment of independent bitemporal lobe epilepsy defined by invasive recordings. *Journal of Neurology, Neurosurgery, and Psychiatry*, 80, 533–538.

Campanini, I., Merlo, A., & Farina, D. (2009). Motor unit discharge pattern and conduction velocity in patients with upper motor neuron syndrome. *Journal of Electromyography and Kinesiology*, 19, 22–29.

Cosi, V., & Versino, M. (2006). Guillain-Barre syndrome. *Neurological Sciences*, 27(1), S47–S51.

Denke, N. J. (2008). Brain injury in sports. *Journal of Emergency Nursing*, 34(4), 363–364.

Dirks, R. P., & Valovich McLeod, T. C. (2008). Sport-related mild traumatic brain injury. *Clinician Reviews*, 18(9), 18–24.

Eliopoulos, C. (2010). *Gerontological nursing* (7th ed.). Philadelphia: Lippincott Williams & Wilkins.

Fick, D. M., & Mion, L. C. (2008). Delirium superimposed on dementia. *American Journal of Nursing*, 108(1), 52–60.

Gilman, S. (1998). Imaging the brain: First of two parts. *New England Journal of Medicine*, 338, 812–820.

Gilman, S. (1998). Imaging the brain: Second of two parts. *New England Journal of Medicine*, 338, 889–896.

Goldberg, M. S. (2007). *CBO testimony. Statement of Matthew S. Goldberg, Deputy Assistant Director for National Security: Projecting costs to care for veterans of U. S. military operations in Iraq and Afghanistan*. Washington, D. C.: Congressional Budget Office.

Huether, S., & McCance, K. (2008). *Understanding pathophysiology* (4th ed.). St. Louis: Mosby Elsevier.

Ignatavicius, D. D., & Workman, M. L. (2010). *Medical-surgical nursing: Patient-centered collaborative care* (6th ed.). St. Louis: Saunders Elsevier.

Krupp, L. B., Christodoulou, C., Melville, R. N., Scherl, W. F., McAllister, W. S., & Elkin, L. E. (2004). Donepezil improved memory in multiple sclerosis in a randomized clinical trial. *Neurology*, 63, 1579–1585.

Luggen, A. S. (2009). Epileptic seizures in older adult patients, part I. *The Clinical Advisor*, 12(3), 23–26.

Luggen, A. S. (2009). Epileptic seizures in older adult patients, part II. *The Clinical Advisor*, 12(4), 26–28, 32–35.

Marrie, R. A., Horwitz, R., Cutter, G., Tyry, T., Campagnolo, D., & Vollmer, T. (2009). Comorbidity delays diagnosis and increases disability at diagnosis in MS. *Neurology*, 72, 117–124.

Martin, E. M., Lu, W. C., Helmick, K., French, L., & Warden, D. L. (2008). Traumatic brain injuries sustained in the Afghanistan and Iraq wars. *American Journal of Nursing*, 108(4), 40–47.

Olson, D. (2008). Paroxysmal events: Differentiating epileptic seizures from nonepileptic spells. *Consultant*, 48(11), 857–859, 863–864, 866–867.

Osborn, K. S., Wraa, C. E., & Watson, A. B. (2010). *Medical-surgical nursing: Preparation for practice*. Upper Saddle River, NJ: Pearson.

Patton, K. T., & Thibodeau, G. T. (2010). *Anatomy and physiology* (7th ed.). St. Louis: Mosby Elsevier.

Peiffer, K. M. Z. (2007). Brain death and organ procurement. *American Journal of Nursing*, 107(3), 58–66.

Peskind, E. R., Tangalos, E. G., & Grossberg, G. T. (2005). A case-based approach to Alzheimer's disease. *Clinical Advisor*, June, 34–46.

Porth, C. M., & Matfin, G. (2009). *Pathophysiology: Concepts of altered health states* (8th ed.). Philadelphia: Lippincott Williams & Wilkins.

Rossom, R., Adityanjee, & Dysken M. (2004). Efficacy and tolerability of memantine in the treatment of dementia. *American Journal of Geriatric Pharmacotherapy*, 2, 303–312.

Sherwood, P. R., Crago, E. A., Spiro, R. M., & Okonkwo, D. (2007). Cervical spine injuries: Preserving function, improving outcomes. *American Nurse Today*, 2(9), 26–29.

Skirton, H. (2005). Huntington disease: A nursing perspective. *Medsurg Nursing*, 14, 167–172.

Smith, C., & Hale, L. (2007). The unique nature of fatigue in multiple sclerosis: Prevalence, pathophysiology, contributing factors and subjective experience. *Physical Therapy Review*, 12, 43–51.

Soares, D. P., & Law, M. (2009). Magnetic resonance spectroscopy of the brain: Review of metabolites and clinical applications. *Clinical Radiology*, 64, 12–21.

Stone, M. B. (2009). Ultrasound diagnosis of papilledema and increased intracranial pressure in pseudotumor cerebri. *American Journal of Emergency Medicine*, 27, 376e1–376e2.

Stowe, R., Ives, N., Clarke, C. E., van Hilten, Ferreira, J., Hawker, R. J., et al. Dopamine agonist therapy in early Parkinson's disease. *Cochran Database of Systemic Reviews* 2008, Issue 2. Art. No.: CD006564. DOI: 10.1002/14651858.CD006564.pub2.

Trapp, B. D., Peterson, J., Ransohoff, R. M., Rudick, R., Mork, S., & Bo, L. (1998). Axonal transection in the lesions of multiple sclerosis. *New England Journal of Medicine*, 338, 278–285.

Tseng, B. P., Kitazawa, M., & LaFerla, F. M. (2004). Amyloid beta-peptide: The inside story. *Current Alzheimer Research*, 1, 231–239.

Umeda, S., Akine, Y., Kato, M., Muramatsu, T., Mimura, M., Kandatsu, S. et al. (2005). Functional network in the prefrontal cortex during episodic memory retrieval. *Neuroimage*, 26, 932–940.

Webber, K. M., Perry, G., Smith, M. A., & Casadesus, G. (2007). The contribution of luteinizing hormone to Alzheimer disease pathogenesis. *Clinical Medicine and Research*, 5(3), 177–183.

Wolf, C. A., Wijdicks, E. F., Bamlet, W. R., & McClelland, R. L. (2007). Further validation of the FOUR score coma scale by intensive care nurses. *Mayo Clinic Proceedings*, 82(4), 435–438.

The Endocrine System

The endocrine system, along with the nervous system, is a chemical communication and coordination system. There are three components to the endocrine system: endocrine glands that secrete chemical messengers into the bloodstream; the chemical messengers themselves, called hormones; and the target cells or organs that respond to the hormones (see Table 9-1). The major functions of the endocrine system include:

- Regulation of digestion
- Storage and use of nutrients
- Electrolyte and water metabolism
- Growth and development
- Reproduction
- Synthesis, storage, and secretion of hormones.

● Physiologic Concepts

ENDOCRINE GLANDS

Endocrine glands are organs that synthesize, store, and secrete hormones into the bloodstream. There are many endocrine glands in the body, including the hypothalamus, pituitary gland, adrenal glands, gonads, pineal gland, thymus, pancreas, thyroid, and parathyroid. Other hormone-secreting organs include the kidneys (erythropoietin), heart (atrial natriuretic factor), and gut (peptide hormones). The endocrine glands reviewed in this chapter are the hypothalamus,

Gland	Hormone(s)	Target Cells
Hypothalamus	Thyrotropin-releasing hormone (TRH)	Anterior pituitary
	Corticotropin-releasing hormone (CRH)	Anterior pituitary
	Gonadotropin-releasing hormone (GnRH)	Anterior pituitary
	Growth hormone–releasing hormone (GHRH)	Anterior pituitary
	Somatostatin	Pituitary, pancreas, GI tract
	Dopamine	Anterior pituitary
Anterior pituitary (adenohypophysis)	Growth hormone (GH)	Systemic
	Adrenocorticotropic hormone (ACTH)	Adrenal cortex
	Thyroid-stimulating hormone (TSH)	Thyroid
	Follicle-stimulating hormone (FSH)	Ovaries, testes
	Luteinizing hormone (LH)	Ovaries
	Prolactin	Mammary glands
	Melanocyte-stimulating hormone	Skin, hair
Posterior pituitary (neurohypophysis)	Antidiuretic hormone (ADH)	Kidney
	Oxytocin	Breast, uterus, testes
Thyroid gland	Thyroxine (T_4)	Systemic
	Triiodothyronine (T_3)	Systemic
	Thyrocalcitonin (calcitonin)	Bone
Parathyroid gland	Parathyroid hormone (PTH)	Bone, kidney, intestine
Adrenal glands (cortex)	Mineralocorticosteriods (mainly aldosterone)	Kidneys
	Glucocorticoids (mainly cortisol)	Most tissues have receptors
	Adrenal androgens	Gonads
Adrenal glands (medulla)	Epinephrine	Cardiac muscle, smooth muscle, glands

TABLE 9-1 Endocrine Glands, Hormones, and Target Cells

table continues on page 308

TABLE 9-1 Endocrine Glands, Hormones, and Target Cells (continued)		
Gland	**Hormone(s)**	**Target Cells**
	Norepinephrine	Sympathetic nervous system
Pancreas	Insulin	Muscles, tissues
	Glucagon	Liver
	Somatostatin	
Gonads (males)	Androgens (testosterone)	Gonads, muscle tissue
Gonads (females)	Inhibin	Ovaries, pituitary, placenta
	Oestrogens (estrogen)	Breasts, uterus
Corpus luteum	Testosterone	Endometrium
	Progesterone	Endometrium
Placenta	Human chorionic gonadotropin (HCG)	Endometrium
	Human placental lactogen (hPL)	Placenta
	Progesterone	Placenta
	Corticotropin-releasing hormone (CRH)	Placenta
Kidneys	Calcitriol (1,25-dihydroxy-vitamin D)	Intestine
	Renin	Kidneys
	Erythropoietin (EPO)	Bone marrow
Gastrointestinal tract	Gastrin	Stomach
	Enterogastrone	Stomach
	Secretin	Liver, pancreas
	Pancreozymin	Pancreas
	Ghrelin	Pituitary
	Cholecystokinin (CCK)	Gallbladder
Liver	Insulin-like growth factor	Nerve, muscle, other cells
	Angiotensinogen	Vascular, brain, kidneys, adrenals
	Thrombopoietin	Bone marrow, platelets
Brain	Peptide hormones	Brain, nervous system
Heart	Atrial-natriuretic peptide (ANP)	Heart

Gland	Hormone(s)	Target Cells
Adipose tissue	Leptin	Brain, nervous cells
	Resistin	Adipose cells
Bones	Osteocalcin	Pancreas, fat cells
Skin	Calciferol (Vitamin D)	Kidneys, intestines, bones

the anterior and posterior pituitary glands, and the glands that function as target organs for the pituitary hormones.

The Hypothalamus

The hypothalamus is a small area of the brain located in the section of the forebrain called the diencephalon. The hypothalamus is a neural and an endocrine organ functioning to maintain homeostasis in the body's internal environment. The hypothalamus is also essential in controlling behavior and allowing appropriate responses to multiple incoming stimuli. It continually receives information from the central and peripheral nervous systems concerning temperature, pain, pleasure, feeding, hunger, body mass, and metabolic status. It also receives input from other hormones of the body and receives neural extensions from other areas of the brain.

The hypothalamus, in turn, responds to all the incoming stimuli by sending neural projections throughout the brain and by synthesizing and secreting its own hormones. Nerve cell bodies in the ventral hypothalamus synthesize several hormones and send them in axon projections to be released into the blood and delivered to the anterior pituitary gland. Other nerve cell bodies in the hypothalamus synthesize hormones that are sent down via axon projections to the posterior pituitary, where they are stored until they are eventually released into the bloodstream. Regulatory hormones include thyrotropin-releasing hormone (TRH), gonadotropin-releasing hormone (GnRH), growth hormone–releasing hormone (GHRH), growth hormone–inhibiting hormone (GHIH) somatostatin, corticotropin-releasing hormone (CRH), prolactin-inhibiting hormone (PIH), and melanocyte-inhibiting hormone (MIH). The two routes by which the hypothalamus controls hormone release by the anterior and posterior pituitary are shown in Figure 9-1.

The Anterior Pituitary

The anterior pituitary, also called the adenohypophysis, is composed of non-neural tissue. It is anatomically separate from the hypothalamus, but functionally connected to it through its blood supply. The anterior pituitary receives its blood through venous drainage from the hypothalamus. When blood flowing in a vein breaks into another capillary network instead of flowing back to the vena cava,

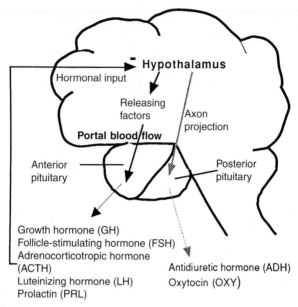

FIGURE 9-1 The hypothalamic–pituitary system. The hypothalamus is connected through the blood to the anterior pituitary while the posterior pituitary is a neural outgrowth.

the system is called a portal venous system. Thus, the hypothalamus and the anterior pituitary are connected by the **hypothalamic–anterior pituitary portal blood flow system**. Because this blood has already been used by the hypothalamus, it is poorly oxygenated but rich in hormonal messages put out by the hypothalamus into the median eminence (see later). The anterior pituitary is, therefore, a major target organ for hypothalamic hormones and responds to these hormones with the release of its own hormones that stimulate various glands or produces a primary effect on cells with mediation of other endocrine glands.

The Posterior Pituitary

The posterior pituitary, also called the neurohypophysis, is true neural tissue derived embryologically from the hypothalamus. There are three parts to the posterior pituitary: the median eminence (sometimes considered hypothalamic tissue), into which the hypothalamus secretes the anterior pituitary–releasing hormones; the infundibular stem connecting the hypothalamus with the posterior pituitary; and the infundibular process, which is the terminal end of the posterior pituitary.

Nerve cell bodies in the supraoptic and paraventricular nuclei of the hypothalamus synthesize two hormones: antidiuretic hormone (ADH), also called vasopressin, and oxytocin. The hypothalamus sends these hormones in axon projections through the infundibular stem to the infundibular process. They are stored there until the hypothalamus stimulates them to be released into the general circulation. Thus, the hormones released by the posterior pituitary are hypothalamic in origin and depend on the hypothalamus for their release.

Target Glands

The third group of endocrine glands discussed in this chapter consists of those outside the brain that respond to the anterior and posterior pituitary hormones with the release of their own hormones. These glands are the target organs of the pituitary hormones and include the thyroid gland, the adrenal gland, and the testes and ovaries. The pancreas, which secretes insulin, is also an endocrine gland and is discussed in Chapter 16.

HORMONES

A hormone is a chemical messenger released by an endocrine gland into the circulation. Once released, a hormone travels in the bloodstream and affects only cells in the body that have receptors (binding sites) specific to it. Cells that respond to a particular hormone are called **target cells** for that hormone. Many hormones may be necessary to initiate a single function and conversely, a single hormone may influence many different tissues in the body.

Typically, a hormone is released in bursts from an endocrine gland in a pattern that often follows an inherent daily (diurnal) rhythm. The burst of hormone release can be increased or decreased above or below baseline level by various inputs to the gland. Inputs that affect hormone release involve: (1) stimulation by another hormone or neurotransmitter, or (2) stimulation caused by a decrease or increase in a certain ion or nutrient. Examples of hormones that cause an increase or decrease in another hormone's release include all the hypothalamic hormones affecting the anterior pituitary. Examples of neurotransmitters affecting a hormone's release include the release of insulin in response to epinephrine and norepinephrine stimulation. Ions that influence the release of a hormone include calcium ion's effect on parathyroid hormone, and sodium ion's effect on aldosterone. Nutrients that affect the release of hormones include the amino acids that stimulate the release of insulin and growth hormone (GH). Frequently, one endocrine gland is stimulated simultaneously by several different inputs.

There are three broad categories of hormones: peptide, steroid, and amino acid. Most hormones, including all the hypothalamic and pituitary hormones, are peptide hormones. The steroid hormones are made from cholesterol and are soluble across the cell membrane. The amino acid hormones are made from the amino acid tyrosine. A fourth category, the fatty acid derivatives, includes the retinoids and eicosanoids.

Peptide Hormones

Peptide hormones range in size from a few amino acids to relatively large protein complexes. Peptide hormones circulate in the plasma to their target organs and exert their effects by binding to specific receptors present on the outside of target cell membranes. By binding to its receptor, a protein hormone changes the cell's permeability to water, electrolytes, or organic molecules such as glucose, or causes the activation of intracellular messengers, which then causes enzyme activation or protein synthesis. Examples of intracellular messengers include the G proteins, which many protein hormones first activate during receptor binding, and the second messengers such as cyclic adenosine monophosphate (cyclic AMP) and calcium, which are subsequently activated by the G proteins. Peptide hormones include hypothalamic-releasing and -inhibiting hormones and factors, anterior pituitary protein hormones, posterior pituitary hormones, hormones of digestion and metabolism (Chapters 15, 16), hormones of blood pressure and electrolyte balance (Chapters 13, 19), hormone for red blood cell development (Chapters 12, 19), and hormone to modulate stress and pain (Chapters 6, 8, 9).

Steroid Hormones

Steroid hormones are cholesterol-based, lipid-soluble molecules produced by the adrenal cortex and the sex organs. Because steroid hormones are lipid-soluble, they can cross the cell membrane and bind to receptors or carriers inside the cell. Once inside a cell, the steroid hormone travels to the cell nucleus, where it influences the cell by affecting DNA replication, transcription of DNA into RNA, or translation of RNA into proteins. Because this is a lengthy process, steroid hormone responses typically take longer to occur than responses caused by nonsteroid hormones. Steroid hormones are discussed in this chapter and in Chapter 20. Steroid hormones include gonadal hormones, estrogens, progesterones, androgens, and hormones of the adrenal cortex.

Amine Hormones

The amine hormones are derivatives of the amino acid tyrosine and include thyroid hormone (TH) and the catecholamines (epinephrine, norepinephrine, and dopamine). Epinephrine, norepinephrine, and dopamine also act as neurotransmitters in the central and peripheral nervous systems. The catecholamine hormones travel in the blood to their target cell and bind to the plasma membrane at specific receptor sites. Binding of catecholamine activates the cyclic AMP second messenger system and alters enzyme activity or membrane permeability. TH travels in the blood mostly bound to carrier proteins with a smaller amount circulating free. Once at the target cell, free TH crosses the cell membrane and binds to the nuclear DNA, directly affecting DNA transcription. Therefore, free hormone, although lesser in quantity, is the active hormone. Amine hormones include aldosterone, glucocorticoids, androgens, and estrogens.

FEEDBACK

In the endocrine system, feedback refers to the response of a target tissue after stimulation by a specific hormone which then influences the continued release of that hormone. Each hormone is stimulated to be released by a specific signal. Once released, a hormone affects its target organ, causing a response that usually reduces further hormone release. This type of feedback, shown in Figure 9-2, is called negative feedback, and allows tight control over hormone levels. Positive feedback is uncommon and occurs when the response by a target

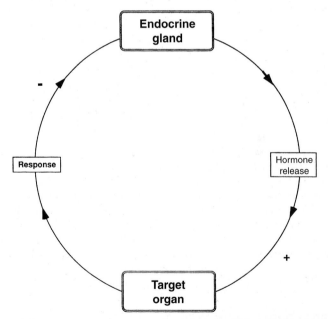

F I G U R E   9 - 2 A typical negative feedback cycle in which an endocrine gland releases a hormone, which then stimulates (+) its target organ to respond in such a way that further secretion of the hormone by the endocrine gland is reduced (–).

tissue to hormonal stimulation increases the further release of that hormone. The feedback mechanism is a series of reactions that work to achieve homeostasis by neuroregulatory mechanisms. The central nervous system (CNS) receives input that is transmitted to the hypothalamus. The hypothalamus then produces and releases either releasing or inhibiting factors that are transported to the pituitary. In the pituitary, releasing or inhibiting factors release or inhibit specific hormones. The anterior pituitary responds by controlling secretion of hormones from target organs or tissues.

FACTORS CONTROLLING HORMONE SECRETION

Factors Controlling Anterior Pituitary Hormone Secretion

The stimuli that control the secretion of the pituitary hormones (except melanocyte-stimulating hormone) are the hormones secreted by the hypothalamus that travel in the portal blood to the anterior pituitary. These hormones are hypothalamic-releasing or hypothalamic-inhibiting hormones, depending on whether they increase or decrease the release of the pituitary hormone they control. When a hypothalamic-releasing hormone is secreted, its corresponding anterior pituitary hormone is released. When a hypothalamic-inhibiting hormone is secreted, it inhibits synthesis and release of the anterior pituitary hormone over which it has control. Once secreted, the pituitary hormones act to stimulate another target organ or cell to perform a function or release a hormone of its own.

The pituitary hormone and the subsequent response to it by its target organ may feed back on the hypothalamus to decrease further release of the hypothalamic hormone. The target organ response may also inhibit further release of the pituitary hormone.

Factors Controlling Hypothalamic Hormone Secretion

For the hypothalamic–pituitary hormonal system, the hypothalamus ultimately determines whether a hormone will be secreted. The hypothalamic-releasing or -inhibiting hormones are secreted at a baseline level that can be increased or decreased as a result of the integration of many neural inputs to the hypothalamus. The inputs are related to stress, pain, body weight, temperature, emotions, and various hormones released by target organs. All these influences can be excitatory or inhibitory for each releasing or inhibiting hormone.

TARGET ORGAN HORMONES

Thyroid Hormone

TH is an amine hormone synthesized and released from the thyroid gland. It is made when one or two iodine molecules are joined to a large glycoprotein called thyroglobulin, which is synthesized in the thyroid gland and contains the amino acid tyrosine. These iodine-containing complexes are called iodotyrosines. Two iodotyrosines then combine to form two types of circulating TH, called T_3 (triiodothyronine) and T_4 (thyroxine). T_3 and T_4 differ in the total number of iodine molecules they contain (three for T_3 and four for T_4). Approximately 90% of the TH released into the bloodstream is T_4, but T_3 is physiologically more potent. A diet adequate in iodine and protein is necessary for T_3 and T_4 to be produced in adequate amounts. TH is stored in the thyroid gland as a colloid compound until needed. In passage through the liver and kidney, most T_4 is converted to T_3. T_3 and T_4 are carried to their target cells in the blood bound to a plasma protein, but enter the cell as free hormone. T_3 and T_4 collectively are referred to as TH.

Effects of Thyroid Hormone

Target cells for TH include almost all cells of the body. Effects of TH are listed below.

- Stimulates metabolic rate of all target cells by increasing the metabolism of protein, fat, and carbohydrate (primary function).
- Stimulates the rate of the sodium–potassium pump in its target cells.
- Increases utilization of energy by the cells, thereby increasing basal metabolic rate (BMR), burning calories, and increasing heat production by each cell (as a result of the two effects listed above).
- Increases sensitivity of target cells to catecholamines, thus increasing heart rate and causing heightened emotional responsiveness.
- Increases rate of depolarization of skeletal muscle, which increases the speed of skeletal muscle contractions, often leading to a fine tremor.
- Essential for normal growth and development of all cells of the body and is required for the function of GH.
- Increases red blood cell production.

Factors Controlling Thyroid Hormone Secretion

The stimulus for the secretion of TH is thyroid-stimulating hormone (TSH), released into the bloodstream from the anterior pituitary. The stimulus for the release of TSH is thyroid-releasing hormone (TRH), secreted from the hypothalamus into the portal bloodstream. TH appears to act in a negative feedback manner on the hypothalamus, to decrease the further release of TRH, and on the pituitary, to decrease the release of TSH. TSH may also act on the hypothalamus to decrease further release of TRH.

Factors Controlling Thyroid-Releasing Hormone Secretion

The stimuli responsible for increasing TRH secretion include exposure of the body to cold temperature, physical and perhaps psychological stress, and low

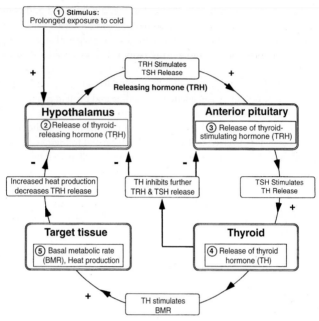

FIGURE 9-3 Feedback: thyroid hormone.

levels of TH. When the secretion of TRH is stimulated by cold temperature, the result is an increase in TH, which increases BMR, thereby increasing body heat and reducing the demand for a further increase in TRH (Fig. 9-3). This is an example of negative feedback.

Glucocorticoids

Glucocorticoids are steroid hormones released from the cortex (outer layer) of the adrenal gland that affect many aspects of metabolism, especially glucose metabolism. In humans, the main glucocorticoid is cortisol. The glucocorticoids also affect many other systems of the body, including the cardiovascular and immune systems. Glucocorticoids are released in a diurnal (daily) manner, peaking in the early morning hours.

Effects of the Glucocorticoids

The major effects of glucocorticoids are listed below. Many of these glucocorticoid effects are essential in times of trauma and stress. They allow one to survive blood loss, periods of hunger or starvation, or prolonged exposure to environmental extremes.

- Increase the level of blood glucose by stimulating gluconeogenesis (conversion in the liver of fats and proteins into glucose).
- Increase blood glucose levels by stimulating muscle, adipose (fat), and lymphatic tissues to use free fatty acids for energy instead of glucose.
- Stimulate protein breakdown and inhibit protein synthesis in all body cells.
- Stimulate hunger, promote fat buildup in the trunk and face, and inhibit growth by suppressing GH and antagonizing the effects of GH on protein synthesis.
- Increase the effect of GH on adipose tissue and increase the effect of TH on its target tissues.
- Increase the effects of the catecholamines, causing increased heart rate and blood pressure.
- Nonmetabolic effect that occurs with high circulating levels of cortisol include inhibition of immune and inflammatory functions by blocking almost every component of the immune and inflammatory responses including depressed cytotoxic T-cell function and suppression of the production, release, and activation of many chemical mediators of inflammation, including interleukins, prostaglandins, and histamine. Levels of cortisol high enough to inhibit immune and inflammatory function may be reached with pharmacologic administration of cortisol for immunosuppression, with tumors of the adrenal gland, or with long-term stress.
- Major effect on emotional stability and mood.

Factors Controlling Glucocorticoid Release

Glucocorticoids are released from the adrenal gland in response to circulating adrenocorticotropic hormone (ACTH) from the anterior pituitary. ACTH is released in response to CRH carried in the portal blood from the hypothalamus. CRH also stimulates the release of endorphins by the anterior pituitary and perhaps elsewhere. When released, glucocorticoids feed back on the hypothalamus and on the anterior pituitary to decrease the further release of CRH and ACTH, respectively.

Factors Controlling Corticotropin-Releasing Hormone

CRH is secreted from the hypothalamus in a diurnal pattern that sets the subsequent release pattern of ACTH and cortisol. Stimuli for an increase in CRH include stress, hypoglycemia (low blood glucose), and decreased circulating levels of glucocorticoids. The feedback cycle of CRH release in response to hypoglycemia is shown in Figure 9-4.

Other Effects of Adrenocorticotropic Hormone

Adrenal androgens are released in response to ACTH stimulation of the adrenal gland. Adrenal androgens are the primary source of androgens in women and

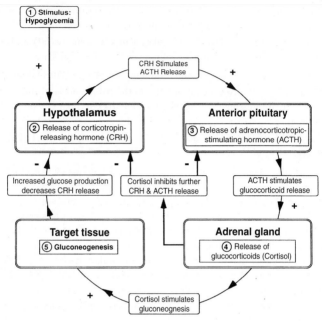

FIGURE 9-4 Feedback: glucocorticoids.

children. High levels of ACTH can result in masculinization of women and children. ACTH is similar in structure to another anterior pituitary hormone, melanin-stimulating hormone (MSH), which causes the cells of the skin to produce the tanning substance melanin. High levels of ACTH can have crossover effects on the skin and cause bronzing. A limited amount of ACTH appears essential for the synthesis of another adrenal cortical hormone, aldosterone. Without aldosterone, salt wasting and death occur.

Growth Hormone

GH, also called somatotropin, is a protein hormone released in a diurnal pattern over 24 hours. Approximately 70% of daily secretion occurs in a burst 1 to 4 hours after the onset of sleep. Accelerated GH release occurs during puberty and pregnancy.

Effects of Growth Hormone

GH effects are listed below.

- Increases protein synthesis in all cells of the body, especially muscle cells.
- Stimulates the growth of cartilage and activity of osteoblasts, the bone-producing cells of the body.

- Essential for longitudinal bone growth and for the continual remodeling of bone which occurs throughout life. Effects of GH on bone and cartilage occur through intermediary peptides, called somatomedins or insulin-like growth factors (IGFs), released from the liver in response to GH.
- Directly stimulates the growth of almost all other organs of the body, including the heart muscle, skin, and endocrine glands.
- Causes breakdown of fats and subsequent use of fatty acids for energy. Because fats are being used as an energy source, GH results in increased circulating blood glucose.
- Induces insensitivity to insulin. With decreased sensitivity to insulin, most cells will not transport glucose intracellularly, further increasing plasma glucose levels.

Factors Controlling Growth Hormone Release

GH is released from the anterior pituitary in response to a balance between two hypothalamic hormones: growth hormone–releasing hormone (GHRH) and growth hormone–inhibiting hormone, also called somatostatin. GH acts in a negative feedback manner on the hypothalamus to decrease further release of GHRH.

Factors Controlling Growth Hormone–Releasing Hormone

Increased GHRH occurs in response to increased levels of circulating amino acids, hypoglycemia, fasting or starvation, physical and emotional stress, and decreased GH. Exercise stimulates the release of GHRH, directly or through the effects of hypoglycemia and physical stress. The reproductive hormones (estrogen and testosterone) appear to increase secretion of GH, either by acting directly on the pituitary or through stimulation of GHRH. The feedback pattern of GHRH secretion in response to increased plasma amino acids is shown in Figure 9-5.

Factors Controlling Somatostatin Release

The hypothalamus releases an inhibitory hormone for GH, called somatostatin. Somatostatin is released in response to high blood glucose, free fatty acids, obesity, and cortisol. Emotional influences—including stress—stimulate somatostatin, most likely through increased cortisol, thereby reducing growth.

Gonadotropins

The gonadotropins include two anterior pituitary hormones: follicle-stimulating hormone (FSH) and luteinizing hormone (LH). Target tissues of FSH and LH are the ovary in women and the testis in men (Chapter 20).

Effects of the Gonadotropins

In response to FSH and LH in women, the ovary secretes the steroid hormones estrogen and progesterone. Estrogen feeds back on the hypothalamus and

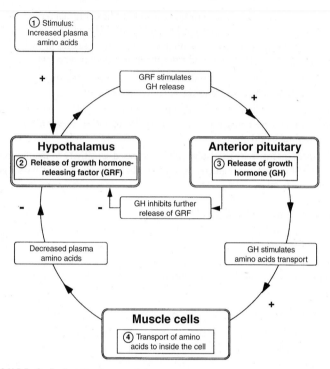

FIGURE 9-5 Feedback: growth hormone.

anterior pituitary in a complicated manner, with a negative effect on increasing the release of FSH and a positive effect on the release of LH, ultimately resulting in ovulation (the rupture of an ovarian follicle). With ovulation, the egg, also called the ovum, is released (Chapter 20) and becomes available for fertilization by a sperm. Progesterone appears to feed back on the anterior pituitary to limit secretion of FSH and LH.

In men, FSH stimulates cells of the testis to initiate and support spermatogenesis (production of sperm). The cells of the testis predominantly affected by FSH in the male are the Sertoli cells. Sertoli cells make up the inner lining of the seminiferous tubules, the site of spermatogenesis, and are important in providing nutrients to the developing sperm (Chapter 20). A hormone produced by Sertoli cells, inhibin, influences the production of testosterone by acting directly on the pituitary gland to decrease the release of FSH.

LH is also released from the anterior pituitary in men. LH causes interstitial cells of the testes to produce and secrete testosterone. Estrogen and testosterone are also synthesized by the adrenal gland, in men and women, in response to stimulation by ACTH.

Factors Controlling Gonadotropin Release

The gonadotropins are released from the pituitary in response to GnRH from the hypothalamus. It appears that one hypothalamic hormone controls the release of both of the pituitary gonadotropins. GnRH is sometimes referred to as luteinizing hormone–releasing hormone (LHRH). An increase in GnRH synthesis and release causes the onset of puberty.

Factors Controlling Gonadotropin-Releasing Hormone

Before puberty, circulating GnRH is very low. With maturation of the hypothalamus and perhaps attainment of a certain body mass, GnRH increases and initiates puberty. After sexual maturation has been established, the circulating level of GnRH is controlled in a negative feedback manner by estrogen and testosterone. Stress, starvation, and fear may affect the release of GnRH at any time, influencing the release of estrogen and progesterone in females and testosterone in males, and altering reproductive function.

Estrogens

Estrogens are steroid hormones that affect their target tissues by altering the rate of DNA replication, DNA transcription, or RNA translation. Although the effects of estrogens are most apparent in females, males also produce and are affected by estrogens. There are three main types of estrogens in humans: estrone, estradiol, and estriol.

Effects of estrogens include the following:

- Development in utero of female internal and external sex organs.
- Female distribution of body fat.
- Pigmentation of the nipples.
- Stimulation of breast development during pregnancy.
- Stimulation of growth of the endometrial lining of the uterus each month to prepare for implantation of the embryo.
- Maintenance of pregnancy.
- Stimulation of lactation.
- Stimulation of bone formation throughout life in males and females.
- Limiting bone resorption (breakdown) by direct action on bone or by limiting bone response to parathyroid hormone in males and females.
- Affecting liver protein production of lipoproteins (stimulates HDL, decreases LDL), coagulation factors, and carrier molecules for steroid hormones and thyroxine in males and females.
- Acting to reduce the risk of coronary artery disease, most likely as a result of increasing HDL, in males and females.
- Stimulating the kidneys to retain sodium in males and females.

- Influencing brain neural signaling in males and females, affecting behavior and mood.
- Estrogen excess in men can cause gynecomastia (breast enlargement).

Progesterone

Progesterone, like estrogen, is a steroid hormone. In women, progesterone is synthesized by thecal cells of the developing follicle, and later the corpus luteum, in response to stimulation by LH and, to a lesser extent, FSH.

Effects of progesterone include the following:

- Progesterone is released from an ovarian follicle after the follicle has ruptured during ovulation. It causes the endometrial lining of the uterus to become secretory in anticipation of fertilization of the ovum and embryo implantation, with the result that blood vessels in the endometrium begin to branch and glands begin secreting a thin glycogen-rich fluid. The ruptured follicle becomes the corpus luteum, which continues progesterone secretion.
- If the ovum is fertilized and the embryo implants in the uterus, the corpus luteum and later the placenta maintain the pregnancy by secreting progesterone. If progesterone decreases, the pregnancy terminates.
- If pregnancy does not occur, the corpus luteum degenerates over the next 14 days, progesterone levels decline, and menstruation (sloughing off of the uterine lining) occurs.
- Progesterone works with estrogen and prolactin to stimulate breast development during puberty and pregnancy.
- Progesterone relaxes smooth muscles, including the uterus and the vascular smooth muscle of the arterioles.
- Progesterone appears to be protective against some cancers.

Testosterone

Testosterone, also a steroid hormone, is the most abundant of the powerful androgen hormones. Testosterone synthesis occurs in specialized cells of the testes called Leydig cells, and in the adrenal gland in women.

Effects of testosterone include the following:

- Development in utero of male internal and external sex organs.
- Maintenance of sperm production throughout a man's lifetime.
- Stimulation and maintenance of male distribution of muscle.
- Stimulation of bone formation throughout life in males and females.
- Stimulation of red blood cell formation in males and females.
- Stimulation of anabolism (buildup) of proteins in males and females.

- Involvement in brain neural signaling, affecting behavior and mood, in males and females.
- Testosterone excess in women can cause clitoral enlargement, voice deepening, and beard development.

Prolactin

Prolactin is a protein hormone released from the anterior pituitary. It is also known as a lactogenic hormone.

Effects of Prolactin

When a girl reaches puberty, prolactin acts in concert with estrogen, progesterone, and GH to promote breast tissue development. Each of these hormones increases dramatically during pregnancy, resulting in further stimulation of breast development. After the birth of an infant, prolactin acts on the breast to stimulate lactation (milk production), allowing the infant to breastfeed. In postpartum women, the posterior hypothalamic hormone oxytocin works in concert with prolactin and is required for successful breastfeeding.

In nonpregnant women, high prolactin levels inhibit the release of two other anterior pituitary hormones: FSH and LH. Because FSH and LH are essential for ovulation and pregnancy, high prolactin in women who breastfeed full time may offer some protection against another pregnancy occurring.

The role of prolactin in men has not been identified, although recent evidence suggests that, in men and women, prolactin may affect the immune system, possibly by modulating the release of certain cytokines.

Factors Controlling Prolactin Release

The secretion of prolactin from the anterior pituitary is controlled by release of a prolactin-inhibitory hormone (PIH) from the hypothalamus, recently identified as the catecholamine dopamine. A decrease in the release of dopamine stimulates prolactin release. There may also be a prolactin-stimulating hormone released from the hypothalamus, although it is yet to be identified.

Stimulation for increased prolactin during pregnancy appears to be an estrogen-dependent decrease in the hypothalamic release of PIH. The suckling of the mother's nipple during breastfeeding by the infant stimulates prolactin release after pregnancy—stimulation of the nipple by suckling appears to cause increased prolactin by decreasing the hypothalamic release of PIH.

The major hypothalamic and anterior pituitary hormones and their target organ effects are listed in Figure 9-6.

Antidiuretic Hormone

ADH is a protein hormone made in the supraoptic nuclei of the hypothalamus and stored in and released from the posterior pituitary. It is also called vasopressin, which means vascular tensor.

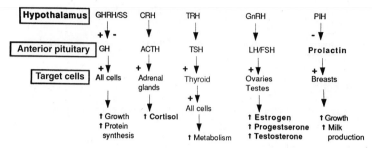

FIGURE 9-6 The major hypothalamic and anterior pituitary hormones. Note that decreased PIH increases prolactin release.

Effects of Antidiuretic Hormone

ADH causes the cells of the renal collecting ducts to become more water permeable. This increases the reabsorption of water into the blood, decreasing urine diuresis (flow). This is the antidiuretic effect of ADH (Chapter 18). At very high levels, ADH causes vascular smooth muscle contraction, increasing total peripheral resistance and blood pressure (Chapter 13). This is the major vasoactive effect.

Factors Controlling Antidiuretic Hormone Release

The major stimulus for ADH release is increased plasma osmolality (increased solute concentration). Increased plasma osmolality is sensed by osmoreceptors in the hypothalamus. Normal plasma osmolality is approximately 280 mOsm/kg. ADH-induced antidiuresis returns a high plasma osmolality toward normal by diluting the plasma (increasing its water concentration), as shown in Figure 9-7.

Other stimuli for ADH release include decreased blood pressure (sensed by the carotid and aortic baroreceptors), stress, pain, and exercise. ADH secretion is inhibited by decreased plasma osmolality, increased blood pressure, and alcohol.

Oxytocin

Oxytocin is a protein hormone made in the paraventricular nuclei of the hypothalamus and stored in and released from the posterior pituitary.

Effects of Oxytocin

Oxytocin stimulates contraction of the smooth muscle lining of the milk ducts of the breast, causing increased intramammary pressure and subsequent letdown of stored milk into the nipples.

Oxytocin also stimulates contraction of the uterine smooth muscle. Its exact role in initiating labor in a pregnant woman is unclear. However, it causes

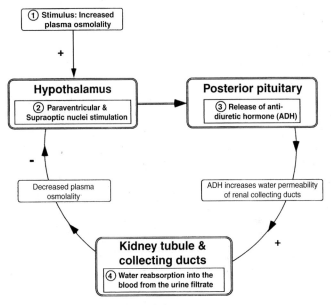

FIGURE 9-7 Feedback: antidiuretic hormone.

increased intensity of uterine contractions as labor progresses and delivery approaches. The drug Pitocin is a derivative of oxytocin and is used clinically to initiate and speed labor.

Factors Controlling Oxytocin Release

The primary stimulus for the release of oxytocin is suckling on the nipple of the breast in women. As shown in Figure 9-8, suckling leads to milk let-down, which allows the infant to feed. As the drive for suckling is reduced, the stimulus for oxytocin release is decreased and milk letdown slows; this is a clear example of negative feedback. Stress or fear may inhibit synthesis of oxytocin.

● Pathophysiologic Concepts

HYPOPITUITARISM

Hypopituitarism refers to the low secretion of any anterior pituitary hormone. Panhypopituitarism refers to low secretion of all anterior pituitary hormones. Clinical manifestations include reproductive malfunction, growth failure, de-creased bone density, and morbid obesity. It can be misinterpreted as child

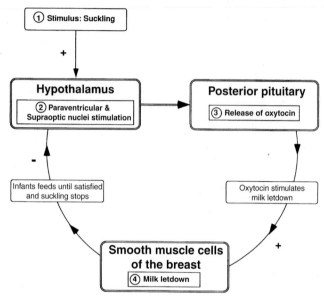

FIGURE 9-8 Feedback: oxytocin.

abuse or neglect. Hypopituitarism can result from malfunction of the pituitary gland or the hypothalamus. Causes include:

- Infection or inflammation.
- Autoimmune disease.
- A tumor (adenoma). Typically, a tumor of one type of hormone-producing cell expands to the point that it begins to interfere with the function of other hormone-producing cells, leading to reduced secretion of one or more other hormones.
- Feedback from a malfunctioning target organ; for example, reduced secretion of TSH from the pituitary would occur if a diseased thyroid gland were secreting excessively high levels of TH.
- Hypoxic necrosis (death caused by lack of oxygen) of the pituitary or hypothalamus resulting from decreased blood flow or decreased oxygenation. Hypoxia can destroy any or all of the hormone-producing cells. An example of this is Sheehan syndrome, which develops following maternal hemorrhage during or after birth.
- Trauma. A traumatic brain injury, surgery, or radiation of the pituitary may damage the gland.
- Genetic abnormalities.

HYPERPITUITARISM

Hyperpituitarism is the excess secretion of an anterior pituitary hormone. Hyperpituitarism typically involves just one of the pituitary hormones; the other pituitary hormones are often secreted in reduced levels. Prolactin-producing tumors are the most common and result in problems with fertility and lactation. Hyperpituitarism can result from malfunction of the pituitary gland or the hypothalamus. Causes include:

- A primary adenoma of one type of hormone-producing cell, usually GH, ACTH, or the prolactin-producing cells.
- A lack of feedback from a target gland; for example, increased TSH may occur in response to decreased or absent secretion of TH by the thyroid gland.

● Conditions of Disease or Injury

HYPOTHYROIDISM

Hypothyroidism results from decreased levels of circulating TH. Hypothyroidism is characterized by myxedema, the nonpitting, boggy edema that develops around the eyes, feet, and hands and infiltrates other tissues as well. Hypothyroidism may result from malfunction of the thyroid gland, the pituitary, or the hypothalamus. If it results from thyroid gland malfunction, low TH levels are accompanied by high TSH and high TRH because of the lack of negative feedback on the pituitary and hypothalamus by TH. If hypothyroidism results from pituitary malfunction, low levels of TH are caused by low TSH. TRH from the hypothalamus is high because there is no negative feedback on its release by TSH or TH. Hypothyroidism caused by hypothalamic malfunction results in low TH, low TSH, and low TRH. Medically induced hypothyroidism may follow previous thyroid therapy or surgery, radioiodine therapy, or drugs such as cytokines, amiodarone, and lithium. Other causes may include radiation, thyroidectomy, congenital hypothyroidism, thyroid gland atrophy, discontinuation of hormone therapy, or aging.

Diseases of Hypothyroidism

- Hashimoto disease, also called autoimmune thyroiditis, results from autoantibody destruction of thyroid gland tissue. This results in decreased TH, with increased TSH and TRH levels caused by minimal negative feedback. The cause of autoimmune thyroiditis is unknown, but there appears to be a genetic tendency to develop the disease.
- Endemic goiter is hypothyroidism caused by a dietary deficiency of iodide. A goiter is an enlargement of the thyroid gland. Goiter occurs with a

deficiency of iodide because the thyroid cells become overactive and hypertrophic (larger) in an attempt to sequester all possible iodide from the bloodstream. Low TH levels are accompanied by high TSH and TRH because negative feedback is minimal.

- Thyroid carcinoma may cause hypothyroidism or hyperthyroidism. Treatment of this rare cancer may include thyroidectomy, TSH suppression drugs, or radioactive iodine therapy to destroy thyroid tissue. All of these treatments may result in hypothyroidism. Exposure to radiation, especially during childhood, is a cause of thyroid cancer. Iodine deficiency may also increase the risk of developing thyroid cancer because it stimulates thyroid cell proliferation and hyperplasia.

Clinical Manifestations

- Sluggishness, slow thinking, and clumsy, slow movements.
- Bradycardia, enlarged heart (myxedemic heart), and decreased cardiac output.
- Bogginess and edema of the skin, especially under the eyes and in the ankles.
- Intolerance to cold temperatures.
- Decreased metabolic rate, decreased caloric requirements, decreased appetite and nutrient absorption across the gut.
- Constipation.
- Weight gain (mild to moderate).
- Change in reproductive function.
- Dry, flaky skin and brittle, thin body and head hair.
- Depression.
- Decreased TH and increased TSH.

Diagnostic Tools

- A good history and physical examination will help diagnose hypothyroidism.
- Blood tests measuring levels of TH (both T_3 and T_4), TSH, and TRH will allow diagnosis of the condition and localization of the problem at the level of the CNS or the thyroid gland. Decreased T_3 and T_4 with an elevated TSH indicate a problem with the thyroid gland while low levels of T_3, T_4, and TSH would suggest a pituitary gland problem.
- Unbound thyroxine (FT_4) in the blood is the best indicator of thyroxine levels.
- Thyroid scanning with a radioactive isotope to evaluate nodules, most of which are benign.
- Ultrasound to evaluate the size, shape, and consistency of nodules.
- Fine-needle biopsy to determine if the nodule is benign or malignant.

Complications

- Myxedema coma is a life-threatening situation characterized by exacerbation (worsening) of all symptoms of hypothyroidism, including hypothermia without shivering, hypotension, hypoglycemia, hypoventilation, and a decrease in consciousness resulting in coma.
- Elevated cholesterol and triglycerides and atherosclerosis may occur.
- Death can occur without TH replacement and stabilization of symptoms.
- There are also risks associated with the treatment of thyroid deficiency. These risks include hormone over-replacement, anxiety, muscle wasting, osteoporosis, and atrial fibrillation.

Treatment

The goal of treatment is to return the patient to a euthyroid state.

- Treatment includes replacement of TH with synthetic thyroxine.
- For endemic goiter, iodide replacement may relieve symptoms.
- If the cause of hypothyroidism is related to a CNS tumor, it may be treated with chemotherapy, radiation, or surgery.

HYPERTHYROIDISM

Hyperthyroidism refers to excessive levels of circulating TH that may produce the clinical syndrome called thyrotoxicosis. Hyperthyroidism can result from dysfunction of the thyroid gland, pituitary, or hypothalamus. Thyroid dysfunction may include nodules, thyroiditis, thyroid follicular cell hyperfunction, thyroid follicular cell destruction, or excessive ingestion of iodine or TH replacement. Increased TH caused by malfunction of the thyroid gland is accompanied by decreased TSH and TRF, as a result of the negative feedback on their release by TH. Hyperthyroidism caused by malfunction of the pituitary results in high TH and high TSH. TRF is low because of negative feedback from TH and TSH. Hyperthyroidism caused by malfunction of the hypothalamus shows high TH accompanied by excess TSH and TRH.

Diseases of Hyperthyroidism

Graves disease, the most common cause of hyperthyroidism, is an autoimmune disorder usually characterized by production of autoantibodies that mimic the action of TSH on the thyroid gland. These IgG autoantibodies, termed thyroid-stimulating immunoglobulins, turn on the production of TH, but are not inhibited by rising levels. TSH and TRH levels are low because they are inhibited by high TH. The cause of Graves disease is unknown; however, there appears to be a genetic predisposition to autoimmune disease. Women in their

20s and 30s are most often diagnosed, although the disease may start during the teen years.

Nodular goiter is an increase in the size of the thyroid gland caused by increased demand for TH. Increased demand for TH occurs during periods of growth or excess metabolic demand such as puberty or pregnancy. In these cases, increased TH is caused by metabolically driven activation of the hypothalamus, and therefore is accompanied by increased TRH and TSH. When the demand for TH is lessened, the thyroid gland usually returns to its previous size. Occasionally, irreversible changes may have occurred and the gland does not regress. The enlarged thyroid may continue to produce excess TH. If the individual remains hyperthyroid, the condition is referred to as a toxic nodular goiter. Pituitary adenomas of TSH-producing cells or hypothalamic diseases rarely occur.

Clinical Manifestations

- Tachycardia and palpitations.
- Increased muscle tone, tremors, irritability, increased sensitivity to catecholamines.
- Increased BMR and heat production, intolerance to heat, excess sweating.
- Weight loss, increased hunger.
- Hyperactivity.
- Fatigue and weakness.
- Insomnia.
- Altered concentration.
- A staring appearance.
- Exophthalmos (bulging of the eyes) may develop.
- Increased number of bowel movements.
- Goiter (usually), which is an increase in the size of the thyroid gland.
- Changes in skin and hair condition may occur.
- Amenorrhea or scant menses, reproductive irregularities.

Diagnostic Tools

- A good history and physical examination will help diagnose hyperthyroidism.
- Blood tests measuring levels of TH (both T_3 and T_4), TSH, and TRH will allow diagnosis of the condition and localization of the problem at the level of the CNS or the thyroid gland. Undetectable TSH is the best indicator of primary hyperthyroidism. T_3 and T_4 are elevated.
- Decreased serum lipids may accompany hyperthyroidism.
- Decreased sensitivity to insulin, which may result in hyperglycemia.

Complications

- Arrhythmias are common in patients with hyperthyroidism and may be the presenting symptom of the disorder. Any person complaining of arrhythmia should be evaluated for thyroid disorder.
- A life-threatening complication of hyperthyroidism is thyrotoxic crisis (thyroid storm), which may develop spontaneously in patients with hyperthyroidism undergoing therapy or during surgery on the thyroid gland, or may occur in undiagnosed patients with hyperthyroidism. The result is a large burst of TH release that causes tachycardia, agitation, tremors, hyperthermia (up to 106°F), and, if untreated, death.

Treatment

Treatment depends on the site and cause of hyperthyroidism.

- If the problem is at the level of the thyroid gland, treatment usually involves antithyroid drugs that block TH production or beta-blocking drugs to decrease sympathetic hyperresponsiveness. Drugs that destroy thyroid tissue may also be used. For instance, radioactive iodine (I^{131}) administered in oral form is actively taken up by hyperactive thyroid cells. Once incorporated, I^{131} destroys the cells. This is a permanent treatment for hyperthyroidism and frequently results in the individual becoming hypothyroid and requiring lifelong TH replacement.
- Partial or total thyroidectomy may be a treatment choice. Total thyroidectomy results in hypothyroidism, as may partial thyroidectomy.
- Percutaneous ethanol injection of the thyroid is used for patients with benign thyroid nodule and those with increased surgical risk due to cardiac or pulmonary diseases, advanced age, multimorbidity, or dialysis.
- Beta-blockers may be given to treat the symptoms.

ADRENAL INSUFFICIENCY

Adrenal insufficiency is a decrease in the circulating level of the glucocorticoids. The mineralocorticoid aldosterone may also be reduced. Adrenal insufficiency may be caused by dysfunction of the adrenal gland, called primary adrenal insufficiency. Dysfunction of the pituitary or hypothalamus or chronic corticosteroid therapy may cause secondary adrenal insufficiency.

Primary adrenal insufficiency is characterized by low levels of glucocorticoids, especially cortisol, accompanied by high ACTH and high CRH because there is no negative feedback on their release. Adrenal androgens and aldosterone levels may be normal, increased, or decreased depending on the cause of the glucocorticoid deficiency.

If the entire adrenal gland is destroyed or malfunctioning, adrenal androgens and aldosterone will be low. If only the glucocorticoid-secreting cells are malfunctioning, the high ACTH levels that accompany primary adrenal insufficiency will cause high levels of circulating adrenal androgens. Aldosterone secretion is primarily determined by the renin–angiotensin system, but may be slightly increased by elevated ACTH.

If the cause of adrenal insufficiency is secondary to a pituitary dysfunction, low glucocorticoids will be accompanied by low ACTH and high CRH. In this case, adrenal androgens will also be low. If there is zero ACTH, aldosterone levels will be reduced. If adrenal insufficiency is caused by a hypothalamus malfunction, the glucocorticoids, ACTH, and CRH will be low.

Diseases of Adrenal Insufficiency

Primary adrenal insufficiency, called Addison disease, occurs from destruction of the adrenal cortex. The disease is usually autoimmune, and results from IgG antibodies directed against all or part of the adrenal gland. Addison disease may also result from infections such as tuberculosis. Tuberculosis of the adrenal gland is a common cause of adrenal insufficiency in developing countries and does not typically resolve with treatment of the infection. Destructive adrenal gland tumors may also lead to adrenal insufficiency. Because it is a chronic metabolic condition, lifelong hormone replacement therapy (HRT) is required.

Addison disease is characterized by low glucocorticoid levels accompanied by high ACTH and high CRH. Total loss of the adrenal gland results in the loss of adrenal androgens and aldosterone as well. Aldosterone deficiency leads to increased loss of sodium in the urine, resulting in hyponatremia (decreased sodium in the blood), dehydration, and hypotension (because water loss in the urine frequently accompanies the loss of sodium). Decreased potassium excretion in the urine will lead to hyperkalemia (increased potassium concentration in the blood).

Secondary adrenal insufficiency can occur as a result of hypopituitarism or hypothalamic dysfunction. With secondary adrenal insufficiency, ACTH is not released, so the adrenals do not secrete glucocorticoids or androgens. Aldosterone synthesis may also be affected.

Secondary adrenal insufficiency can occur if cortisol is used therapeutically for anti-inflammatory purposes. When one takes pharmacologic levels of corticosteroids, the pituitary secretion of ACTH is inhibited in a negative feedback manner. If the prescribed medication is abruptly discontinued, the pituitary remains in a refractory period and does not secrete ACTH for an extended period of time. Even a few weeks of oral glucocorticoid therapy can result in the suppression of ACTH, and hence secondary adrenal insufficiency, for several months. Judicious treatment of inflammatory illnesses with glucocorticoids for fewer than approximately 10 days will not result in pituitary suppression.

Clinical Manifestations

- Depression, because cortisol levels influence mood and emotions.
- Severe and chronic fatigue, related to hypoglycemia, and decreased gluconeogenesis.
- Anorexia, vomiting, diarrhea, nausea, and weight loss.
- Hyperpigmentation of the skin if ACTH levels are high (primary adrenal insufficiency) as a result of ACTH having MSH-like effects on the skin.
- Sparse body hair in women, if the adrenal cells producing androgens are destroyed or if ACTH levels are very low.
- Altered menstrual cycles.
- Inability to respond to stressful situations, perhaps leading to severe hypotension and shock.
- Mineralocorticoid deficiency → urinary loss of sodium, chloride, water → hyponatremia, extracellular fluid loss, decreased cardiac output, hyperkalemia.
- Salt craving.
- Orthostatic hypotension.
- Lethargy, weakness, and fever.

Diagnostic Tools

- A good history and physical examination will help diagnose glucocorticoid deficiency.
- Blood tests measuring levels of CRH, ACTH, and different glucocorticoids will allow diagnosis of the condition and localization of the problem at the level of the CNS or adrenal gland.
- The most specific test is the short ACTH stimulation test. Inability to respond to synthetic cortisol is indicative of insufficiency.
- Abdominal CT scan of the adrenal glands may be helpful in determining the cause.
- 24-hour urine to detect alterations in the biosynthesis of adrenal cortical hormones.
- Hyponatremia, hyperkalemia, and hypotension may be present if the adrenal cells that produce aldosterone are destroyed or if ACTH levels are undetectable.

Complications

- Adrenal crisis may occur after physical or mental stress in an affected individual. This can be life-threatening and is characterized by volume depletion, hypotension, and vascular collapse.

Treatment

- Glucocorticoid replacement such as the use of hydrocortisone or cortisone acetate is required.
- Health providers should monitor the history of glucocorticoid dose adjustments; potential adverse events including any crisis since last visit; the individual's ability to cope with daily stressors; the individual's body weight; and signs that suggest over-replacement or under-replacement.
- Monitoring blood pressure, peripheral edema, serum sodium, serum potassium, and plasma renin activity provides clues to treatment efficacy.
- Aldosterone replacement (only in primary adrenal insufficiency) may be necessary.
- Glucocorticoid administration may need to be increased during periods of stress, including infection, trauma, and surgery. Morbidity and mortality are high without treatment.
- If the cause of adrenal insufficiency is related to a pituitary tumor, it may be treated with chemotherapy, radiation, or surgery.
- Androgen replacement may improve libido, sexual satisfaction, and overall sense of well-being in females with Addison disease.

GLUCOCORTICOID EXCESS

Glucocorticoid excess refers to any condition in which there are very high levels of circulating glucocorticoids. The cause of glucocorticoid excess may reside at the level of the adrenal gland or at the pituitary/hypothalamic level. If the cause of glucocorticoid excess is primary adrenal gland hypersecretion, there is usually an adrenal tumor present. In this situation, low ACTH and low CRH levels will be present as a result of negative feedback from high glucocorticoids. Adrenal androgen levels will be low because ACTH is low. Bronzing of the skin will not occur.

If glucocorticoid excess results from an adenoma of the pituitary cells producing ACTH, elevated ACTH will also cause excess adrenal androgen production. Bronzing of the skin will occur because of crossover effects between ACTH and MSH. CRH levels will be low as a result of negative feedback from ACTH and the glucocorticoids.

Excess ACTH may also occur as a result of the production of ACTH by a tumor outside of the pituitary or hypothalamus. This is referred to as an ectopic (abnormal) source of ACTH. Many tumors demonstrate ectopic production of ACTH, especially lung tumors. Excess adrenal androgens and skin bronzing will accompany ACTH-secreting tumors.

High levels of glucocorticoids also may result from chronic administration of high-dose corticosteroids, especially cortisol, for treatment of inflammatory conditions. Disease states in which long-term administration of corticosteroids occurs include asthma and several different autoimmune diseases.

Diseases of Excess Glucocorticoids

- Cushing's syndrome refers to any condition of high glucocorticoids and includes glucocorticoid excess caused by therapeutic administration of corticosteroids.
- Cushing disease refers to high glucocorticoid levels caused specifically by the malfunction of the anterior pituitary resulting in excess ACTH.

Clinical Manifestations

- Altered fat metabolism leading to fat pads on the back (subclavian buffalo hump), moon face, protruding abdomen with thin extremities, and stretch marks on breasts, thighs, and abdominal surface. Muscle weakness from protein breakdown.
- Acne and purple striae on the face.
- Hypertension as a result of increased catecholamine responsiveness. Eventually left ventricular hypertrophy will occur.
- Weight gain resulting from strong appetite stimulation. Because of effects on hepatic gluconeogenesis, a reversible form of diabetes mellitus may result.
- Inhibition of immune and inflammatory reactions, leading to poor wound healing.
- Extreme emotional swings (lability), sometimes causing psychosis and occasionally resulting in suicide.
- Masculinization of women and children as a result of adrenal androgen stimulation if ACTH levels are high.
- Bronzing of the skin if ACTH levels are high.
- Muscle wasting and pathologic fractures.

Diagnostic Tools

- A good history and physical examination will help diagnose glucocorticoid excess.
- Blood tests measuring levels of CRH, ACTH, and different glucocorticoids will allow diagnosis of the condition and localization of the problem at the level of the CNS or adrenal gland.
- Loss of normal diurnal (morning) pattern of cortisol release.
- Hyperglycemia, hypernatremia, and hypokalemia may be present because of aldosterone-like properties of the glucocorticoids. This can contribute to hypertension and cardiac and neural irregularities.

- A dexamethasone challenge test is commonly used in clinical practice to evaluate states of glucocorticoid excess. In healthy individuals, a low dose of dexamethasone will suppress ACTH secretion; in those with Cushing syndrome, suppression does not occur.
- 24-hour urine to detect free cortisol levels.
- CT scan or MRI to determine if a tumor is the cause.

Complications

- There are many complications of excess glucocorticoid levels. Morbidity and mortality are high without treatment and approximately 50% of individuals die within 5 years. Causes of death include suicide, overwhelming infections, and coronary artery disease from severe hypertension.
- Insulin resistance and hypertension may develop in those with glucocorticoid excess. These may be due to abnormal changes in hepatic fatty acid metabolism.

Treatment

- Correction of high glucocorticoid levels depends on the cause of the problem.
- Surgery for tumors of the adrenal, pituitary, or other tissue (e.g., the lung) is frequently performed. Radiation therapy is done if a tumor is present.
- Drugs that block steroid synthesis may be used if the tumor is inoperable.
- Discontinue corticosteroid therapy, by weaning down, if the syndrome is caused by medication.

CONGENITAL ADRENAL HYPERPLASIA

Congenital adrenal hyperplasia, also referred to as the adrenogenital syndrome, is the total or relative unresponsiveness of the adrenal glucocorticoid-producing cells to ACTH during gestation, resulting in very low levels of glucocorticoids and masculinization of the genitalia in a female fetus. Female masculinization occurs because the androgen-producing cells of the adrenal gland respond to the continuously high levels of ACTH resulting from little or no negative feedback on ACTH release. Congenital adrenal hyperplasia occurs as a result of an autosomal-recessive genetic alteration whereby there is a deficiency in one or more of the five enzymes needed to produce cortisol. Mineralocorticoid production (aldosterone) may be affected. The most common enzyme deficiencies are of 21-hydroxylase or 11β-hydroxylase. Enzyme deficiencies may be partial or total. Carriers of the disorder do not appear to be affected.

Clinical Manifestations

- Masculinization of the female infant is apparent at birth and may include ambiguous genitalia with an enlarged clitoris, fused labia, and malformation of the urogenital area. The degree of abnormality is variable. Male fetuses are usually normal at birth or have slightly enlarged genitalia.

- If aldosterone production is blocked, salt wasting, dehydration, vomiting, hyperkalemia, and hypotension develop.
- In the rare case of enzyme 11-deoxycorticosterone deficiency, mineralocorticoid levels increase, resulting in salt retention, hypokalemia, and hypertension.

Diagnostic Tools

- Physical examination at or soon after birth will help diagnose the condition in females.
- Blood tests will demonstrate enzyme deficiency in either sex.

Complications

- Because cortisol is essential to surviving even relatively minor stresses, illnesses or surgeries in the newborn period may be fatal if the diagnosis of congenital adrenal hyperplasia has not been made.
- Psychological distress to the child and family may result from delayed diagnosis.

Treatment

- Cortisol, and possibly aldosterone, replacement therapy will be required throughout life. Therapy must be monitored and adjusted appropriately for growth and in times of excess physical stress.
- Mineralocorticoid replacement for salt losers.
- Masculinized females may require reconstructive surgery. With successful treatment, sexual functioning and fertility will be unaffected.

PHEOCHROMOCYTOMA

A rare, but potentially dangerous tumor of the adrenal medulla is known as pheochromocytoma. It is a tumor of chromaffin tissue and can occur in other locations such as the sympathetic ganglia. The excessive production and secretion of catecholamines (epinephrine and norepinephrine) in response to sympathetic stimuli results in a hypermetabolic state with episodic or long-term hypertension which could be fatal.

Clinical Manifestations

- Hypertension accompanied by profuse sweating and nausea.
- Headache, palpitations, tachycardia.
- Nervousness, tremor, facial pallor, fatigue, and generalized gastrointestinal complaints may occur.

- Fever, weight loss, polyuria, and polydipsia caused by the hypermetabolic state.

Diagnostic Tools

- Classic triad of hypertension, headache, and tachycardia are highly indicative.
- 24-hour blood and urine to monitor catecholamine metabolites,
- Free or unconjugated catecholamine assays.
- CT scan or MRI to assess tumor size and location.

Complications

- Hypertensive episodes may be triggered by stress, medications, foods, tobacco, physical activity, excitement, or abdominal pressure.
- Uncontrolled hypertension can lead to organ damage or stroke.

Treatment

- Surgical removal of the tumor. If both adrenals are removed, treatment for adrenocorticoid insufficiency is necessary.
- Catecholamine blocking medications when surgery is not an option.

GROWTH HORMONE DEFICIENCY

GH deficiency is a decrease in circulating levels of GH and affects most cells of the body. GH deficiency is usually clinically recognized only in children. When an infant is born with midline craniocerebral defects such as cleft lip or cleft palate, GH deficiency should be ruled out because the development of the pituitary gland and the midline structures occur at the same stage of fetal development.

Typically, GH deficiency is caused by a pituitary adenoma of another anterior pituitary hormone–producing cell type. Other possible causes are listed below.

- It can be a result of hypoxic necrosis (death caused by lack of oxygen) and inflammation of the pituitary.
- The cause may be at the hypothalamic level, resulting from malnutrition, sleep deprivation, or stimulation of somatostatin released during periods of prolonged physical or emotional stress. For example, some studies suggest that growth potential may be reduced in adolescent female athletes as a result of intense physical exercise and reduced nutritional intake caused by dieting. Low estrogen levels are frequently seen in female athletes, which may also affect growth.
- GH deficiency may result from genetic abnormality, from defects of the brain present congenitally or following infection or trauma, or from cranial irradiation used in treatment for a brain tumor or for leukemia prophylaxis.

Diseases of Growth Hormone Deficiency

- Dwarfism.
- A reduction of growth potential may occur in children.
- Alteration in metabolic functioning, including insulin resistance and abnormal lipid profile, may occur in children and adults.

Clinical Manifestations

- In children, GH deficiency results in proportional short stature (below the third percentile for their age). Affected children have decreased muscle mass, increased subcutaneous fat stores, immature facial features, delayed skeletal maturation, and are typically bright mentally.
- Short stature different from predicted based on familial patterns may be observed if a reduction in growth potential occurs.
- If GH deficiency occurred in utero, boys may have micropenis and undescended testicles.
- Delayed onset of puberty may accompany GH deficiency, especially if abnormalities in the gonadotropins occur concomitantly.
- Delayed dental eruption, thin hair, and delayed nail growth.
- Adult-onset GH deficiency may result in nonspecific changes in functioning, including alterations in physical and mental well-being, cardiac function, and metabolic parameters.
- Adults with GH deficiency may experience lower levels of energy and libido.

Diagnostic Tools

- A good history and physical examination will help diagnose GH deficiency.
- Blood tests measuring decreased levels of GH will support diagnosis of the condition.
- Neuroimaging tests to identify pituitary tumors can improve diagnosis.
- Lack of responsiveness to GH provocation will assist in confirming GH deficiency.
- The best indicator of GH reserve is insulin-induced hypoglycemia.

Complications

- Increased arterial intima-media thickness, atherosclerotic plaques, and endothelial dysfunction.
- Increased cardiac mortality in adults with decreased GH.
- Associated cardiovascular and metabolic syndrome risk factors including central adiposity, increased visceral fat, dyslipidemia, and insulin resistance.
- Elevated C-reactive protein (CRP) and interleukin-6.

Treatment

- Treatment of GH deficiency in children involves subcutaneous injections of recombinant GH several times per week during the pubertal years or earlier. Success is greater in children treated early.
- GH deficiency in adults may also be treated with GH injections.

GROWTH HORMONE EXCESS

GH excess is the increase in circulating levels of GH. Increased levels of GH stimulate the liver to produce IGF-1. Together, these two hormones cause the upregulation of bone, cartilage, and other tissues. Direct effects of GH on the breakdown of carbohydrates and on protein synthesis also occur. GH excess is usually caused by a benign somatotropic tumor in the pituitary gland.

Diseases of GH Excess

- Gigantism, a disease of excess longitudinal growth of the bones of the skeleton, is seen as a result of GH excess before puberty.
- Acromegaly, a disease of connective tissue proliferation, is seen in adults with GH excess. Because skeletal epiphyses have closed, long bone growth has stopped in adults, and GH excess cannot cause growth of the skeleton. It is associated with growth of the cartilage of the hands, feet, nose, jaw, chin, and facial bones. Connective tissue proliferation of internal organs, including the heart, also occurs.

Clinical Manifestations

- Tall stature with gigantism. Accelerated growth velocity, exceeding the 95th percentile on the growth chart.
- Thickening of the fingers, jaw, forehead, hands, and feet with acromegaly. Increased ring and shoe size, prominent brow, overgrowth of jaw with prominent underbite, and coarse facial features.
- Goiter and cardiomyopathy due to soft tissue hypertrophy.
- Deep voice due to vocal cord thickening.
- Sleep apnea due to thickening of the tongue.
- Because GH excess is usually caused by an aggressively growing adenoma, other hormone-secreting cells of the anterior pituitary are frequently destroyed. Thus, symptoms of GH excess often include those associated with deficiencies of other hormones. For example, if the growing tumor displaces the gonadotropin-secreting cells of the anterior pituitary, decreased reproductive function may occur. If the tumor affects any other hormone-producing cells, manifestations particular to that hormone will prevail.

Increased intracranial pressure can also occur with a growing tumor. Symptoms include headache, vomiting, and papilledema (swelling where the optic nerve enters the eye chamber).

Diagnostic Tools

- A good history and physical examination will help diagnose GH excess.
- Blood tests measuring increased levels of GH will support diagnosis of gigantism or acromegaly.
- Increased blood glucose levels may be present with either condition.
- The secretory pattern of GH release is no longer predictable and is unrelated to sleep with either condition.

Complications

- Complications of acromegaly include cardiac hypertrophy and hypertension.
- Diabetes mellitus can occur from the tendency of GH to increase blood glucose and decrease cellular insulin sensitivity.
- Headaches and visual disturbances due to increased intracranial pressure with pituitary tumor growth.

Treatment

- Treatment of GH excess is usually by surgical excision of the GH-secreting tumor. Radiation therapy may also be applied.
- Somatostatin analogs produce feedback GH inhibition.
- GH receptor antagonists bind to GH receptors on the cell surface and block binding of endogenous GH thus interfering with GH signal and resulting in decreased IGF-1 levels.
- Dopamine agonists to decrease GH levels.

GONADOTROPIN DEFICIENCY

Gonadotropin deficiency is a decrease in circulating levels of FSH and LH. Gonadotropin deficiency is usually caused by pressure exerted on the gonodotropin-producing cells by a pituitary tumor of another hormone-producing cell type. Oversecretion of the target gland hormones estrogen, progesterone, or testosterone can also act in a negative feedback manner to cause gonadotropin deficiency. Prolactin is known to inhibit pituitary secretion of the gonadotropins, and prolactin-secreting tumors can cause gonadotropin deficiency. Finally, the hypothalamus may decrease its secretion of GnRHs under periods of physical stress, obesity, starvation, or emotional trauma.

Clinical Manifestations

- Amenorrhea (lack of menstrual periods), vaginal, uterine, and breast atrophy in women.
- Testicular atrophy and reduction in beard growth in men.
- Patients with hypogonadotropic hypogonadism manifest decreased testosterone levels and interruption of spermatogenesis.

Diagnostic Tools

- Blood tests measuring the levels of estrogen, testosterone, and the gonadotropins will allow diagnosis of the condition and localization of the problem at the level of the CNS or the ovary or testicle.

Treatment

- Surgery if a tumor is present.
- Gonadotropin, estrogen, or testosterone replacement may be considered.
- Stress reduction, weight gain, or weight loss.

HYPOPROLACTEMIA

Hypoprolactemia is a decrease in circulating levels of prolactin. Hypoprolactemia may occur as a result of hypothalamic dysfunction leading to increased release of PIH. It may also occur because of dysfunction of the prolactin-secreting cells of the pituitary. Dysfunction of pituitary cells may be caused by increased pressure from a pituitary tumor of another cell type. More commonly, hypoprolactemia is diagnosed after an episode of pituitary ischemia and necrosis.

Diseases of Hypoprolactemia

Sheehan syndrome is a condition of hypopituitarism resulting from an intrapartum or postpartum hemorrhage (during or after delivery of an infant). With a significant loss of blood volume during the birth process, blood flow to the anterior pituitary may be reduced. Complicating the problem further is that during pregnancy the anterior pituitary grows and becomes very active metabolically. This is especially true for cells that produce prolactin, TSH, and GH. The result is a very high oxygen demand. In addition, anterior pituitary blood flow is venous blood coming from the hypothalamus through the hypothalamic–pituitary portal system, and is therefore relatively deoxygenated. Thus, the anterior pituitary is particularly susceptible to ischemic damage with a birth hemorrhage. Sheehan syndrome may manifest after delivery of the infant when the woman experiences an inability to breastfeed. Other pituitary hormones may also be deficient.

Clinical Manifestations

- Inability to breastfeed in women.
- In Sheehan syndrome, other symptoms will depend on which hormone-producing cells were affected by the ischemia.

Diagnostic Tools

- Blood tests measuring decreased levels of prolactin will allow diagnosis of the condition.

Treatment

- Treatment is related to needs of the individual and may involve HRT.

HYPERPROLACTEMIA

Hyperprolactemia is an increase in circulating levels of prolactin. Hyperprolactemia may be caused by a decrease in secretion of PIH by the hypothalamus, or as a result of a prolactin-secreting tumor of the pituitary (prolactinoma). Certain phenothiazine drugs, used to treat psychosis, sometimes cause hyperprolactemia, probably by affecting the hypothalamus. It may also occur with pregnancy and during hypothyroidism.

Clinical Manifestations

- Infertility, hypogonadism, anovulation, and amenorrhea in women as a result of prolactin-mediated decreases in LH or FSH secretion by the pituitary. This may result in osteopenia.
- Galactorrhea (lactation not associated with childbirth or nursing) may develop.
- No clinical signs are apparent in men.

Diagnostic Tools

- Blood tests measuring the increased level of prolactin will allow diagnosis of the condition.
- Imaging of the sella turcica may provide evidence of tumor.

Treatment

- A prolactin-secreting tumor may be surgically resected.
- If the condition is drug related and the patient is concerned about her reproductive status, further use of the drug should be evaluated.

- Dopamine agonists (cabergoline and bromocriptine) to inhibit prolactin secretion may be prescribed.

SYNDROME OF INAPPROPRIATE ANTIDIURETIC HORMONE (ADH)

Syndrome of inappropriate ADH (SIADH) is characterized by the increased release of ADH from the posterior pituitary in the absence of normal stimuli for ADH release. Increased ADH release usually occurs in response to increased plasma osmolality (a decrease in plasma water concentration) or, to a lesser extent, decreased blood pressure. With SIADH, *ADH remains high even when the plasma osmolality is low*. Plasma osmolality continues to decrease because of ADH stimulating water reabsorption by the kidneys. Release of ADH continues without feedback control, in spite of low osmolality and increased blood volume. The end result is significant water retention and dilutional hyponatremia. Left untreated, this condition is life-threatening.

SIADH is most commonly induced by drugs. Other causes of SIADH include disease, injury, or tumors of the CNS, pain, stress, and temperature extremes. Surgery may result in a transient occurrence of SIADH. Tumors outside the CNS, especially bronchogenic carcinomas, frequently produce ADH ectopically. Other possible causes include cancer of lymphoid tissue, prostate and pancreas, positive-pressure breathing in which baroreceptors are activated, pulmonary tuberculosis, severe pneumonia, some medications such as chlorpropamide, and possible genetic factors.

Clinical Manifestations

- Water retention and weight gain.
- Decreased urinary output.
- Nausea and vomiting worsening with the degree of water intoxication.
- Headache, anorexia, thirst, oliguria, muscle cramps, weakness, and fatigue due to water intoxication.
- Irritability, mental confusion, and disorientation progressing to seizures or coma as hyponatremia increases.

Diagnostic Tools

- Blood tests measuring increased levels of ADH with decreased plasma osmolality and hyponatremia (decreased sodium concentration, mild: serum sodium decreased to 130 mEq/L; severe: serum sodium below 126 mEq/L) will allow diagnosis of the condition.
- BUN and hematocrit will be low due to increased extracellular fluid volume.
- Urine osmolality and specific gravity.

Complications

- Neurologic symptoms may range from headache and confusion to muscle twitching, seizures, coma, and death as a result of hyponatremia and water intoxication.
- Cerebral edema may result if hyponatremia is corrected too quickly.

Treatment

- For mild cases, fluid restriction is adequate to control symptoms until the syndrome spontaneously regresses.
- If the condition is more severe, diuretics and drugs that block ADH action on the collecting tubules will be administered. A hypertonic solution of sodium chloride may occasionally be used to increase plasma sodium concentration.
- Identify and treat the cause. If ADH is arising from ectopic tumor production, treatment will be aimed at eliminating the tumor.

DIABETES INSIPIDUS

Diabetes insipidus is a disease of decreased ADH production, secretion, or function. The term diabetes insipidus refers to the quantity and quality of the urine: the disease is associated with copious amounts of dull, or tasteless, urine. Without ADH, the renal-collecting tubules cannot reabsorb water and cannot concentrate the urine. Central diabetes insipidus may result from a partial or total lack of ADH production by the hypothalamus, or decreased release of ADH from the posterior pituitary. These deficits may result from a tumor or head injury. Alcohol and medications such as phenytoin may suppress the release of ADH. Diabetes insipidus may also result from the kidney not responding to circulating ADH because of a receptor or second messenger deficit. This type of diabetes insipidus is called nephrogenic, that is, originating in the kidney. Causes of nephrogenic diabetes insipidus include a genetic, X-linked recessive trait, kidney disease, hypokalemia, and hypercalcemia.

Clinical Manifestations

- Polyuria (large volumes of dilute urine) and polydipsia (excessive thirst) are the hallmark findings.
- Decreased urine specific gravity.
- Hypertonic dehydration and increased serum osmolality.

Diagnostic Tools

- Blood tests measuring decreased levels of ADH with increased plasma osmolality and hypernatremia (>145 mEq/L) will allow diagnosis of the condition.

- Water deprivation test to differentiate between central DI and nephrogenic DI. Urine osmolality will increase after the administration of vasopressin if it is a central problem and there will be little or no response if the problem is nephrogenic.
- MRI of the pituitary–hypothalamic area.

Complications

- Severe dehydration may occur if large volumes of drinking water are unavailable.

Treatment

- Drugs are available that mimic the action of ADH. The most commonly used drug of this category, desmopressin, was previously offered only as a nasal spray for home use but is now available in pill form.
- Oral antidiabetic agent chlorpropamide may be used to stimulate ADH release, but it has the potential to cause hypoglycemia.
- For nephrogenic diabetes insipidus, thiazide diuretics are administered. These seem to work by decreasing glomerular filtration rate, allowing increased amounts of fluid to be reabsorbed at the proximal, rather than collecting, tubule.

PEDIATRIC CONSIDERATIONS

- Children release more of their GH in the nocturnal burst than do adults. In children, GH is essential for the longitudinal bone growth that occurs throughout gestation, infancy, childhood, and puberty. Infants and children suffering emotional or physical neglect may develop failure to thrive syndrome, characterized by a decrease in longitudinal growth and weight gain. It has been suggested that a stress-induced increase in the release of somatostatin as a result of neglect may play a role in failure to thrive syndrome.
- Estrogen acts during puberty to cause the development of female secondary sex characteristics, including the development of breasts and growth of axillary and pubic hair. Estrogen also acts along with GH and the androgens to cause skeletal growth during puberty, and causes the closure of the epiphyseal bone plates to halt growth in males and females at the end of puberty. Estrogen can pathologically affect children, causing precocious (early) onset of menstruation in girls and breast development in girls and boys.
- Testosterone acts during puberty to cause the development of male secondary sex characteristics, including growth of the penis and scrotum and the development of male axillary and pubic hair patterns. Testosterone is also important for skeletal growth during puberty, especially in males. Excess testosterone in girls can cause voice deepening, acne, male pattern muscle development, and clitoral enlargement.

- Infants born without a thyroid gland or with defects in TH synthesis will develop congenital hypothyroidism, a disease sometimes referred to as cretinism. Congenital hypothyroidism is characterized by low TH, with high TSH and TRF. TH is permissive (necessary) for functioning of all cells of the body, including cells of the CNS. Development of the CNS occurs in utero and for approximately 1 year after birth. Because an infant with congenital hypothyroidism was exposed to maternal TH in utero, it will be born neurologically intact. If the condition is unrecognized after birth and TH is not replaced pharmacologically, further development of infant CNS will be compromised and severe mental retardation will result. Growth will be stunted and skeletal deformity will develop. Many states require measurement of TH levels at birth. With thyroxine replacement, CNS damage can be avoided. Hypothyroidism at birth may also occur if maternal antithyroid antibodies attack the fetal thyroid during pregnancy. Likewise, if a pregnant woman is severely deprived of iodide, her infant may also have hypothyroidism after birth. Long-term neurologic prognosis for either of these conditions depends on the extent of thyroid deficit.

- Most children with short stature do not have an endocrine or genetic abnormality, but rather have a normal genetic predisposition to be short (i.e., short parents). However, any child who presents with short stature should be carefully assessed to rule out underlying illnesses, including renal, cardiac, or gastrointestinal disease, and certain genetic abnormalities such as Turner syndrome. Medications should be assessed, since, for example, oral steroids used to treat chronic asthma and medications used to treat attention-deficit disorder have been reported to reduce growth. The term constitutional short stature is used to describe children who are shorter than others of their age, and those growing at a reduced pace without a known cause. Under certain circumstances, treatment with exogenous GH may be used to increase final growth in this population as well. In general, GH treatment appears to be safe for most children without other contraindications. Patients who have GH insensitivity syndrome (e.g., receptor defects) do not respond to exogenous GH treatments.

- Elevated growth in children may occur as a result of a normal genetic predisposition (i.e., tall parents) or may accompany certain genetic abnormalities such as Marfan syndrome and Klinefelter syndrome. The term constitutional tall stature is used to describe children who are taller than others their age, and those growing at an accelerated velocity. Occasionally, treatment may involve the judicial administration of sex hormones (birth control pills in girls) to retard excess growth.

 GERIATRIC CONSIDERATIONS

- Normal endocrine changes associated with aging include:
  - Atrophy of thyroid gland → decreased BMR, decreased radioactive iodine uptake, decreased secretion and release of thyrotropin
  - Decreased ACTH secretion → decreased secretion of estrogen, progesterone, androgen, glucocorticoids
  - Decreased pituitary gland volume → reduced somatotropic GHs in the blood

- Inadequate insulin release from beta cells, decreased tissue sensitivity to insulin, decreased ability to metabolize glucose.

- Menopause is considered to have occurred when a woman has not experienced a menstrual period for a year. Menopause happens when aging ovaries no longer respond to the signals of the gonadotropins to synthesize and secrete estrogen. As estrogen levels decrease, LH, FSH, and GnRH levels increase because any negative feedback by estrogen has been removed. Although menopause is a normal developmental stage, lack of estrogen in postmenopausal women causes decreased bone density, increased risk of cardiovascular disease, drying of skin and vaginal membranes, and hot flashes or flushes. Most women in developed countries experience menopause in their late 40s or early 50s. Hormonal and cytotoxic treatments used for breast cancer may induce early menopause in some women. Several randomized clinical trials carefully investigated the safety of HRT in postmenopausal women, including estrogen given both alone and in combination with progesterone. Results indicated that combination hormone therapy was associated with an increased risk of breast cancer, cardiovascular disease, and stroke among postmenopausal women. The effect of estrogen alone is still being investigated, although estrogen alone is contraindicated for women with an intact uterus due to an increased risk of endometrial cancer. As a result of these studies, which have been termed the Women's Health Initiative, clinical experts recommend that HRT either not be prescribed at all or be prescribed for as short a period of time as necessary to control menopausal symptoms.

- The testes continue to respond to the gonadotropins as a man ages, albeit at a reduced level. Testosterone synthesis and release by the testes continues, as does sperm production, throughout a man's lifetime, albeit at some declining rate. Testosterone levels adequate to maintain sperm production and muscle mass continue into a man's seventh decade, at least.

- Myxedema coma is usually seen in elderly persons who are not being adequately treated for hypothyroidism. It is more common in older women with autoimmune thyroiditis. It may also occur after an acute illness in this population. Prolonged exposure of an elderly individual to cold weather may precipitate the disorder.

- Hyperthyroidism is often mistaken as depression when the older adult reports insomnia, weight loss, fatigue, and impaired cognition and memory.

- Because thyroid antibodies normally increase with age, it is difficult to determine when an increased level indicates thyroiditis.

SELECTED BIBLIOGRAPHY

Adler, J. T., Sippel, R. S., Schaefer, S., & Chen, H. (2008). Preserving function and quality of life after thyroid and parathyroid surgery. *Lancet Oncology, 9,* 1069–1075.

Arlt, W., & Allolio, B. (2003). Adrenal insufficiency. *Lancet, 361,* 1881–1893.

Arlt, W., Walker, E. A., Draper, N., Ivison, H. E., Ride, J. P., Hammer, F., et al. (2004). Congenital adrenal hyperplasia caused by mutant P450 oxidoreductase and human androgen synthesis: Analytical study. *Lancet, 363,* 2128–2135.

Buck, M. L. (2009). Levothyroxine use in infants and children with congenital or acquired hypothyroidism. *Pediatric Pharmacotherapy*, 14(10), 90–94.

Cameron, D. R., & Braunstein, G. D. (2004). Androgen replacement therapy in women. *Fertility and Sterility*, 82, 273–289.

Cinemre, H., Bilir, C., Gokosmanoglu, F., Akdemir, N., Erdogmus, B., & Buyukkaya, R. (2009). Predictors of time to remission and treatment failure in patients with Graves' disease treated with propylthiouracil. *Clinical Investigative Medicine*, 32(3), E199–E205.

Cook, L. K. (2009). Pheochromocytoma. *American Journal of Neurology*, 109(2), 50–53.

Copstead, L. C., & Banasik, J. L. (2010). *Pathophysiology* (4th ed.). St. Louis, MO: Saunders Elsevier.

Dattani, M., & Preece, M. (2004). Growth hormone deficiency and related disorders: Insights into causation, diagnosis, and treatment. *Lancet*, 363, 1977–1987.

Daub, K. F. (2008). Pheochromocytoma: Not your everyday diagnosis. *American Nurse Today*, 3(7), 9–11.

Dubey, P., Raymond, G. V., Moser, A. B., Kharkar, S., Bezman, L., & Moser, H. W. (2005). Adrenal insufficiency in asymptomatic adrenoleukodystrophy patients identified by very long-chain fatty acid screening. *Journal of Pediatrics*, 146, 528–532.

Ehrmann, D. A. (2005). Polycystic ovary syndrome. *New England Journal of Medicine*, 352, 1223–1236.

Eliopoulos, C. (2010). *Gerontological nursing* (7th ed.). Philadelphia, PA: Lippincott Williams & Wilkins.

Falkenstern, S. K., & Bauer, L. A. (2009). Growth failure. *The Nurse Practitioner*, 34(3), 31–41.

Laurberg, P., Andersen, S., Pedersen, I. B., & Carle, A. (2005). Hypothyroidism in the elderly: Pathophysiology, diagnosis and treatment. *Drugs and Aging*, 22, 23–38.

Minhtri, K., & Nguyen, I. K. (2005). An analysis of current quantitative approaches to the treatment of severe symptomatic SIADH with intravenous saline therapy. *Clinical Experimental Nephrology*, 9, 1–4.

Osborn, D. A., & Hunt, R. (2007). Prophylactic postnatal thyroid hormones for prevention of norbidity and mortality in preterm infants. *Cochrane Database of Systemic Reviews*, Issue 1. Art. No.: CD005948. DOI: 10.1002/14651858.CD005948.pub2.

Osborn, K. S., Wraa, C. E., & Watson, A. B. (2010). *Medical-surgical nursing: Preparation for practice*. Upper Saddle River, NJ: Pearson.

Petraglia, F., Musacchio, C., Luisi, S., & De Leo, V. (2008). Hormone-dependent gynaecological disorders: A pathophyiological perspective for appropriate treatment. *Best Practice and Research Clinical Obstetrics and Gynaecology*, 22(2), 235–249.

Porth, C. M., & Matfin, G. (2009). *Pathophysiology: Concepts of altered health states* (8th ed.). Philadelphia, PA: Lippincott Williams & Wilkins.

Raparia, K., Min, S. K., Mody, D. R. Anton, R., & Amrikachi, M. (2009). Clinical outcomes for "suspicious" category in thyroid fine-needle aspiration biopsy: Patient's sex and nodule size are possible predictors of malignancy. *Archives of Pathology Laboratory Medicine*, 133, 787–790.

Tabloski, P. A. (2010). *Gerontological nursing*. Upper Saddle River, NJ: Pearson.

Thibodeu, G. A., & Patton, K. T. (2010). *The human body in health and disease* (5th ed.). St. Louis, MO: Mosby Elsevier.

The Musculoskeletal System

Skeletal muscles and bones support and move the body and protect soft tissues and the internal organs. Bones serve as a calcium reservoir and some contain hematopoietic connective tissue that is vital to the formation of blood cells. Muscles are responsible for vascular tone, gut contractions, genitourinary function, and the beating of the heart. Life is impossible if the cardiac or respiratory muscles are destroyed. Some muscles function relatively independently of neural or hormonal stimulation, whereas other muscles are active only in response to neural stimulation. Bones and muscles are joined at the joints by tendons and ligaments. Diseases or injuries to the muscles and bones make movements difficult or painful and have the potential to result in long-term disability.

● Physiologic Concepts

There are three types of muscles: skeletal, cardiac, and smooth. The basic processes of contraction are similar in all three types, but important differences exist. Although the focus of this chapter is the skeletal–muscular system, the unique characteristics of the cardiac and smooth muscles will be presented briefly.

SKELETAL MUSCLE

Skeletal muscles are connected to bones through tendons. Tendons move the bones by contraction of the skeletal muscles, which is controlled by lower motor neurons from the spinal cord. One motor neuron may innervate several muscle fibers. A motor neuron and all the muscle fibers it innervates are called a **motor unit**. In general, the muscles over which we have fine control have only a few muscle fibers innervated by a single motor neuron. Muscles that do not need fine control (i.e., the support muscles of the back) are composed of many muscle fibers per motor neuron.

Skeletal muscle cells are highly differentiated cells whose growth during embryogenesis and later in life is under the control of growth factors, hormones, and physical stimuli. During embryogenesis, skeletal muscle cells undergo both hyperplasia (increase in cell number) and hypertrophy (increase in cell size). After embryogenesis, skeletal muscle cells continue to undergo hypertrophy in response to certain stimuli, including exercise, but no longer undergo hyperplasia. The protein myostatin, also known as "growth and differentiating factor-8," has been identified as playing a key role in the regulation of skeletal muscle growth before and after birth, by limiting the growth and reproduction of muscle cell fibers. In animals that lack the gene coding for myostatin, muscle hypertrophy and hyperplasia occur both before and after birth, resulting in increased muscle mass and strength.

Skeletal Muscle Structure

Each skeletal muscle is made up of many muscle cells, called **muscle fibers**. A given muscle may have a few hundred or several thousand fibers. The more muscle fibers present in a muscle, the greater the potential strength of that muscle.

Skeletal muscle is called striated muscle because of the banding that can be seen throughout the muscle with a light microscope. The striations reflect the subunits of each muscle fiber: the myofibrils. A single muscle cell is made up of many myofibrils. The myofibrils are composed of smaller subunits called myofilaments; myofilaments are the functional units of the muscle cell. They are composed of thick and thin contractile proteins, grouped together into a repeating pattern, called a **sarcomere**.

The Sarcomere

Three sarcomeres are aligned together as shown in Figure 10-1. Each sarcomere contains thick and thin filaments. The thick filaments are located in the central region of the sarcomere, and are composed of several hundred copies of the contractile protein **myosin**. The thin filaments are attached to the edges of the sarcomere and are composed of the proteins **actin**, **tropomyosin**, and **troponin**.

The area of the sarcomere where only thick filaments are present is called the H zone. The area where only thin filaments are present is termed the I zone. The A band is the section where the thin and thick filaments overlap. The Z lines are the borders of the sarcomere, where the actins attach. Each sarcomere spans from one Z line to the next.

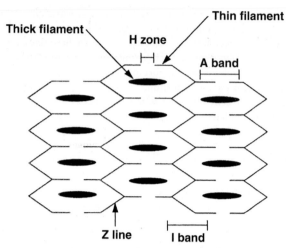

FIGURE 10-1 The sarcomere.

Cross-Bridges

Each myosin molecule is composed of six peptide chains: two heavy chains that twist together to form a long tail with two globular heads, and four light chains that group, two to a head, with the myosin heads. The heads form small projections that extend from the myosin filament. These projections are called **cross-bridges**. When a muscle is relaxed, the myosin cross-bridges are unattached in the sarcomere. During this relaxed state, an adenosine triphosphate (ATP) molecule binds to myosin and is split into ADP and a high-energy phosphate (P). The ADP and P remain bound to the myosin, without releasing the energy generated by the splitting of ATP.

Muscle Contraction

Contraction of a muscle occurs when the myosin cross-bridges bind to specific sites on the actin proteins. When this occurs, energy that has been stored in the myosin head from the previous splitting of an ATP molecule is released. The released energy is used to swing the cross-bridges, causing the actin and myosin filaments to slide over each other. This shortens and contracts the muscle. With cross-bridge swinging, the remaining ADP and P release from myosin.

During muscle contraction, the lengths of the actin and myosin filaments do not change, but the I band and the H zone shorten. The different regions of the sarcomere are described in Table 10-1; the thick filaments, myosin heads, and thin filaments are shown in Figure 10-2. Each muscle contraction involves several repeated cycles of filament sliding to provide the tension necessary for the muscle to do work.

Region	Filament	Composition	Condition with Contraction
H zone	Thick	Myosin	Shortens
I zone	Thin	Actin, troponin, tropomyosin	Shortens
A band	Thick and thin overlap	Myosin, actin, troponin, tropomyosin	No change
Z line	Borders of sarcomere	Actin attachments	No change

TABLE 10-1 Sarcomere Composition and Changes During Contraction

Excitation–Contraction Coupling

Because skeletal muscle contraction only occurs in response to neural stimulation and the subsequent release of intracellular calcium, myosin, and actin cannot always bind to each other so the cross-bridges cannot always swing. This prevents constant muscle contraction.

The process of muscle contraction is summarized below. When an action potential is delivered by a motor neuron to a skeletal muscle fiber, the neuron releases acetylcholine (ACh) into the neuromuscular junction. ACh diffuses to

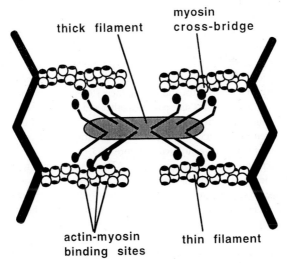

thick filament

myosin
cross-bridge

actin-myosin
binding sites

thin filament

FIGURE 1 0 - 2 Diagrammatic representation of myosin molecules lined up in thick filaments with globular heads extending in to form cross-bridges with overlying and underlying actin molecules.

a specialized area of the muscle cell, called the end plate. Muscle cell end plates are concentrated with receptors for ACh. ACh binds to the receptors causing the opening of sodium channels present in the muscle cell. With the opening of these channels, sodium ions rush into the cell, depolarizing (making the cell positively charged on the inside) and initiating an action potential. The action potential passes along the entire muscle fiber, depolarizing the fiber. Depolarization spreads into the fiber through small tubules, called transverse (T) tubules, which run along the juncture between the A and I bands. When the inside of the cell becomes positive, calcium ion is released from intracellular bags of calcium (called lateral sacs) that lie adjacent to the T tubules. The lateral sacs are outpouchings of a large intracellular calcium storage compartment: the **sarcoplasmic reticulum** causes high levels of intracellular calcium released from the sarcoplasmic reticulum to initiate muscle contraction.

The Role of Intracellular Calcium in Initiating Muscle Contraction

When a skeletal muscle fiber is at rest, the myosin heads are prevented from binding to the actin molecules by the presence of the other two proteins of the thin filaments: tropomyosin and troponin. Without myosin binding to actin, energy from ATP cannot be released, cross-bridges cannot swing, and the muscle cannot contract. Elevated intracellular calcium changes the interaction of these proteins and causes contraction.

At rest, tropomyosin is attached to the actin molecules in such a way that it blocks the sites on actin where the myosin cross-bridges would bind. Troponin attaches to both the actin and the tropomyosin molecules. It also has a binding site for calcium. When calcium concentration inside the cell increases, calcium binds to troponin, causing troponin to shift its position on the tropomyosin molecule. This causes tropomyosin to shift its position on actin, uncovering the binding site for myosin. Once the binding site on actin is uncovered, the myosin heads immediately bind actin and release their stored energy, and the cross-bridges swing. The filaments slide past each other and the muscle contracts. The greater the number of cross-bridges connected and swinging at one time, the greater the tension produced by the muscle. Excitation–contraction coupling and the role of calcium are outlined in Figure 10-3.

After each cross-bridge swinging, a new ATP molecule binds to the myosin molecule (the old ADP and P have already been released). This causes the myosin cross-bridges to separate from actin and the fiber to relax. Once relaxed, the new ATP molecule is split, and its energy is again stored in the myosin head. If calcium is still high intracellularly, the myosin cross-bridge will again bind actin, and this energy will be released, leading to a second contraction. Excitation–contraction coupling occurs when intracellular calcium levels increase from a resting molar concentration of less than 10^{-7} to approximately 10^{-5}. During a typical action potential, calcium concentration is approximately 2×10^{-4} molar; this is approximately 10 times the level required to maximally contract the muscle.

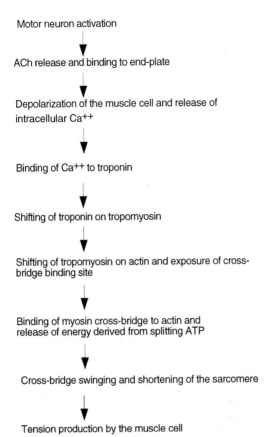

Motor neuron activation

ACh release and binding to end-plate

Depolarization of the muscle cell and release of intracellular Ca^{++}

Binding of Ca^{++} to troponin

Shifting of troponin on tropomyosin

Shifting of tropomyosin on actin and exposure of cross-bridge binding site

Binding of myosin cross-bridge to actin and release of energy derived from splitting ATP

Cross-bridge swinging and shortening of the sarcomere

Tension production by the muscle cell

FIGURE 10-3 Flow diagram showing excitation–contraction coupling in a muscle cell, initiated by release of ACh from a motor neuron.

Muscle Fiber Summation

Each calcium pulse lasts approximately 1/20th of a second and produces what is called a single muscle twitch. **Summation** occurs if calcium is maintained in the intracellular compartment by repeated neural stimulation of the muscle. Summation means individual twitches are added together, causing increased contraction strength. If stimulation is prolonged, the individual twitches blend together until the strength of contraction is at a maximum. At this point, the muscle is said to have reached **tetany**, which is characterized by a smooth, continued contraction. Summation and tetany in an individual muscle fiber are shown in Figure 10-4.

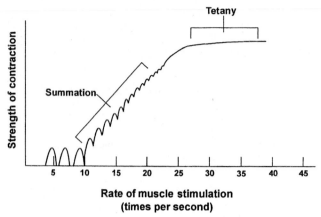

FIGURE 10-4 Summation and tetany.

Whole-Muscle Summation: Multiple-Fiber Summation

The total amount of tension produced by an entire muscle is the result of the summation of the tension produced by each muscle fiber. An increase in the number of fibers stimulated to contract will increase the amount of tension produced by the entire muscle. This is called multiple-fiber summation. Multiple-fiber summation occurs when additional motor units are activated, leading to the contraction of more muscle fibers.

Relaxation of the Muscle

Muscle fibers relax when calcium is pumped out of the cytoplasm back into the sarcoplasmic reticulum. Calcium pumping is an active process occurring in the membrane of the sarcoplasmic reticulum. This process uses energy derived from splitting a different ATP molecule. When calcium levels decrease to approximately 10^{-7} molar, troponin returns to its original position on the tropomyosin molecule, and tropomyosin again inhibits the binding of actin and myosin, which causes muscle contraction to stop.

Muscle Metabolism and Muscle Fatigue

Muscle contraction depends on the production of ATP from one of three sources: (1) creatinine phosphate (CP) stored in the muscle, (2) oxidative phosphorylation of foodstuffs stored in or delivered to the muscle, and (3) anaerobic glycolysis. Muscle fatigue results when the use of ATP in a muscle becomes excessive.

When a muscle first starts contracting, it begins to use its stores of CP to drive contraction. CP contains a high-energy phosphate molecule that it transfers to ADP to produce ATP: CP + ADP = C + ATP.

This source of ATP is rapidly accessed, but is limited by the amount of CP present in the cell at the start of contraction. After several seconds, the muscle begins to rely mostly on oxidative phosphorylation. Sources of fuel for oxidative phosphorylation include glycogen stored in the muscle and, later, glucose and fatty acids delivered to the muscle in the blood supply. This source of energy is available for 30 minutes or so, depending on the intensity of contraction. If the intensity of exercise is very high, or the duration is very long, the muscle begins to rely increasingly on anaerobic glycolysis. Anaerobic glycolysis produces a limited amount of ATP from the metabolism of muscle glycogen and circulating blood glucose. A muscle using anaerobic glycolysis for a large part of its ATP production rapidly fatigues. Muscle fatigue can be predicted experimentally by depletion of glycogen stored in the muscle. Lactic acid is a byproduct of anaerobic glycolysis and may accumulate in the muscle and blood with intense or prolonged muscle contraction, contributing to fatigue. Lactic acid may also contribute to the muscle pain felt a day or two after intense exercise.

Length–Tension Relationship

The resting length of a muscle fiber determines the maximum amount of tension it can produce. This relationship is shown in Figure 10-5. Muscle fiber length affects tension production as a result of stretching of the sarcomere. If

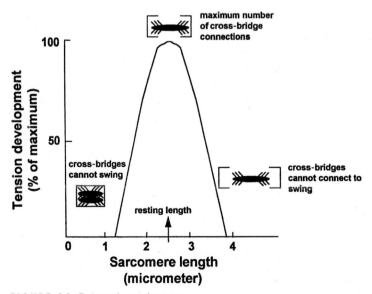

FIGURE 10-5 Length–tension curve.

a sarcomere is stretched beyond an optimum length, as shown on the right side of the figure, some myosin cross-bridges will be too far away to connect with the actin sites and therefore will not swing. This will reduce total tension. In contrast, if the sarcomere is less than optimally stretched, as shown on the left side of the figure, the cross-bridges will be bunched too closely together to be able to swing freely, thus limiting filament sliding and again reducing total tension. In a normal skeletal muscle, muscle length at rest will produce the maximum amount of tension.

Isometric Contraction

Isometric contractions are those in which cross-bridge swinging occurs and tension is produced without shortening of the muscle. An isometric contraction occurs when an individual is trying to lift a load that requires greater tension than can be produced by the muscle. No mechanical work is performed. Tension is produced, but the muscle does not change in length.

Isotonic Contraction

Isotonic contractions occur when a muscle shortens against a constant load. Work is done to lift the load. An example of an isotonic contraction is when a weightlifter lifts a barbell. The tension remains the same, but the muscle length changes. Most muscle contractions include both isotonic and isometric periods.

Series Elastic Elements

There is typically a delay between excitation of a muscle and an isotonic contraction. A delay occurs because the elastic components of the muscle, including the tendons and the attachments of the sarcomeres, must be shortened before the muscle itself shortens. The elastic components of a muscle are called the **series elastic elements**. If a second contraction of the muscle occurs before the series elastic elements relax, there is no delay, and muscle tension can be increased immediately. This concept of the series elastic element may be easier understood by picturing a spring connected to an object. Before the object can be lifted by pulling the spring, the spring must first be stretched. This delays lifting of the object.

Fast-Twitch and Slow-Twitch Fibers

Different muscles contain different types of muscle fibers, depending on the range of jobs performed. Muscles that must function continually, such as those of the respiratory system, must have long endurance and an ample supply of oxygen. Others function briefly and intensely and then relax; these muscles must be able to produce short bursts of high energy. Usually, a muscle will contain a mixture of fiber types, with one fiber type predominating but not exclusively. Two main divisions of muscle fibers are fast-twitch and slow-twitch fibers.

Fast-twitch fibers release calcium rapidly from the sarcoplasmic reticulum, and rapidly split ATP to ADP on the myosin head. This causes the rate of cross-bridge swinging to be fast. Fast-twitch fibers may depend primarily on either oxidative phosphorylation or anaerobic glycolysis for energy, depending on what type of work they typically perform.

Fast-twitch fibers that frequently produce large amounts of energy for quick bursts of tension have large stores of glycolytic enzymes and produce a great deal of their ATP from anaerobic glycolysis. These are usually large fibers and require less vascularization because they rely less on oxidative phosphorylation; therefore, they appear white. These fibers are called *fast-glycolytic fibers*. Fast-glycolytic fibers tire rapidly and predominate in the muscles of weightlifters and sprinters.

Fast-twitch fibers that rely mostly on oxidative phosphorylation, called *fast-oxidative fibers*, are well vascularized and contain elevated stores of the muscle protein myoglobin. Myoglobin combines in the muscle with oxygen, serving as an oxygen storage bank. Fast-oxidative fibers tire less rapidly and predominate in muscles of longer distance runners.

Slow-twitch fibers are small, highly vascularized fibers that depend predominantly on oxidative phosphorylation for the production of ATP. Muscles with slow-twitch fibers look red because of their high vascularity and the presence of the protein myoglobin. Slow-oxidative fibers have long endurance and predominate in muscles required to produce tension for prolonged periods, such as back muscles.

Stretch Reflex

Many skeletal muscles contain special muscle fibers that act as stretch receptors, called **muscle spindle fibers**. Muscle spindle fibers are fibers wrapped by afferent nerve endings, which increase their rate of firing when the muscle is stretched. The impulses are transmitted to the spinal cord by an afferent neuron. In the spinal cord, the afferent neuron synapses directly on the motor neuron supplying the muscle (a monosynaptic reflex) or on an interneuron, which then stimulates the motor neuron (a multisynaptic reflex). Activation of the motor neuron causes the muscle to contract, thus removing the stretch on the muscle spindles and returning the nerves' firing rate to normal. This process is called the stretch reflex. The opposite occurs if stretch on the spindles is suddenly reduced (called the negative stretch reflex). The result of either type of stretch reflex is maintenance of the muscle at a resting length. Voluntary muscle movement involves simultaneous contraction of regular muscle fibers and muscle spindle fibers. This contraction allows movements to be fluid. The afferent neurons that innervate the muscle spindle fibers are called gamma

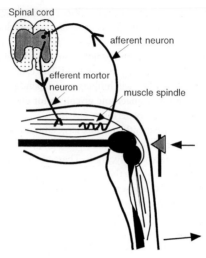

FIGURE 10-6 The knee-jerk reflex occurs when a muscle spindle fiber is stretched artificially. This sends a signal to the spinal cord leading to rapid contraction of the muscle.

neurons. The monosynaptic stretch reflex that results in the knee-jerk response is shown in Figure 10-6.

CARDIAC MUSCLE

Myocardial cells (myocytes) are long, narrow fibers. Cardiac muscle contraction is similar to skeletal muscle contraction, with the following differences:

- Cardiac cells are capable of spontaneous contraction; that is, contraction without neural stimulation. Neural stimulation can increase or decrease the rate of cardiac contraction.
- Cardiac muscle fibers are connected to each other through areas of low resistance, called intercalated disks. The plasma membrane of adjacent cardiac fibers connects in this area. Intercalated disks allow depolarization, beginning in one cardiac muscle fiber, to pass rapidly to neighboring fibers, ensuring simultaneous contraction of all cardiac muscle fibers at one time. Simultaneous contraction is required for the maintenance of cardiac output and blood pressure.
- Two sources of calcium are involved in producing a cardiac muscle cell contraction. In cardiac muscle, as in skeletal muscle, calcium ions are released intracellularly from the sarcoplasmic reticulum, but they also enter the cell from the extracellular fluid through sodium–calcium channels present in

the T tubules. These channels are also voltage sensitive but are slow to open and thus prolong the duration of the cardiac action potential. The strength of cardiac contraction, therefore, is highly dependent on extracellular calcium level. In contrast, skeletal muscle contraction does not depend on extracellular calcium.

- Because of the slow calcium channels, cardiac muscle cell contraction lasts approximately 10 times as long as skeletal muscle contraction. As a result, *cardiac muscle is unable to fire action potentials rapidly and does not undergo summation or tetany.* If the cardiac muscle were to achieve a state of maintained contraction, the heart would be unable to fill with blood.

- At rest, cardiac muscle cells are stretched less than is required to produce maximum tension, which allows the heart to increase tension when it is stretched during times of increased filling (e.g., during exercise).

SMOOTH MUSCLE

Smooth muscle contraction and skeletal muscle contraction have some similarities and some important differences. Smooth muscle contraction is not the same in all smooth muscles. Some characteristics of smooth muscle contraction include the following:

- Smooth muscle is innervated and stimulated by the sympathetic and parasympathetic nerves of the autonomic nervous system. These nerves do not innervate the smooth muscle at specific end plates, but branch over the muscle cells and diffusely release transmitter substances onto the fibers.

- Some smooth muscles function as a unit composed of millions of fibers. These fibers contract in response to action potentials produced from mechanical stretch, local chemical mediator release, or neural or hormonal stimulation. Spontaneous firing of action potentials can also occur. In this type of smooth muscle, action potentials generated from any source pass from one cell to another across gap junctions. This type of smooth muscle is called **single-unit smooth muscle**. It is found in the gut, throughout the genitourinary tract, and in many blood vessels.

- Some smooth muscle fibers contract individually and only in response to neural stimulation. These fibers are usually innervated by one neuron that releases ACh or norepinephrine. These fibers depolarize and contract, but usually do not fire action potentials. This type of smooth muscle is called **multi-unit smooth muscle**. It is found in the muscles of the eyes and in the muscles that surround hair follicles. When contracted, these muscles cause the hair to stand up on the skin.

- Although smooth muscle contains actin and myosin and splits ATP to produce tension, the thin filaments in smooth muscle fibers do not contain troponin. When intracellular calcium levels increase in smooth muscle fibers, calcium binds to a protein called calmodulin, resulting in phosphorylation of one of the light chains of the myosin heads. Phosphorylation of the light chain allows the myosin head to bind to actin and split ATP.

- The sarcomeres of smooth muscle do not show striations under the microscope, but are more diffuse and less regular in pattern, allowing the muscle to contract over a wide range of lengths. There are many more actin molecules than myosin molecules in smooth muscle fibers, although maximal tension production is similar.

- In smooth muscle, most calcium enters from the extracellular fluid through voltage-sensitive calcium channels. Some calcium is released from the sarcoplasmic reticulum. In some smooth muscles, intracellular calcium levels always are sufficient to maintain a low level of cross-bridge connection. This results in a resting muscle tone in these muscles.

- The speed of cross-bridge cycling and muscle contraction is reduced in smooth muscle compared to skeletal muscle, most likely because myosin heads contain less ATPase. Therefore, it takes longer for ATP to be split, prolonging the amount of time myosin is attached to actin. A longer period of attachment results in increased production of tension. The slow speed of the calcium pumps in smooth muscle also prolongs contraction.

- A latch mechanism in smooth muscle allows muscle contraction to be maintained for long periods of time at a fraction of the energy expenditure of skeletal muscle. This mechanism is probably related to the length of time myosin remains attached to actin.

TENDONS

Tendons are bundles of collagen fibers that anchor the muscles to the bones. Tendons transmit force generated by the contracting muscle to the bone and thereby move the bone. The collagen fibers are considered connective tissue and are produced by fibroblast cells. The dense fibrous connective tissue forming tendons gives them great strength.

LIGAMENTS

Ligaments are cords of strong fibrous connective tissue that join bone to bone, usually at joints. Ligaments grow out of the periosteum and allow and limit joint movement.

BONES

Bone Structure

Mature bone is composed of 30% organic (living) material and 70% salt deposits. The organic material is called the matrix, and is composed of more than

90% collagen fibers and less than 10% proteoglycans (proteins plus polysaccharides). The salt deposits are primarily calcium and phosphate, with small amounts of sodium, potassium carbonate, and magnesium ions. The salts cover the matrix and are bound to the collagen fibers by the proteoglycans. The organic matrix gives bone its tensile strength (resistance to being pulled apart). The bone salts give bone its compressional strength (ability to withstand compression).

Exchangeable Calcium

Some calcium ion in bone is noncrystallized. This noncrystalline salt is considered exchangeable calcium, in that it can rapidly move between the bone, interstitial fluid, and blood.

Bone Formation

Bone formation is ongoing and can involve the lengthening and thickening of the bone. The rate of bone formation changes throughout the lifespan. Bone formation is determined by hormonal stimulation, dietary factors, and the amount of stress put on a bone, and results from activities of the bone-forming cells, the osteoblasts.

Osteoblasts are found on the outer surface and on the inside of bones. Osteoblasts respond to various chemical signals to produce the organic matrix. When the organic matrix is first produced, it is called the osteoid. Within a few days, calcium salts begin to precipitate on the osteoid and the bone hardens over the next several weeks or months. Some osteoblasts remain part of the osteoid, and are called osteocytes or true bone cells. As the bone forms, osteocytes in the matrix send out projections to each other, forming a system of microscopic canals (canaliculi) in the bone.

Osteoblast activity is affected by diet, hormonal stimulation, and exercise. These factors interact and are dynamic, resulting in different rates of bone formation throughout a lifetime.

Exercise and Osteoblast Activity

Osteoblastic activity is stimulated by exercise and weight-bearing, as a result of the electrical currents produced when stress is applied to the bone. Bone fracture dramatically stimulates osteoblast activity, but the exact mechanism is unclear.

Hormonal Stimulation and Osteoblast Activity

Estrogen, testosterone, and growth hormone enhance osteoblast activity and bone growth. Bone growth is accelerated during puberty as a result of surging levels of these hormones. Estrogen and testosterone eventually cause the long bones to stop growing by stimulating closure of the epiphyseal plate (growing end of the bone). When estrogen levels decrease after menopause, osteoblastic activity is reduced. Deficiencies in growth hormone impede bone formation.

Diet and Osteoblast Activity

An adequate diet during childhood and adolescence is essential for maximal bone growth. Calcium ion deficiency during adolescence will result in bones that are less dense than optimum later in life. Most of the calcium present in bones in an individual's lifetime is deposited before the age of 20.

Vitamin D Control of Osteoblast Activity

Vitamin D stimulates bone calcification directly by acting on the osteoblasts, and indirectly by stimulating calcium absorption across the gut. Increased calcium absorption increases blood calcium concentration, which promotes bone calcification. Thus, vitamin D is essential in order to ensure adequate calcium absorption across the gut. Very large amounts of vitamin D, however, may increase bone breakdown in an attempt to liberate calcium in order to increase serum calcium levels. Large amounts of vitamin D without adequate calcium in the diet actually can promote bone resorption.

Bone Breakdown

Bone breakdown, called resorption, occurs simultaneously with bone formation and is also ongoing throughout life. Bone resorption results from the activity of cells called osteoclasts. Osteoclasts are multinucleated, large phagocytic cells derived from monocytes (white blood cells) present in the bone. Osteoclasts secrete various acids and enzymes that digest the bone and allow for its phagocytosis. Osteoclasts also secrete various cytokines that further stimulate resorption. Osteoclasts are usually present in only one small section of bone at a time, and phagocytize the bone section by section. Once they finish in one area, the osteoclasts disappear and osteoblasts arrive. The osteoblasts begin to fill in the clear section with new bone. This process allows old, weakened bone to be replaced with new, stronger bone.

Factors that control osteoclast activity include parathyroid hormone and calcitonin. Parathyroid hormone tends to increase the number and resorptive capacity of osteoclasts while calcitonin reduces the number and resorptive capacity of osteoclasts.

Parathyroid Hormone and Osteoclastic Activity

Osteoclast activity is primarily controlled by parathyroid hormone, which is released by the parathyroid glands located directly behind the thyroid gland. Parathyroid hormone release increases in response to decreased serum calcium levels. Parathyroid hormone increases osteoclastic activity and stimulates bone breakdown, liberating free calcium into the blood. Increased serum calcium acts in a negative feedback manner to reduce further release of parathyroid hormone. It has been hypothesized that estrogen reduces bone resorption by inhibiting the effect of parathyroid hormone on osteoclasts; the mechanism of this is unknown.

Other Effects of Parathyroid Hormone

Parathyroid hormone maintains serum calcium levels by:

- Initiating calcium release from the bones.
- Simulating tubular reabsorption of calcium.
- Enhancing intestinal absorption of calcium through vitamin D activation.
- Increasing renal excretion of phosphate ion $\rightarrow$ decreasing blood phosphate levels.

Calcitonin and Osteoclastic Activity

Calcitonin is a hormone secreted by the thyroid gland in response to high serum calcium. It has a weak effect on inhibiting osteoclastic activity and formation. Calcitonin causes calcium to be sequestered in bone cells and decreases renal tubular reabsorption of calcium and phosphate. These effects increase bone calcification, thereby reducing serum calcium levels.

Remodeling

The balance between osteoblast and osteoclast activity continually remodels, or renews, the bone. In children and teenagers, osteoblastic activity outpaces osteoclastic activity, leading to thickening and lengthening of the skeleton. Osteoblastic activity also outpaces osteoclastic activity in bones healing from fracture. In a young adult, osteoblastic activity and osteoclastic activity are typically in equilibrium, resulting in a constant total amount of bone mass. By middle age, osteoclastic activity outpaces osteoblastic activity and bone density begins to decrease. Osteoclastic activity is also accelerated in immobilized bones. By the seventh or eighth decade of life, dominance of osteoclastic activity may cause the bones to become brittle, leading to increased fractures. Osteoclastic activities are controlled by several physical and hormonal factors.

Types of Bones

Bone is classified as long, short, flat, or irregular. Long bones are found in the extremities, whereas short bones are found in the ankles and wrists. Flat bones are found in the skull and rib cage. Irregular bones include the vertebrae, the bones of the face, and the jaw.

A long bone consist of a long, thick shaft, called the diaphysis, and two ends, called the epiphyses. Proximal to each epiphysis is the metaphysis. In between the epiphysis and the metaphysis is an area of growing cartilage, called the epiphyseal or growth plate. Long bones grow by means of the accumulation of cartilage at the epiphyseal plate. Cartilage is replaced by the osteoblasts, and the bone elongates. By the end of the teen years, the cartilage is used up, the epiphyseal plate fuses, and the bones stop growing. Growth hormone, estrogen, and testosterone stimulate growth of long bones. Estrogen, in conjunction with testosterone, stimulates fusion of the epiphyseal plates. The shaft of a long bone is hollowed out along the medullary canal, which is filled with bone marrow.

Bone Marrow

Bone marrow consists of cells involved in blood cell formation (red marrow) and fat cells (yellow marrow). Marrow is found in long and flat irregular bones. Bone marrow biopsy is performed on flat bones.

JOINTS

Joints are areas of the body where two bones come together. A joint may be freely movable, called a **diarthrodial joint**, or may be immobile, called a **synarthrodial joint**.

In a diarthrodial joint, the two ends of the bone are not connected directly, but come together in a fibrous joint capsule that surrounds and supports the joint. There are two layers of the joint capsule: an outer layer and an inner membrane layer called the synovium or *synovial membrane*. The synovial membrane secretes a slippery fluid, called *synovial fluid*, which lubricates the joint. The synovial membrane also covers the tendons that connect the bone to muscle, and the ligaments that connect the bones to each other. There is a well-developed vascular supply to the synovium, which may be damaged with joint trauma, leading to swelling, bruising, and pain surrounding the joint. In some joints, the synovial membrane forms a closed sac external to the joint, called a *bursa*. Bursae are found in areas where the bones are physically close together, or where a tendon runs over the bone. Bursae too may become inflamed, a condition called *bursitis*. Most joints in the body are diarthrodial joints, including the sacroiliac joint, the interphalangeal joints, the hip and knee joints, and the shoulder and elbow joints. Although all diarthrodial joints are considered movable, some of these joints move more than others (i.e., the sacroiliac joint is nearly fixed, whereas the shoulder joint is capable of moving in several different directions).

In synarthroses, the bones are held together by connective tissue, cartilage, ligaments, or other bones; thus, their positions are, to a large degree, fixed. Examples of synarthroses are the joints of the skull bones, ribs, and intervertebral disks.

● Pathophysiologic Concepts

ATROPHY

Atrophy is the decrease in size of a cell or tissue. Muscle atrophy may result from muscle disuse or severing of the nerve supplying the muscle. With muscular atrophy, the size of the myofibrils is reduced. Although bones do not atrophy, bone density can decrease with disuse or metabolic deficiencies or disease.

STRAINS

A strain is trauma to a muscle or tendon, usually occurring when the muscle or tendon is stretched beyond its normal limit. Strains may involve tissue tears or ruptures. Inflammation occurs with injury to muscles or tendons, leading to pain and swelling of tissue. Healing may take several weeks.

SPRAINS

A sprain is trauma to a joint, usually related to a ligament injury. In a severe sprain, the ligament may be completely torn or ruptured. Sprains lead to inflammation, swelling, and pain. Healing may take several weeks.

JOINT DISLOCATION

Dislocation of a joint occurs when a bone is displaced from its position in a joint. A *subluxation* is a partial dislocation of the joint in which the ends of the bone remain in partial contact with each other. Joint dislocation typically occurs after a severe trauma, which disrupts the ability of the ligament to hold the bone in place. Dislocation of a joint may also occur congenitally; for example, dislocation of the hip is sometimes seen in a newborn (developmental hip dysplasia). Pathologic dislocations may follow long-term problems such as infection, arthritis, paralysis, or neuromuscular disease. For a trauma-induced dislocation, there is associated marked pain, swelling, deformity, and loss of range of motion of the joint. Sometimes a popping noise may be heard or felt at the time of occurrence or during physical examination; in the newborn examination, manipulation of the joint to reproduce the sound or feeling of dislocation is used to diagnose the condition. Dislocation of a joint will usually be apparent on a radiograph and is treated by manipulation or surgical repair followed by immobilization until the joint structures are healed.

RHABDOMYOLYSIS

Rhabdomyolysis is a potential complication of toxic myopathy (muscle damage secondary to drugs or toxins). Acute muscle fiber necrosis causes muscle protein to leak into the bloodstream and eventually spill over into the urine. The presence of large amounts of muscle protein (myoglobin) in the urine can lead to acute renal failure if the myoglobin gets trapped in the delicate capillaries or tubules of the kidney, interfering with renal blood flow. Rhabdomyolysis usually occurs after major muscle trauma, especially a muscle crush injury. Long-distance running, certain severe infections, and exposure to electrical shock can cause extensive muscle damage and excessive release of myoglobin. Other potential causes include overexertion, narcotics, sedatives, hypolipidemic agents, antifibrinolytics, or drugs that induce hypokalemia.

OSTEOPENIA

Osteopenia is a reduction in bone mass greater than expected for age, race, or sex and is common to all metabolic bone diseases. It is the result of decreased bone formation, inadequate bone mineralization, or excessive bone deossification. Possible causes include osteoporosis, osteomalacia, malignancies, and endocrine disorders. The majority of hip fractures are the result of osteopenia.

RIGOR MORTIS

Rigor mortis is stiffening or contraction of muscles that occurs several hours after death. The condition results from ATP depletion in the muscle cells. Without ATP to bind to myosin, the actin–myosin cross-bridges that are connected in the muscle at the time of death cannot disengage, and the muscle stays contracted. Within a day, muscle proteins are destroyed by local enzymes released as cells degenerate, causing the muscles to relax.

● Conditions of Disease or Injury

MUSCULAR DYSTROPHY

Muscular dystrophy is a group of inherited disorders characterized by progressive muscular atrophy. The disorders involve an enzymatic or metabolic defect in which the muscle cells die and are phagocytized by cells of the inflammatory system, resulting in scar tissue buildup and loss of muscle function. There are several types of muscular dystrophy some of which can be fatal. Only the most common type will be discussed here.

Duchenne Muscular Dystrophy

The most common and most severe form of muscular dystrophy is Duchenne muscular dystrophy, a sex-linked disorder passed on the X chromosome and seen almost exclusively in males. In approximately 50% of cases, the disease shows a clear family history and is passed from mother to son. The other 50% occur as spontaneous mutations on the X chromosome before or during conception. Because males have only one X chromosome, the defective gene that causes the disease is not compensated for by a healthy gene on another X chromosome.

Duchenne muscular dystrophy results from a defect in the gene that produces the protein dystrophin. Dystrophin appears to act as an anchor for the actin filaments; without it, the muscle fiber is literally pulled apart with repeated contractions. Without dystrophin the cell membrane weakens, allowing extracellular fluid to leak into the cell. Activation of proteases and inflammatory processes result in muscle cell necrosis and phagocytosis. Necrotic muscle cells are replaced with fat and connective tissue.

Muscle cell weakness begins in the pelvic region by the time an affected child is approximately 2 or 3 years old. The weakness spreads to the legs and upper body within 3 to 5 years. When the muscle cells die, scar tissue and fat cells replace the dead cells, causing the muscles (especially the calf muscles) to appear strong and well muscled (called pseudohypertrophy), when in actuality they are weak and poorly functioning. Eventually, the skeleton begins to deform and the child becomes progressively immobile and finally restricted to a wheelchair. Cardiac muscle is often involved, and approximately 50% of affected children develop heart failure. Respiratory effort is progressively compromised, related to dysfunction of the diaphragm and other respiratory muscles as well as the inability to expand the chest because of severe kyphosis. Smooth muscle dysfunction may cause GI disturbance. Mental retardation may also be present. Death usually occurs as a result of respiratory or cardiac complications in the 20s or younger.

Clinical Manifestations of Duchenne Muscular Dystrophy

- Clumsiness, waddling gait, and frequent falls in toddlers.
- Walking on toes because of anterior tibial weakness.
- Decreased deep tendon reflexes.
- Pseudohypertrophy of the calf muscles.
- Gowers' maneuver, whereby the child uses his arms to push up onto his legs when standing up from the floor, is seen during the toddler years.
- Immobility and confinement to a wheelchair by the early teens.
- Curvature of the spine (kyphoscoliosis) caused by weakness of the postural muscles.
- Frequent respiratory infections from a failure to fully expand the lungs.

Diagnostic Tools

- Serum levels of the muscle enzyme creatine kinase (CK) are elevated, even before symptoms develop. CK may be elevated in female carriers who are asymptomatic for the disease.
- Elevated serum alanine transaminase and aspartate transaminase, which tend to correlate with CK levels.
- Muscle biopsy will demonstrate cell death, scar tissue, fatty infiltration, and little or no dystrophin, but is typically only performed if genetic testing is negative.
- Electromyography recordings (measurements of electrical signals in a muscle) will be reduced.
- Molecular genetic testing is now becoming the gold standard for diagnosis. Analysis of polymerase chain reaction (PCR) of genomic DNA obtained from leukocytes in a blood sample reveal large deletions of the gene.

- Because the gene for dystrophin has been identified, prenatal testing for the disorder is possible.

Complications

- Family stress, feelings of guilt or blame, anger, and grief are common.
- Dysphagia; coughing and choking while eating.
- Scoliosis will eventually develop in most cases.
- Constipation, behavioral issues, intellectual disability in approximately 30%.
- Increased risk of malignant hyperthermia.
- Usually wheelchair bound by 12 years of age.
- Respiratory or cardiac failure and death are likely before adulthood.

Treatment

- Support groups and family counseling are important to improve family coping.
- Nonstrenuous exercises are recommended to maintain mobility and function as long as possible. Strenuous exercise may hasten muscle deterioration.
- Corticosteroids tend to increase muscle strength temporarily.
- Experimental studies involving intramuscular injection of dystrophin, or the gene for dystrophin, are under way in animal models. Insertion of the gene for dystrophin may be accomplished by producing a genetically engineered virus that will carry the correct gene into host muscle cells.
- Experimental studies are under way in which healthy, immature muscle cells are taken from the fathers of young male children with muscular dystrophy and injected into the muscles of their sons. Whether significant improvement in muscle function will occur in the children is unclear.
- The discovery that the protein myostatin limits skeletal muscle growth suggests that inhibition of the myostatin pathway may someday offer a potential treatment for muscular dystrophy.

BONE FRACTURE

A bone fracture is a break in a bone. Terms and descriptions of various types of bone fractures are included in Table 10-2.

Causes of Bone Fractures

The most frequent cause of bone fracture is trauma, especially in children and young adults. Falls and sports injuries are common causes of traumatic

TABLE 10-2   Types of Bone Fractures

Fracture Type	Description
Complete	Fracture that extends through the bone
Incomplete	Fracture that extends partially through the bone
Closed (formerly simple)	Fracture that does not cause a break in the skin
Open (formerly compound)	Fracture that causes a break in the skin
Comminuted	Multiple fractures of the bone
Linear	Fracture is parallel to long axis of the bone
Oblique	Fracture at an angle to long axis of the bone
Spiral	Fracture encircles bone
Transverse	Fracture perpendicular to long axis of bone
Impacted	Fracture fragments pushed into each other
Greenstick	Break in cortex of bone with splintering of inner bone surface

fractures. In a child, abuse must be considered when evaluating a fracture, especially if there is a previous history of fractures or if the history of the current fracture is unconvincing.

Some fractures may result after minimal trauma or slight pressure if the bone is weak. These are called **pathologic fractures**. Pathologic fractures often occur in elderly persons who suffer from osteoporosis, or in individuals with bone tumors, infections, or other diseases.

Stress fractures may occur in normal bone as a result of prolonged or repeated low-level stress. The two types of stress fractures are **fatigue fracture** and **insufficiency fracture**. Stress fractures usually accompany a rapid increase in the training level of an athlete, or the beginning of a new physical activity. Because muscle strength increases more rapidly than bone strength, an individual may feel capable of performing beyond a previous level even though the bones may be incapable of supporting the added pressure. The disconnect between muscles and bone development results in microfractures in the cortex. Fatigue fractures are most common in those who pursue endurance sports such as long-distance running. Insufficiency fractures typically occur in bones with an altered ability to deform and recover. They may occur in weakened bone in response to normal weight-bearing or only a slight increase in activity level. Individuals suffering a stress fracture should be encouraged to follow a bone-healthy diet and be screened for reduced bone density.

Effects of a Bone Fracture

When a bone breaks, bone cells die. Bleeding typically occurs around the site and into the soft tissues surrounding the bone. The soft tissues are usually damaged by the injury. An intense inflammatory reaction follows the break. White cells and mast cells accumulate, causing increased blood flow to the area. Phagocytosis and removal of dead cell debris begin. A fibrin clot (fracture hematoma) forms at the break and acts as a meshwork to which new cells can adhere. Osteoblastic activity is immediately stimulated and immature new bone, called **callus**, is formed. The fibrin clot is soon reabsorbed, and the new bone cells are slowly remodeled to form true bone. The true bone replaces the callus and is slowly calcified. Healing takes several weeks to a few months (fractures in children heal faster). Healing can be delayed or impaired if the fracture hematoma or callus is disrupted before true bone is formed, or if the new bone cells are disrupted during calcification and hardening. A summary of the process from injury to healing is included in Figure 10-7.

Clinical Manifestations

- Numbness initially followed by intense and often incapacitating pain.
- Pain usually accompanies a traumatic bone break and soft tissue injury. Muscle spasm may follow a bone break and contribute to the pain. With a stress fracture, the pain typically accompanies activity and is relieved by rest. Pathologic fractures may not be associated with pain.
- An unnatural position of the bone or a limb may be obvious.
- Swelling around the site of a fracture will accompany the inflammatory processes.
- Impaired sensation or tingling may occur, signaling nerve damage. Pulses distal to the fracture should be intact and equal to the nonfractured side. A loss of distal pulse may indicate compartmental syndrome (see later), although the presence of a pulse does not rule out this disorder.
- Crepitus (a grating sound) may be heard with movement, as the broken ends of the bone move across each other.

Diagnostic Tools

- Radiograph can reveal a bone fracture.
- Bone scan can reveal a stress fracture.

Complications

- Nonunion, delayed union, or malunion of the bone may occur, leading to deformity or loss of function.

Break in the bone

Disruption of periosteum, blood vessels in the cortex, marrow and surrounding soft tissue

Bleeding from bone ends and soft tissue

Clot formation within medullary canal between fractured ends of bone and beneath periosteum

Death of bone tissue adjacent to fracture

Intense inflammatory response with vasodilation, exudation of plasma & leukocytes and infiltration by inflammatory leukocytes, growth factors and mast cells

Decalcification of fractured bone ends - within 48 hours: vascular tissue invades fracture area

Increased blood flow

Stimulation of bone-forming cells in periosteum, endosteum and marrow

Production of subperiosteal procallus along outer surface of shaft and over broken ends of the bone – osteoblasts within procallus synthesize collagen and matrix

Mineralization to form callus

Remodeling

Trabeculae formed along lines of stress

FIGURE 10-7 From fracture to healing.

- Compartment syndrome may occur. Compartment syndrome is characterized by nerve and blood vessel damage or destruction that results from swelling and edema in the area of a fracture. With intense interstitial swelling, pressure exerted on blood vessels supplying the area may cause them to collapse. This leads to tissue hypoxia and may cause death of the nerves supplying the area. Typically, pain is intense. The individual may be unable to move his or her fingers or toes. Compartment syndrome usually occurs in limbs that have tight volume restrictions, such as the arms. The risk of developing compartment syndrome is greatest if muscle trauma has occurred with the break because swelling will be pronounced. Casting of a fractured limb too early or too tightly may cause increased pressure in the limb compartment, and permanent loss of function or loss of the limb may result. A cast must be immediately removed and sometimes the skin of the limb must be split. Frequent neurovascular assessments will facilitate early identification of developing compartment syndrome. Assessing for pain, pallor, paresthesias, pulselessness, and paralysis is imperative.
- Fat embolism syndrome involves a set of clinical manifestations caused by fat droplets in small blood vessels of the lungs or other organs. It may occur after the breakage of a bone, especially a long bone or as the result of major trauma. A bone fracture → disruption of venous sinusoids and fat cells → entrance of fat globules into the venous circulation → particles lodge in pulmonary capillaries or go to general circulation. Fat embolus may be generated from exposure of the bone marrow, or may result from activation of the sympathetic nervous system leading to stimulation of free fatty acid mobilization after the trauma. Typical findings associated with a fat embolism include respiratory failure, cerebral dysfunction, and skin petechiae, typically on the anterior chest. Fat emboli may be present, however; only a small percentage of patients develop fat embolism syndrome.
- Complex regional pain syndrome in which pain is out of proportion to the injury.
- Decreased mobility may result in thromboemboli and/or muscle weakness and atrophy.
- Infection (see osteomyelitis).

Treatment

- A fracture should be immediately immobilized to allow formation of a fracture hematoma and minimize damage.
- Realignment of the bone (reduction) is important to allow recovery of normal positioning and range of motion. Most reduction can be performed without surgical intervention (closed reduction). If surgery is required for fixation (open reduction), pins or screws may be inserted to maintain realignment. Traction may be required to maintain reduction and stimulate healing.

- Long-term immobilization after reduction is important to allow formation of callus and new bone. Long-term immobilization is usually accomplished by casting or the use of splints.
- Traction.

ACUTE OSTEOMYELITIS

Osteomyelitis is an acute infection of the bone that may occur from the spread of a blood-borne infection (hematogenous osteomyelitis) or, more commonly, after contamination of an open fracture or surgical reduction (exogenous osteomyelitis). A puncture wound to the soft tissue or bone, resulting from an animal or human bite or a misplaced intramuscular injection, may cause exogenous osteomyelitis. Bacteria are the usual cause of acute osteomyelitis, but viruses, fungi, and other microorganisms may be involved. The invading organism causes an intense inflammatory response with vascular engorgement, edema, leukocyte activity, and abscess formation. Small terminal vessels begin to thrombose, causing exudates to be sealed in the bone's canaliculi. Exudates begin to extend into the metaphysis, narrow cavity, and through small metaphysical openings into the cortex. Infection disrupts and weakens the cortex.

Osteomyelitis is a difficult disease to treat because local abscesses may develop. A bone abscess typically has a poor blood supply; therefore, delivery of immune cells and antibiotics is limited. Intense pain and lifelong disability may result if a bone infection is not treated immediately and aggressively.

Clinical Manifestations

- Symptoms of hematogenous osteomyelitis in children may include fever, chills, and a reluctance to move a particular limb. In adults, symptoms may be vague and include fever, fatigue, and malaise. A urinary, respiratory tract, ear, or skin infection frequently precedes hematogenous osteomyelitis.
- Exogenous osteomyelitis typically presents with evidence of injury and inflammation at the site of pain. Fever and regional lymph node enlargement occur.

Diagnostic Tools

- Bone scan using injected radiolabeled nucleotides may show an inflammatory bone site. Magnetic resonance imaging (MRI) may allow for increased diagnostic sensitivity.
- Blood analysis may demonstrate elevation in complete blood count (CBC) and erythrocyte sedimentation rate, suggesting an active infection is in progress.

Complications

- Chronic osteomyelitis may develop, characterized by unrelenting, severe pain, and decreased function of the affected body part.

Treatment

- Antibiotics may be prescribed to an individual suffering a bone break or puncture wound to the soft tissue surrounding a bone before a sign of infection develops. If a bone infection occurs, aggressive antibiotic therapy is required. Antibiotic-impregnated bioabsorbable beads.
- Debridement.
- Wound irrigation.
- Bone biopsy.
- Hyperbaric oxygen therapy to stimulate healing by suppressing proinflammatory cytokines and prostaglandins.
- Joint implants may need to be removed.

OSTEOPOROSIS

Osteoporosis is a metabolic bone disease characterized by a severe reduction in bone density, leading to easy bone fracture and is the most common metabolic bone disease. Osteoporosis occurs when the rate of bone resorption greatly exceeds the rate of bone formation. Bone that is produced is normal; however, because there is too little of it, the bones are weak. All bones can be affected by osteoporosis, although osteoporosis usually develops in the bones of the hips, pelvis, wrists, and vertebral column. See Figures 10-8, 10-9, and 10-10 for illustrations relating to osteoporosis.

The National Osteoporosis Foundation estimates that more than 10 million people in the United States have osteoporosis and another 33.6 million have osteopenia of the hip (http://www.nof.org). Although currently seen most frequently in Caucasian women, it is predicted that in the next 20 years, the number of men and minorities with osteoporosis will increase significantly as a result of demographic changes. The American College of Physicians now recommends conducting a risk assessment for all older men.

Causes of Osteoporosis

The rate of bone formation decreases progressively with age, beginning at approximately age 30 or 40. The denser the bones are before that time, the less likely that osteoporosis will occur. As people age into their 70s and 80s, osteoporosis becomes a common disease.

Although bone resorption begins to outpace formation by the fourth or fifth decade of life, in women the most significant thinning of the bones occurs during and after menopause. The postmenopausal decrease in estrogen appears to

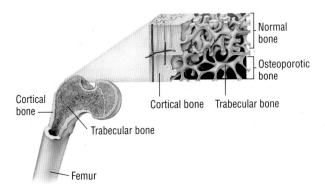

FIGURE 10-8 Osteoporosis is a metabolic bone disease characterized by a severe reduction in bone density leading to easy bone fracture. Osteoporosis occurs when the rate of bone resorption greatly exceeds the rate of bone formation. Bone that is produced is normal; however, because there is too little of it, the bones are weak.

be primarily responsible for this development in the elderly female population. Although the mechanism by which estrogen acts to preserve bone density is unclear, it is thought that estrogen stimulates osteoblastic activity and limits the osteoclastic-stimulating effects of parathyroid hormones. Therefore, a loss of

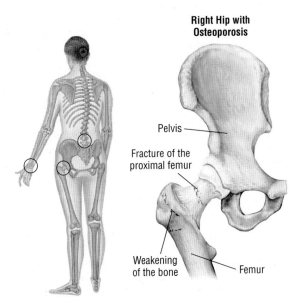

FIGURE 10-9 All bones can be affected by osteoporosis, although it usually develops in the bones of the hips, pelvis, wrists, and vertebral column.

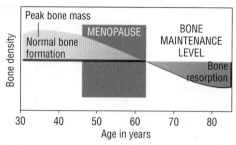

FIGURE 10-10 Although bone resorption begins to outpace bone formation by the fourth or fifth decade of life, in women the most significant thinning of the bones occurs during and after menopause. The postmenopausal decrease in estrogen primarily appears to be responsible for this development. Although the mechanism by which estrogen acts to preserve bone density is unclear, it is thought that estrogen stimulates osteoclastic activity and limits the osteoclastic-stimulating effects of parathyroid hormones. Therefore, a loss of estrogen causes a pronounced shift toward osteoclastic activity, dropping overall bone mass below the maintenance density level and risking fracture.

estrogen causes a pronounced shift toward osteoclastic activity. Thin women, fair-haired women, and women who smoke are especially prone to osteoporosis because their bones are less dense before menopause than those of heavier, dark-haired, nonsmoking women. Although elderly men may be less prone to osteoporosis because they typically have denser bones than women (by approximately 30%), and reproductive hormone levels remain high until a man is in his 80s, the risk is still significant. However, elderly men have less dense bones than younger men.

For men and women, other causes of osteoporosis include reduced physical activity and the ingestion of certain drugs, including corticosteroids and some aluminum-containing antacids that increase calcium elimination. It has been shown that even very elderly men and women can significantly increase bone density by participating in moderate forms of weight-bearing activity. Family history also plays a role in determining an individual's future risk. Bone density has been shown to decrease in breastfeeding women, although a return to near-normal density occurs after weaning. Other risk factors include weight loss, low body weight, smoking, alcohol or caffeine use, and low vitamin D and calcium intake.

Clinical Manifestations

- Although insidiously advancing, osteoporosis may not be associated with any clinical manifestations unless a bone break occurs. Pain and deformity usually accompany a break.
- With weakness and collapse of the vertebral bodies, an individual may shrink in height or develop kyphosis (sometimes called dowager hump).

- In 2004, the U.S. Surgeon General identified a low trauma fracture as a sentinel event indicating poor bone health that should be considered an indication for bone density screening, even in young people or others not considered at high risk of osteoporosis.

Diagnostic Tools

- A careful family and personal history will identify patients at risk of developing osteoporosis. Physical examination identifying kyphosis and a demonstrable reduction in height will assist diagnosis.
- Bone-mineral content of the whole body, and bone-mineral density of specific bones such as the lumbar spine, femoral neck, and shaft of the femur, tibia, fibula and distal radius, are often assessed using dual-energy radiograph absorptiometry (DEXA). This measurement offers an accurate reading of bone mass and allows a clinician to chart the rate of bone decay. Bone density testing that reveals a bone density of fewer than two standard deviations below normal (based on average of young women) is considered abnormal.

Complications

- Fractures of the hips, wrists, vertebral column, and pelvis.
- Hospitalization, placement in a nursing home, and loss of ability to perform activities of daily living may occur after an osteoporotic fracture.

Treatment

- Prevention of osteoporosis begins in childhood and the teen years with the formation of lifelong habits of good nutrition and physical exercise to strengthen bones.
- Weight-bearing exercise, even in the very elderly (>85 years), has been shown to increase bone density and muscle mass and improve balance and physical endurance. The effects of high-impact exercise, such as jumping and running, on maintaining bone health in children are being studied more closely. The use of vibration to maintain bone health in children and elders with limited mobility is being studied as well.
- Dietary supplements of vitamin D and calcium reduce the development of osteoporosis in the elderly and are essential components of prevention.
- Cigarette smoking should be avoided.
- Estrogen–progesterone replacement therapy or selective estrogen receptor modulators (SERMs) taken during and after menopause can reduce the development of osteoporosis in women. Contraindications for estrogen replacement include a family or personal history of breast cancer or a personal history of blood clots.
- Drugs known as bisphosphonates (e.g., alendronate, risedronate, and ibandronate) have been shown to decrease bone resorption and prevent bone loss.

These drugs, in combination with vitamin D and calcium supplements, are used for treatment and prevention of osteoporosis. The bisphosphonates significantly increase bone density in the hip and spine especially, and can be used in postmenopausal and drug-induced (glucocorticoid) osteoporosis. They are also used as chemotherapeutic adjuvants in cancer therapy because of their potential to prevent bone metastasis. Bisphosphonates are not easily absorbed by the body, so must be taken on an empty stomach with a full glass of water. The patient must remain upright and refrain from eating for a certain period afterward, to ensure absorption and prevent gastrointestinal side effects. Adherence to bisphosphonates therefore is often problematic. A once-a-month oral preparation that may improve adherence has been approved by the FDA. Another alternative, intravenous ibandronate, bypasses the gastrointestinal tract and is administered once every 3 months. Intravenous zoledronic is given once every 12 months. Both medications can be administered in an out-patient setting.

- Patients who do not respond positively to other strategies may be given teriparatide, a synthetic parathyroid hormone that helps build bone.
- Calcitonin may also be prescribed for those suffering from severe osteoporosis. Intranasal administration has recently become available, increasing patient usage.
- Testosterone therapy may reduce osteoporosis in men.
- Teriparatide, a parathyroid compound, has been found to increase bone density.
- Guidelines for preventative treatment are currently in progress by groups such as the World Health Organization.

HYPERPARATHYROIDISM

Hyperparathyroidism is a disorder of bone mineralization and muscle weakness caused by high levels of circulating parathyroid hormone. Usually, the elevated parathyroid hormone results from a tumor of the parathyroid gland or another gland. With excess parathyroid hormone, bone resorption is stimulated, resulting in high serum calcium levels. Low serum phosphate accompanies high levels of parathyroid hormone. The bones become brittle and weak.

Secondary hyperparathyroidism can occur with states of hypocalcemia, caused by vitamin D deficiency or renal failure. Calcium levels remain low even with elevated parathyroid hormone.

Clinical Manifestations

- Multiple pathologic fractures, diffuse bone demineralization, cystic bone lesions.
- Kyphosis of the spine and vertebral compression fractures.
- Fatigue and weakness because high serum calcium leads to decreased nerve and muscle cell excitability.

Diagnostic Tools

- Serum assay will demonstrate elevated serum calcium levels (normal 8.6 to 10.5 mg/dL).
- Serum phosphate levels will be low (normal 2.5 to 4.5 mg/dL).
- Serum parathyroid hormone levels.

Complications

- Calcium-based kidney stones may develop, causing pain and inflammation of the urinary tract.
- Electrocardiogram (ECG) (Chapter 13) abnormalities may develop, including premature ventricular contractions (PVCs) and sinus tachycardia, related to the effects of high serum calcium on cardiac muscle depolarization.

Treatment

- Treatment depends on the cause and severity of the disease.
- Fluids are essential in management.
- Oral phosphate may be administered.
- Specific drugs to treat hypercalcemia, including steroids and calcium-losing diuretics, may be used.
- Surgical excision of the parathyroid glands may be required.

OSTEOMALACIA AND RICKETS

Osteomalacia is a metabolic bone disease seen in adults. It is caused by decreased mineralization of the osteoid as a result of a deficiency of calcium, phosphate, or both. Decreased mineralization results in soft, malleable bone. Osteomalacia usually results from a vitamin D deficiency or insensitivity or from renal disease.

Vitamin D is required for the maintenance of calcium absorption in the gut. With vitamin D deficiency or insensitivity, decreased serum calcium develops, which in turn stimulates parathyroid hormone release. Increased parathyroid hormone stimulates bone breakdown to liberate calcium and increases renal excretion of phosphate. Without adequate mineralization of the bone, the bone becomes thinner. Abnormal amounts of noncrystallized osteoid accumulate and coat the channels of the inner bone, which leads to bone deformity.

Renal failure is associated with osteomalacia because of two factors: the inability of the kidney to activate vitamin D and the decreased ability to excrete phosphate in the urine. Increased serum phosphate also stimulates parathyroid secretion, and hence bone breakdown. Other causes of osteomalacia not directly related to dietary deficiency include the malabsorption of dietary calcium seen in Crohn disease, malabsorption syndrome, and cystic fibrosis.

Rickets is a bone disease in children caused by vitamin D deficiency, inadequate absorption of calcium, and impaired bone mineralization. Rickets causes disorganization of the bone, especially at the growth or epiphyseal plates, retarding growth and distorting bone development. Frank rickets is uncommon in the United States, but may be seen in cases of extreme poverty or neglect, or may be subtle in presentation.

Clinical Manifestations

- Osteomalacia
  - May be symptomless until a fracture occurs.
  - Pain, tenderness, fracture.
  - Muscle weakness in severe cases.
  - Vertebral collapse is common, with associated changes in posture and height.
  - May be accompanied by compensatory or secondary hyperparathyroidism as a result of low serum calcium levels.
- Rickets is characterized by permanent skeletal deformity, including bowed legs, lumbar lordosis (convexity of the spine), and rib and skull deformity. Children may be unable to walk without support. They may also show poor dentition.

Diagnostic Tools

- Radiograph evaluation can demonstrate reduced bone ossification.
- Measurements of serum calcium and phosphate will be low in severe cases.
- Serum parathyroid hormone and vitamin D.
- Bone density studies or bone biopsy.

Treatment

Treatment is targeted at identifying and treating the underlying cause.

- Nutritional: Vitamin D therapy with calcium supplementation is required.
- If osteomalacia or rickets is caused by another disease, that disease will require treatment.

OSTEOARTHRITIS

Osteoarthritis is a degenerative bone disease characterized by loss of articular (joint) cartilage and abnormal formation of new bone (bone spurs). The process involves low-grade inflammation, articular cartilage calcification, genetic alterations, and metabolic disorders. Cytokines, matrix molecules, growth factors, and enzymes play a role in the degenerative process. Without cartilage buffering, the underlying bone is irritated, leading to degeneration of the joint. Osteoarthritis may develop idiopathically (for no known reason) or may occur after trauma, with repeated stress such as that experienced by a long-distance runner or ballerina, or in association with a congenital deformity. Individuals with hemophilia or other conditions characterized by chronic joint swelling and edema may develop osteoarthritis. Osteoarthritis is common in the elderly, affecting more than 70% of men and women older than the age of 65. The occurrence in males and females is about equal, but females tend to have more severe cases. Obesity can worsen the condition.

Clinical Manifestations

- Pain and stiffness in one or more of the joints, commonly the hands, wrists, feet, knees, upper and lower spine, hips, and shoulders. Pain may be worse with weight-bearing.
- Pain may be associated with tingling or numbness, especially at night.
- Swelling of the affected joints, with a decreased range of motion. Joints may appear deformed. Crepitus or grating sound with movement.
- Heberden nodes, bony growths on the distal interphalangeal joints of the fingers, and Bouchard nodes on the proximal interphalangeal joints, may develop.

Diagnostic Tools

- Arthroscopy (visualization of the joint through a fiber-optic instrument), MRI, and CT scan may support the clinical diagnosis.

Treatment

- A balance between resting and exercising the joints, geared toward minimizing inflammation but preserving range of motion, is helpful.
- Assistive devices to ease weight-bearing.
- Weight loss for those overweight.
- Analgesics and anti-inflammatory drugs to reduce swelling and inflammation.
- Nutraceuticals such as glucosamine and chondroitin may slow progression and ease pain.
- Intra-articular injections of high-molecular-weight viscose supplements.
- Surgery may be required to correct a deformity or replace a joint.

RHEUMATOID ARTHRITIS

Rheumatoid arthritis (RA) is a systemic, chronic, inflammatory disease that causes degeneration of connective tissue. According to the National Institute of Arthritis and Musculoskeletal and Skin Disorders (2006), it affects about 2.1 million people in the United States. Unlike other forms of arthritis, RA typically occurs in a symmetrical pattern. Women are two to three times more likely than men to develop RA. The peak incidence is during the fourth and fifth decades. The connective tissue usually destroyed first is the synovial membrane, which lines the joints. In RA, the inflammation becomes unrelenting and spreads to the surrounding structures of the joint, including the articular cartilage and the fibrous joint capsule. Eventually, the ligaments and tendons become inflamed. The inflammation is characterized by white blood cell accumulation, complement activation, extensive phagocytosis, and scarring. With chronic inflammation, the synovial membrane undergoes hypertrophy and thickens, occluding blood flow and further stimulating cell necrosis and the inflammatory response. The thickened synovium becomes covered by inflammatory granular tissue called **pannus**. Pannus may spread throughout the joint, leading to further inflammation and scarring. These processes slowly destroy the bone and cause great pain and deformity.

Causes of Rheumatoid Arthritis

RA is an autoimmune disease that develops in susceptible individuals after an immune response against an unknown triggering agent. The triggering agent may be a bacterium, mycoplasma, or virus that infects the joints or resembles the joint antigenically. Typically, the original antibody response to the microorganism is IgG mediated. Although this response may successfully destroy the microorganism, individuals who develop RA begin to produce other antibodies, usually IgM or IgG, against the original IgG antibody. These self-directed antibodies are called rheumatoid factors (RFs). The RFs persist in the joint capsule, causing chronic inflammation and destruction of the tissue. RA is thought to result from a genetic predisposition to autoimmune disease. Women are more often affected than men. There is strong evidence to suggest that various cytokines, especially tumor necrosis factor alpha (TNF-α), contribute to the cycle of inflammation and joint destruction.

Clinical Manifestations

- Onset of RA is characterized by general symptoms of inflammation, including fever, fatigue, body aches, and joint swelling. Joint tenderness and stiffness develop, first because of acute inflammation and then from scar formation. The metacarpophalangeal joints and the wrists are usually first involved. Stiffness is worse in the morning and affects joints bilaterally. Episodes of inflammation are interspersed with periods of remission.
- Decreased range of motion, joint deformity, and muscular contractions.
- Extrasynovial rheumatoid nodules develop in approximately 20% of individuals with RA. These swellings consist of white blood cells and cell debris that present at areas of trauma or increased pressure. Usually, nodules develop in the subcutaneous tissue over the elbows and fingers.

Diagnostic Tools

- Elevated serum RF in 80% of cases. Presence of antibodies against cyclic citrullinated peptide (anti-CCP antibody). Presence of RF and CCP together may indicate a more aggressive disease process.

- Elevation of inflammatory markers such as C-reactive protein and erythrocyte sedimentation rate. Hypergammaglobulinemia, thrombocytosis, and hypochromic microcytic anemia may also be present.
- Radiograph changes including bony decalcification of the joints.
- Synovial fluid aspiration may show white blood cells in a sterile culture.
- Swan-neck deformity due to contractures of intrinsic muscles and tendons.
- The American Rheumatism Association (1987) revised criteria for the classification of RA. At least four of the seven criteria must be present and criteria 1 to 4 must be present for at least 6 weeks:

1. Morning stiffness in and around joints that takes at least 1 hour to achieve maximal improvement.
2. Soft tissue swelling of at least three joint areas (right and left proximal PIP, metacarpophalangeal, wrist, elbow, knee, ankle, metatarsophalangeal joints).
3. Swelling of at least one wrist, MCP, or PIP joint.
4. Simultaneous symmetric swelling in joints listed in #2.
5. Subcutaneous rheumatoid nodules.
6. Positive RF.
7. Radiographic erosions and/or periarticular osteopenia of hand and/or wrist joints (Arnett et al., 1987).

Complications

- Extrasynovial rheumatoid nodules may develop on cardiac valves or in the lungs, eyes, or spleen. Respiratory and cardiac function may be affected. Glaucoma may result if nodules that block outflow of ocular fluid develop in the eye.
- Vasculitis (inflammation of the vascular system) may lead to thrombosis and infarction.
- Loss of ability to carry out activities of daily living, depression, and family stress may accompany exacerbations of the disease.

Treatment

The goals of treatment include: (1) relief of pain and swelling, (2) prevention of structural damage, and (3) retention of function.

- Rest of the inflamed joints during exacerbations.
- Rest periods each day.
- Alternating hot and cold packs.
- Physical therapy.
- Diet high in calories and vitamins.

- Aspirin, other nonsteroidal anti-inflammatory drugs (NSAIDs), or systemic steroids. Other therapies such as gold treatments, antimalarial agents, or combination therapies may be tried.
- Disease-modifying antirheumatic drugs (DMARDs) such as methotrexate.
- Anti-TNF medications are being used to block cytokine-mediated inflammation.
- Surgery to remove the synovial membrane or to correct deformity.
- Herbal remedies with anti-inflammatory properties have been used for generations to reduce the symptoms of RA. These include cat's claw (*Uncaria tomentosa*), devil's claw (*Harpagophytum procumbens*), and the Chinese herb lei gong teng (*Tripterygium wilfordii*). Practitioners should ask patients if they are using these or other over-the-counter medications, and should counsel patients regarding the lack of scientific evidence on the mechanism of action and clinical effectiveness of these herbs.

GOUT

Gout is a disorder of purine metabolism in which high blood levels of uric acid cause precipitation of urate crystals in the joints resulting in acute inflammation. Primary gout is the result of excessive production of uric acid or decreased urate excretion by the kidney. Secondary gout is due to medications or disease processes that cause overproduction or impair elimination of uric acid. The prevalence is higher in males than females and there is a familial tendency. Obesity, chronic alcohol ingestion, and excessive intake of high purine foods also tend to increase the risk. Joints most often involved include the metatarsophalangeal joint of the big toe and joints in the heels, ankles, knees, fingers, wrists, or elbows.

Clinical Manifestations

- Sudden, severe pain in a single joint.
- Systemic signs of inflammation such as elevated temperature, malaise, headache, and chills.
- With chronic gout, tophi (hard, painless nodules) is a hallmark finding.

Diagnostic Tools

- Thorough history and physical examination.
- Serum uric acid level is often elevated.
- Definitive diagnosis is by synovial fluid analysis of the involved joint that will contain uric acid crystals.

Complications

- Limited range of motion in the affected joint leading to deformity.

Treatment

Acute and chronic gout are treated differently. The goal of treatment for acute gout is pain relief while the goal of treatment for chronic gout is threefold: (1) preventing future attacks, (2) decreasing presence of tophi, and (3) minimizing the risk for renal involvement.

- Acute
  - Rest the joint and apply ice to reduce discomfort.
  - NSAIDs to decrease pain and inflammation.
  - Uric acid inhibitors to block accumulation of uric acid in the blood and uric acid crystal formation within the joints.
  - Glucocorticoids administered orally or intraarticularly.
- Chronic
  - Identify and avoid trigger foods.
  - If obese, encourage weight loss with the reduction of fat, cholesterol, and sodium.
  - Moderate exercise program.
  - Xanthine oxidase inhibitors to block uric acid formation.
  - Uricosuric agents to block renal reabsorption of uric acid and increase excretion.

LOW BACK PAIN

Low back pain is one of the most common reasons for health care visits. The associated pain and disability are a major health care cost as well as the reason for many days of missed work. The back protects the spinal cord and provides support for muscles and tendons. Most low back pain is idiopathic in nature. Possible causes include injury, infection, muscle strain, lumbar disk herniation, degenerative disk disease, spondylolysis, spinal stenosis, and bone disease (i.e., osteoarthritis).

Clinical Manifestations

- Pain in the back that may radiate.
- Muscle tension and tightness.

Diagnostic Tools

- Thorough history and physical.
- X-ray, CT scan, MRI.
- Myelogram, nerve-conduction studies, diskography, and epidurography.

Complications

- Disability and subsequent depression.

Treatment

- Bed rest.
- Heat or cold.
- Analgesics, anti-inflammatory drugs, muscle relaxants.
- Strengthening exercises and physical therapy.
- Education about proper lifting.
- Spinal surgery.

CARPAL TUNNEL SYNDROME

Carpal tunnel syndrome is one of the most common nerve entrapment syndromes. Decreased tunnel size or increased volume exerts pressure on the median nerve causing pain and paresthesia. The carpal bones and transverse carpal ligament form the carpel tunnel. Inflammation or fibrosis of the tendon sheaths that pass through the carpal tunnel cause edema and compress the median nerve. The compression neuropathy causes sensory and motor changes in the median distribution of the hand and impairs sensory transmission to the thumb, index finger, second finger, and inner aspect of the third finger. Possible causes include repetitive wrist motion, wrist injury, pregnancy, and birth-control medications. It may also accompany some systemic conditions such as RA, diabetes, or acromegaly.

Clinical Manifestations

- Pain, paresthesia, weakness, burning, tingling, and/or numbness of the thumb, index finger, second finger, and inner aspect of the third finger.
- Wrist and hand pain that is worse at night and in the morning. Vasodilation, stasis, and prolonged wrist flexion during sleep contribute to compression of the carpal tunnel.
- Weakness in precision grip.

Diagnostic Tools

- Positive Phalen (acutely flexed wrists for 60 seconds elicits numbness and tingling) and Tinel test (tapping over the inflamed nerve elicits paresthesia).
- Electromyography.
- Nerve-conduction studies.

Complications

- Pain may interfere with work duties and activities of daily living.

Treatment

- Identify and eliminate the cause (repetitive movements).
- Avoid movements that cause nerve compression.
- Splinting.
- Anti-inflammatory medication.
- Corticosteroid injections into the carpal tunnel to decrease inflammation and swelling.
- Surgery to divide volar carpal ligaments to relieve pressure on the nerve.

FIBROMYALGIA

Fibromyalgia is one of the most common rheumatologic conditions in all ethnic groups. While the pathology is not totally understood, the chronic, widespread pain and fatigue can be disabling. Family history, infection, trauma, stress, anxiety, and depression may be contributing factors. Several theories related to the pathogenesis are listed below.

- Altered sympathetic nervous system (chronic sympathetic activation) and hypothalamic–pituitary–adrenal axis responses.
- Altered muscle activity and pain-processing mechanisms.
- Research has shown increased levels of nerve growth factor and the *substance P* (a chemical signal) in spinal fluid and decreased levels of serotonin. Nerve growth factor and *substance P* initiate and perpetuate pain and low serotonin levels impair pain-killing endorphins thus amplifying pain sensitivity.
- Accelerated loss of gray matter in the brain.
- Deficient hypothalamic corticotrophin-releasing hormone function, delayed adrenocorticotropic-hormone release, and increased norepinephrine response with exposure to interleukin-6. An increase in inflammatory markers has also been noted.

Clinical Manifestations

- Increased pain response.
- Pain in the back, neck, forearms, and knees.
- Numbness and tingling of hands and feet.
- Headaches.
- Inability to sleep.

- Fatigue, generalized weakness, dizziness, memory loss.
- Alternating constipation and diarrhea.

Diagnostic Tools

- Thorough history and physical to rule out other conditions.
- Widespread pain for at least 3 months and pain in 11 of 18 tender points. Because symptoms may be cyclic, 11 points may not be painful at the exact time of examination so this must be considered. Tender points include occipital, low cervical trapezius, supraspinatus, rib, epicondyle, gluteal area, knee area.

Complications

- Because the symptoms are vague and no physical explanation can be seen, many people are misdiagnosed or not taken seriously and may become depressed.

Treatment

- Cognitive-behavioral therapy and operant behavior therapy to decrease subjective perception of pain.
- Physical exercises.
- Patient education and support groups.
- Acupuncture.
- Muscle relaxants.
- Pregabalin decreases release of several neurotransmitter in the CNS resulting in decreased hyperexcitability.
- Dual serotonin norepinephrine reuptake inhibitors (duloxetine, venlafaxine) to treat pain, sleep problems, cognitive impairment, depression, and mood changes.
- Tricyclic antidepressants have been effective in some cases, but are not FDA-approved for this use.

OSTEOGENESIS IMPERFECTA

Osteogenesis imperfecta (OI), also referred to as "brittle bone disease" is a genetic disease characterized by a defect in the synthesis of connective tissue. It results in thin, poorly developed bones that fracture easily. There are a variety of genetic mutations that may result in this disease, all of which result in an abnormality in the production of procollagen proteins.

There are four general categories of OI, separated based on clinical manifestations and genetic analysis. OI is usually inherited as an autosomal-dominant disorder, meaning that an individual heterozygous for the trait will express the disease. The expression of the disease is variable. In other cases, the genetic disorder is inherited as an autosomal-recessive disease. In this case, the child is homozygous for the genetic error and the resultant pathology is more severe. These children typically die before, during, or soon after birth from fractures sustained in utero or during delivery.

Clinical Manifestations

- For the autosomal-dominant condition, children may appear healthy until they begin to walk and fall as toddlers. At this time, frequent fractures with poor healing may occur. Some cases may be investigated as child abuse before the condition is diagnosed.
- Osteopenia.
- Children will be of short stature and may have deformed cranial structure and limbs.
- Thin skin, with bluish sclera of the eye, indicates reduced collagen deposits.
- Tooth development and enamel are abnormal.
- Deafness frequently develops as the child ages because of bone deformity and scarring of the middle and inner ear.

Diagnostic Tools

- Elevation of serum alkaline phosphatase levels. Alkaline phosphatase is released with cell injury and is high during periods of rapid bone formation.
- Fibroblast analysis in a skin culture will demonstrate reduced quantity of connective tissue–producing cells.
- Prenatal diagnosis of OI is possible.

Complications

- Infants homozygous for the autosomal-recessive condition are frequently stillborn or die within the first year of life.
- Vascular deformities such as aortic aneurysm because type I collagen is a main component of blood vessels.

Treatment

- Treatment is aimed at reducing the number of fractures by teaching safety measures.
- Secure stabilizing of fractures with internal fixation is frequently performed.
- Moderate levels of growth hormone supplementation may improve growth outcome and reduce fracture occurrence.

- Current research is indicating a positive response to biphosphates, which decrease osteoclastic activity resulting in inhibition of bone resorption. Studies are also under way to determine the effectiveness of increasing calcium and vitamin D intake.

SCOLIOSIS

Scoliosis is curvature of the spine. It may result from an actual structural deformity of the vertebral column that is present at birth (congenital) or may develop as a result of a neuromuscular disease such as cerebral palsy or muscular dystrophy. Some structural scoliosis may develop for no known reason (idiopathic) or as a result of poor posture. Scoliosis results in deformity, and occasionally in pain. If the condition is untreated, respiratory and pulmonary function may be compromised.

Clinical Manifestations

- Abnormality of the usual concave–convex–concave vertebral presentation seen in descent from shoulder to buttocks.
- Prominence of the ribs on the convex side.
- Unevenness in the height of the iliac crest, which may cause one leg to be shorter than the other.
- Asymmetry of the thoracic cage and misalignment of spinal vertebrae will be apparent when the individual bends over.

Diagnostic Tools

- Physical examination and screening may allow for early diagnosis.
- Lateral deviation of the vertebrae can be confirmed by radiograph.

Complications

- Back pain may develop. Respiratory, cardiac, and GI complications may develop from thoracic or lumbar deformity.

Treatment

- Postural scoliosis is treated by passive and active exercises. An external brace may be used to encourage compliance and speed recovery.
- Structural scoliosis is treated with surgical intervention, which may include placing a flexible rod down the back to reverse the curve of the vertebral column. Fusion of the spine at different levels to correct a deformity may be performed in severe cases.

PAGET DISEASE

Paget disease is a bone disorder characterized by accelerated patterns of bone remodeling. Repeated episodes of rapid bone breakdown are followed by short periods of bone formation. The new bone is thickened and rough, and the process eventually leads to structural deformity and weakness. Blood flow to bones affected by Paget disease is increased to support high metabolic demands. The long bones and the bones of the cranium, spine, and pelvis are most commonly affected. Paget disease is usually seen in those older than 70 years of age and is slightly more common in males than females. There is no known cause of the disease and it is the second most common metabolic bone disease.

Clinical Manifestations

- Changes in the shape of the skull, with associated headaches, hearing abnormalities, and sometimes mental deterioration.
- Pain in the long bones, spine, or pelvis.
- Frequent pathologic fractures.

Diagnostic Tools

- Radiographs demonstrate bone deformity and will support a clinical diagnosis.
- Elevation of serum alkaline phosphatase (biochemical marker of bone turnover) supports the diagnosis.
- Bone biopsy can rule out infection or tumor.
- Radionuclide bone scan.

Complications

- Heart failure may occur because of the high blood flow demands of remodeling bones (high-output failure).
- Respiratory failure may occur if thoracic bones are affected and deformed.
- Secondary problems may include arthritic pain, dental problems, weakness, numbness, paresthesia, hearing and visual problems.
- Paget disease is a risk factor for sarcoma (bone cancer), perhaps related to the rapid rate of cell cycling seen with the disease.

Treatment

- Calcitonin may be administered to slow the rate of bone breakdown.
- Anti-inflammatory agents may reduce the pain associated with growing deformity. These drugs will reduce the constant inflammation that accompanies cell breakdown. The disease has no known cure.

- Oral or intravenous bisphosphates. The newest drug, zoledronic acid, has a high affinity for bone mineral so the effect is longer lasting.

TALIPES EQUINOVARUS

Talipes equinovarus, also called clubfoot, is a congenital abnormality characterized by deformity of the bones and soft tissue of the foot. The front portion of the foot is abducted (turned in) whereas the rear of the foot is inverted. The foot is usually pointed down (in equinus). The individual typically walks on tiptoes. Clubfoot results from the abnormal development of the foot during gestation (fetal growth). This leads to abnormality of the muscles and joints and soft tissue contracture. There may be a genetic tendency for this disorder, and other associated structural malformations may be present.

Clinical Manifestations

- Clubfoot is apparent at birth.

Treatment

- Casting of foot (or feet) immediately after birth with cast replacement weekly for several months.
- Corrective shoes may be necessary during the toddler years.
- Surgery may be performed, usually between 6 and 9 months of age.

DEVELOPMENTAL HIP DYSPLASIA

Developmental hip dysplasia is dislocation of the hip present at birth (congenital) or occurring within the first year of life. The hip may be out of the hip joint or present in the joint but easily displaced. The acetabulum (joint cavity) may be abnormally shaped, which allows the head of the femur to slip. The cause of hip dysplasia is unknown, but a genetic tendency toward the disorder is apparent. Breech birth is a strong risk factor for hip dysplasia, as is any condition that limits space for the fetus in the uterus, such as multiple fetuses, abnormalities in the anatomy of the uterus, or amniotic fluid deficiency. Early diagnosis of developmental dysplasia of the hip may decrease the need for surgical intervention.

Clinical Manifestations

- Asymmetry in leg length, leading to gait abnormality.
- Asymmetry in folds of the gluteus (buttocks).
- Hyperlaxity of the hip.
- Forefoot adduction.

Diagnostic Tools

- A thorough examination of the hips is performed during each physical examination in the newborn period and up until 18 months of age. This examination includes visual inspection of the limbs for differences in length and physical manipulation of the hip joints. In one procedure, the infant is placed on his or her back with his or her legs splayed outward. Pressure is then exerted downward on the knees, and the observer watches and feels for hip dislocation; a positive response is called Barlow sign. A second maneuver follows in which the practitioner gently reduces the hip back into the joint, producing a telltale click, called Ortolani's sign.
- Ultrasound or radiograph is used to confirm the diagnosis.

Complications

- Limping and leg pain and deformity may result without treatment. In older children, undiagnosed hip instability may be a cause of delayed standing and walking.

Treatment

- Early treatment is essential and may involve bracing or casting depending on the child's age and the severity of the defect. Surgery may be required for late diagnosis or if the casting or braces are ineffective.

OSGOOD–SCHLATTER DISEASE

Osgood–Schlatter disease is a condition in which there is partial separation of the epiphysis of the tibia from the tibial tuberosity (joint area of the knee). This occurs as a result of physical stress placed on the knee during periods of rapid growth in early puberty. The stress is usually associated with sports such as running, biking, climbing, or hiking. This condition is especially common in teenage boys from the ages of 11 to 15, and girls from 8 to 13 years of age. Inflammation of the patellar tendon (tendonitis) occurs, as does the development of ossified cartilage in the tibial tuberosity. This condition is usually self-limited and symptoms resolve on closure of the tibial growth plate at the end of puberty. Occasionally, minor symptoms may continue in adulthood.

Clinical Manifestations

- Pain and swelling at the front of the knee, especially during physical activity or kneeling.

Diagnostic Tools

- A thorough history and physical examination is used to diagnose Osgood–Schlatter disease. MRI or radiography may be used to rule out other causes of pain.

Complications

- The condition is usually self-limited. Occasionally pain may continue past puberty.

Treatment

- Treatment is usually limited to the use of anti-inflammatory medications and ice packs after exercise. Rest and refraining from sports may be required during a flare-up. Knee supports or braces may be of some use.
- Occasionally, surgery may be performed if the condition is severe or seems complicated by the development of bony fragments in the patellar tendon.

BONE TUMORS

Bone tumors may be cancerous or benign. Bone cancer may occur as a primary disease (originating in the bone) or more commonly as a result of metastasis from another tumor.

Primary bone cancer may begin in any cell of the bone. Cancers of the bone marrow lead to leukemia or myeloma. Leukemia and myeloma are discussed in Chapter 12. Primary cancer of the osteoblast or osteocyte is called osteogenic sarcoma. Osteogenic sarcoma often occurs in a long bone, especially the femur (thigh), or in the knee. Cancers of the cartilage are called chondrosarcoma. Chondrosarcoma usually occurs in the femur or pelvis.

Clinical Manifestations

- Pain related to inflammation with swelling in and around the bone.
- Pathologic fracture.

Diagnostic Tools

- MRI will identify tumors of the bones.
- Bone biopsy will identify the neoplasm and the involved tissue.

Complications

- Amputation of the limb is common.
- Anxiety, fear, and family stress often accompany the diagnosis of cancer, especially in children.

Treatment

For osteosarcoma and chondrosarcoma:

- Resection of the diseased part of the bone may allow successful treatment of the cancer without amputation.
- Amputation of the limb may be required.
- Chemotherapy is administered.
- Bone marrow cancers are treated with chemotherapy and radiation.

PEDIATRIC CONSIDERATIONS

- Proper nutrition to maximize bone health begins very early in life, as suggested by studies in which vitamin D supplementation during infancy was associated with increased bone density years later.

- Stress fractures are becoming increasingly common in younger athletes, as the pressure to perform in sports at an early age is increasing. Girls and young women are especially affected, perhaps because of the combined pressures for thinness and athletic excellence.

- At particular risk for future development of osteoporosis are children and teenagers who do not consume adequate calcium or vitamin D during their bone-forming years. This is especially, but not exclusively, true of diet-conscious girls who frequently limit caloric and milk intake. Young women athletes in particular may have measurably less dense bone than their peers. This phenomenon appears related to low estrogen levels, which often accompany high or moderate physical exercise and may sometimes lead to amenorrhea (absent or infrequent menstrual cycling). Athletic women may also be thinner than their peers, as a result of the high intensity of their exercise patterns combined with an often reduced caloric intake. These women may experience severe osteoporosis in later years. The combination of amenorrhea, reduced bone mineralization, and disordered eating in young women athletes is known as the "female athlete triad." In addition, the increased consumption of carbonated soda drinks by both boys and girls increases later risk of osteoporosis. Not only do these drinks often replace milk in the diet, but they may contribute to bone resorption indirectly by affecting calcium handling.

- Juvenile idiopathic arthritis is a chronic autoimmune inflammatory disease involving joints and other tissues. It is usually diagnosed before 16 years of age and occurs more frequently in females. In approximately 70% of the cases the disease process becomes inactive. Gene-expression studies are currently under way with the hope that one day a more individualized treatment regimen will improve outcomes.

GERIATRIC CONSIDERATIONS

- Muscle mass, muscle strength, and bone density decrease in the elderly, usually as a result of disuse. Decreased muscle mass, muscle strength, and bone density can be reversed, even in the very elderly (those 85 years or older), with moderate, regular weight-bearing exercise. Weight-bearing exercise coupled with mild aerobic exercise such as walking also improves balance and coordination in the elderly and may help prevent falling. Safety is a major concern.

- Fractures resulting from even minor falls are a major cause of disability in the elderly. A large percentage of the elderly who suffer a fracture, especially a hip fracture, do not regain the same level of functioning as before the fall. When an elderly person suffers a fracture, loss of independence frequently follows, which often results in the individual being cared for in a nursing home at high cost to both the patient and society. Many frail elderly never recover from a fracture. A fear of falling is a significant concern for many elderly individuals, even those who have never fallen.

SELECTED BIBLIOGRAPHY

Alexander, I. M. (2009). Pharmacotherapeutic management of osteoporosis and osteopenia. *The Nurse Practitioner*, 34(6), 30–40.

American College of Physicians. (2008). Screening for osteoporosis in men: A clinical practice guideline from the American Academy of Physicians. *Annals of Internal Medicine*, 148, 680–684.

Arnett, F. C., Edworthy, S. M., Bloch, D. A., Mcshane, D. J., Fries, J. F., Cooper, N. S., et al. (2005). The American Rheumatism Association 1987 revised criteria for the classification of rheumatoid arthritis. *Arthritis and Rheumatism*, 31(3), 315–324.

Berarducci, A. (2008). Stopping the silent progression of osteoporosis. *American Nurse Today*, 3(5), 18–22.

Copstead, L. C., & Banasik, J. L. (2010). *Pathophysiology*. St. Louis, MO: Saunders Elsevier.

Coughlin, M. (2008). Improving patient outlook in rheumatoid arthritis: Experience with abatacept. *Journal of the American Academy of Nurse Practitioners*, 20(10), 486–495.

Cummings, S.R., Browner, W. S., Baurer, D., Stone, K., Ensrud, K., Jamal, S., et al. (1998). Endogenous hormones and the risk of hip and vertebral fractures among older women. *New England Journal of Medicine*, 339, 733–738.

D'Arcy, Y. (2008). Treating osteoporotic compression fractures. *The Nurse Practitioner*, 33(12), 8–10.

D'Arcy, Y. (2009). Is low back pain getting on your nerves? *The Nurse Practitioner*, 34(5), 10–17.

FitzGibbons, J. (2007). Be a myth-buster: Stop the misconceptions about fibromyalgia. *American Nurse Today*, 2(9), 40–44.

Frazier, M. S., & Dzymkowski, J. W. (Eds.). (2009). *Essentials of human diseases and conditions* (4th ed.). St. Louis, MO: Saunders.

Giske, L., Vollestad, N. K., Mengshoel, A. M., Jensen, J., Knardahl, S., & Roe, C. (2008). Attenuated adrenergic responses to exercise in women with fibromyalgia—A controlled study. *European Journal of Pain*, 12, 351–360.

Guyton, A.C., & Hall, J.A. (2006). *Textbook of medical physiology* (11th ed.). Philadelphia, PA: W.B. Saunders.

Hanayama, K., Liu, M., Higuchi, Y., Fujiwara, T., Tsuji, T., Hase, K., et al. (2008). Dysphagia in patients with Duchenne muscular dystrophy evaluated with a questionnaire and videofluorography. *Disability and Rehabilitation*, 30(7), 517–522.

Huether, S. E., & McCance, K. L. (2008). *Understanding pathophysiology* (4th ed.). St. Louis, MO: Mosby Elsevier.

Kasper, R. W., Allen, H. D., & Montanaro, F. (2009). Current understanding and management of dilated cardiomyopathy in Duchenne and Becker muscular dystrophy. *Journal of the American Academy of Nurse Practitioners*, 21, 241–249.

Kessenich, C. (2008). Postmenopausal osteoporosis: The role of intravenous bisphosphonates. *Advance for Nurse Practitioners*, 16(11), 59–62.

Kuchinad, A., Schweinhardt, P., Seminowicz, D. A., Wood, P. B., Chizh, B. A., & Bushnell, M. C. (2007). Accelerated brain gray matter loss in fibromyalgia patients: Premature aging of the brain. *The Journal of Neuroscience*, 27(15), 4004–4007.

McClung, B., & Brown, J. P. (2008). Paget's disease: A therapy update. *American Nurse Today*, 3(6), 20–22.

Montgomery, M. (2008). Gout: Tips on diagnosis, treatment, and patient education. *The Nurse Practitioner*, 33(12), 28–32.

Napoli, M. (2009). The marketing of osteoporosis: How a risk factor became a disease. *American Journal of Neurology*, 109(4), 58–61.

National Guideline Clearing House. (2008). Adult low back pain. [Online]. Retrieved May 14, 2009 from http://www.guideline.gov/summary/summary.aspx?view_id=1& doc_id=13479.

National Institute of Arthritis and Musculoskeletal and Skin Diseases. http://www.niams.nih.gov/.

National Osteoporosis Foundation. http://www.nof.org.

Obermair, G.J., Kugler, G., Baumgartner, S., Tuluc, P., Grabner, M., & Flucher, B.E. (2005). The Ca^{2+} channel $\alpha 2G$-1 subunit determines Ca^{2+} current kinetics in skeletal muscle but not targeting of $\alpha_1\sigma$ or excitation–contraction coupling. *Journal of Biological Chemistry*, 280, 2229–2237.

Osborne, K. S., Wraa, C. E., & Watson, A. B. (2010). *Medical-surgical nursing: Preparation for practice*. Upper Saddle River, NJ: Pearson.

Patton, K. T., & Thibodeau, G. A. (2010). *Anatomy and physiology* (7th ed.). St. Louis, MO: Mosby.

Porth, C. M., & Matfin, G. (2009). *Pathophysiology: Concepts of altered health states* (8th ed.). Philadelphia, PA: Lippincott Williams & Wilkins.

Rouff, G. E. (2008). Gout: Clues to clinical diagnosis. *Consultant*, 48(13), 1010–1012, 1014–1015.

Ruoff, G. E. (2009). Gout: Update on therapy. *Consultant*, 49(1), 49–53.

Rubin, R., & Strayer, D. S. (Eds.). (2008). *Rubin's pathology: Clinicopathologic foundations of medicine* (5th ed.). Philadelphia, PA: Lippincott Williams & Wilkins.

Sherman, C. (2008, August). Keep low back pain patients out of surgery. *The Clinical Advisor*, 11(8), 29–32.

Sherman, C. (2009, June). Osteoporosis: No gender gap for therapy. The Clinical Advisor, 12(6), 19–20.

Southern California/RAND Evidence-based Practice Center. (2007, December). *Comparative effectiveness of treatments to prevent fractures in men and women with low bone density or osteoporosis.* Rockville, MD: Agency for Healthcare Research and Quality; Number 12. Available at http://effectivehealthcare.ahrq.gov/repFiles/LowBoneDensityFinal.pdf.

Stein-Zamir, C., Volovik, I., Rishpon, S., & Sabi, R. (2008). Developmental dysplasia of the hip: Risk markers, clinical screening and outcome. *Pediatrics International*, 50, 341–345.

Thibodeau, G. A., & Patton, K. T. (2010). *The human body in health and disease* (5th ed.). St. Louis, MO: Mosby Elsevier.

Wehrens, X. H. T., Lehnart, S. E., & Marks, A. R. (2005). Intracellular calcium release and cardiac disease. *Annual Review of Physiology*, 67, 69–98.

Wilson, D., Curry, M. R., & Hockenberry, M. J. (2009). The child with musculoskeletal or articular dysfunction. In M. J. Hockenberry & D. Wilson (Eds.). *Wong's essentials of pediatric nursing* (8th ed.) (pp. 1106–1144). St. Louis, MO: Mosby Elsevier.

Yiu, E. M., & Kornberg, A. J. (2008). Duchenne muscular dystrophy. *Neurology India*, 56(3), 236–247.

The Senses

The special sense organs of hearing, vision, taste, and smell, along with touch, play a vital role in protecting the human body. These organs also facilitate meaningful interaction with the environment. Each sense allows us to respond to subtle and not-so-subtle stimuli with precision and recognition. Because of the way our senses bring the external environment to us, the day-to-day implications of losing a sense are enormous.

● Physiologic Concepts

SIGHT

Stimulation of light-sensitive receptors in the eye, called **photoreceptors**, leads to the sense of sight. The response of the photoreceptors is transmitted to the brain by way of electrical signaling that passes through several levels of increasingly complex cell networks. Once the signals reach the brain, they are interpreted as a particular visual image based on the complexity of firing patterns, the rate of firing frequency, and the coding of color. Therefore, to have the sense of sight, one needs:

- a functioning eye to receive a stimulus,
- cells capable of coding the stimuli electrically,
- intact neural pathways to transmit the electrical signal, and
- a cerebral cortex capable of interpreting the signal as a meaningful image.

Structure of the Eye

The eye is composed of three layers including the sclera, the choroid, and the retina. A diagrammatic representation of the eye is presented in Figure 11-1. The outermost (anterior) portion of the eye consists of tough white connective tissue covering the eyeball, called the **sclera**. At the center of the eye, the sclera becomes a transparent membrane, the **cornea**. Light rays enter the eye through the cornea. By way of its natural curvature, the cornea bends the rays, causing the light to become less scattered and more focused on the underlying tissue. The image projected through the cornea is upside down and reversed right to left where it strikes the back of the eye. A venous sinus, the **canal of Schlemm**, lies at the junction of the sclera and cornea.

The **choroid**, a darkly pigmented and highly vascular membrane lying under the sclera, helps reduce light scatter. Directly under the cornea, the choroid becomes the **iris**. The iris is a colored membrane that gives the eye its tint. At the center of the iris is an area without pigment: the **pupil**. The cornea focuses light rays on the pupil. The diameter of the pupil is controlled by smooth muscles that innervate the iris. These muscles cause the pupil to constrict in the light and dilate in the dark. The muscles controlling the diameter of the pupil are innervated by parasympathetic and sympathetic nerves.

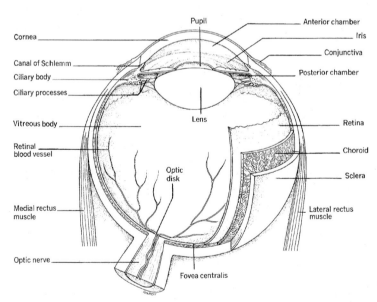

FIGURE 11-1 Transverse section of the eyeball. (From Porth, C. (2005). *Pathophysiology: Concepts of altered health states* (7th ed.). Philadelphia, PA: Lippincott Williams & Wilkins.)

Parasympathetic stimulation causes the pupil to constrict, and sympathetic stimulation causes it to dilate. Varying pupil diameter determines the amount of light that passes deeper into the eye.

Posterior to the iris and pupil is the **lens**. The lens is a curved transparent structure that further bends the light rays. By passage through the lens, light rays are focused exactly on the most posterior and sensitive portion of the eye, the **retina**. The shape of the lens is controlled by a muscle that allows the lens to focus both distant and close objects precisely on the retina. The retina contains the photoreceptors of the eye, the **rods** and **cones** that change light rays into the electrical messages that the brain interprets as vision. In the center of the retina is the **macula**, the site of the most acute and finely detailed vision. The retina also contains the cells that join together to form the **optic nerve**— the pathway by which the visual signal travels to the brain. The **fovea centralis** is a depression in the macula corresponding to the point of central vision. Between the lens and the retina, the eyeball is filled with blood vessels and a gelatinous fluid, called **vitreous fluid**.

Cells of the Retina

The structures of the eye anterior to the retina function primarily to focus the light rays scattered by a particular image exactly on the retina. Once the light rays strike the retina, the cells there have the job of changing the light signal into an electrical signal and then passing the signal to the brain. The cells of the retina that receive and transform the signal are the photoreceptors: the **rods** and the **cones**. The second class of cells in the pathway is the **bipolar cells**; bipolar cells receive the electrical signal from the rods and the cones and pass that signal to the third class of cells in the retina: the **ganglion cells**. The axons of the ganglion cells travel to the central nervous system as the optic nerve.

Rods and Cones

Rod-shaped photoreceptors are heavily concentrated on the periphery of the retina. Each rod is connected by way of a chemical synapse to a bipolar cell. The rods contain the photosensitive chemical rhodopsin, which is one of the four photopigments present in the retina (the other three are found in the cones). Rhodopsin decomposes when struck by light. When rhodopsin is decomposed, sodium permeability in the rod is reduced, leading to a hyper-polarization of the rod (i.e., the inside becomes more negative). Hyperpolar-ization *decreases* the firing rate of the rod on the bipolar cell. Normally, the rod inhibits the firing of the bipolar cell. When the rod is hyperpolarized by light, bipolar cell inhibition is removed, and the bipolar cell depolarizes. Depolar-ization of the bipolar cell causes an action potential to fire in the ganglion cell. Action potentials produced by the ganglion cells are sent to the brain via the optic nerve. Rods fire even with low levels of light and so function to provide night vision. They do not provide information regarding color.

Cone photoreceptors are heavily concentrated in the center of the eye. They are the only photoreceptors present in the fovea, an area located at the center of the macula. Each cone cell contains one of the other three photopigments, which, like rhodopsin, decompose when struck by light. As in a rod cell, decomposition of the photopigment in the cone cell hyperpolarizes the cone cell, removing its inhibitory influence from the bipolar cell and causing an action potential to fire in the bipolar cell. As before, the bipolar cell transmits this action potential to a ganglion cell that sends the signal to the brain via the optic nerve. Unlike rods, cones are insensitive to faint light and so contribute little to night vision. The photopigments present in the cone cells are color sensitive, allowing cone cells to transmit information regarding color, as described below. Vitamin A produces visual pigments and is an important component of both rhodopsin and the cone photopigments.

Reactivation of the Photopigments.

Immediately after decomposition, the original structure of the photopigments is returned. The rods and cones again inhibit the firing of the bipolar cells and are ready to respond to another light signal.

Differences Between Rods and Cones.

Rods are capable of responding to low levels of light; therefore, they provide limited vision in the dark. Many rods usually converge on one bipolar cell. The convergence of many rods on one bipolar cell reduces the acuity of rod vision, but increases its sensitivity. Rods are not color sensitive. Therefore, all stimulation is perceived in shades of gray. Cone stimulation requires higher levels of light and so cones do not fire in the dark or in near dark. Because few cones converge on any one bipolar cell, there is increased acuity of cone vision.

Color Vision.

The different photopigments of the cones allow for color vision because of their sensitivity to the colors red, blue, and green. The ratio of red, blue, and green cones activated at any one time results in color vision. Which cones are stimulated determines which bipolar cells depolarize and which ganglion cells fire action potentials. Ganglion cells may receive information from several different bipolar cells activated by one color-specific cone or a few different color-specific cones. Ganglion cells may be activated by one color, but inactivated by a second color. These variations and levels of stimuli allow for fine discrimination between many shades of color.

Lateral Neurons

Two types of neurons, the horizontal cells and the amacrine cells, lie laterally (sideways) in the retina and fire in such a way that they modify and control the messages being passed from the rods and cones to the bipolar cells and from the bipolar cells to the ganglion cells. Horizontal cells connect rods and cones to each other and to bipolar cells. Horizontal cells fine-tune the transmission of signals to the bipolar cells, thereby refining visual acuity. The amacrine cells fine-tune signals between the ganglion cells, functioning to sharpen transient responses. Given the large number of lateral neurons in the retina, their importance in fine visual discrimination must be great indeed, although their exact mechanism of action is poorly understood.

Optic Nerve

Ganglion cell axons join together to form the eye's optic nerve (cranial nerve II). The optic nerve leaves the eye as a bundle through an area of the retina called the **optic disk**. The optic disk lacks rods or cones; therefore, it does not participate in the response to light (i.e., it is a blind spot). The central artery of the retina enters the eye through the optic disk. An area called the physiologic cup is at the center of the optic disk.

When the optic nerve reaches the brainstem, some fibers from the left eye cross and project to the right side of the brain. At the same time, some fibers from the right eye cross and project to the left side of the brain. This crossing at the optic chiasma allows both cerebral hemispheres access to information from each eye. Other fibers do not cross sides. The optic nerves terminate in the thalamus, in an area called the dorsal lateral geniculate nucleus, and there activate other neurons that then project to the occipital lobe. It is in the occipital lobe—the area of the brain that interprets the electrical signals as a meaningful visual image—that the visual cortex of the brain resides (Fig. 11-2). The integrity of the image from the dorsal lateral geniculate nucleus to the occipital lobe is ensured because each cell in the dorsal lateral geniculate nucleus passes the information in the same exact spatial arrangement to the visual cortex. The pathway of vision is shown in Figure 11-3.

Descending Inhibition to the Dorsal Lateral Geniculate Nucleus

Descending fibers from higher brain centers can influence the transmission of signals from the dorsal lateral geniculate nucleus to the visual cortex. These inhibitory and excitatory fibers come from the visual cortex itself and from areas of the brainstem. Descending stimulation can limit or accentuate what visual information is allowed to pass into consciousness.

Integration of the Visual Pathways

Integration of the pathways of vision occurs at each level of the retina: between the rods and the cones, at the horizontal cells, at the amacrine cells, at the bipolar cells, and at the ganglion cells. At each level, some cells fire with certain stimuli, such as specific on–off fields or various horizontal and vertical patterns, while the same stimuli turn off the firing of other cells. Ganglion cells have a complex pattern of firing that depends on the various on–off firing patterns of the bipolar cells and the amacrine cells. Bipolar cells are activated by unique combinations of the firings of rods, cones, and horizontal cells.

☐ Frontal lobe ☐ Parietal lobe ☐ Temporal lobe ☐ Occipital lobe

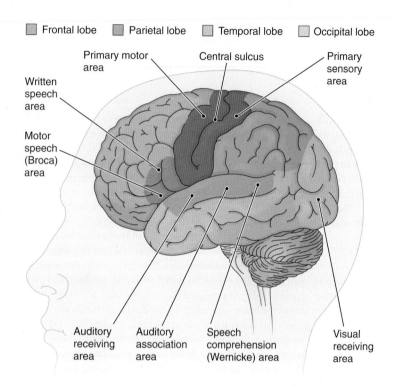

FIGURE 11-2 Primary sensory areas of the cerebral cortex.

Continued integration of signals in the brain further refines the original, simple photoreceptor decomposition that initiated the cascade.

Optics of Vision

It is essential that the cornea and lens direct the light rays exactly toward the cells of the retina so that well-focused images can appear. Although the cornea must bend the rays initially, it is by changing the shape of the lens that the image is made to land exactly on the retina. This process is called **accommodation**. Accommodation occurs by the contraction and relaxation of the muscles that control the shape of the lens. A progressive loss in the ability of the lens to accommodate and focus the light rays occurs by approximately the fifth decade of life and is responsible for the loss of near vision in middle age (called **presbyopia**). Accommodation, pupil size, and eye movements are controlled by cranial nerves II, III, IV, and VI.

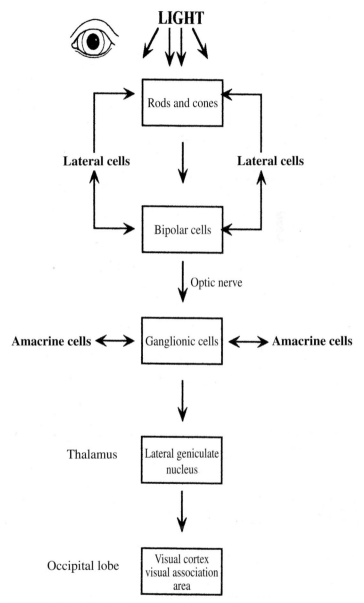

FIGURE 11-3 Pathway of vision.

Intraocular Pressure

Pressure in the chamber of the eye is called intraocular pressure (IOP). IOP is tightly controlled at approximately 15 millimeters of mercury (mm Hg). The pressure is determined by the amount of a fluid, called **aqueous humor**, which fills the space between the lens and the retina. Aqueous humor is formed by a small gland, the **ciliary body**, located behind the iris. Once formed, aqueous humor flows through the eye, bathing all structures and providing nutrients to the lens and other cells. The aqueous humor then exits the eye through a venous channel between the cornea and the iris. This venous channel, the canal of Schlemm, joins extraocular veins that carry blood and fluid away from the eye.

External Structures of the Eye

The lacrimal glands (tear ducts), conjunctiva (mucous membrane layer on the outside of the eye), and eyelids make up the external structures of the eye. These structures protect the eye from irritants and injury. Tears also contain antimicrobial chemicals.

HEARING

The sense of hearing occurs when sound waves enter the external structure of the ear, pass through the middle ear to the inner ear, and stimulate specific receptor cells in the inner ear that fire action potentials, which in turn are carried to the brain. The action potentials are transmitted via the cochlear nerve (part of cranial nerve VIII) to the auditory cortex, a structure located in the temporal lobe of the brain (see Fig. 11-2), where they are interpreted as sounds. A diagrammatic representation of the ear is presented in Figure 11-4.

External Ear

The external ear consists of the **auricle** (outside cartilage) and the **external ear canal**. The auricle gathers the sound waves and projects them into the external canal. The external ear canal is a tube through which the sound waves travel to the middle ear. Separating the external ear from the middle ear is the **tympanic membrane**, also called the eardrum. A part of the temporal bone, the mastoid process, lies behind and below the external canal.

Middle Ear

The tympanic membrane is stretched tightly across the end of the external canal. When sound waves strike the eardrum, it is pushed in, or bowed, toward the middle ear. The degree of bowing of the eardrum depends on the loudness of the sound. After one sound wave, the eardrum returns to its previous position. The eardrum can be pushed in again and again if the sound waves

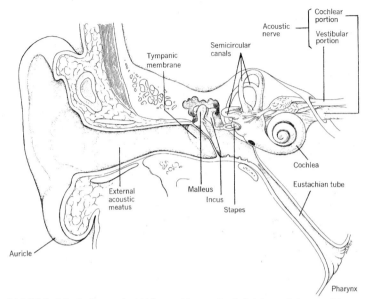

FIGURE 11-4 External, middle, and internal subdivisions of the ear. (From Porth, C. (2005). *Pathophysiology: Concepts of altered health states* (7th ed.). Philadelphia, PA: Lippincott Williams & Wilkins.)

continue, causing the drum to vibrate. The frequency with which the eardrum vibrates depends on the frequency of the sound waves.

The middle ear has three bony processes, which are connected in series to the eardrum: the **malleus** (hammer), the **incus** (anvil), and the **stapes** (stirrup). Vibrations of the eardrum are transmitted from one small bone to the next, eventually striking the **oval window**. The oval window is a small membrane at the entrance to the inner ear. Because the oval window is smaller than the tympanic membrane, the force of the sound waves on the oval window per unit of area is significantly magnified.

The middle ear is connected to the nose and throat via the **eustachian tube**. Although normally closed, the eustachian tube opens with yawning or swallowing. This opening allows the pressure in the middle ear to remain equal to atmospheric pressure.

Inner Ear

The inner ear is a complex organ consisting of two mazelike structures: the outer **bony labyrinth** and the inner **membranous labyrinth**. The bony labyrinth is separated from the membranous labyrinth by a thick fluid called the perilymph. The membranous labyrinth is filled with a slightly different fluid called endolymph. The bony labyrinth contains the **cochlea**, the **vestibule**, and the **semicircular canals**. The cochlea is the organ responsible for changing sound waves to action potentials. The vestibule and the semicircular canals maintain equilibrium and balance, which is a major function of the inner ear.

Cochlea

The cochlea is a shell-shaped organ, filled with perilymph. The cochlea is separated down the middle by a structure called the **basilar membrane**. On the basilar membrane is a blanket of hair cells that, together with the basilar membrane, compose the **organ of Corti**, which is the organ of hearing. The hair cells on the basilar membrane depolarize when deformed or bent. Each hair cell synapses upon an afferent neuron, the axons of which make up the acoustic nerve. Depolarization of a hair cell initiates a receptor potential, which, if large enough, stimulates an action potential in the afferent neuron. The hair cells are covered by an overhanging membrane, called the **tectorial membrane**. It is against the tectorial membrane that the hair cells bend when a sound wave is passed into the inner ear.

Sound Wave Transmission

When a sound wave strikes the oval window, a pressure wave is generated in the fluid-filled inner ear. The pressure wave causes a wavelike displacement of the basilar membrane against the overhanging tectorial membrane. As the hair cells rub against the tectorial membrane, they are bent. This bending leads to the depolarization of the hair cell and the production of a receptor potential. With significant deformation, the afferent nerves synapsed upon by the hair cells are stimulated to fire action potentials and the signal is transmitted to the auditory cortex. The pathway of hearing is shown in Figure 11-5.

The frequency of the pressure wave determines which hair cells are displaced and, consequently, which afferent neurons fire action potentials. For instance, the hair cells lying on the part of the basilar membrane nearest to the oval window are most displaced by high-frequency sounds, whereas the hair cells lying on the basilar membrane farthest from the oval window are most displaced by low-frequency sounds. The brain interprets the pitch of a sound by which neurons are activated. The brain interprets the intensity of a sound by the frequency of neuronal impulses and the number of afferent neurons firing.

Vestibular System and Equilibrium

The vestibule and the semicircular canals also contain hair cell receptors that are sensitive to movement and position. The **crista ampullaris** is located in the canals and each time the head is moved, nerve impulses are generated. When the head is turned, the hair cells are bent as they pass through the thick endolymph surrounding them. As in the organ of Corti, bending of a hair cell in the vestibule and semicircular canals causes depolarization of the cell and the firing of an action potential. Action potentials initiated in the vestibule and semicircular canals are carried via the vestibular nerve to the parietal lobe of the brain, converging

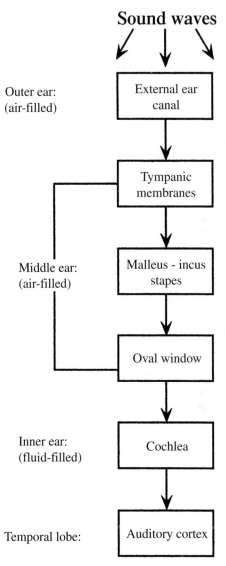

Sound waves

Outer ear:
(air-filled)

External ear
canal

Middle ear:
(air-filled)

Tympanic
membranes

Malleus - incus
stapes

Oval window

Inner ear:
(fluid-filled)

Cochlea

Temporal lobe:

Auditory cortex

FIGURE 11-5 Pathway of hearing.

near the somatosensory area, where information on joint and muscle position is integrated (see Fig. 11-2). The semicircular canals and the vestibular apparatus work together with other tactile and visual systems to determine the current position of the body and any change in motion or direction.

TASTE

Chemical receptors that generate impulses resulting in taste are called **taste buds**. Taste buds are located in a pattern on the tongue and are depolarized in response to specific chemical stimulation. **Gustatory cells** in the taste buds are the sensory receptor cells responsible for generating nerve impulses. Depolarization of the taste buds leads to action potentials and the firing of cranial nerves V, VII, IX, and X. These nerves send their information to the taste cortex in the parietal lobe (Fig. 11-2), where the sensation is identified. The pathway of taste is shown in Figure 11-6.

There are specific taste buds for many different taste sensations, some of which are as yet unidentified. Known taste receptors are usually divided into those which respond to sweet, bitter, salty, and sour tastes. Research is suggesting that the metallic taste and a "meaty" or "savory" flavor activated by amino acid glutamate may also be considered primary tastes. Activation of different receptors to varying degrees by substances found in food allows for a wide range of tastes. The sense of taste initiates digestion and provides a stimulus to eat. There can be adaptation (decreased firing) of the taste buds if exposure to a chemical stimulus is prolonged. Certain drugs, including nicotine, may sensitize some receptors while desensitizing others, causing taste sensations to change. Another important component influencing the sense of taste is smell.

OLFACTION

The sense of smell is provided by receptor cells, called olfactory cells, which line the membranes of the nasal mucosa. The olfactory cells contain cilia

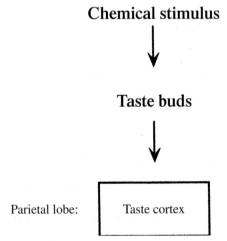

FIGURE 11-6 Pathway of taste.

that depolarize when bound by certain chemicals corresponding to specific odors in the air. A few types of cilia hyperpolarize in response to any one specific odor. Significant depolarization or hyperpolarization of the cilia leads to the firing of action potentials in the neurons of the olfactory nerve (cranial nerve I) that terminate in the olfactory bulbs of the frontal lobe. From there, the signal is passed to the olfactory cortex in the limbic system of the brain (see Fig. 11-2). The olfactory receptor cells adapt rapidly to a continuing smell. The pathway of smell is shown in Figure 11-7. Progressive reduction in the sense of smell can occur from the pollutants of tobacco smoke as well as the aging process.

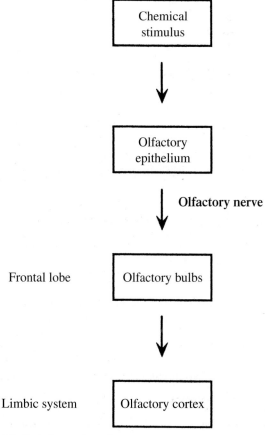

FIGURE 11-7 Pathway of smell.

TOUCH

Tactile sensations include the body's recognition of touch, pressure, and vibration. Each of these sensations appears to be mediated by receptors that vary only in location; touch receptors are located in or near the skin, whereas pressure receptors are found deeper in the tissues. Vibration is sensed as rapidly repeating stimuli activating both touch and pressure receptors.

Tactile Receptors

There are several types of tactile receptors spread over the body. Tactile receptors are **mechanoreceptors**, cells that respond to physical deformation and compression with depolarization, causing a receptor potential. If the depolarization is great enough, the nerve fiber attached to the receptor fires an action potential and transmits the information to the spinal cord and the brain. Different tactile receptors vary in sensitivity and in the velocity with which they send their impulses. They also vary as to which type of nerve fiber transmits their signal to the spinal cord and the brain.

Peripheral Nerve Fibers that Transmit Tactile Information

Tactile sensation is carried to the spinal cord by one of three types of sensory neurons: large type A beta (β) fibers, smaller type A delta (δ) fibers, and small type C fibers. Both types of A fibers are myelinated, transmitting action potentials rapidly; the larger fibers transmit faster than the smaller fibers. Tactile information carried in the A fibers is typically well-localized and pinpoint. The small C fibers are unmyelinated, transmitting action potentials to the spinal cord much more slowly than the A fibers. Tactile information carried in the C fibers is poorly localized.

Transmission of Tactile Information in the Spinal Cord

Virtually all information on touch, pressure, and vibration enters the spinal cord via the dorsal roots of the corresponding spinal nerve. After synapsing in the spine, highly localized information carried in the fast-firing A fibers (both β and δ) is sent to the brain by way of the dorsal column–lemniscal system. Nerve fibers in this system cross over left to right in the brainstem and travel through the thalamus before synapsing in the somatosensory cortex (see Fig. 11-2). Information on temperature and poorly localized touch is carried to the spinal cord by way of the slow-firing C fibers. This information is sent to the reticular area of the brainstem and then to higher centers via fibers carried in the anterolateral system. Pain and some sexual sensations are transmitted in the anterolateral tracts.

Types of Tactile Receptors

There are six basic types of tactile receptors: free nerve endings, Meissner corpuscles, expanded-tip tactile receptors, hair end-organ receptors, Ruffini end-organ receptors, and Pacinian corpuscles. These six types of tactile receptors are discussed individually in the following sections.

Free Nerve Endings

Receptors that respond to touch are found all over the skin and are called free nerve endings. Most send their information to the spinal cord via the small type A δ fibers. From the spinal cord, information from the free nerve endings is sent through the thalamus to the somatosensory area (parietal lobe) of the cortex. Some free nerve endings send their information to the cord via the slow type C fibers. Free nerve endings respond to stimuli perceived as painful.

Meissner Corpuscles

Touch receptors found on areas of the body not covered with hair, especially the fingertips and lips, are called Meissner corpuscles. These receptors allow for precise discrimination concerning the location of a touch. Information from Meissner corpuscles is carried to the spinal cord via fast-firing type A β nerve fibers. From the spinal cord, information from Meissner corpuscles is sent through the thalamus to the somatosensory area of the cortex.

Expanded-Tip Tactile Receptors

The expanded-tip tactile receptors are present in association with Meissner corpuscles, as well as on areas of the body that do have hair. These receptors provide information on continuous touch, responding with a strong signal when a touch is initiated and continuing with a weak signal for as long as the touch remains. These receptors send their information to the spinal cord via the type A β fibers, allowing for fine discrimination concerning the location and the quality of the touch. From the spinal cord, information is delivered through the thalamus to the somatosensory area of the cortex.

Hair End-Organ Receptors

Each hair follicle on the body has a nerve fiber at its base that acts as a touch receptor. When a hair is bent, the nerve fires an action potential. The hair receptors send their information to the spinal cord via type A β fibers and then on through the thalamus to the somatosensory area of the cortex.

Ruffini End Organs

Nerve fibers located deep in the skin and underlying tissues are known as Ruffini end organs. These receptors fire continuously in response to deformation. Ruffini end organs are present in the joints and provide information on joint position and movement. They send their information to the spinal cord via type A β fibers and then on through the thalamus to the somatosensory area of the cortex.

Pacinian Corpuscles

Pacinian corpuscles are rapidly adapting fibers located under the skin and in other body tissues such as the penis, clitoris, and nipples. These corpuscles fire quickly with the onset of a touch, especially one involving deep pressure or high-frequency vibration, and then adapt. They send information via type A β fibers to the spinal cord and then on through the thalamus to the somatosensory area of the cortex. The pathways of touch are shown in Figure 11-8.

Temperature Sensation

Temperature is sensed by specific warm and cold receptors located immediately under the skin. There are more cold receptors than warm receptors. Pain receptors also participate in temperature sensation.

Warm receptors are poorly understood but appear to be free nerve endings that depolarize with a warm stimulus. Cold receptors have been identified as free nerve endings of the small type A δ fibers. From the spinal cord, nerves carrying temperature information pass through the reticular activating system on their way to the thalamus. A few fibers continue to the somatosensory area of the cortex. Temperature receptors are not mechanoreceptors. They are activated chemically by substances produced by cells after temperature-induced changes in metabolic activity.

Position Sensation

Perception of body movement and position, also known as proprioception, is mediated by proprioceptive receptors located mainly in muscles, tendons, and joint capsules and also in the inner ear. Signals are transmitted through the dorsal column–medial lemniscus pathway to the thalamus where they are processed before reaching the cerebral cortex. Intact functioning is vital for equilibrium, coordination, and muscular contraction.

● Pathophysiologic Concepts

AMBLYOPIA

The loss of visual acuity in an eye that appears to be structurally intact is known as amblyopia. With amblyopia, the central nervous system becomes unable to identify visual stimuli; that is, the signals are sent from the eye but are not recognized in the brain. Often, amblyopia develops from the disuse of one eye (lazy eye), due to conditions of abnormal binocular interaction (e.g., strabismus or infantile cataracts). Amblyopia occurs under these conditions because normal development of the visual areas of the thalamus and the visual cortex require binocular visual stimuli during a critical period of development (0 to 5 years of age). Occasionally, amblyopia may result from ingestion of toxins

Pressure-vibration-touch Temperature

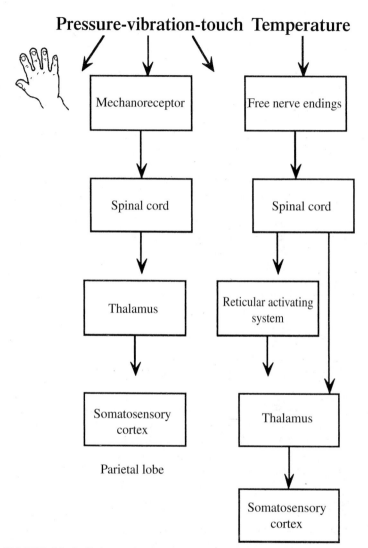

FIGURE 11-8 Pathway of touch.

such as alcohol or tobacco or may be associated with a systemic disease such as renal failure or diabetes mellitus. Other possible causes include psychological problems such as hysteria, nutritional deficits such as insufficient vitamins A or B, or physical obstructions such as cataracts. Diagnosis is confirmed when all organic causes of decreased visual acuity have been ruled out. Although amblyopia may be irreversible, in some cases intensive visual retraining may allow even adults to obtain some vision in the eye. Atropoine drops to blur vision or occlusion of the unaffected eye may be helpful in forcing the affected eye to assume proper functioning.

STRABISMUS

The condition called strabismus is a deviation in the position of the eyes relative to each other due to a weak or hypotonic eye muscle. The deviation may be superior, inferior, medial, or lateral and may cause the eyes to appear crossed. An individual who has strabismus often complains of double vision.

Strabismus may result from a congenital inability to use both eyes together. This condition is called nonparalytic strabismus and is treated by patching the eye that can fix on an object (the good eye). Patching forces the deviating eye to focus. Without treatment, ambylopia develops and visual activity in the deviating eye is lost by approximately 6 years of age.

Paralytic strabismus usually occurs later in life after paralysis of one or more of the muscles controlling eye movement. Tumor, injury, or infection may cause paralytic strabismus. Strabismus occurring in adulthood may be treated with eye exercises to retrain eye focus, botulinum toxin to minimize overactive eye muscles, prism eyeglasses to correct double vision, or more commonly, eye muscle surgery to loosen or tighten muscles around the eye to minimize misalignment.

NYSTAGMUS

The involuntary, rhythmic movement of one or both eyes is called nystagmus. The movement may be jerking, rotating, or pendular. Causes of nystagmus include damage to the vestibular system; injury of cranial nerves III, IV, or VI; cerebellar disturbance; and drug intoxication. Rotating nystagmus is frequently associated with dizziness and nausea. Miners exposed to years of working in the dark may develop pendular nystagmus.

MYOPIA

Myopia, also called nearsightedness, occurs when the eye is unable to accommodate sufficiently to objects that are far away. Myopia may result from developmental elongation of the eyeball that causes the image to be focused in front of the retina. Myopia has a genetic predisposition and frequently develops in late childhood. It is especially common in children who read extensively, perhaps as a result of changes in the length of the eyeball after prolonged focusing on near objects. Myopia is treated with a concave lens in eyeglasses or contact lenses. A surgical procedure, laser-assisted in situ keratomileusis (LASIK), also can significantly improve myopia. LASIK surgery involves the use of a laser to permanently change the shape of the cornea to improve vision, thereby reducing or eliminating the individual's need to wear corrective lenses.

HYPEROPIA

Hyperopia, also called farsightedness, occurs when the eye is unable to accommodate sufficiently to close objects, causing the object to be focused past the retina. Hyperopia may be present early in life or may develop later, typically after the fourth decade of life (presbyopia). In older persons, hyperopia occurs due to inflexibility of the aging lens. Hyperopia is treated with convex eyeglasses or contact lenses. LASIK surgery can significantly improve hyperopia as well.

ASTIGMATISM

In astigmatism, light rays are scattered rather than focused on the retina because of an asymmetric curvature of the cornea. The image is distorted or blurred. Astigmatism may occur with myopia or hyperopia. Specially constructed lenses are required.

COLOR BLINDNESS

Color blindness is usually a sex-linked genetic disorder caused by a deficiency in one of the three photopigments. Color-blind individuals see only colors formed by the activity of the other two types of cones. Color blindness is passed on the X chromosome; therefore, it usually affects males. In extreme cases, more than one color cone can be deficient.

PAPILLEDEMA

Papilledema is the swelling of the optic disk where the optic nerve leaves the eye and enters the brain. Because the optic disk is in communication with the brain, papilledema can occur in any condition that causes severely increased intracranial pressure. Such conditions may include brain tumor, infection, or injury. Papilledema is often an important diagnostic clue in severe brain pathology. Increased intracranial pressure compresses the veins leading to backup of blood and slow arterial flow. As pressure continues to increase, capillary permeability increases causing edema. Unresolved pressure can result in damage to the optic nerve and blindness.

CONDUCTIVE HEARING LOSS

Conductive hearing loss is a decrease in hearing caused by a blockage in the conduction of sound waves in the external or middle ear. Conductive hearing loss may occur if a foreign object is present in the ear or if there is an excessive wax or fluid buildup in the external or middle ear. Middle-ear infections (otitis media) may cause conductive hearing loss. A hearing aid may offer improvement.

SENSORINEURAL HEARING LOSS

Sensorineural hearing loss is usually irreversible and involves higher frequencies. Sound waves reach the inner ear, but are distorted or decreased before reaching the brain. Sensorineural hearing loss is a decrease in hearing caused by dysfunction of the organ of Corti, the auditory nerve, or the brain. The organ of Corti may become damaged from prolonged exposure to high levels of noise or after the use of ototoxic (ear-damaging) drugs. Ototoxic drugs include aminoglycoside antibiotics (gentamicin, neomycin, and streptomycin), analgesics (aspirin), tobacco, and alcohol. Other causes may include systemic diseases such as diabetes mellitus and syphilis, trauma, central nervous system infections such as meningitis, degenerative conditions, or tumors.

TINNITUS

Described as a ringing in one or both ears, tinnitus may accompany ear wax buildup or presbycusis. Aspirin overdose or other drugs may induce tinnitus. Middle-ear infection, Ménière disease, or otosclerosis (irregular ossification of middle-ear bones) may also cause tinnitus.

VERTIGO

The sensation of motion or spinning, often described as a feeling of being off balance, is called vertigo. Vertigo is sometimes accompanied by nausea, weakness, and mental confusion. Inner-ear inflammation, especially of the semicircular canals, is the most common cause of vertigo. Cranial nerve disorders may also cause vertigo. Drugs such as the aminoglycosides, aspirin, and loop diuretics may cause dizziness and imbalance, also related to damaging effects on the inner ear.

HYPOSMIA

A decrease in the sensation of smell is called hyposmia and may be bilateral or unilateral. If all smells are affected, congestion of the nasal passages is most likely the cause. Other causes may include medications, nerve tract damage, frontal-lobe injury or it could be idiopathic. A gradual decrease in the sense of smell is considered to be a normal part of aging. A thorough examination is required to determine the cause. Treatment is focused on the underlying cause.

HYPOGEUSIA

A decrease in taste sensation is called hypogeusia. Those affected may lose sensation of one specific taste or of all tastes. It may indicate damage to one of the cranial nerves innervating either the tongue or the palate. Sometimes tastes previously enjoyed are suddenly perceived as distasteful. This phenomenon is called parageusia and may occur with drug therapy, including chemotherapeutic drugs, or with liver dysfunction. In the elderly, hypogeusia sometimes occurs spontaneously. Cigarette smoking may affect taste.

● Conditions of Disease or Injury

CONJUNCTIVITIS

Inflammation of the conjunctiva of the eye caused by an infectious process, physical irritation, or an allergic response is known as conjunctivitis. With inflammation, the conjunctiva becomes red, swollen, and tender. Conjunctivitis stemming from a bacterial infection is sometimes called pink eye. Pink eye may exist alone, or it may coexist with an ear infection. Viral conjunctivitis is often caused by adenovirus infection. Bacterial and viral conjunctivitis are highly contagious. Allergic conjunctivitis occurs as part of the inflammatory reaction to an environmental allergen and is not contagious. Physical stimulation by a foreign object in the eye will irritate and inflame the conjunctiva as well, causing inflammation and pain.

Clinical Manifestations

- Red, swollen conjunctiva. With infectious or allergic conjunctivitis, both eyes are usually affected.
- Photophobia (an aversion to light).
- A purulent discharge is characteristic of bacterial conjunctivitis. Infection and discharge often begin in one eye and spread to the other. The eyes may be matted shut by a greenish crust.
- A clear, watery discharge is characteristic of viral conjunctivitis. Viral conjunctivitis frequently accompanies an upper respiratory tract infection.
- Burning and itching of the eyes is characteristic of allergic conjunctivitis.
- Conjunctivitis due to a foreign object is associated with discomfort and a feeling of sand or grit in the eye. Usually with a foreign object, only one eye is affected.

Diagnosis

- Diagnosis follows history and physical examination. Cultures may be required in some circumstances.

- A foreign object in the eye should be visualized with the use of fluoroscein dye and a special lamp, called a Wood lamp.

Complications

- Certain bacterial infections (gonorrhea, some types of chlamydial conjunctivitis) and viral infections may cause permanent damage to the eye if untreated.
- A foreign body in the eye may lead to corneal abrasion and scarring.
- Conjunctivitis may be an early symptom of the severe systemic disease **Kawasaki disease**. This disease is one of widespread vasculitis that affects many organs of the body, including the heart, brain, joints, liver, and eyes. It begins acutely with a high fever, followed shortly by bilateral conjunctivitis that is notable for its lack of discharge and its prolonged course. A rash and swelling of hands and feet accompany these early symptoms. Early diagnosis is important to prevent damage to the coronary arteries. Treatment for Kawasaki disease involves the use of aspirin and gamma globulin.

Treatment

- Bacterial conjunctivitis is usually treated with antibiotic eye drops or cream, but it often resolves within approximately 2 weeks, even without treatment. Because it is highly contagious among family members and schoolmates, excellent hand washing techniques and separate towels for infected individuals are required. Family members should not share bed linens or pillows.
- Conjunctivitis coassociated with otitis media is treated with systemic antibiotics.
- Warm compresses placed on the eyes may remove the discharge. Cool compresses may help alleviate discomfort.
- Viral conjunctivitis is usually treated with warm compresses. Excellent hand washing techniques are required to prevent transmission.
- Allergic conjunctivitis is treated by avoidance of the allergen if possible. Antihistamines or steroid-containing eye drops may be used to reduce itching and inflammation.
- Conjunctivitis caused by an irritant is treated by removal of any foreign object, followed by the use of antibacterial medication.

CATARACTS

A cataract is a progressive loss in the transparency of the lens. The lens becomes cloudy or gray-white in color, and visual acuity is reduced. Cataracts occur when proteins in the normally transparent lens break down and coagulate on the lens.

Causes of Cataracts

Most cataracts, called senile cataracts, develop from degenerative changes associated with aging. Exposure to ultraviolet light, oxidative stress, and a hereditary
predisposition contribute to their development. Other causes may include:

- Trauma to the eye which causes rupture and swelling of the lens.
- Eye infections.
- Exposure to radiation or certain drugs such as systemic corticosteroids.
- Fetal exposure to rubella.
- Long-term metabolic diseases such as diabetes mellitus which may impair
  blood flow to the eye and alter handling and metabolism of glucose.
- Cigarette smoking and excessive alcohol intake.

Clinical Manifestations

- Progressively decreased visual acuity.
- Gradual, painless blurring of vision, glaring, and loss of color perception.
- Opacity of the lenses.

Diagnosis

- History and physical examination with an ophthalmoscope or slit lamp, during which whitish opacities on the lens may be seen. As cataracts progress,
  the retina cannot be visualized.
- In infants, there may be an absence of the red reflex on eye examination.

Complications

- Loss of vision may occur if untreated.
- Injuries secondary to poor vision.

Treatment

- Treatment may involve excision of the entire lens and replacement with an
  artificial lens, or fragmentation of the lens by ultrasound or laser, followed
  by aspiration of the fragments and lens replacement.
- Custom intraocular lens implants are now possible to help correct accommodation or astigmatism.

GLAUCOMA

Glaucoma is a condition of the eye usually caused by an abnormal increase in
IOP (to greater than 20 mm Hg). The high pressures, sometimes reaching

60 to 70 mm Hg, cause compression of the optic nerve as it leaves the eyeball, leading to death of the nerve fibers. In some cases, glaucoma may develop even though IOP is normal. This type of glaucoma is associated with other causes of optic nerve damage. Glaucoma is a main cause of blindness in the United States and is the second most common cause of blindness worldwide.

Blindness caused by glaucoma usually develops gradually as IOPs slowly increase, but may occur within a few days if IOPs suddenly become high. Typically, loss of peripheral vision occurs first, followed by loss of central vision. The blindness caused by glaucoma is irreversible. The two main types of glaucoma are **acute angle closure** glaucoma and **primary open angle** glaucoma, which is the most common form.

Causes of Glaucoma

Glaucoma is usually caused by an obstruction of aqueous humor flow out of the eye chamber. Acute angle closure glaucoma is caused by sudden obstruction to flow through the angle between the cornea and the iris, which may occur with infection or injury or even for unknown reasons. In contrast, primary open angle glaucoma develops more gradually, usually from age-related fibrosis of the angle or gradual obstruction of other channels involved in the flow of aqueous humor. In these cases, there is a progressive increase in IOP. Occasionally, an increase in the production of aqueous humor may cause increased IOP. Risk factors for glaucoma include age (10% at age >80), positive family history, Hispanic ethnicity, African Caribbean origin, thin corneas, increased cup-disk ratio, myopia, and genetic mutation.

Clinical Manifestations

- Acute glaucoma
  - Severe eye pain and sudden loss of the visual field.
  - "Halos" of light around objects.
  - Enlargement of the eye may occur.

- Chronic glaucoma
  - Slow decrease in visual acuity and blurring, beginning with peripheral vision.
  - Headache and eye pain may develop as the condition worsens.
  - The eye may be red and tender to the touch.

Diagnosis

- Glaucoma can be diagnosed from history and physical examination.
- Gradual or sudden reductions in visual field may be reported.

- IOP readings will usually be high, however, glaucomatous changes have been seen in individuals with normal pressures. The degree of pressure does not correlate with the degree of optic nerve damage.
- Close inspection of the optic nerve may show characteristic color changes and cupping of the retinal rim.
- Because there is no definitive test with optimal sensitivity and specificity, the American Academy of Ophthalmology (2004) recommends comprehensive eye exams on a routine basis. Comprehensive exams should include visual acuity, IOP measurement with applanation tonometer, visual field, ophthalmoscopic exam, and split-lamp examination.
- Perimetry is used to map responses to light stimuli in the visual field. A new short-wavelength automated perimetry can detect glaucoma type changes about 3 to 5 years earlier than the original perimetry.
- Early diagnosis of glaucoma is essential to reduce the risk of blindness.

Complications

- Optic nerve atrophy.
- Blindness may develop with any type of glaucoma. Acute angle closure glaucoma is a medical emergency.
- Topical agents used to treat glaucoma may have adverse systemic effects, especially in the elderly. These effects may include worsening of cardiac, respiratory, or neurologic conditions.

Treatment

Treatment is aimed at slowing disease progression and preserving vision while minimizing adverse effects of therapy. Stabilization of the optic nerve and retinal nerve fiber layer, stabilization of the visual field, and control of the IOP are the goals of treatment. IOP can be reduced by decreasing the production of aqueous humor and/or increasing the outflow.

- Eye drops are applied to decrease IOP. Prostaglandin analogs are thought to relax the ciliary muscle or remodel the surrounding extracellular matrix thus increasing the outflow of aqueous humor.
  - Beta blockers reduce the production of aqueous humor by blocking beta receptors in the ciliary epithelium.
  - Parasympathomimetic drugs to constrict the pupil and increase the flow of aqueous humor out of the eye.
  - Alpha-2-adrenergic agonists decrease aqueous humor secretion and increase outflow.

- Carbonic anhydrase inhibitors interfere with the enzyme involved in sodium and fluid transport in the ciliary body thus reducing aqueous fluid production. The topical form is recommended and is used in conjunction with other drugs.
- With acute angle closure, diuretics may be used to decrease IOP. Surgery may be required. IOPs should be monitored annually in individuals older than age 40 or anyone who has an increased risk of the disorder.
- Surgery that includes iridectomy for angle closure glaucoma, drainage surgery, or laser trabeculoplasty may be employed to improve aqueous outflow.
- Incision trabeculectomy may be used when laser surgery is unsuccessful. The surgery involves creating a tiny opening in the trabecular meshwork to facilitate drainage of the aqueous humor.
- Other procedures involve creating openings for the flow of aqueous humor into the bloodstream or placement of tube shunts that allow excess fluid to flow into the eye tissue.
- A last resort treatment is laser cycloblation, which involves destruction of the ciliary body to decrease aqueous humor production.

OTHER EYE DISORDERS

Table 11-1 includes a summary of other common eye disorders.

TABLE 11-1	Disorders of the Eye		
	Retinal Detachment	**Diabetic Retinopathy**	**Macular Degeneration**
Description	Separation of sensory retina from pigment epithelium of the retina	One of the leading causes of blindness in the United States; hemorrhages of the retinal blood vessel interfere with oxygen supply to the photoreceptors resulting in new vessels that block vision	Most common cause of blindness in those >65 years of age; atrophy and outer retina degeneration with the dry form
Causes/ risk factors	Age; trauma; myopia	Chronically elevated blood glucose levels; hypertension	Age; injury; infection; exudative macular degeneration; female; Caucasian; cigarette smoking

	Retinal Detachment	Diabetic Retinopathy	Macular Degeneration
Clinical manifestations	Painless visual changes; often described as a curtain coming down; flashing lights or sparks; floaters	Glare; cotton-wool spots; flame-shaped hemorrhages	Loss of central visual field; loss of fine detail discrimination; drusen spots on the retina; in the wet form, choroidal neurovascular membrane is formed with vessels that leak easily thus separating the pigmented epithelium from the neurosensory retina
Treatment	Early detection; immediate bed rest; laser or cryotherapy to seal the tear; scleral buckling	Frequent and comprehensive eye exams and follow-up; photocoagulation with argon laser; vitrectomy	Mostly symptomatic treatment such as magnifying glasses, high-intensity reading lamp; for the wet form, thermal laser photocoagulation, periocular corticosteroid injections or photodynamic laser therapy

OTITIS

Otitis is an inflammation of the ear. Inflammation may be of the external ear canal, called **otitis externa**, or of the middle ear, called **otitis media**.

Otitis externa may develop in susceptible individuals after swimming or following other types of exposure of the external ear to water. Otitis media is divided into two classes: (1) acute otitis media, characterized by recent abrupt onset, fluid in the middle ear space, acute infection with fever, and ear pain, and (2) otitis media with effusion, characterized by fluid within the middle ear space without signs or symptoms of acute infection (see page C9 for illustrations).

Acute otitis media often results from a bacterial infection, usually by *Streptococcus pneumoniae, Haemophilus influenzae,* or *Staphylococcus aureus*. Acute otitis media may also result from a viral infection. Immaturity of the immune system or gastroesophageal reflux disease in young children may be causative as well. Acute otitis media occurs when the eustachian tubes that normally drain middle-ear secretions to the throat become blocked or full, causing middle-ear secretions and fluid to accumulate. When the tubes reopen, pressure in the congested ear can draw contaminated nasal secretions through the eustachian tubes into the middle ear, leading to infection.

Otitis media with effusion refers to the accumulation of fluid in the middle ear that often results from an allergy. In some circumstances, a secondary bacterial infection may develop.

Inflammation of the middle ear for greater than 12 weeks is classified as chronic otitis media. Left untreated, irreversible damage such as tympanic membrane atrophy or perforation may occur. Chronic otitis media may be the result of acute otitis media, trauma, or disease.

Clinical Manifestations

- Pain in the affected ear is the most common symptom of acute otitis media.
- In an infant or toddler, fever, irritability, difficulty sleeping, and pulling on the ear may signify acute otitis media.
- Anorexia, vomiting, and diarrhea may accompany acute otitis media.
- An uncomfortable feeling of fullness in the ear is common with otitis media with effusion.
- Pain with manipulation of the external structures of the ear suggests otitis externa.
- With chronic otitis media, the classical clinical finding is purulent drainage from the ear. Conductive hearing loss may be present.

Diagnostic Tools

- Otoscopic examination provides information on the eardrum that can be used to diagnose otitis media. Acute otitis media presents with a reddened, bulging eardrum when examined otoscopically. Bony landmarks and the light reflex may be obscured. Otitis media with effusion may present as a gray eardrum, either bulging or depressed inward. Otitis externa is diagnosed by the observance of a reddened, inflamed external canal and pain with manipulation of the external ear.
- The use of a pneumonic device with the otoscope (pneumatic otoscope) further assists diagnosis of otitis media. By squeezing an air-filled bulb connected to the otoscope, a small bolus of air can be injected into the external ear. The mobility of the tympanic membrane can be observed by the examiner through the otoscope. With acute otitis media and otitis media with effusion, tympanic mobility is reduced.
- A tympanogram, a test that involves placing a small probe in the external ear and measuring the movement of the tympanic membrane (eardrum) after the presentation of a fixed tone, can also be used to evaluate tympanic

mobility. With acute otitis media and otitis media with effusion, the mobility of the eardrum is reduced.

- Audiologic testing may show a hearing deficit, which is an indication of fluid buildup (infectious or allergic).

Complications

Repeated or untreated otitis media may cause scarring of the eardrum and permanent reduction in hearing acuity.

- Rare complications of acute otitis media include facial paralysis, meningitis, otogenic brain abscess, or infection of the mastoid bone.
- The 2004 American Academy of Pediatrics treatment guidelines for acute otitis media may result in overtreatment. Approximately 90% of cases will resolve spontaneously so treating prematurely with antibiotics may increase resistance.

Treatment

- Pain diagnosis and management with acetaminophen or other analgesics are recommended for acute otitis media.
- Acute otitis media is usually treated with antibiotics, although a period of watchful waiting may be appropriate. Repeated episodes of acute otitis media may lead to insertion of a tympanostomy tube in an attempt to prevent future infections.
- Although otitis media with effusion usually will resolve on its own over 3 to 4 months, close observation by the health care provider is needed. When hearing loss is involved, the patient is referred to an otolaryngologist for evaluation on the use of tympanostomy tube placement.
- Otitis externa is treated with anti-inflammatory drops, antimicrobial drops, or both.

MÉNIÈRE DISEASE

A chronic disorder of the semicircular canals and labyrinths of the inner ear is called Ménière disease. It is named after Dr. Prosper Ménière, who first reported the syndrome in a young girl in 1861. This disease is associated with severe attacks of vertigo (sense of spinning or disequilibrium), often accompanied by nausea. The cause of Ménière disease is unknown, but it appears related to an overproduction of endolymph in the inner ear, which causes distention in the endolymphatic compartment. Elevation in antidiuretic hormone may be involved in some cases. Occurrences of Ménière disease may follow middle-ear infection or head trauma or may be associated with systemic illness such as thyroid disease or adrenal–pituitary insufficiency. The condition may also show a genetic predisposition. Currently, research is being conducted to determine if there is an autoimmune component involved with the disease process. Typically, the disorder begins unilaterally and eventually progresses to both ears.

Clinical Manifestations

- Ménière disease is characterized by the classical triad of extreme vertigo, lasting several minutes to a few hours, tinnitus, and fluctuating hear loss. The episodes come and go, often with several months between attacks.
- Autonomic nervous symptoms such as nausea, vomiting, hypotension, and sweating often occur with attacks.
- Feeling of fullness in the ear.
- Nystagmus may occur during the acute attack.

Diagnosis

- Ménière disease is usually diagnosed from history and physical examination. Tests of vestibular function, including balance testing, and tests of nystagmus eye movements may help confirm the diagnosis.
- Diagnosis needs to rule out other causes of vertigo and tinnitus, including autoimmune disease, auditory nerve damage, or tumor.

Complications

- Ménière disease may progress to nerve deafness.
- Safety is a major issue during acute attacks due to the severe vertigo.

Treatment

- Symptoms may decrease if the patient lies down or sits still, making no sudden movements.
- Treatments to reduce fluid volume, including diuretics and a low-salt diet, are suggested. Vasodilators, antihistamines, and steroid hormones have been used with varying degrees of success.
- Smoking cessation, allergy management, elimination of caffeine, and stress management may minimize symptoms.
- Medications that can reduce nausea are available.
- Surgical placement of a shunt to drain excess endolymph may be performed. Ablation of a portion of the eighth cranial nerve and destruction of the labyrinth may be helpful. Surgery is typically a last resort.
- Prescriptions of vestibulotoxic drugs, including systemic administration of streptomycin or intratympanic delivery of streptomycin and gentamicin, is used for severe cases.

PAIN

Pain is a subjective sensation of unpleasantness usually associated with actual or potential tissue damage. Pain can be protective, in that it causes an individual to back away from a dangerous stimulus, or it can serve no function, as is the case with chronic pain. Pain is sensed when specific pain receptors are activated. Description of pain is subjective and objective, based on the duration, the speed of sensation, and the location.

Receptors for Pain

Pain receptors are called **nociceptors**. Nociceptors include the free nerve endings, which respond to many stimuli, including mechanical pressure, deformation, temperature extremes, and various chemicals. With intense stimuli, other receptors such as the Pacinian corpuscles and Meissner corpuscles also send information perceived as painful. Chemicals that cause or worsen pain include histamine, bradykinin, serotonin, several prostaglandins, potassium ion, and hydrogen ion. Each of these substances accumulates at sites of cellular injury, hypoxia, or death, alerting the individual to these happenings. Although all pain receptors are capable of responding to any type of tactile stimuli, each receptor appears to respond most readily to one specific type of stimulation.

Duration of Pain

Pain may be acute (lasting less than 6 months) or chronic (lasting longer than 6 months). Acute pain can be beneficial, serving to alert the individual to danger. Chronic pain is never beneficial and has the potential to severely interfere with the quality of life.

Speed of Sensation

Fast pain is sensed less than 1 second (usually much less) after the application of a painful stimulus (e.g., touching a hot burner). Fast pain is well localized to the site and is frequently described as pricking or sharp. Fast pain is usually felt on or near the surface of the body. It is transmitted to the spinal cord by the A δ fibers.

Slow pain is felt 1 second or more after the application of a painful stimulus (e.g., pain that continues after a bump to the head). Slow pain is frequently described as dull, throbbing, or burning. It can intensify over the course of several minutes and may occur on the skin or in any deep tissue of the body. Slow pain can become chronic pain and lead to great disability. Slow pain is transmitted to the spinal cord by the slow C fibers. The C fibers are believed to release the neurotransmitter substance P when they synapse in the spinal cord. The neurotransmitter released by the A δ fibers is unknown. The pathways of pain are shown in Figure 11-9.

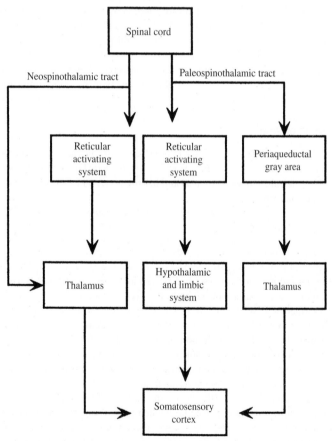

FIGURE 11-9 Pathways of pain.

Location

Cutaneous pain is pain felt on the skin or in subcutaneous tissues (e.g., pain felt with a pinprick or a skinned knee). Cutaneous pain is well localized over a dermatome (an area of the skin innervated by a certain spinal cord segment) and is transmitted rapidly. **Deep somatic** pain is pain arising from bones and joints, tendons, skeletal muscles, blood vessels, and deep nerve pressure. A headache is considered deep somatic pain. Deep somatic pain is slow pain, which may radiate along a nerve route. **Visceral** pain is pain in the abdominal or thoracic cavity. Visceral pain is typically severe and may be well localized at one spot, but it may also be referred to different parts of the body. Visceral pain localizes over embryonic dermatomes and is caused by stimulation of several pain receptors. **Referred** pain is pain perceived in an area other than the location of injury making it difficult to identify the exact origin. Referred pain is typically perceived in the same dermatome as the origin.

Pain Threshold

Pain threshold is the level at which a stimulus is first perceived as pain. In general, humans have similar pain thresholds. An individual's pain threshold varies little over time.

Pain Tolerance

Pain tolerance is an individual's ability to withstand a painful stimulus without demonstrating physical signs of pain. Pain tolerance is unique for each individual. It depends on past experience; cultural, familial, and role expectations; and the individual's current emotional and physical state. In some cultures it is considered weak to show pain, so pain tolerance is high. An individual who is depressed or anxious may have a reduced tolerance for pain. An individual who is distracted, or one who is in the middle of an emergency or an athletic challenge, may show a high tolerance for pain.

Central Nervous System Pathways for Pain

Once in the spinal cord, most pain fibers synapse on neurons in the dorsal horns of the segment they enter. However, some fibers may travel up or down several segments in the cord before synapsing. After activating cells in the spinal cord, information concerning painful stimuli is sent by one of two ascending pathways to the brain—the neospinothalamic tract or the paleospinothalamic tract.

Neospinothalamic Tract

Information carried to the spine in the fast-firing A δ fibers is transmitted ascendingly from the spinal cord to the brain via the fibers of the neospinothalamic tract. Some of these fibers terminate in the reticular activating system, alerting one to the occurrence of pain, but most travel to the thalamus. From the thalamus, signals are sent to the somatosensory cortex where the location of the pain is well localized. Cortical stimulation is required for the conscious interpretation of the pain signal.

Paleospinothalamic Tract

Information carried to the spine in the slowly transmitting C fibers, as well as that carried in a few of the A δ fibers, is transmitted ascendingly to the brain via the fibers of the paleospinothalamic tract. These fibers travel to the reticular area of the brainstem and to an area of the mesencephalon called the **periaqueductal gray area**. Paleospinothalamic fibers that travel through the reticular area go on to activate the hypothalamus and the limbic system, influencing the function of these emotion-controlling areas. The periaqueductal gray area is an important integrating center for pain; the perception of pain is highly modified in this area. Pain carried in the paleospinothalamic tract is poorly localized and is responsible for causing the emotional distress associated with pain.

Gating of Pain in the Spinal Cord and the Brain

Experimental evidence suggests that the likelihood of transmitting painful stimuli from the spinal cord to the brain can be influenced by descending neurons firing on the cells of the spinal cord. Descending input to the spine may increase the transmission of a painful stimulus, or it might decrease the likelihood that a stimulus is perceived as painful. Reduced passage of a painful stimulus is called **analgesia**.

Descending neurons that affect pain transmission come from the cerebral cortex, the hypothalamus, the limbic system, and, especially, the periaqueductal gray area. The ability of upper brain areas to influence transmission of pain in the spinal cord is called **gating**. Gating occurs at each level of pain transmission (across both the neospinothalamic and the paleospinothalamic tracts) and in the brain as well. Fibers from the periaqueductal gray area that diffusely innervate the cerebral cortex, the limbic system, the hypothalamus, and the reticular formation are especially important in influencing pain transmission in the brain.

Interpretation of the Gate Theory

The gate theory of pain offers an explanation of how cultural and personal expectations, mood, and fear can influence an individual's perception and tolerance of pain. By emphasizing the ability of descending pathways to influence pain perception, the gate theory of pain explains how distraction or relaxation techniques may reduce pain, whereas focusing on a painful stimulus may increase the likelihood of the stimulus being passed into consciousness.

The gate theory of pain also explains how gating can occur with peripheral nervous stimulation to the spinal cord. Data suggest that when the large

A β neurons carrying skin tactile information are stimulated at the same time that the A δ and C fibers are transmitting painful stimuli, spinal activation of both the neospinothalamic and the paleospinothalamic tracts is reduced. This reduced activation appears to result from lateral inhibition of the cells in the dorsal spine by the large A β neurons. Rubbing the head or skin after an injury stimulates the large A β fibers and produces some degree of analgesia. This is an example of gating the passage of a painful stimulus.

Endorphins, Enkephalins, and Serotonin

Some of the analgesic responses described above appear to result from the central nervous system production and release of the endogenous opiates: the endorphins and the enkephalins. Serotonin, another neurotransmitter, is also involved in producing analgesia.

Enkephalin is a small peptide released in the spinal cord from neurons descending from the periaqueductal gray area. Enkephalin causes presynaptic inhibition of types C and A δ fibers in the spine. This inhibition reduces the passage of a painful stimulus beyond the spinal cord. Enkephalin is also present in the limbic system and the hypothalamus.

The endorphins and serotonin act as neurotransmitters in the brain to reduce the passage and perception of pain. The pituitary releases endorphin in response to intense exercise and during painful experiences such as labor and delivery. Endorphins also affect mood. Prolonged pain has been shown to deplete endorphin levels; perhaps this contributes to the despair and anguish seen in individuals who have chronic pain. Serotonin is produced in the brain and is released from descending fibers synapsing in the spinal cord. Drugs that increase brain serotonin levels, such as the tricyclic antidepressants, reduce pain perception.

Clinical Manifestations

- Acute pain is characterized by increased heart rate, increased respiratory rate, facial grimacing, withdrawal, and crying. Dilated pupils and sweating occur. Usually, a person suffering acute pain is highly focused on the pain.
- Pain stimulates stress hormones such as aldosterone, antidiuretic hormone, and cortisol resulting in fluid conservation and elevated glucose.
- Chronic pain is associated with a return of heart and respiratory rate to normal. An individual who has chronic pain may appear quiet and subdued. Depression and despair may develop.
- Acute and chronic pain may occur simultaneously.

Diagnostic Tools

- Rating scales from 1 to 10 allow an individual to evaluate pain and may help a clinician recognize the intensity of a person's pain. For children, a diagram showing a range of faces, from happy to very sad and crying, may be used to help identify level of pain.

- Recognizing the subtle cues shown by an individual in pain is important for responding to pain when cultural, linguistic, or age barriers to communication exist.

Complications

- Pain stimulates the stress response. Stress can reduce the functioning of the immune and inflammatory systems, and thus delay or impair healing.
- Acute, severe pain may lead to cardiovascular collapse and shock.

Treatment

Effective pain management requires competent, consistent, compassionate care in a timely manner no matter what treatment modality is used.

- Application of cool compresses may reduce pain associated with inflammation.
- Measures to reduce the discomfort associated with wounds include warming the cleansing solution, careful dressing removal, use of atraumatic dressings, and scheduling changes.
- Comfort measures such as back rubs may reduce pain by stimulating the large A β fibers and by activating descending pathways stimulated by distraction.
- Behavioral techniques, including distraction and imaging, may stimulate descending pathways that block the transmission of painful stimuli to the brain. The Lamaze method of breathing during labor is based on this principle. Other nonpharmacologic therapies may include biofeedback, acupuncture, hypnosis, or relaxation.
- Transcutaneous electrical nerve stimulation (electrodes on the skin) may relieve pain by stimulating the large type A β nerve fibers. Acupuncture may stimulate these fibers and reduce pain as well.
- Analgesics such as acetaminophen can relieve mild pain, most likely by blocking the production of prostaglandins or other substances that sensitize pain receptors.
- Nonsteroidal anti-inflammatory drugs, such as aspirin and ibuprofen, or steroids may be used for mild to moderate pain. These drugs block prostaglandin production both locally at sites of injury and in the central nervous system.
- Local anesthetic agents to block peripheral pain transmission.
- Narcotics, such as morphine, can reduce intense pain. Morphine binds to opiate receptors in the central nervous system and alters pain perception.

- Nerve block by injection of drugs or surgery may occasionally be used to treat severe pain.

PEDIATRIC CONSIDERATIONS

- Amblyopia is the most common cause of decreased vision in the pediatric population. Early diagnosis is difficult, but the outcome is much more positive with early intervention.

- A child who suffers repeated episodes of otitis media may develop a speech deficiency if hearing is reduced during critical periods of language development. Repeated episodes of middle-ear infections may cause scarring of the eardrum and permanent hearing loss.

- Congenital sensorineural hearing loss may occur after fetal exposure to rubella or maternal drug exposure (including to the aminoglycosides). Congenital sensorineural hearing loss may also be inherited.

- Newborns may develop conjunctivitis during the birth process. The causative microorganism is often chlamydia, which may colonize in the mother's cervix, or gonorrhea. Both of these diseases are sexually transmitted. Pregnant women with a sexually transmitted disease should be treated with antibiotics before giving birth. Untreated neonatal eye infections may lead to blindness.

- Otitis media is the most common reason for children needing medical care. Infants and young children are most susceptible to middle-ear infections because their eustachian tubes are shorter and straighter than those of older children and adults. Prevention of acute otitis media in infants includes not putting a baby to bed with a bottle and feeding an infant with the head raised. Young children who have repeated ear infections may have reduced hearing acuity or experience language delays. To prevent this, tubes may be placed in the ear to assist drainage.

- Infants and children acutely feel pain and should never be exposed to painful therapies without pain medication. Infants may express pain differently than older children and adults.

GERIATRIC CONSIDERATIONS

- The center of the lens receives no direct capillary supply. Therefore, as a person ages, the cells at the center of the lens are the oldest and least oxygenated. When the cells in the center of the lens die, they are not replaced. This loss tends to make the lens stiff and less transparent. The lens becomes less able to change its shape to focus an object on the retina, which causes the object to appear out of focus. Visual quality is often reduced in the elderly. The lens may also become opaque (cloudy) with age, a condition known as a cataract. Cataracts further limit visual quality.

- Hearing acuity generally decreases with age. Causes include atherosclerosis and poor blood flow to the structures of the ear, stiffening of the middle-ear bones, and loss of receptor cells in the inner ear. Cerumen (wax) also builds up, which decreases sound transmission. Concomitant systemic disease, such as diabetes mellitus, may reduce hearing as well by compromising blood flow or diminishing neural transmission.

- Loss of taste and smell acuity occur with normal aging. Concomitant disease, including Alzheimer disease and certain medications taken by the elderly may worsen the normal loss of taste and smell. Reduced taste and smell may contribute to the poor appetite seen in some elderly individuals and may partially explain why the elderly often oversalt their food. Interestingly, the perception of sweet taste does not disappear with age, which may contribute to the weight gain seen in some individuals.

- Temperature sensation is decreased in the elderly. Decreased sensation may result in accidental burns from heating pads or hot baths.

- With age, most people experience a decline in color vision caused by yellowing of the lens. The decline in color vision may interfere with visual cues and contribute to falls.

- The basilar membrane of the cochlea stiffens with age, resulting in sensorineural hearing loss called **presbycusis**. Receptor hair cells die and are not replaced. Loss of receptors in the high-frequency range is especially common. Because of these changes, the elderly person is better able to hear deep voices compared to higher-pitched voices.

- Pain may be undertreated in older adults due to the myth that pain is part of aging. Dementia and an altered ability to communicate may also interfere with adequate treatment. Recent studies are showing a link between chronic pain and depression and suicidal risk in the older adult.

SELECTED BIBLIOGRAPHY

American Academy of Ophthalmology Glaucoma Panel. (2005). *Primary open-angle glaucoma*. Preferred Practice Patterns. San Francisco, CA: American Academy of Ophthalmology. Available at http//one.aao.org/asset.axd?id=2e86ca2e-9db0-43c9-b605-c004a82b6ea5.

American Academy of Pediatrics, American Academy of Family Physicians Subcommittee on Management of Acute Otitis Media. (2004). Clinical practice guideline: Diagnosis and management of acute otitis media. *Pediatrics*, 113, 1451–1455.

American Academy of Pediatrics, American Academy of Family Physicians, American Academy of Otolaryngology—Head and Neck Surgery, American Academy of Pediatrics Subcommittee on Otitis Media With Effusion. (2004). Clinical practice guideline: Otitis media with effusion. *Pediatrics*, 113, 1412–1429.

Aoki, M., Ando, K., Kuze, B., Mizuta, K., Hayashi, T., & Ito, Y. (2005). The association of antidiuretic hormone levels with an attack of Meniere's disease. *Clinical Otolaryngology*, 30, 521–525.

Ashley, J. L. (2008). Pain management: Nurses in jeopardy. *Oncology Nursing Forum*, 35(5), E70–E75.

Benbow, M. (2009). A practical guide to reducing pain in patients with wounds. *British Journal of Nursing*, 18(11), S20–S28.

Bickley, L. S., & Szilagyi, P. G. (2007). *Bates' guide to physical examination and history taking* (9th ed.). Philadelphia, PA: Lippincott Williams & Wilkins.

Caprioli, J., & Coleman, A. L. (2008). Intraocular pressure fluctuations: A risk factor for visual field progression at low intraocular pressures in the Advanced Glaucoma Intervention Study. *Ophthalmology*, 115(7), 1123–1129.

Chopra, V., Varma, R., Francis, B., Wu, J., Torres, M., & Azen, S. (2008). Type 2 diabetes mellitus and the risk of open-angle glaucoma: The Los Angeles Latino Eye Study. *Ophthalmology*, 115(2), 227–232.

Copstead, L. C., & Banasik, J. L. (2010). *Pathophysiology* (4th ed.). St. Louis, MO: Saunders Elsevier.

Danforth, D. A. (2008, August). What to do when the "eyes" have it. The *Clinical Advisor*, 11(8), 33–40.

Eliopoulos, C. (2010). *Gerontological nursing* (7th ed.). Philadelphia, PA: Lippincott Williams & Wilkins.

Guyton, A. C., & Hall, J. (2006). *Textbook of medical physiology* (11th ed.). Philadelphia, PA: W.B. Saunders.

Holcomb, S. S. (2009). Get an earful of the new cerumen impaction guidelines. *The Nurse Practitioner*, 34(4), 14–19.

Huether, S. E., & McCance, K. L. (2008). *Understanding pathophysiology* (4th ed.). St. Louis, MO: Mosby Elsevier.

Kirwan, J. F., Rennie, C., & Evans, J. R. (2009). Beta radiation for glaucoma surgery. *Cochran Database of Systemic Reviews*, (2). Art. No.: CD003433. DOI: 10.1002/14651858.CD003433.pub2.

Koch, J., & Sikes, K. (2009). Getting the red out: Primary angle-closure glaucoma. *The Nurse Practitioner*, 34(5), 6–9.

Lee, C. A., Mistry, D., Uppal, S., & Coatesworth, A. P. (2005). Otologic side effects of drugs. *Journal of Laryngology and Otology*, 119, 267–271.

Liu, L., Zhu, W., Zhang, Z. -S., Yang, T., Grant, A., Oxford, G., et al. (2004). Nicotine inhibits voltage-dependent sodium channels and sensitizes vanilloid receptors. *Journal of Neurophysiology*, 91, 1482–1491.

McKinnon, S. J., Goldberg, L., Peeples, P., Walt, J. G., & Bramley, T. J. (2008). Current management of glaucoma and the need for complete therapy. *Journal of Managed Care*, 14(suppl 1), S20–S27.

Medeiros, F. A., Weinreb, R., Zangwill, L., Alencar, P., Sample, C., Vasile, C., & Bowd, C. (2008). Long-term intraocular pressure fluctuations and risk of conversion from ocular hypertension to glaucoma. *Ophthalmoscopy*, 115(6), 934–940.

Meeks, T. W., Dunn, L. B., Kim, D. S., Golshan, S., Sewell, D. D., Atkinson, J. H., et al. (2007). Chronic pain and depression among geriatric psychiatry inpatients. *International Journal of Geriatric Psychiatry*, 23, 637–642.

Megale, S., Scanavini, A., Andrade, E. C., Machado Fernandes, M., & Anselmo-Lima, W. T. (2006). Gastroesophageal reflux disease: Its importance in ear, nose and throat practice. *International Journal of Pediatric Otorhinolaryngology*, 70, 81–88.

Minckler, D., Vedula, S. S., Li, T., Mathew, M., Ayyala, R., & Francis, B. (2006). Aqueous shunts for glaucoma. *Cochrane Database of Systemic Reviews*, (2), Art. No.: CD004918. DOI: 10.1002/14651858. CD004918.pub2.

National Eye Institute. (2006). *Report of the glaucoma panel: Program overview and goals.* Bethesda, MD. Available at http://www.nei.nih.gov/resources/strategicplans/neiplan/frm_glaucoma.asp.

Ng, W. S., Ang, G. S., & Azuara-Blanco, A. (2008) Laser peripheral iridoplasty for angle-closure. *Cochrane Database of Systemic Reviews*, (3), Art. No.: CD0006746. DOI: 10.1002/14651858. CD0006746.pub2.

Patton, K. T., & Thibodeau, G. A. (2010). *Anatomy and physiology* (7th ed.). St. Louis, MO: Mosby Elsevier.

Pediatric Academic Societies (PAS). (2009). Annual Meeting. Abstract 4315.4. Presented May 4, 2009.

Porth, C. M., & Matfin, G. (2009). *Pathophysiology: Concepts of altered health states* (8th ed.). Philadelphia, PA: Lippincott Williams & Wilkins.

Richardson, B. (2006). *Practice guidelines for pediatric nurse practitioners.* St. Louis, MO: Elsevier Mosby.

Rolim de Moura, C., Paranhos, A., & Wormald, R. (2007). Laser trabeculoplasty for open angle glaucoma. *Cochrane Database Syst Rev*, (4), CD003919.

Rubin, R., & Strayer, D. S. (2008). *Rubin's pathology: Clinicopathologic foundations of medicine* (5th ed.). Philadelphia, PA: Lippincott Williams & Wilkins.

Schiffman, S. S., & Graham, B. G. (2000). Taste and smell perception affect appetite and immunity in the elderly. *European Journal of Clinical Nutrition*, 54(suppl 3), S54–S63.

Sharts-Hopko, N. C., & Glynn-Milley, C. (2009). Primary open-angle glaucoma: Catching and treating the 'sneak thief of sight.' *American Journal of Neurology*, 109(2), 40–47.

Steenerson, R. L., Hardin, R. B., & Cronin, G. W. (2008, August). Gentamicin injections for Meniere disease: Comparison of subjective and objective end points. *Ear, Nose and Throat Journal*, 87(8,) 452, 454, 456.

Watson, S. L., Bunce, C., & Allan, B. D. S. (2005). Improved safety in contemporary LASIK. *Ophthalmology*, 112, 1375–1380.

Oxygen
Balance and
Deficiencies

HISTOLOGIC CHARACTERISTICS OF CANCER CELLS

Cancer is a destructive growth of cells, which invades nearby tissues and may metastasize to other areas of the body. Dividing rapidly, cancer cells tend to be extremely aggressive.

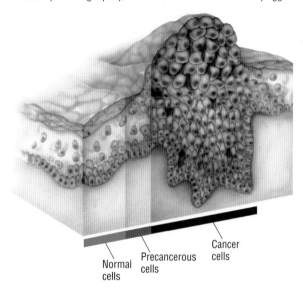

Normal cells
Precancerous cells
Cancer cells

HOW CANCER METASTASIZES

Cancer cells may invade nearby tissues or metastasize to other organs. They may move to other tissues by any or all of the three routes described below.

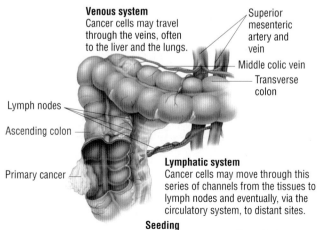

Venous system
Cancer cells may travel through the veins, often to the liver and the lungs.

Superior mesenteric artery and vein

Middle colic vein

Transverse colon

Lymph nodes

Ascending colon

Primary cancer

Lymphatic system
Cancer cells may move through this series of channels from the tissues to lymph nodes and eventually, via the circulatory system, to distant sites.

Seeding
Cancer may penetrate the wall of an organ, move into a body cavity, and spread throughout that area.

The inflammatory response
occurs after tissue injury or
infection. Inflammation may
precede a specific immune
response or be initiated by
one. There are two stages in
an acute inflammatory reaction:
vascular and cellular.

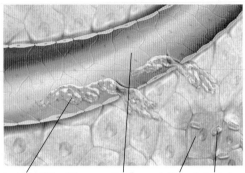

Increased blood flow   Blood vessel Wound Bacterium
carrying plasma proteins
and fluid to injured tissue

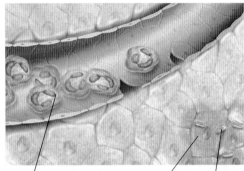

Movement of defensive white   Wound   Bacterium
blood cells to injured tissue

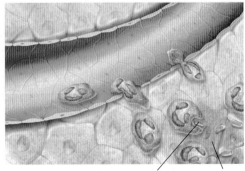

Phagocyte engulfing   Wound
bacterium

Common Skin Lesions

Bulla
Measuring more than 1.0 cm in diameter and filled with watery fluid, a bulla is a large, raised area on the skin. Bullae are large blisters that can occur after a burn.

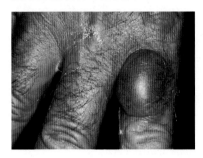

Cyst
An elevated, circumscribed encapsulated lesion in the dermis or subcutaneous layer is called a cyst. It may be filled with liquid or a semisolid substance.

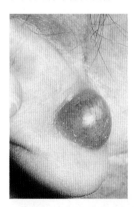

Excoriation
An excoriation is a scratch on the skin with loss of the epidermis (e.g., a skinned knee). It may be a hollowed-out, crusted area with slight bleeding.

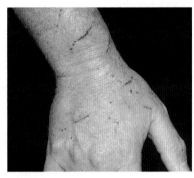

Fissure
A fissure is a linear crack in the skin from the epidermis to the dermis, for example, as seen with athlete's foot. The fissure may be pink or red, dry or moist, and usually there is no bleeding.

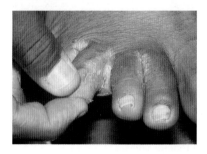

Keloid
A keloid is a scar formation on the skin, occurring after a trauma, injury, or piercing, that is out of proportion to the injury. Keloids are caused by excessive collagen formation during the healing process. They appear raised, red, and firm.

Common Skin Lesions

Macule

A macule is a flattened area of the skin, characterized by a change in color. A macule (e.g., a freckle or a flat mole, also called a nevus) is typically smaller than 1.0 cm in diameter.

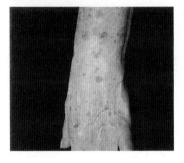

Papules

A papule is a solid, elevated mass, smaller than 1.0 cm in diameter. Examples of papules include elevated moles and warts.

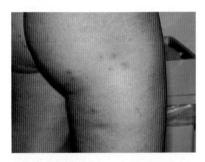

Urticaria/Wheals

Urticaria, also known as hives, consists of raised edematous plaques (wheals) associated with intense itching (pruritus). Urticaria results from the release of histamine during an inflammatory response to an allergen to which the individual has become sensitized. A wheal is a raised area of skin edema that exists only temporarily and itches (e.g., the area surrounding a mosquito bite or an area of the skin during an occurrence of urticaria [hives]). The center of a wheal is pink or red, with a surrounding circle of paler skin.

Pustules

A pustule is an elevated vesicle filled with pus. Examples of pustules are the lesions of impetigo or acne.

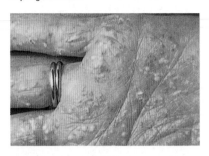

Petechia/Purpura

A deep red spot of pinpoint hemorrhage under the skin is called petechia. Petechiae may signify a bleeding disorder or fragility of the capillaries and may accompany a serious infection. A purpuric lesion is a large patch of purple discoloration under the skin associated with hemorrhage. It may result from a variety of causes, including thrombocytopenia (decreased platelets), trauma (a "black and blue mark"), or an allergic response.

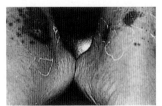

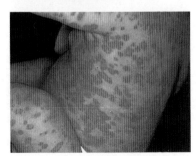

From Bickley, L. (2007). *Bates' guide to physical examination and history taking* (9th ed.). Philadelphia, PA: Lippincott Williams & Wilkins.

Keratoses
A horny overgrowth or abnormal growth of keratinocytes.

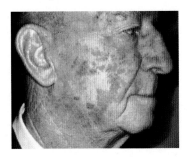

Vitiligo
Vitiligo (leukoderma) is a localized loss of melanocytes in the skin and hair. White patches of skin with definite borders may appear on the face, neck, axillae, or extremities.

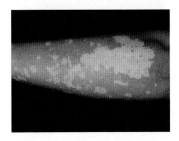

Contact dermatitis
Contact dermatitis is an acute or chronic inflammation of the skin caused by exposure to an irritant (irritant dermatitis) or allergen (allergic dermatitis). The location of the dermatitis on the skin corresponds to the site of exposure.

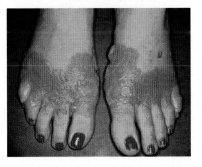

Atopic dermatitis
Atopic dermatitis (atopic eczema) is an inflammation of the skin involving overstimulation of T lymphocytes and mast cells. Histamine from the mast cells causes itching and erythema. Water loss from the epidermis and decreased skin lipid levels cause the skin to be dry. Scratching can cause skin breakdown.

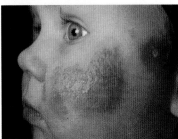

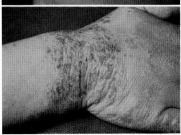

Herpes simplex 1
Herpesviruses cause characteristic skin and mucous membrane lesions and are passed by viral shedding from the lesions. The incubation period is approximately 2 to 24 days after infection. A prodromal period often precedes the appearance of lesions.

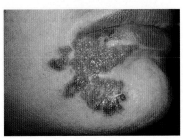

Chicken pox

Chicken pox is a common childhood communicable disease caused by the varicella zoster virus.

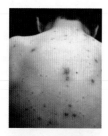

Rubeola

Rubeola, also called measles or red measles, is an upper respiratory tract infection caused by the paramyxovirus.

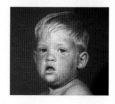

Rubella

Rubella, also called German measles or 3-day measles, is a viral infection of the respiratory tract caused by the rubella virus. There is a 14- to 21-day incubation period after infection, followed by prodromal symptoms lasting 1 to 4 days. A rash then develops.

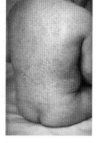

Impetigo

A superficial skin infection, usually caused by staphylococcus or group A beta-hemolytic streptococcal infection, is known as impetigo. There are two types of impetigo: vesicular and bullous.

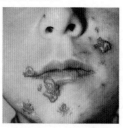

Cellulitis

Cellulitis is a bacterial infection of the dermis or subcutaneous layer of the skin. Cellulitis typically occurs after a surface wound, bite, or untreated carbuncle or furuncle.

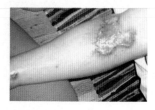

Acne

Acne is a common inflammatory disease of a sebaceous gland associated with a hair follicle, called the pilosebaceous unit. There are two types of acne: inflammatory and noninflammatory.

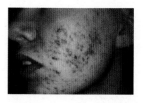

Psoriasis

Psoriasis is a chronic, autoimmune, inflammatory skin disease that affects approximately 2.6 million Americans. Psoriasis is characterized by rapid turnover of epidermal cells, leading to abnormal proliferation of the epidermis and the dermis. The skin demonstrates red, raised scaly plaques that can cover any body surface.

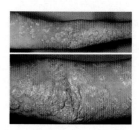

From Porth, C., & Matfin, G. (2009). *Pathophysiology, concepts of altered health states* (8th ed.). Philadelphia, PA: Lippincott Williams & Wilkins.

Decubitus ulcers, also called pressure ulcers or bed sores, are lesions on the skin that occur after the breakdown of the epidermis, the dermis, and occasionally, the subcutaneous tissue and underlying bone. The severity of an ulcer is based on the depth of erosion into the tissue.

Stage I
Reddened area

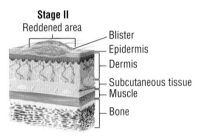

- Epidermis
- Dermis
- Subcutaneous tissue
- Muscle
- Bone

A Stage I pressure ulcer is an observable pressure-related alteration of the intact skin. The ulcer appears as a defined area of persistent redness in lightly pigmented skin; in darker skin, the ulcer may appear with persistent red, blue, or purple hues.

Stage II
Reddened area

- Blister
- Epidermis
- Dermis
- Subcutaneous tissue
- Muscle
- Bone

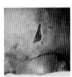

A Stage II pressure ulcer is characterized by partial-thickness skin loss involving the epidermis or dermis. The ulcer is superficial and appears as an abrasion, blister, or shallow crater. These wounds heal within a few weeks.

Stage III

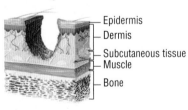

- Epidermis
- Dermis
- Subcutaneous tissue
- Muscle
- Bone

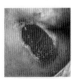

A Stage III pressure ulcer is characterized by full-thickness skin loss involving damage or necrosis of subcutaneous tissue, which may extend down to, but not through, the underlying fascia. The ulcer appears as a deep crater with or without undermining of adjacent tissue.

Stage IV

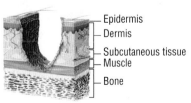

- Epidermis
- Dermis
- Subcutaneous tissue
- Muscle
- Bone

A Stage IV pressure ulcer is characterized by full-thickness skin loss with extensive destruction, tissue necrosis, or damage to muscle, bone, or support structures (e.g., tendon or joint capsule).

A cerebral vascular accident (CVA), often called a stroke or brain attack, is a brain injury related to an obstruction in brain blood flow. There are two general classifications of CVAs: ischemic and hemorrhagic. Ischemic CVAs develop from a prolonged blockage in arterial blood flow to a part of the brain. Hemorrhagic CVAs may occur as a result of bleeding into the brain.

Ischemic Stroke

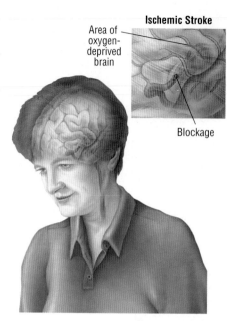

Area of oxygen-deprived brain

Blockage

Intracerebral hemorrhage

Bleeding within the brain tissue itself is known as intracerebral hemorrhage and is primarily caused by hypertension.

Hemorrhagic Stroke

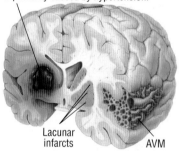

Lacunar infarcts

AVM

When a stroke occurs due to small vessel disease, a very small infarction results, sometimes called a lacunar infarction, from the French word "lacune" meaning "gap" or "cavity."

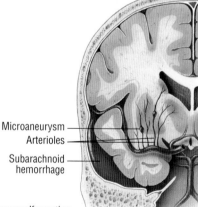

Microaneurysm
Arterioles
Subarachnoid hemorrhage

An arteriovenous malformation (AVM) is an abnormality of the brain's blood vessels in which arteries lead directly into veins without first going through a capillary bed. The pressure of the blood coming through the arteries is too high for the veins, causing them to dilate in order to transport the higher volume of blood. This dilation can cause them to rupture.

Classifications

Otitis media—inflammation of the middle ear—is divided into two classes: acute otitis media and otitis media with effusion. Acute otitis media is characterized by recent abrupt onset, fluid in the middle ear space, acute infection with fever, and ear pain. Otitis media with effusion is characterized by fluid within the middle ear space without signs or symptoms of acute infection.

Otoscopic view

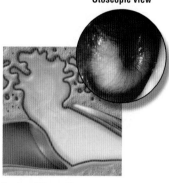

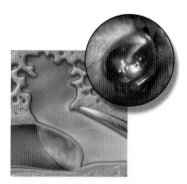

Acute otitis media
- Infected fluid in middle ear
- Rapid onset and short duration

Otitis media with effusion
- Relatively asymptomatic fluid in the middle ear
- May be acute, subacute, or chronic in nature

Complications

Complications of otitis media include atelectasis and perforation.

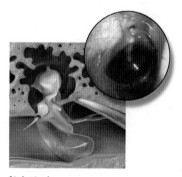

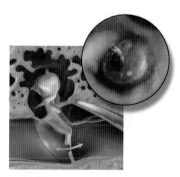

Atelectasis
- Thinning and potential collapse of tympanic membrane

Perforation
- A hole in the tympanic membrane caused by chronic negative middle ear pressure, inflammation, or trauma

Hypertension, or high blood pressure, is characterized by an elevation in diastolic or systolic blood pressure. Hypertension is the major cause of stroke, heart disease, and kidney failure.

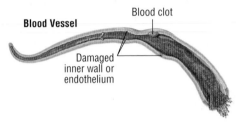

Blood Vessel
Blood clot
Damaged inner wall or endothelium

In hypertension, severely elevated blood pressure damages the inner layer of small vessels, resulting in fibrin (a whitish protein) accumulation in the vessels, local edema (swelling) and, possibly, intravascular clotting (clotting within the blood vessels).

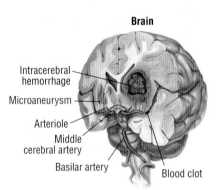

Brain
Intracerebral hemorrhage
Microaneurysm
Arteriole
Middle cerebral artery
Basilar artery
Blood clot

Cerebrovascular accident (stroke)
Hypertension is the major cause of stroke. The harmful effects of hypertension in the brain may be caused by blood clots stopping blood flow to parts of the brain.

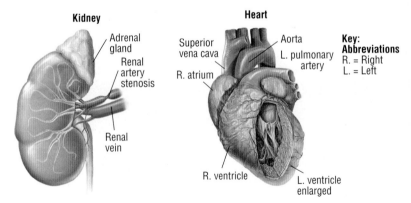

Kidney
Adrenal gland
Renal artery stenosis
Renal vein

Heart
Superior vena cava
R. atrium
Aorta
L. pulmonary artery
R. ventricle
L. ventricle enlarged

**Key:
Abbreviations**
R. = Right
L. = Left

Renovascular hypertension
If blood pressure rises because of narrowing (stenosis) of the major renal arteries or because of atherosclerosis of their branches, renovascular hypertension occurs.

Left ventricular hypertrophy
Due to increased blood pressure, the left ventricle may become enlarged and thickened.

Adult Respiratory Distress Syndrome (ARDS)

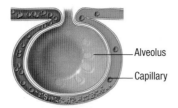

— Alveolus
— Capillary

Phase I
Injury reduces normal blood flow to the lungs. Platelets aggregate and release histamine (H), serotonin (S), and bradykinin (B).

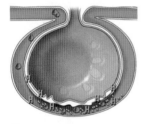

Phase II
Those substances, especially histamine, inflame and damage the alveolocapillary membrane, increasing capillary permeability. Fluids then shift info the interstitial space.

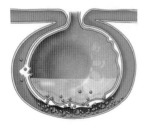

Phase III
As capillary permeability increases, proteins and fluids leak out, increasing interstitial osmotic pressure and causing pulmonary edema.

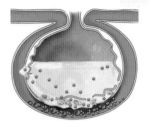

Phase IV
Decreased blood flow and fluids in the alveoli damage surfactant and impair the cell's ability to produce more. As a result, alveoli collapse, impeding gas exchange and decreasing lung compliance.

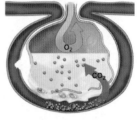

Phase V
Sufficient oxygen can't cross the alveolocapillary membrane, but carbon dioxide can and is lost with every exhalation. Oxygen and carbon dioxide levels decrease in the blood.

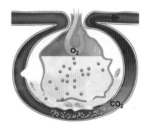

Phase VI
Pulmonary edema worsens, inflammation leads to fibrosis, and gas exchange is further impeded.

From Anatomical Chart Company. (2010). *Atlas of pathophysiology* (3rd ed.). Philadelphia, PA: Lippincott Williams & Wilkins.

Asthma is a progressive respiratory disease characterized by inflammation of the respiratory tract and spasm of airway bronchiolar smooth muscle. This results in excess mucus production and accumulation, hypertrophy of the bronchial smooth muscle, obstruction to airflow, and a decrease in ventilation of the alveoli.

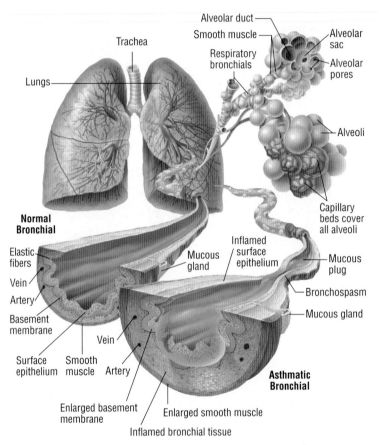

Alveolar duct

Smooth muscle

Trachea

Respiratory bronchials

Alveolar sac

Alveolar pores

Lungs

Alveoli

Capillary beds cover all alveoli

Normal Bronchial

Elastic fibers

Vein

Artery

Basement membrane

Surface epithelium

Smooth muscle

Artery

Vein

Inflamed surface epithelium

Mucous gland

Mucous plug

Bronchospasm

Mucous gland

Asthmatic Bronchial

Enlarged basement membrane

Enlarged smooth muscle

Inflamed bronchial tissue

Type 1 diabetes mellitus refers to hyperglycemia caused by an absolute lack of insulin. Insulin is needed to transport glucose from the bloodstream to the cells in order to supply energy to the body.

2. Cellular View of Pancreas
The pancreas contains two types of secretory tissues. The exocrine portion secretes digestive juices, while the endocrine portion releases hormones. The endocrine portion consists of cells arranged in groups called the **islets of Langerhans.** The islets contain hormone-secreting cells such as alpha cells and beta cells. It is believed that the body's immune system attacks and destroys the insulin-producing beta cells.

1. Digestive System
As food enters the digestive system, it is broken down into glucose. It is either stored in the liver or absorbed into the bloodstream, where it is used by the body for energy.

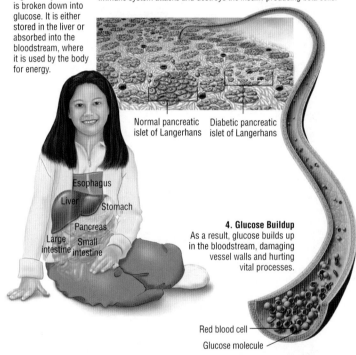

Normal pancreatic islet of Langerhans

Diabetic pancreatic islet of Langerhans

Esophagus

Liver

Stomach

Pancreas

Large intestine

Small intestine

4. Glucose Buildup
As a result, glucose builds up in the bloodstream, damaging vessel walls and hurting vital processes.

Red blood cell

Glucose molecule

3. Normal Cells versus Diabetic Cells
Normally, insulin molecules bind to muscle cell receptors, preparing the cells to absorb glucose from the blood. When activated by insulin, portals open to allow glucose to enter the cells, where it is converted to energy.

Without insulin, portals are not opened. As a result, glucose is not able to enter the cells to be converted to energy.

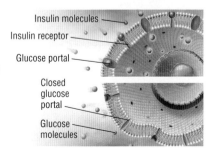

Insulin molecules

Insulin receptor

Glucose portal

Closed glucose portal

Glucose molecules

From Anatomical Chart Company. (2002). *Women's health and wellness: An illustrated guide* (1st ed.). Philadelphia, PA: Lippincott Williams & Wilkins.

Type 2 diabetes mellitus refers to hyperglycemia caused by cellular insensitivity to insulin. In addition, there is a corresponding insulin secretory defect that results in the pancreas being incapable of secreting enough insulin to maintain normal plasma glucose.

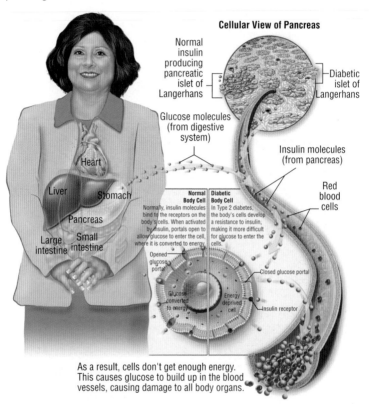

Cellular View of Pancreas

Normal insulin producing pancreatic islet of Langerhans

Diabetic islet of Langerhans

Glucose molecules (from digestive system)

Insulin molecules (from pancreas)

Red blood cells

Heart

Liver

Stomach

Pancreas

Large intestine

Small intestine

Normal Body Cell	Diabetic Body Cell
Normally, insulin molecules bind to the receptors on the body's cells. When activated by insulin, portals open to allow glucose to enter the cell, where it is converted to energy.	In Type 2 diabetes, the body's cells develop a resistance to insulin, making it more difficult for glucose to enter the cells.

Opened glucose portal

Closed glucose portal

Glucose converted to energy

Energy deprived cell

Insulin receptor

As a result, cells don't get enough energy. This causes glucose to build up in the blood vessels, causing damage to all body organs.

From Anatomical Chart Company. (2002). *Women's health and wellness: An illustrated guide* (1st ed.). Philadelphia, PA: Lippincott Williams & Wilkins.

Glomerulonephritis is an inflammation of the glomerulus. Types of glomerulonephritis include acute, rapidly progressive, and chronic. Acute glomerulonephritis occurs when there is a sudden inflammation of the glomerulus initiated by deposition of antibody–antigen complexes in the glomerular capillaries.

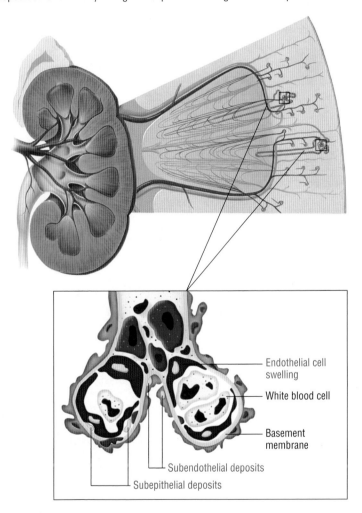

Endothelial cell swelling

White blood cell

Basement membrane

Subendothelial deposits

Subepithelial deposits

Genital Herpes

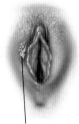

Herpetic lesions on labia majora

Herpetic lesions on penis

Genital Warts

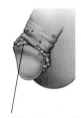

Genital warts on penis

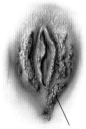

Genital warts on perineum

Syphilis

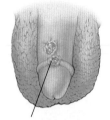

Chancre of syphilis

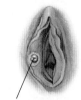

Chancre of syphilis

Mucopurulent Cervicitis with Chlamydia and Gonorrhea

Trichomoniasis

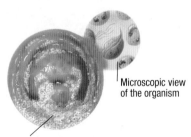

Microscopic view of the organism

Greenish-gray cervical dischargae (trichomonal vaginitis)

From Anatomical Chart Company. (2010). *Atlas of pathophysiology* (3rd ed.). Philadelphia, PA: Lippincott Williams & Wilkins.

12

The Hematologic System

The hematologic system includes all the blood cells, the bone marrow in which the cells mature, and the lymphoid tissue where the cells are stored when not in circulation. The hematologic system is designed to:

- carry oxygen and nutrients,
- transport hormones,
- remove waste products,
- deliver cells to prevent infection, stop bleeding, and promote healing,
- allow the body to feed and heal itself, and
- allow the body to communicate between sites.

● Physiologic Concepts

COMPOSITION OF THE BLOOD

The blood is made up of approximately 45% formed elements and 55% plasma. The formed elements are the red blood cells (erythrocytes), the white blood cells (leukocytes), and the platelets (thrombocytes). The red blood cells account for 99% of the formed elements; the white blood cells and platelets constitute the other 1%. The plasma is 90% water, with the other 10% made up of plasma proteins, electrolytes, dissolved gases, various waste products of metabolism, nutrients, vitamins, and cholesterol. Plasma water is responsible for transporting oxygen from the lungs and nutrients from the gastrointestinal tract to the cells of the body and for delivering waste products to the appropriate excretory organs. The plasma proteins include albumin, the globulins, and fibrinogen. **Albumin** is the most abundant plasma protein and helps maintain the plasma osmotic pressure and blood volume. The **globulins** bind insoluble hormones and other plasma constituents to make them soluble. This allows these important substances to be transported in the blood from their site of production to their site of action. Examples of substances that are carried bound to plasma proteins include thyroid hormone, iron, phospholipids, bilirubin, steroid hormones, and cholesterol. Other globulin proteins, the immunoglobulins, are the antibodies that travel in the blood to fight infection. **Fibrinogen** is a key element in blood clotting.

HEMATOPOIESIS

Red blood cells, white blood cells, and platelets are formed in the liver and spleen in the fetus, and in the bone marrow after birth. The process of blood-cell formation is called **hematopoiesis**.

Hematopoiesis begins in the bone marrow with pluripotential (meaning "many possible") stem cells. Stem cells are the source of all blood cells. These cells continually self-renew and differentiate throughout a lifetime; their supply is endless and they are often described as immortal. After several stages of differentiation, a stem cell becomes committed to forming just one type of blood cell. This cell, called a progenitor cell, remains in the marrow and, when instructed by specific growth factors, differentiates into a red blood cell, a white blood cell, or a platelet. The development of the blood cells from original pluripotential stem cells to differentiated cells is shown in Figure 12-1.

Control of Progenitor Cell Differentiation

Progenitor cells are stimulated to proliferate and differentiate by a variety of hormones and locally produced agents that collectively are called **hematopoietic growth factors**. Each progenitor cell responds only to some of these growth factors, but many growth factors may be acting nonspecifically on

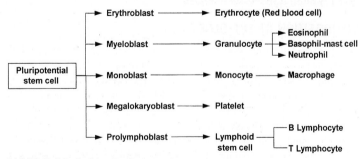

FIGURE 12-1 Blood cell maturation.

several progenitor cells. Many hematopoietic growth factors are cytokines. Cytokines are released from immune and inflammatory cells and communicate to the progenitor cells the need for more cells to fight infection or help the body heal. Hematopoietic growth factors specific to the line of cells they stimulate are called **colony-stimulating factors**. For example, granulocyte colony-stimulating factor stimulates the production of white blood cells known as granulocytes (see later), whereas monocyte–macrophage colony-stimulating factor increases the proliferation of monocytes and macrophages. An example of an important colony-stimulating growth factor for red blood cells is the hormone **erythropoietin**, which is produced by the kidney in response to low oxygen concentration in the blood. Other nonspecific cytokines may act on cells less differentiated than the progenitor cells, stimulating the production of a variety of blood cells.

THE RED BLOOD CELL

The red blood cell (erythrocyte) contains no nucleus, mitochondria, or ribosomes. It cannot reproduce or undergo oxidative phosphorylation or protein synthesis. The red blood cell contains the protein hemoglobin, which carries oxygen from the lungs to all cells of the body. Hemoglobin takes up most of the red blood cell's intracellular space. Red blood cells are produced in the bone marrow in response to hemopoietic growth factors, especially erythropoietin, and require iron, folic acid, and vitamin B_{12} for their synthesis. Once a red blood cell nears maturity, it is released from the bone marrow, completes its maturation in the bloodstream, and lives out its approximately 120-day life span. It then disintegrates and dies. Dying red blood cells are replaced with new ones released from the bone marrow. If red blood cell death is excessive, a larger than normal number of immature red blood cells, called *reticulocytes*, will be released from the bone marrow; elevated levels of circulating reticulocytes are suggestive of certain types of anemia.

Characteristics of Red Blood Cells

Red blood cells are small, biconcave (two-sided) disks shaped like donuts without holes. Their high surface area allows for rapid diffusion of oxygen and carbon dioxide, while their small size (7 μm in diameter) and relative flexibility allows them to squeeze through even the smallest of capillary beds without damage. In a blood sample, the percentage of the blood that is taken up by red blood cells is called the **hematocrit**, which usually ranges from approximately 36% to 52% depending on age and sex. The concentration of hemoglobin in a blood sample (grams per 100 mL) usually is approximately one third of the hematocrit. Red blood cells are described clinically by their size and by the amount of hemoglobin present in the cell. The suffix "cytic" refers to size, and the suffix "chromic" refers to the concentration of hemoglobin in the cell. The mean corpuscular volume (MCV) is a measure in cubic microns of the volume occupied by a single red cell. The MCV is the most commonly used index for identifying whether a cell is of normal, small, or large size and is used clinically to categorize an anemia.

- Normocytic: cells of normal size (MCV 87 to 103 fL/red cell or μm^3/red cell)
- Microcytic: cells too small in size (MCV < 87 μm^3/red cell)
- Macrocytic: cells too large in size (MCV > 103 μm^3/red cell)
- Hypochromic: cells with too little hemoglobin
- Normochromic: cells with normal amounts of hemoglobin
- Hyperchromic: cells with too dense hemoglobin

Red Blood Cell Antigens

The red blood cell has a variety of specific antigens present on its cell membrane that are not found on other cells. The most important of these antigens are known as A and B and Rh.

ABO Antigens

An individual carries two alleles (genes), each coding for the A antigen, the B antigen, or neither antigen, which is designated O. One allele is received from each parent. The A and B antigens are codominant. Individuals with both the A and B antigen (AB) will have AB blood. Those with two A antigens (AA), or one A and one O (AO), will have A blood. Those with two B antigens (BB), or one B and one O (BO), will have B blood. Individuals with neither antigen (OO) will have O blood. Individuals who have AB blood will accept A, B, or O blood. However, an immune response will develop if an individual without an A or a B antigen is exposed to that antigen in a blood transfusion.

Rh Antigens

Rh antigens are the other main antigen group on the red blood cell and are also passed as genes from each parent. The main Rh antigen is called the Rh factor. An individual who carries the Rh antigen is considered Rh positive (Rh⁺). An individual who lacks the Rh antigen is considered Rh negative (Rh⁻). The Rh-positive gene is dominant; therefore, an individual must have two negative Rh factors to be Rh negative. Individuals who are Rh positive will accept Rh-negative blood, but those who do not have the Rh antigen will develop an immune response if exposed to Rh-positive blood.

Universal Blood Recipients and Donors

Universal blood recipients are those with AB-positive blood because their immune system will recognize as self the A or B antigen and the Rh-positive antigen. Therefore, they will accept blood with any ABO or Rh profile. Universal blood donors are those with O-negative blood. Although their immune systems will attack blood containing the A or B antigen or the Rh factor, their blood can be given for transfusion to any recipient in an emergency (see Table 4-3). Other, weaker antigens on red blood cells exist, however, and may provoke an immune reaction in a recipient.

Hemoglobin

Hemoglobin consists of an iron-containing substance called heme and the protein globulin. There are approximately 300 hemoglobin molecules in each red blood cell. Each hemoglobin molecule contains four binding sites for oxygen. Oxygen bound to hemoglobin is called oxyhemoglobin. Hemoglobin in the red blood cell may be partially or completely bound with oxygen on all four sites. Fully saturated hemoglobin is completely bound with oxygen, while partially saturated or deoxygenated hemoglobin is less than 100% saturated. Systemic arterial blood from the lungs is fully saturated with oxygen. Because hemoglobin releases oxygen to the cells, the hemoglobin saturation in venous blood is approximately 60%. The final job of the hemoglobin is to pick up carbon dioxide and hydrogen ions and carry them to the lungs, where they are exhaled to the air. There are at least 100 types of abnormal hemoglobin molecules that have been recognized in humans, resulting from a variety of different mutations. Most of these mutations cause the hemoglobin molecule to carry oxygen more poorly than normal.

Breakdown of the Red Blood Cell

When the red blood cell begins to disintegrate at the end of its lifetime, hemoglobin is released into the circulation. Hemoglobin is broken down in the liver and spleen. The globulin molecule is converted into amino acids that are used again by the body. The iron is stored in the liver and spleen until it is reused. The rest of the molecule is converted to bilirubin, which is excreted in the stool as bile or in the urine. Normally, the rate of red cell breakdown is equal to the rate of synthesis. In certain conditions, either synthesis or breakdown may outpace the other.

WHITE BLOOD CELLS

White blood cells are formed in the bone marrow from committed progenitor cells. On further differentiation, the progenitor cells become non-granular-appearing T and B lymphocytes, monocytes, and macrophages, or granular-appearing neutrophils, basophils, and eosinophils. The job of the white blood cells is to recognize and fight microorganisms in immune reactions, and to assist in the inflammation and healing processes. The platelets, which are fragments of bone marrow cells, are essential in the control of bleeding. In addition, they often function with the white blood cells in the inflammatory and healing processes.

Types of White Blood Cells

B lymphocytes develop in the bone marrow and then circulate in the blood until they encounter the antigen to which they are programmed to respond. At this point, B lymphocytes mature further, become plasma cells, and begin secreting antibody, as described later.

T lymphocytes leave the bone marrow and develop during migration through the thymus. After leaving the thymus, they circulate in the blood or reside in the lymphatic tissue until they encounter an antigen to which they are programmed to respond. Once stimulated by an antigen, they produce chemicals to destroy the microorganism and alert other white blood cells that an infection is occurring, as described later.

Monocytes are formed in the bone marrow and enter the bloodstream in an immature form. At the site of injury or infection, the monocytes leave the blood and mature into macrophages in the tissues. Macrophages may remain stored in the tissues, or may be used in an inflammatory reaction as soon as they mature.

Neutrophils, basophils, and eosinophils are granular-appearing white blood cells that assist in the inflammatory response. Macrophages, neutrophils, and eosinophils function as phagocytes, cells that destroy and digest microorganisms and accumulated cell debris. Although the exact function of the basophils is unclear, they appear to act like circulating mast cells (Chapter 4) that release vasoactive peptides that stimulate the inflammatory response.

THE SPLEEN

The spleen is a small organ located in the upper left abdominal cavity. It is considered a secondary lymphoid organ, as opposed to the bone marrow and thymus, which are primary lymphoid organs. Like all lymphoid organs, the spleen is involved in the formation and storage of the blood.

The spleen is the site of hematopoiesis in the fetus. After birth, the spleen contains tissue macrophages and aggregates of lymphocytes. The spleen is well supplied with blood vessels that branch off from the splenic artery, which is a branch of the abdominal aorta. The intricate vasculature of the spleen circulates blood containing microorganisms, dead cells, and other debris past the macrophages and lymphocytes, where they can be acted on or destroyed. After flowing through the splenic capillary networks, the blood vessels rejoin into venules, and blood is delivered to the liver through the hepatic portal blood flow system.

As blood passes through the spleen, residing macrophages act as phagocytes to clear the blood of cell debris (including lysed red blood cells) and digest microorganisms. The macrophages present pieces of digested microorganisms to nearby B and T cells, initiating an immune response. Individuals who have lost their spleen (usually after trauma, although some individuals may have their spleen removed surgically when platelet count is low and cannot be corrected) are at a disadvantage in fighting certain infections compared to those with a functioning spleen.

The spleen also serves as a reservoir for blood, capable of holding a few hundred milliliters in the adult. With a decrease in blood pressure, the spleen can expel this blood into the venous circulation to help return pressure. It also serves as a storage site for iron released during the catabolism of hemoglobin. Iron is stored in splenic macrophages until required for production of new red blood cells. Iron deficiency may occur without the spleen. The spleen also stores senescent (aged) red blood cells.

LYMPH NODES

Lymph nodes are small capsules of lymphoid tissue interspersed throughout the lymphatic system, near the lymphatic veins. Lymph flowing in the lymphatic vessels is filtered through many nodes.

Lymph nodes contain many lymphocytes, monocytes, and macrophages. These cells proliferate in the nodes and some are released into the circulation during infection or inflammation. Residing white blood cells filter, detect, entrap, and phagocytize microorganisms that are delivered by the lymph flow, cleansing the lymph before it is returned to the general circulation. The lymph node closest to an infection is exposed to the highest number of microorganisms, which causes the macrophages and lymphocytes to proliferate and the node to enlarge. An active node may become tender and palpable as it fights to contain infection.

HEMOSTASIS

The human body experiences frequent small capillary tears and occasional large blood vessel cuts. While unable to control large vessel bleeding without external support, the body is able to stop small vessel bleeding. Control of bleeding occurs in two steps—the formation of a platelet plug followed by the formation of a blood clot. These processes are interdependent and occur one after the other in rapid succession. The control of bleeding is called hemostasis.

Role of the Platelets in Hemostasis

Platelets play an important role in both steps of hemostasis. Platelets normally circulate throughout the bloodstream without sticking to vascular endothelial cells. However, within seconds after damage to a blood vessel, platelets are drawn to the area in response to exposed collagen on the subendothelial layers of the damaged blood vessel. Platelets attach to proteins (called von Willebrand factors [vWF]) expressed on the damaged surface of a blood vessel, and release several vasoactive chemicals, including serotonin and adenosine diphosphate (ADP). Serotonin causes vasoconstriction, helping to reduce blood flow to the area and limit bleeding. Serotonin and other chemicals, including ADP, also cause the platelets to change shape and become sticky, beginning the formation of what is called a platelet plug inside the damaged blood vessel. Other platelets are drawn to the area and further build up the plug. **Thromboxane A$_2$** is produced by the platelets and contributes to the attraction of more platelets to the area. **Fibrinogen**, a circulating plasma protein, connects between exposed sites on the platelets, serving like a bridge to add stability to the plug. The platelet plug effectively seals the damaged area. Deficiencies in any of the involved factors will result in excessive bleeding of even small capillary tears.

Limits on Platelet Function

Unimpeded platelet aggregation could cause a prolonged decrease in blood flow to the tissue or result in a plug becoming so enlarged that it may break off from the original site and travel downstream as an embolus, blocking downstream flow. To prevent either of these occurrences from happening, neighboring *undamaged* endothelial cells release other substances that limit the extent of platelet aggregation. The main substances released by neighboring endothelial cells to limit platelet aggregation are prostaglandin I$_2$, also called **prostacyclin**, and **nitric oxide**, an important vasodilator.

Ultimately, the balance between proclotting and anticlotting factors serves to keep the platelets active at the site of injury while preventing excessive platelet aggregation and spread of the platelet plug to uninjured vascular tissue. Platelet aggregation and the production of the platelet plug are shown in Figure 12-2.

Blood Clot

The platelet plug becomes a true clot as it enlarges and traps circulating red cells and macrophages. The entire clot is stabilized and strengthened by a network of fibrin strands, produced from the fibrinogen bridges mentioned earlier. The production of stabilized fibrin is the final step in the other essential component of hemostasis, the coagulation cascade.

Coagulation Reactions

Coagulation reactions involve a series of coagulation factors or proteins activated in domino fashion, leading to the coagulation (clotting) of the blood. There are a total of 13 proteins involved in the coagulation pathways; some of these are activated in what is called the *intrinsic pathway* and some are activated in the *extrinsic pathway*. Under most physiologic conditions, coagulation occurs first through the extrinsic pathway; activation of the extrinsic pathway then turns on the more powerful intrinsic pathway. Both pathways ultimately

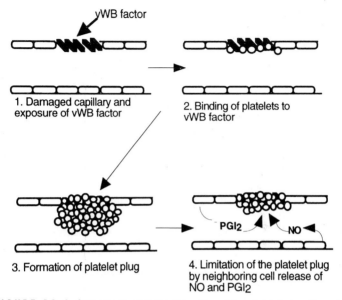

FIGURE 12-2 Steps involved in the formation of the platelet plug. The role of von Willebrand (vWB) factor, platelets, and prostaglandin I2 (PGI2) and nitric oxide (NO) released from neighboring endothelial cells is emphasized.

merge and function by activating one protein, factor X; the merging of the intrinsic and extrinsic pathways at factor X is called the final common pathway. Factor X is responsible for converting the plasma protein prothrombin to **thrombin**. Thrombin is the key catalyst that drives the conversion of fibrinogen to fibrin and causes coagulation. Thrombin also acts in a positive feedback manner to stimulate the proteins involved in its own production, furthering the coagulation cascade. Both pathways are shown in Figure 12-3.

The intrinsic pathway begins with the activation of the circulating coagulation factor, factor XII, also called the Hageman factor. Factor XII is activated when it comes into contact with damaged vascular tissue. Ultimately, activation of factor XII leads to the conversion of prothrombin to thrombin. Factors XI and IX are important intermediate steps in the cascade, and factors V and VIII are important cofactors. Lack of any of these factors could interfere with coagulation.

The extrinsic pathway, the usual way of stimulating coagulation, begins when damaged vascular endothelial cells release factor III, also called tissue factor or thromboplastin, into the circulation. When tissue factor encounters another coagulation factor circulating in the plasma, factor VII (also called serum prothrombin conversion factor), the extrinsic cascade is stimulated, again resulting in the production of factor X. The extrinsic pathway also can turn on the intrinsic pathway through the activation of factor IX.

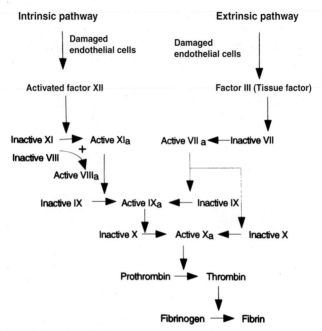

FIGURE 12-3 Simplified diagram of the intrinsic and extrinsic pathways of coagulation. Factor VII is highlighted to identify its pivotal role as a coenzyme in the intrinsic pathway. Letter "*a*" designates an activated factor.

The blood does not continually and excessively clot even though factors XII and VII are always present in the circulation because healthy endothelial cells are smooth and intact. Therefore, they do not directly activate factor XII or produce tissue factor and activate factor VII. Healthy vascular endothelium repels coagulation factors and platelets. It is only when the endothelium is damaged by trauma, infection, forces of chronic hypertension, or accumulation of fat and cholesterol (Chapter 13) that a clot begins to develop.

Because several coagulation factors are produced in the liver in reactions involving vitamin K, liver disease or vitamin K deficiency can impair the production of coagulation factors and cause bleeding.

Anticoagulants

Anticoagulants are present in the blood to prevent clots from developing. For example, antithrombin proteins are released by undamaged endothelial cells and function to inactivate thrombin. The most important of these, antithrombin III, is itself activated by heparin, an anticoagulant produced by mast cells and basophils in response to tissue injury and inflammation. Other substances, called tissue factor inhibitors, circulate in the plasma and bind to tissue factor (factor III), directly blocking its activation and interfering with the extrinsic pathway. Finally, as mentioned earlier, nondamaged endothelial cells secrete prostacyclin and nitric oxide, which limit platelet aggregation and thus reduce coagulation.

Anticoagulation drugs are available and include the prostaglandin inhibitor aspirin, which in low doses inhibits the production of thromboxane A_2 but not prostaglandin I_2, and oral anticoagulants such as warfarin. Other drugs are available that do not prevent clotting, but serve to break down previously formed clots. Examples of these drugs, called thrombolytic agents, include streptokinase and t-PA; thrombolytic agents play an important role in the early treatment of myocardial infarct and thrombotic stroke.

LABORATORY TESTS OF THE BLOOD

The Complete Blood Count with Differential and Platelet Count

The blood is frequently tested for adequacy of cell number and function. The most common test is the complete blood count (CBC), which provides information on the number, concentration, and physical characteristics of red blood cells, white blood cells, and platelets present in a venous blood sample. The CBC with differential is age dependent and, to a lesser extent, sex dependent. Exercise, reproductive status, and many drugs may cause test deviations. The CBC with differential is used as part of well physical examinations, to screen for specific conditions, and to determine preoperative health. The CBC is also used to evaluate treatment success.

A description of red cell size as indicated by the mean corpuscular volume (MCV) and mean corpuscular hemoglobin concentration (MCHC) provides additional information when evaluating patients with anemia. Red cells also are described by the red cell size distribution width (RDW) in a blood sample. If the RDW is high, it means there is a wide range of RBC sizes in the sample. The RDW is useful in distinguishing between similar types of anemia. For example, a patient with microcytic (small) red cells who has a normal RDW may have a hemoglobin abnormality such as thalassemia, while a patient with similarly microcytic cells but a high RDW is more likely experiencing iron deficiency. Other combinations of red cell values provide different clues to the etiology of blood disorders.

Other common blood tests include blood typing of ABO and Rh antigens and tests to identify the presence of microorganisms and antibody titers. The erythrocyte sedimentation rate (SED rate) is a test that evaluates the tendency of red blood cells to settle out of unclotted blood in 1 hour. This test is based on the fact that inflammation and similar processes stimulate the liver to release an increased number of proteins into the blood, which cause red cells to aggregate together, becoming heavier and thus settling to the bottom of a container. Because of this, the SED rate is often increased nonspecifically with inflammatory disease.

The Normal CBC with Differential and Platelet Count (Adult)

- Red blood cell count: 4.0 to 5.5 million/mL of blood
- White blood cell count: 5000 to 10,000/mL of blood
- Platelet count: 140,000 to 400,000/mL of blood
- Hematocrit (% of red blood cells): 42% to 52% for males; 36% to 48% for females
- Hemoglobin: 14.0 to 17.5 g/100 mL for males; 12.0 to 16.0 g/100 mL for females
- Neutrophils: 50% to 62%
- Eosinophils: 0% to 3%
- Basophils: 0% to 1%
- Lymphocytes: 25% to 40%
- Monocytes: 3% to 7%

Tests of Red Blood Cell Size and Hemoglobin (Adult)

- MCV: 82 to 98 fL/red cells
- MCHC: 32 to 36 g/dL
- RDW: 11.5 to 14.5 coefficient of variation of red cell size

Sedimentation Rate

- SED rate: 0 to 20 mm/hour

Bleeding Time

Bleeding time refers to the length of time bleeding occurs after a standardized puncture wound to the skin. Bleeding time is measured in minutes and indicates the functioning status of the platelets, specifically the effectiveness of the platelet plug. Bleeding time should not exceed 15 minutes (normal: 3.0 to 9.5 minutes) for a forearm stick.

Partial Thromboplastin Time/Prothrombin Time

Partial thromboplastin time (PTT) and prothrombin time (PT) detect deficiencies in the activity of various clotting factors. Both tests evaluate clotting in a venous blood sample.

PTT especially demonstrates the effectiveness of the intrinsic pathway of coagulation and should not exceed 90 seconds (normal: 30 to 45 seconds). This test is important in determining the effectiveness and safety of heparin therapy.

PT demonstrates the effectiveness of the vitamin K–dependent coagulation factors, especially the extrinsic and common pathways of coagulation.

PT should not exceed 40 seconds, or 2 to 2.5 times a control level (normal: 11 to 13 seconds). PT is used to determine the effectiveness of warfarin (Coumadin) therapy.

The international normalized ratio (INR) is a worldwide standard for evaluating the extrinsic pathway of coagulation. This test allows for standardization regardless of the reagents, unlike the PT, which may vary depending on the laboratory reagent. The INR should be less than 2.0 for anyone not taking anticoagulants. For patients receiving anticoagulant therapy, values up to 3.5 are considered in the normal range depending on the reason for therapy (venous thrombosis, mechanical heart valve, recurrent systemic embolus).

Pathophysiologic Concepts

ANEMIA

Anemia is a decrease in the quantity of circulating red blood cells, an abnormality in the hemoglobin content of red blood cells, or both. Anemia can be caused by a disorder in red blood cell production or an elevated loss of red blood cells through chronic bleeding, sudden hemorrhage, or excessive lysis (destruction). All anemias result in decreased values for hematocrit and hemoglobin but may vary in values of MCV, MCHC, and RDW. For example, using the MCV as an index, a microcytic anemia has a MCV < 82 fL/red cell; a normocytic anemia has a MCV between 82 and 98 fL/red cell; and a macrocytic anemia has a MCV > 98 fL/red cell. The symptoms associated with anemia depend on its duration, its severity, and the host's age and prior health status. All symptoms ultimately relate to a reduction in the delivery of oxygen to host cells and organs, thereby interfering with function and compromising health. Clinical manifestations may include tachycardia, orthostatic hypotension, murmurs, dyspnea, tachypnea, headache, lightheadedness, fatigue, pallor, and intermittent claudication.

Anemia Caused by a Disorder in Red Cell Production

Anemias that result from a disorder in red cell production occur if there is inadequate or inaccessible iron, or a lack of folic acid, vitamin B_{12}, or globulin. Red blood cell production may also be insufficient if there is bone marrow disease, as would occur in leukemia, after radiation exposure, or with other diseases of the marrow. A deficiency in erythropoietin, as would occur in renal failure, would also lead to a decrease in red cell production. Anemias due to disorders in RBC production may result in a red cell that is too small (microcytic) or too large (macrocytic), and hemoglobin content that is abnormally low (hypochromic).

TABLE 12-1 Common Anemias

Common Type of Anemia	Causes	Laboratory Findings
Normocytic	Acute hemorrhage Sickle cell anemia Malaria Aplastic anemia Thalassemia Anemia of chronic disease	↓ Hct ↓ Hemoglobin No change MCV No change MCHC Normal iron Normal ferritin
Microcytic	Iron-deficiency Slow chronic hemorrhage Anemia of pregnancy	↓ Hct ↓ Hemoglobin ↓ Iron status (except sideroblastic) ↓ Ferritin ↓ MCV ↓ Or no change MCHC
Megaloblastic anemia	Folic acid deficiency Vitamin B deficiency	↓ Hct ↓ Hemoglobin ↑ MCV Normal MCHC

Anemia Caused by Sudden or Chronic Hemorrhage or Lysis

Anemias caused by sudden hemorrhage, a slow chronic hemorrhage, or lysis result in a decrease in the total number of circulating red cells. This type of anemia may be associated with an increased percentage of circulating immature red cells (reticulocytes). Normal red blood cells live approximately 120 days. Red cell destruction or loss occurring before 100 days is abnormal. Common anemias, their causes, and laboratory profiles are shown in Table 12-1, and some are discussed more fully in the final section of this chapter.

POLYCYTHEMIA

Polycythemia is an increase in the number of red blood cells. Primary polycythemia (polycythemia vera) is characterized by an increase in platelets and granulocytes as well as red blood cells, and is believed to be the result of a precursor cell abnormality.

Polycythemia may occur secondarily to chronic hypoxia. Chronic hypoxia causes increased release of the renal hormone erythropoietin, which stimulates the production of red blood cells. Individuals who live at high altitude or suffer from chronic lung disease frequently experience secondary polycythemia.

Athletes who blood dope, meaning they accept self-transfusions of previously collected packed red cells, demonstrate polycythemia. And finally, poly-cythemia may be relative, rather than absolute. During dehydration, for in-stance, a decrease in plasma volume is reflected as an increase in the concentration of red cells. Polycythemia from any cause is associated with an increased risk of thrombus formation and an increase in the workload of the heart. Clinical manifestations are the result of increased blood viscosity and may include hypertension, headache, inability to concentrate, and impaired hearing and vision secondary to decreased cerebral blood flow.

LEUKOPENIA

Leukopenia is an absolute decrease in the number of white blood cells. Leukopenia may be caused by a variety of conditions, including prolonged stress, viral infection, bone marrow disease or destruction, radiation, or chemotherapy. Severe systemic diseases such as lupus erythematosus, thyroid disease, and Cushing syndrome may cause a decrease in white blood cells. All or one type of white cells may be affected although neutrophils, as the most prominent type of granulocytes, are most often affected. Leukopenia may predispose the individual to infection.

LEUKOCYTOSIS

Leukocytosis is an increase in the number of circulating white blood cells. Leukocytosis is a normal response to infection or inflammation. It can be seen after emotional disturbance, after anesthesia or exercise, and during pregnancy. Abnormal leukocytosis is observed in certain malignancies and bone marrow disorders. Usually, only one type of white blood cell is affected. For example, allergic responses and asthma are specifically associated with increased num-bers of eosinophils. Leukemia is characterized by an abnormally high level of one type of white cell and deficiencies in the others.

SHIFT TO THE LEFT

Shift to the left is a term used to describe an increased proportion of immature leukocytes (usually neutrophils) seen in the blood of an individual fighting an infection. In a shift to the left, neutrophils will be released from the bone mar-row before their final maturation, when the demand for white blood cells is excessive. The immature neutrophils are frequently referred to as bands or stabs. As the infection or inflammation begins to recede, the release of imma-ture neutrophils stops and the blood is said to show a return shift to the right, as mature neutrophils again dominate a blood smear. The returning mature neutrophils are frequently referred to as segmented neutrophils.

THROMBOCYTOPENIA

Thrombocytopenia is a decrease in the number of circulating platelets. It is associated with increased risk of severe bleeding, even with small injuries or small spontaneous bleeds. Thrombocytopenia is characterized by small spots of subcutaneous bleeding, called *petechiae*, or larger areas of subcutaneous bleeding, called *purpura*. Ecchymosis (bruising) may also be present. Primary thrombocytopenia, also referred to as immune thrombocytopenic purpura, may occur idiopathically (for unknown reasons) or as a result of an autoimmune disorder characterized by antibodies built against the platelets. Secondary causes of thrombocytopenia include bone marrow–damaging chemotherapeutic drugs and radiation, and certain viral infections, including HIV. Thrombocytopenia also develops in the serious condition disseminated intravascular coagulation (DIC), in which, after periods of extensive clotting, platelets begin to be consumed, leading to extensive bleeding and high mortality.

THROMBOCYTHEMIA

Thrombocythemia is an increase in the number of circulating platelets. Thrombocythemia is associated with increased risk of thrombosis (clotting) in the vasculature. Depending on the site of clot formation or trapping, stroke, myocardial infarct, or respiratory distress may develop.

Primary thrombocythemia may occur with malignancy, polycythemia vera, and other diseases of the bone marrow. Secondary causes of thrombocythemia include acute infection, exercise, stress, and ovulation. Secondary thrombocythemia caused by these conditions is usually short lived. However, prolonged secondary thrombocythemia may occur after removal of the spleen because this organ normally stores some platelets until they are needed in the circulation. Inflammatory diseases such as rheumatoid arthritis may also be associated with prolonged thrombocythemia.

LYMPHADENOPATHY

Lymphadenopathy, or lymphoid hyperplasia, is the enlargement of the lymph nodes in response to a proliferation of B or T lymphocytes. Lymphadenopathy typically occurs after infection by a microorganism.

Regional lymphadenopathy indicates a localized infection. Generalized lymphadenopathy usually indicates a systemic infection such as AIDS or an autoimmune disorder such as rheumatoid arthritis or systemic lupus erythematosus. Occasionally, lymphadenopathy of either type may indicate a malignancy.

SPLENOMEGALY

Splenomegaly is enlargement of the spleen. It is usually a result of lymphocyte proliferation in the spleen, caused by an infection elsewhere in the body.

Splenomegaly caused by macrophage proliferation occurs if there are excessive numbers of dead cells (especially red blood cells) needing to be cleared from the circulation.

Splenomegaly may also occur as a result of engorgement of the spleen with blood. This is usually a complication of portal hypertension. Splenic tumors or cysts may also cause splenomegaly. Splenomegaly in response to an infection is usually associated with lymphadenopathy; other causes of splenomegaly are not.

● Conditions of Disease or Injury

CLASSIC SYMPTOMS OF ALL TYPES OF ANEMIA

Classic systemic signs of anemia are common to all of the anemias described in this chapter and include the following:

- Increased heart rate as the body attempts to deliver more oxygen to the tissues.
- Increased respiratory rate as the body attempts to provide more oxygen to the blood.
- Dizziness caused by decreased brain blood flow.
- Fatigue caused by decreased oxygenation of various organs, including cardiac and skeletal muscles.
- Skin pallor caused by decreased oxygenation.
- Nausea caused by decreased gastrointestinal and central nervous system blood flow.
- Decreased hair and skin quality.

APLASTIC ANEMIA

Aplastic anemia, also referred to as hypoplastic anemia, is a normocytic, normochromic anemia caused by dysfunction of the bone marrow such that dying blood cells are not replaced. Aplastic anemia may be characterized by **pancytopenia** (deficiency in red blood cells, white blood cells, and platelets), although rarely it may affect only the red cells.

Aplastic anemia may be hereditary due to defects in DNA repair or it may be acquired. There are many causes of acquired aplastic anemia, including cancers of the bone marrow, autoimmune destruction of bone marrow, vitamin deficiency, ingestion of many different drugs (i.e., chloramphenicol, phenytoin, clozapine) or chemicals (i.e., benzene, insecticides, kerosene), and high-dose radiation or chemotherapy. There tends to be a higher incidence in Asians and individuals of European descent. Aplastic anemia may also develop after various viral infections, including mononucleosis, cytomegaloviruses, hepatitis, and AIDS. Frequently, the cause is unknown.

Although the exact pathophysiology is not totally understood, T cells tend to attack the hematopoietic stem cell and cause apoptosis which impairs reproduction and differentiation of the stem cells. Aplastic anemia induced by drugs is most likely the result of a deficiency in a protein required to remove drug metabolites from cells. The elevated levels of drug metabolites in cells interfere with normal cell function.

Clinical Manifestations

- Classic symptoms of all types of anemia.

In aplastic anemia, if platelets and white blood cells are involved, additional symptoms include:

- Bleeding from the gums and teeth; easy bruising, including petechia and purpura.
- Low-grade fever.
- Recurrent infection.
- Ulceration and hemorrhaging in the mouth, nose, and gastrointestinal tract.
- Pale, waxy skin tones.
- Poor healing of skin and mucosal sores.
- Elevated iron stores.

Diagnostic Tools

- CBC with differential and platelet count, MCV, and MCHC will diagnose anemia (Hgb <7 g/dl).
- Peripheral blood smears (absence of reticulocytes).
- Bone marrow biopsy will determine involved cells. Fatty deposits may replace hypocellular marrow space and hematopoietic stem cells will be absent.

Complications

- Heart failure and death as a result of cardiac overload can occur with severe anemia.
- Death from infection and hemorrhage if white blood cells or platelets are involved.

Treatment

- Treat underlying disorder if known or remove causative agent.
- Transfusions to reduce symptomatology.
- Bone marrow transplant.
- Immunosuppression therapy to minimize T cell affect on hematopoietic stem cells.

- Drugs to stimulate bone marrow function may be effective.
- Prophylactic antibiotics and/or antifungals for the patient who is severely neutropenic.
- Chelation therapy to reduce iron stores.
- Stem cell transplant is considered curative.

Hemolytic Anemia

Hemolytic anemia is a decrease in red blood cell number caused by excessive destruction of red cells or hemolysis. Remaining red cells are normocytic and normochromic. Red blood cell production in the bone marrow will increase to replace destroyed cells, and the advancement into the blood of immature red cells, or reticulocytes, will be accelerated.

Hemolytic anemia can occur from many different causes, such as a genetic defect in the red blood cell that accelerates its destruction, or the idiopathic development of autoimmune destruction of the cells. A severe burn, infection, incompatible blood exposure, or exposure to certain drugs or toxins may also cause hemolytic anemia. Depending on the cause, hemolytic anemia may occur once or repeatedly. Specific causes of hemolytic anemia that are discussed in detail include sickle cell anemia, malaria, hemolytic disease of the newborn, and transfusion reaction.

Sickle Cell Anemia

Sickle cell anemia is an autosomal recessive disorder caused by inheritance of two copies of a defective hemoglobin gene, one from each parent. The defective hemoglobin, called hemoglobin S (HbS), becomes rigid and elongated and forms a sickle shape when exposed to low oxygen. Oxidative stress also triggers the production of circulating advanced glycation end products that aggravate the vascular pathology in individuals with sickle cell anemia. The sickled red blood cell loses its ability to move easily through narrow vascular spaces and becomes trapped in the microvasculature. This causes a blockage in blood flow to downstream tissues, leading to painful tissue ischemia. Although sickling is reversible if oxygen saturation of the hemoglobin returns, the sickled cells are especially fragile and many are destroyed in the microvasculature, leading to anemia. Destroyed cells are filtered and removed from the circulation in the spleen; this places an extra demand on splenic function. Scarring and sometimes infarction (cell death) of various organs, especially the spleen and bone, may occur. Multiorgan dysfunction is common after many years.

Stimuli for sickling include hypoxia, anxiety, fever, and exposure to the cold. Because the spleen is an important immune organ, infections, especially of bacterial origin, are common and frequently stimulate a sickle cell crisis.

At birth, signs of sickle cell anemia may not be apparent because all infants have a high level of a different type of hemoglobin, fetal (F) hemoglobin. Fetal hemoglobin does not sickle, but only lasts until approximately 4 months after birth. It is at this time that signs of disease become apparent. These signs include the classic symptoms of anemia, as well as signs related to the painful occlusions characteristic of the disorder.

Individuals with sickle cell anemia carry two defective genes and thus have only HbS. Individuals who are heterozygous for the sickle cell gene (carry one defective gene) are said to carry the sickle cell trait. Heterozygotes usually express HbS in approximately 30% to 40% of their red cells, with normal hemoglobin carried in the rest of the red cells. These individuals are typically asymptomatic unless exposed to low oxygen levels, especially while exercising. Approximately 80,000 people in the United States have sickle cell disease while as many as 12 million have the sickle cell trait.

The demographic roots of sickle cell anemia may be traced to malaria-endemic areas. The sickle cell trait has been shown to offer protection against the destruction of the red blood cell after an infection by the microorganism responsible for malaria. It is thought that this protection allowed the sickle cell gene to survive during evolution in areas with endemic (widespread) malaria, such as equatorial Africa. Thus, in the United States, sickle cell anemia primarily affects individuals who trace their ancestry to this area of Africa: up to approximately 10% of African Americans carry the trait, and approximately one child in every 375 African American live births has the disease. Figure 12-4 shows a chi square diagram of the genetic inheritance of sickle cell anemia.

Clinical Manifestations

- Classic symptoms of all types of anemia.
- Jaundice.
- Intense pain caused by vascular occlusion in a sickling episode.
- Serious bacterial infections caused by inadequate splenic filtering of microorganisms.

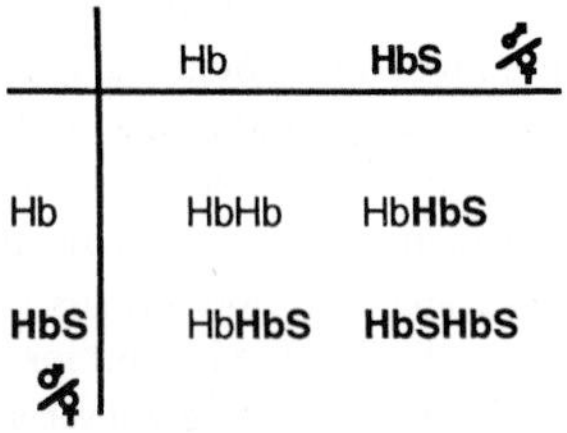

	Hb	HbS
Hb	HbHb	Hb**HbS**
HbS	Hb**HbS**	**HbSHbS**

FIGURE 12-4 A chi square diagram showing the transmission of the sickle cell hemoglobin (HbS). There is 25% chance the offspring will not have the trait or the disease (HbHb); 50% chance the offspring will have the trait (Hb**HbS**); and 25% chance the offspring will have sickle cell disease (**HbSHbS**).

• Splenomegaly as the spleen removes the dead cells, sometimes leading to an acute crisis.

Diagnostic Tools

• Hemoglobin electrophoresis is used to identify the presence of sickle cell hemoglobin and confirm the disease. As of 2006, screening newborns for sickle cell disease is mandated in all 50 states, the District of Columbia, Peurto Rico, the U.S. Virgin Islands, and Guam.

• High performance liquid chromatography or DNA analysis may also be used.

• Serial blood tests demonstrate decreased hematocrit, hemoglobin, and red cell count.

• Prenatal testing identifies the presence of the homozygote state in the fetus.

Complications

• Anemia that varies from mild to severe.

• Vaso-occlusive events leading to tissue infarct may cause intense pain and disability.

• Febrile illness and infection. Infection is a leading cause of morbidity and mortality.

• A sudden trapping of blood in the spleen, called splenic sequestration, may lead to hypovolemia, shock, and possibly death. The cause of splenic sequestration is unknown, but it may occur with fever and pain. Frequently the spleen will be removed after an occurrence. Loss of the spleen compromises the individual's subsequent responses to infection.

• Stroke leading to weakness, seizures, or inability to speak may occur from occlusion of the cerebral vessels.

• Acute chest syndrome which is characterized by fever, cough, worsening anemia, chest pain, and in children, wheezing. It may be the result of fat embolism, pulmonary infarction, or infection.

• Pulmonary hypertension.

• Cholelithiasis secondary to chronic hemolysis.

• Aplastic crisis, during which the bone marrow temporarily stops erythropoiesis, may occur.

• Avascular necrosis of the long bones of the leg or arm may occur from occlusion. Hip replacement is a common sequela of severe disability.

• Priapism, prolonged and painful erection, may occur with vaso-occlusion of the vessels of the penis; this may lead to impotence in some circumstances.

• Other complications may include retinopathy, chronic renal insufficiency, and chronic leg ulcers.

Treatment

- Newborn screening for sickle cell anemia has dramatically improved the prognosis of infants with the disease. All identified infants are given prophylactic antibiotics (penicillin or erythromycin) to prevent infections, from birth until at least 5 years of age.

- If at any time a fever or other sign of infection develops, the child should be evaluated immediately and parenteral antibiotics should be provided. Most children with a fever should be admitted to the hospital.

- Ibuprofen or acetaminophen should be administered to relieve minor pain, and more potent pain medication should be provided if needed.

- All childhood immunizations should be administered on schedule, with the addition of the pneumococcal vaccine in the first 2 years of life and a booster dose at 5 years of age. This will reduce the main cause of mortality in children with sickle cell anemia: infection leading to sepsis. Annual influenza vaccines are also recommended.

- Increased hydration by at least 1.5 to 2 times normal requirements may reduce the severity of a vaso-occlusive event.

- Avoidance of low oxygen situations or oxygen-demanding activities.

- Therapeutic drugs, including hydroxyurea (an S-phase cytotoxic drug), are available for use. Hydroxyurea has a direct effect on increasing cell volume and increasing fetal hemoglobin production. Not only does fetal hemoglobin not sickle, it also has an increased affinity for oxygen compared to adult hemoglobin. Other drugs with similar mechanisms of action are available as well.

- Use of ion channel blockers, anti-adhesion and anti-inflammatory agents that interfere with injurious red cell–endothelial interactions, limits the vascular damage associated with the disorder.

- Red blood cell transfusions are frequently required but should be limited when possible to reduce the risk of transmission of infectious agents.

- Bone marrow transplant with an HLA-matched donor may eliminate the production of sickled cells, but will not improve already damaged organs, and requires the subsequent lifelong use of immunosuppressants to block rejection.

- Nitric oxide inhalation may be used to prevent pulmonary hypertension associated with sickle cell anemia.

- Genetic counseling for families allows for future informed childbearing decisions.

Malaria

Malaria is a cause of hemolytic anemia related to an infection of the red blood cells by a protozoan of the genus *Plasmodium* that is transmitted to humans in the saliva of a mosquito. When the mosquito sucks the blood of an infected person the parasite goes to the gut and grows until it ruptures. After it ruptures, the parasite migrates to the mosquito's salivary glands where it stays until the mosquito bites another human. Blood-borne transmission by transfusion of blood from an infected individual has also occurred.

Malaria is endemic in tropical and subtropical environments of the world; although due to world travel, more cases are being reported in the United States. It is an acute disease that can become chronic, with repeated episodes of debilitation. More than 1 million people die annually from malaria, most of whom are infants and children.

The *Plasmodium* microorganism first infects the cells of the liver and then passes into the erythrocytes. Infection causes massive hemolysis of the red blood cells. At this point, more parasites are released into the circulation and subsequent cycles of infection occur. Red cell hemolysis leads to acute and chronic anemia. Cycles of infection typically occur approximately 72 hours apart. The host response to infection includes activation of the immune system, including production of various cytokines designed to increase the immune response. These cytokines, including tumor necrosis factor and interleukins 1 and 6, are key in fighting against the parasite, but also are responsible for most of the clinical manifestations of the disease, especially fever and myalgia (muscle aches). Individuals usually recover, but may relapse.

Clinical Manifestations

- Classic symptoms of all types of anemia.
- Cyclic (usually every 72 hours) fever spikes.
- Chills and sweating with fever.
- Headache, nausea, and vomiting.
- Hot, dry skin.
- Bounding pulse.
- Myalgia.
- Hepatomegaly and splenomegaly.
- Jaundice may occur from excessive red blood cell lysis and release of bilirubin.

Diagnostic Tools

- Blood analysis will demonstrate the occurrence of anemia and the presence of red blood cell parasites.
- Peripheral blood smear to confirm diagnosis and identify the parasite.
- Rapid lab antigen test followed by microscopic confirmation.
- Stool culture for ova and parasites.

Complications

- With severe disease, hypoglycemia, respiratory distress, shock, and coma may develop.
- Some strains of the parasite are becoming resistant to traditional drug therapy.

Treatment

- Prophylactic therapy against malaria is advised for travelers to endemic areas.
- Prevention in endemic areas involves elimination of standing sources of water and the use of insecticides, mosquito nets, and repellents.
- The placement of mosquito-repellent nets around the sleeping areas of all those living in endemic areas, especially children, is advised.
- Antimalarial drugs are available to treat the disease if contracted, although resistance to all available drugs, including the chloroquine-related drugs, is high.
- Blood transfusions are occasionally performed; however, this has resulted in transmission of HIV in endemic areas.
- Vaccines against malaria are being developed, including DNA vaccines that may stimulate the immune response to infection. Some vaccines in use do not prevent infection by the parasite, but may reduce the severity of the disease.
- The mosquito-killing fungi *Beauveria bassiana* and *Metarhizium anisopliae* are being investigated with the hope that they will become new, environmentally friendly weapons against malaria.
- Although NOT approved in the United States, a Chinese treatment involving artemisinin has been shown to be effective in individuals with multidrug resistant malaria. A combination drug of artesunate and amodiaquine is also being researched as a possible cost-effective treatment.

Hemolytic Disease of the Newborn

Hemolytic disease of the fetus and newborn, also known as erythroblastosis fetalis, is a normocytic, normochromic anemia seen in an Rh-positive fetus or an infant born to an Rh-negative mother who has previously been exposed to Rh-positive blood, and has therefore developed antibodies to the Rh antigen. The development of antibodies usually occurs only after multiple maternal exposures to the antigen; these may occur during previous pregnancies, abortions, miscarriages, or during amniocentesis. The maternal antibodies, usually IgG, are transferred to the fetus through the placenta and attack fetal red blood cells, leading to excessive red cell lysis and anemia. If the condition is mild, the maternal circulation effectively eliminates the waste products of hemoglobin metabolism, including bilirubin, for the fetus, and it suffers few ill effects in utero. Occasionally, maternal destruction of the fetal cells may be excessive, leading to a severe anemia and *hydrops fetalis*, a fatal condition characterized by massive edema and heart failure.

After delivery in the less-affected infant, clinical signs of anemia may occur. More significant in the neonatal period is the development of severe jaundice, as the breakdown products of hemoglobin are ineffectively cleared by the infant's immature liver. A dramatic elevation in bilirubin can lead to a significant neurologic disorder, called **kernicterus**, as the unconjugated bilirubin precipitates out in the infant's brainstem, causing brain damage.

Hemolytic disease of the newborn in response to Rh incompatibility is uncommon and has become rarer with fewer pregnancies experienced by each woman and important prophylactic interventions (see later). As a result of these factors, the incidence of hemolytic disease of the newborn has dropped by at least 80% in the last few decades. More common than Rh incompatibility is ABO incompatibility. In this condition, maternal antibodies are produced as a result of ABO incompatibility, even during a first pregnancy. The presence of antibodies against the A or B antigens seldom leads to full-blown newborn hemolytic disease. Hemolytic disease of the newborn is described further in Chapter 17.

Clinical Manifestations

- Mild hemolytic disease may be relatively asymptomatic, with slight hepatomegaly and minimally elevated bilirubin.
- Moderate and severe disease manifests with pronounced signs of anemia.
- Hyperbilirubinemia, resulting from excessive red cell lysis, may occur, leading to jaundice.

Complications

- Kernicterus.
- Severe anemia may cause heart failure.
- *Hydrops fetalis.* Affected fetuses often abort spontaneously at approximately 17 weeks' gestation.
- In one study, 10% of school-aged children who had received in utero transfusions for severe Rh incompatibility showed neurologic abnormalities, most likely related to asphyxia and anemia at birth.

Treatment

- Prevention of Rh-induced hemolytic disease begins with the prenatal visit and documentation of a woman's Rh-negative status and the presence or absence of Rh antibodies. Women who are confirmed Rh negative and who do not show Rh-positive antibodies are administered an anti-Rh antibody preparation called RhoGAM at 28 weeks' gestation, or at the time of a miscarriage, abortion, or amniocentesis. If, after birth, the infant is deemed to be Rh positive and the woman is still Rh negative, she is again given RhoGAM within 72 hours. The RhoGAM injection provides passive immunity to the woman such that she does not develop her own antibodies against the Rh factor. A woman who is found to be Rh positive at any time is not given RhoGAM, but she and her fetus are observed closely during pregnancy and after delivery.

- If a woman becomes Rh positive during pregnancy, the fetus is observed by serial amniocentesis to determine bilirubin level. Mildly affected fetuses are delivered at term; moderately affected fetuses may be delivered before term; severely affected fetuses may receive an intrauterine transfusion and be delivered before term.
- In the newborn with hemolytic disease, exchange blood transfusions may be required. Transfusion is with Rh-positive blood not containing Rh antibody. Treatment should begin within 24 hours of birth and be repeated until twice the blood volume of the infant has been exchanged.
- In mild cases, phototherapy to reduce the levels of unconjugated bilirubin may be sufficient.

Transfusion Reaction

A transfusion reaction is an immune-mediated destruction of incompatible red blood cells received in a blood transfusion. Transfusion reactions against donated white blood cells occur more frequently, but are typically mild. Although host and donor blood antigens are always identified (typed) for ABO and Rh compatibility before a transfusion is given, an error in red blood cell typing or a mix-up in the blood supplies may occur. Transfusion reactions may also develop as a result of an immune reaction to bacteria transferred in contaminated blood products.

Clinical Manifestations

Immediate, life-threatening reactions occur with ABO incompatibility. Manifestations include:

- Classic triad of fever or chills, flank pain, and reddish or brown urine.
- Immediate flushing of the face.
- A feeling of warmth in the vein receiving the blood.
- Chest or low back pain.
- Abdominal pain with nausea and vomiting.
- Decreased blood pressure with increased heart rate.
- Dyspnea (a sensation of breathing difficulty).
- Transfusion reactions against white blood cells are milder and usually include fever and occasionally chills.

Complications

- Renal failure may result from red blood cell casts and hemoglobin obstruction of the nephrons.
- Shock, cardiopulmonary arrest, and death.

Treatment

- Prevention is the key. To decrease the risk of human error, the correct blood product and the correct patient should be verified. Also, a thorough assessment of the patient is necessary.
- The transfusion must be stopped immediately.
- Fluids may be given to reduce the risk of renal damage.
- Ensure a patent airway. Support blood pressure, cardiac output, and urine output.
- Anaphylactic responses are treated by anti-inflammatory drugs, including antihistamines and steroids.
- Leukocyte-cleansed blood is available, which will eliminate reactions to white blood cells.

POSTHEMORRHAGIC ANEMIA

Posthemorrhagic anemia is a normocytic, normochromic anemia that results from sudden loss of blood in an otherwise healthy individual. The hemorrhage may be obvious or hidden.

Blood pressure decreases with sudden hemorrhage. Reflex responses to decreased blood pressure and tissue hypoxia include increased activation of the sympathetic nervous system. This results in increased vascular resistance, heart rate, and stroke volume, all of which serve to return blood pressure toward normal. Respiratory rate increases to improve oxygenation. Renal responses to decreased blood pressure include decreased urine output and increased release of the hormone renin. Salt and water reabsorption in the kidney increase, serving to return blood pressure toward normal. Renal secretion of erythropoietin is stimulated, leading to increased red cell production.

Clinical Manifestations

- Classic symptoms of all types of anemia.
- Increased heart rate and respiratory rate, with a decrease in blood pressure. Consciousness may be impaired.
- The cause of the hemorrhage will present with individual clinical manifestations.

Diagnostic Tools

- Reduction in red cell count, hematocrit, and hemoglobin on the CBC as interstitial fluid moves into the vascular compartment in an attempt to increase blood volume.

Complications

- Hypovolemic shock with the possibility of renal failure, respiratory failure, or death.

Treatment

- Identify and treat the underlying cause of blood loss.
- Restore blood volume with intravenous infusion of plasma or type-matched whole blood (or O negative). Saline, dextran, or albumin may also be infused.

PERNICIOUS ANEMIA

Pernicious anemia is a megaloblastic anemia characterized by abnormally large red blood cells with immature (blastic) nuclei. Pernicious anemia is caused by a deficiency of vitamin B_{12} in the blood. Vitamin B_{12} is essential for DNA synthesis in red blood cells and for neuronal functioning. It is provided in the diet and absorbed across the stomach into the blood. A gastric hormone, *intrinsic factor*, is essential for absorption of vitamin B_{12}. Intrinsic factor is secreted by the parietal cells of the gastric mucosa. Most causes of pernicious anemia result from intrinsic factor deficiency, but dietary deficiency of vitamin B_{12} may occur. Usually, B_{12} deficiency is a slowly developing disorder, and frequently goes unnoticed until symptoms are severe. Typically, patients affected are elderly; it is rare for an individual younger than 30 to suffer pernicious anemia unless it is present at or soon after birth.

Intrinsic factor deficiency may occur congenitally or may develop after atrophy or destruction of the gastric mucosa as a result of chronic gastric inflammation. It may be the result of an autoimmune disease in which antibodies against gastric parietal cells are produced. There appears to be a genetic susceptibility to autoimmune causes. Surgical removal of all or part of the stomach will also result in intrinsic factor deficiency.

Clinical Manifestations

- Vague symptoms such as infections, mood swings, weakness, fatigue.
- Paresthesia of fingers and feet.
- Neurologic symptoms such as ataxia, loss of vibration sense, loss of position, spasticity, memory loss.

- Abdominal pain, loss of appetite, beefy red tongue.
- Pale yellow skin.
- Hepatomegaly.
- Hemoglobin 7 to 8 g/dL.

Diagnostic Tools

- Blood analysis will demonstrate anemia characterized by macrocytic cells with normal hemoglobin (significantly elevated MCV > 103, normal MCHC).
- Schilling test to identify problems with absorption.
- A decrease in serum B_{12} (<100 pg/mL) will confirm the disease.

Complications

- Severe anemia may cause heart failure, especially in the elderly.
- Safety is an issue with altered mental status.

Treatment

- Lifelong intramuscular or subcutaneous injections of vitamin B_{12}. Research is under way to determine if oral replacement may be just as effective if given at the appropriate doses.

FOLATE-DEFICIENCY ANEMIA

Folate (folic acid)–deficiency anemia is a megaloblastic anemia characterized by enlarged red cells with immature nuclei. Folic acid deficiency is caused by a lack of the vitamin folate. Folate is essential for red blood cell production and maturation. It is also important for DNA and RNA synthesis and for the function of several DNA proofreading enzymes (Chapter 2). Folic acid is provided in the diet, but deficiency is relatively common, especially in young women, malnourished individuals, and alcohol abusers. Folic acid absorption occurs across the small intestine and does not require intrinsic factor. Because of widespread folic acid deficiency and its recognized importance in maintaining health, folic acid supplementation of cereals and other grains is soon to be initiated in the United States. Folic acid supplementation is especially important for pregnant women, as described later.

Clinical Manifestations

- Classic symptoms of all types of anemia.
- Stomatitis and tongue ulcerations.
- Dyphagia, flatulence, watery diarrhea.

Diagnostic Tools

- Blood analysis will demonstrate anemia characterized by macrocytic cells with normal hemoglobin (elevated MCV > 98, normal MCHC). Typically, the MCV will be elevated less than in pernicious anemia, and there will be no vitamin B deficiency.
- Serum folate level < 5 ng/mL.

Complications

- Maternal deficiencies in folic acid are associated with an increased risk of fetal malformations, especially neural tube defects.
- Adult deficiency may be associated with an increased risk of cardiovascular disease.

Treatment

- Dietary counseling and vitamin supplementation.
- Administration of oral folate. Women intending to become pregnant should begin vitamin supplementation at least 3 months before conception. It is important not to confuse folate-deficiency anemia with pernicious anemia because treatment with folic acid is contraindicated in pernicious anemia.
- Blood transfusions may be required in severe cases.

IRON-DEFICIENCY ANEMIA

Iron-deficiency anemia is a microcytic-hypochromic anemia that results from a diet deficient in iron, from the slow, chronic loss of blood, or from malabsorptive disorders. It is the most common cause of anemia worldwide. Iron is an essential component of the hemoglobin that makes up a large part of the red blood cell. Iron deficiency is a problem in toddlers and children with increased growth demands. Pregnant women are frequently iron-deficient because of the iron demands of the growing fetus. Menstruating women also tend to be iron deficient because of iron loss each month and diets that may be deficient in iron. Menstruating women who exercise are at increased risk because exercise increases the metabolic demands of muscle cells. In men, iron deficiency usually occurs with an ulcer or liver disease characterized by bleeding. Iron deficiency develops slowly. Decreased red blood cell numbers prompt the bone marrow to increase the release of abnormally small, hemoglobin-deficient red cells.

Clinical Manifestations

- Classic symptoms of all types of anemia.
- In adults, systemic signs of anemia are present once hemoglobin decreases to less than 12 g/100 mL. Individuals usually do not seek treatment for symptoms until hemoglobin decreases to 8 g/100 mL or below.

- Shortness of breath and activity intolerance.
- Cold intolerance.
- Headache.
- Pale palms, pale conjunctivae, and pale earlobes may be present.
- In severe cases, pica (ingesting typically nonedible substances such as clay), eating ice, stomatitis, glossitis, gastric atrophy, leg cramps.

Diagnostic Tools

- Blood analysis demonstrates anemia characterized by microcytic cells (MCV < 87) and decreased serum iron, serum ferritin, and serum transferrin. Iron-binding capacity in the blood is high because proteins that bind iron are in less demand. Erythrocyte count is decreased.
- Stool test for occult blood may be positive, suggesting a GI bleed or carcinoma.
- A definitive diagnosis is based on bone marrow aspiration which reveals absent iron stores in the marrow.

Complications

- A hemoglobin value of less than 5 g/100 mL can lead to heart failure and death.

Treatment

The goals of treatment are threefold: treat the immediate distress, identify, and treat the underlying cause, and replace iron as necessary.

- An iron-rich diet containing red meat and dark green vegetables, such as spinach.
- Oral or parenteral iron supplementation depending on the severity of the anemia.
- Treat the cause of abnormal bleeding if known.

SIDEROBLASTIC ANEMIA

Sideroblastic anemia is a microcytic-hypochromic anemia characterized by the presence of abnormal red cells (sideroblasts) in the circulation and the bone marrow. Sideroblasts carry iron in the mitochondria rather than in the hemoglobin molecules, and thus are unable to transport oxygen to the tissues. There is no iron deficiency.

Poor transport of oxygen causes hypoxia. This is sensed by erythropoietin-secreting kidney cells. Erythropoietin stimulates new red cell production in the bone marrow, which causes the marrow to become congested and increases the production of sideroblasts, worsening the anemia.

Hereditary sideroblastic anemia can occur as a result of a rare genetic defect on the X chromosome (primarily seen in males) or may occur spontaneously, especially in the elderly. Acquired sideroblastic anemia is more common and may be caused by certain drugs (e.g., some chemotherapeutic agents), lead ingestion, alcoholism, copper deficiency, or hypothermia.

Clinical Manifestations

- Classic symptoms of all types of anemia.
- Bronze-colored skin.
- Iron accumulation results in hepatomegaly and splenomegaly.

Diagnostic Tools

- Blood analysis demonstrates anemia characterized by microcytic hypochromic cells, with elevated plasma iron and normal iron-binding capacity.
- A bone marrow examination demonstrates the presence of iron accumulations, sideroblasts, and phagocytic macrophages.

Complications

- Some cases progress to myelodysplastic syndrome and acute myeloblastic leukemia (AML).
- Heart rhythm disturbances.
- Congestive heart failure.

Treatment

- The cause of the disease, if related to a drug, is removed.
- The drug pyridoxine may successfully treat the disease, especially in persons with no evidence of neutropenia or thrombocytopenia. Iron is not given.

ACUTE INFECTIOUS MONONUCLEOSIS

Mononucleosis is an acute infection of the B lymphocytes, usually caused by the Epstein–Barr virus (EBV) or, less frequently, by the cytomegalovirus. Most adults were exposed to these viruses in early childhood and at that time successfully fought off active infection to gain lifelong immunity. Usually, individuals who develop mononucleosis are children who do not fight off the infection, or teenagers and young adults who are exposed to the virus for the first time. Transmission of the virus occurs primarily through oral secretions and appears to require repeated exposures. In the teenage to young adult years, the immune system may be less active or depressed by poor dietary and sleep habits, making those age groups especially susceptible to infection.

Clinical Manifestations

- Malaise, chills, and anorexia typically precede the onset.
- The classic triad of symptoms of mononucleosis includes: severe sore throat, fever, and swelling of the cervical lymph nodes.
- Overwhelming or mild fatigue may be present.
- Swelling of all lymphoid tissues, including spleen, tonsils, and other neck nodes, may be present. The lymph nodes are usually tender.
- The liver and spleen may be enlarged and tender.

Diagnostic Tools

- The liver may be palpable and liver function tests are abnormal in 95% of cases. Jaundice is rare in young people.
- Laboratory findings demonstrate a brief leukopenia followed by proliferation first of the infected B cells, and then immunoactive T cells. Many white cells are atypical.
- Blood tests, especially the Monospot agglutination test, demonstrate antibodies to the EBV.
- Presence of heterophil antibodies produced when the B cells harbor the EBV.

Complications

- Complications are rare, but may include hepatitis, meningitis, encephalitis, transverse myelitis, cranial nerve palsies, and Guillain–Barré syndrome. Rarely, Burkitt lymphoma or B-cell lymphoma may develop.

Treatment

- Mononucleosis is usually self-limiting. Treatment is supportive and encourages adequate rest and hydration.
- It is important to avoid contact sports so as not to injure or rupture the spleen.
- Ibuprofen and acetaminophen may be given. Aspirin is not recommended because of its association with Reye syndrome.

LEUKEMIA

Leukemia is a cancer of one class of white blood cells in the bone marrow, which results in the proliferation of that cell type to the exclusion of other types.

Leukemia appears to be a clonal disorder, meaning one abnormal cancerous cell proliferates without control, producing an abnormal group of daughter cells. These cells prevent other blood cells in the bone marrow from developing normally, causing them to accumulate in the marrow. Because of these factors, leukemia is called an accumulation and a clonal disorder. Eventually, leukemic cells take over the bone marrow. This reduces blood levels of all nonleukemic cells, causing the many generalized symptoms of leukemia.

Classification of Leukemia

Leukemia is typically classified as acute or chronic and lymphocytic or myelocytic. It is described as acute or chronic, depending on the suddenness of appearance and how well the cancerous cells are differentiated. The cells of acute leukemia are poorly differentiated, whereas those of chronic leukemia are usually well differentiated. Lymphocytic leukemia involves immature lymphocytes and their progenitors, which infiltrate the lymph nodes. Myelocytic leukemias involve pluripotent myeloid stem cells in the bone marrow that impair maturation of all other blood cells.

Leukemia is also described based on the proliferating cell type. For instance, acute lymphoblastic leukemia (ALL), the most common childhood leukemia, describes a cancer of a primitive lymphocyte cell line. Granulocytic leukemias are leukemias of the eosinophils, neutrophils, or basophils. Leukemia in adults is usually chronic lymphocytic (CLL) or acute myeloblastic (AML). Chronic myelobalstic leukemia (CML) occurs most often in adults 25 to 60 years of age. Long-term survival rates for leukemia depend on the involved cell type, but range to more than 75% for childhood acute lymphocytic leukemia, which is a remarkable statistic for what was once a nearly always fatal disease.

Risk Factors for Developing Leukemia

Risk factors for leukemia include a genetic predisposition coupled with a known or unknown initiator (mutating) event. Siblings of children with leukemia are two to four times more likely to develop the disease than other children. Certain abnormal chromosomes are seen in a high percentage of patients with leukemia. Likewise, individuals with certain chromosomal abnormalities, including Down syndrome, have an increased risk of developing leukemia. Exposure to radiation, some drugs that depress the bone marrow, and various chemotherapeutic agents have been suggested to increase the risk of leukemia. Environmental agents such as pesticides and certain viral infections also have been implicated.

Previous illness with a variety of diseases associated with hematopoiesis (blood cell production) has been shown to increase the risk of leukemia. These diseases include Hodgkin lymphoma, multiple myeloma, polycythemia vera, sideroblastic anemia, and myelodysplastic syndromes. Chronic leukemia may sometimes transform into acute leukemia.

Clinical Manifestations

Acute leukemia has marked clinical manifestations. Chronic leukemia progresses slowly and may have few symptoms until advanced.

- Pallor and fatigue from anemia.
- Frequent infections caused by a decrease in white blood cells.
- Bleeding and bruising caused by thrombocytopenia and coagulation disorders.
- Bone pain caused by accumulation of cells in the marrow, which leads to increased pressure and cell death. Unlike growing pains, bone pain related to leukemia is usually progressive.
- Weight loss caused by poor appetite and increased caloric consumption by neoplastic cells.
- Lymphadenopathy, splenomegaly, and hepatomegaly caused by leukemic cell infiltration of these lymphoid organs may develop.
- Central nervous system symptoms may occur.

Diagnostic Tools

- Laboratory findings include alterations in specific blood cell counts, with overall elevation or deficiency in white blood cell count variable, depending on the type of cell affected.
- Bone marrow tests demonstrate clonal proliferation and blood cell accumulation.
- Cerebral spinal fluid is examined to rule out central nervous system involvement.

Complications

- Children who survive leukemia have an increased risk of developing a new malignancy later on in life when compared to children who have never had leukemia, most likely related to the aggressiveness of chemotherapeutic (or radiological) regimens.
- Treatment regimens, including bone marrow transplant, are associated with temporary bone marrow depression, and increase the risk of developing a severe infection that could lead to death.
- Even with successful treatment and remission, leukemic cells may still persist, suggesting residual disease. Implications for prognosis and cure are unclear.

Treatment

- Multiple drug chemotherapy.
- Antibiotics to prevent infection.

- Transfusions of red blood cells and platelets to reverse anemia and prevent bleeding.
- Bone marrow transplant may successfully treat the disease. Blood products and broad spectrum antibiotics are provided during bone marrow transplant procedures to fight and prevent infection.
- Immunotherapy, including interferons and other cytokines, is used to improve outcome.
- Therapy may be more conservative for chronic leukemia.
- The treatments described earlier may contribute to the symptoms by causing further bone marrow depression, nausea, and vomiting. Nausea and vomiting may be controlled or reduced by pharmacologic and behavioral intervention.
- Anthocyanins (chemicals with known antioxidant and liver protecting properties) isolated from the plant *Hibiscus sabdariffa* are being studied as chemopreventive agents in that they cause cancer cell apoptosis (death) in human promyelocytic leukemia cells.

HODGKIN LYMPHOMA (HODGKIN DISEASE)

Hodgkin lymphoma, formerly called Hodgkin disease, is a cancer of the lymphoid tissue, usually the lymph nodes and spleen. It is one of the most common cancers in young adults, especially young males. There is a second peak in incidence in the sixth decade of life.

Hodgkin lymphoma is a clonal disorder, arising from one abnormal cell. The abnormal cell population appears to be derived from a B cell or, less frequently, a T cell or monocyte. Neoplastic cells of Hodgkin lymphoma are large, atypical, mononuclear cells and are called Reed–Sternberg cells. These cells intersperse among normal lymph tissue present in the lymph organs. Because of its B-cell and clonal nature, in 2005, Hodgkin disease was reclassified by the World Health Organization as a lymphoma and renamed Hodgkin lymphoma.

There are four major classifications of Hodgkin lymphoma, based on the cells involved and whether the neoplasms are nodular in form. Staging of Hodgkin lymphoma is important because it guides treatment and strongly influences outcome. The early stages of the disease, stages I and II, are usually curable. Cure rates for stages III and IV are approximately 75% and 60%, respectively.

The cause of Hodgkin lymphoma is unknown. However, individuals with the disease and in remission from it demonstrate reduced T-cell–mediated immunity. In addition, exposure to carcinogens and sporadic case clusters suggest that a virus, perhaps one of the herpes strains, especially the EBV, may be involved. There is likely a genetic tendency to develop the disease.

Clinical Manifestations

- Painless enlargement of lymph nodes, especially in the neck and under the arms (above the level of the diaphragm).

- Mediastinal masses may cause cough, dyspnea, and chest discomfort.
- Evening fevers and night sweats may occur accompanied by pruritus.
- Weight loss accompanies advanced stages of the disease.

Diagnostic Tools

- Lymph node biopsy can diagnose Hodgkin lymphoma. Presence of the Reed–Sternberg cell gives a definitive diagnosis.
- CT scan, lymphangiogram, or PET scan help determine the extent of involvement.

Complications

- Secondary malignancies and cardiotoxicity may develop after aggressive treatment (especially radiation). Because of these and other treatment complications, Hodgkin lymphoma patients have a higher chance of dying from acute and late treatment toxicities than from the disease itself.
- As the disease progresses, impaired cell-mediated responses with increased susceptibility to fungal, viral, and protozoal infections.

Treatment

- Multidrug chemotherapy.
- Radiation therapy.
- Bone marrow transplant.
- Targeted biologically based therapies, such as the use of receptor-specific antibodies, inhibition of antiapoptotic pathways, and induction of specific cytotoxicity, may have better patient tolerability and fewer long-term complications.

NON-HODGKIN LYMPHOMA

Non-Hodgkin lymphomas are cancers of the lymph tissue that are not Hodgkin lymphoma. Non-Hodgkin lymphoma usually occurs in older adults and is typically discovered at a more advanced stage than Hodgkin lymphoma. Non-Hodgkin lymphoma is not confined to a single group of lymph nodes as in Hodgkin lymphoma, but rather is diffusely spread throughout the lymphoid organs, including the lymph nodes, liver, spleen, and occasionally the bone marrow. Disease may also be found in the sinuses. Like Hodgkin lymphoma, non-Hodgkin disease is classified under several divisions, primarily related to whether the neoplastic tissue is nodular or diffuse.

Non-Hodgkin disease appears to develop primarily from a malignancy of the B cells, but T cells and macrophages may also be the original site of the cancer. Causes of non-Hodgkin lymphoma are unclear, but viral infection, including HIV infection, appears to be responsible for at least some cases. Overall, non-Hodgkin lymphoma has a poorer prognosis than Hodgkin lymphoma, but there are multiple types of this disease, with some aggressive and others less so; therefore, prognosis varies greatly.

Clinical Manifestations

- Painless enlargement of lymph nodes.
- Splenomegaly.
- GI complications may occur.
- Fever; fatigue.
- Severe night sweats.
- Weight loss.
- Back and neck pain with hyper-reflexia.

Diagnostic Tools

- Lymph node biopsy can diagnose non-Hodgkin lymphoma.
- Other tools to help with staging may include PET scan, CT scan, MRI, bone marrow biopsy, gallium scan, bone scan, and DNA microarray analysis.

Treatment

- Aggressive chemotherapy is used for advanced disease. Diffuse disease usually requires even more aggressive therapy.
- In current practice, a combination of drugs known as CHOP (cyclophosphamide, doxorubicin, vincristine, and prednisone) plus adjuvant radiotherapy is used. For patients less than 61 years old with localized large B-cell lymphoma, an intensive regimen of another drug combination, ACVBP (doxorubicin, cyclophosphamide, vindesine, bleomycin, prednisone), appears superior to CHOP.
- Monoclonal antibodies such as rituximab offer minimal toxicity and are offering favorable results. The benefits seem to increase when given in combination with chemotherapy.
- Conservative chemotherapy may be used for slow-growing lymphomas and for palliative treatment.
- Radiotherapy is also used, as is surgery to remove large tumors.
- Bone marrow transplant may be performed.

MULTIPLE MYELOMA

Multiple myeloma is a clonal disorder characterized by proliferation of one type of B lymphocyte, and plasma cells derived from that lymphocyte. These cells disperse throughout the circulation and deposit primarily in the bone, causing bone breakdown, inflammation, and pain. Antibodies produced by the plasma cells are usually clonal IgG or IgA. Monoclonal fragments of these antibodies may be found in the urine of patients with the disease. These fragments are called Bence Jones proteins. The cause of multiple myeloma is unknown, but risk factors are believed to include occupational exposures to certain materials and gases, ionizing radiation, and possibly multiple drug allergies. African Americans and males tend to be at a greater risk and the age of onset is typically during or after the sixth decade of life. Survival rate is generally low, although some patients may live a long time with this disease.

Clinical Manifestations

- Bone pain and fracture may occur.
- Weight loss and fatigue may occur.
- Neurologic dysfunction resulting from high blood calcium levels is seen with bone breakdown.
- Bone lesions secondary to bone infiltration with malignant plasma cells and activation of osteoclasts to reabsorb bone. As calcium is released from the bone, lytic lesions develop.
- Proteinuria.
- Recurrent infections from reduced B-cell function are common.

Diagnostic Tools

- Bone biopsy and blood analysis confirm the disease.
- Serum electrophoresis to identify Bence Jones proteins.
- Urine may also be diagnostic with the presence of Bence Jones proteins.
- Osteolytic bone lesions on x-ray.
- Serum immunoglobulin electrophoresis.
- Hypercalcemia may be present when bones are involved.

Complications

- Renal failure may develop as a result of Bence Jones proteins depositing in the renal tubules.
- Patients may become severely anemic due to decreased erythropoiesis.
- Hyperviscosity syndrome.

Treatment

- Chemotherapy may prolong life. One type of chemotherapy involves the use of an old drug, thalidomide, which is an immunomodulator as well as an inhibitor of blood vessel development. Other drug therapies include proteasome inhibitors (bortezomib) and alkylating agents.

- Immunotherapy.
- Corticosteroids.
- Radiation therapy is used to reduce the size of bone lesions and relieve pain.
- Bone marrow transplant may be successful in some patients.

HEMOPHILIA A

Hemophilia A, also called classic hemophilia, is an X-linked recessive disease resulting from an error in the gene coding for coagulation factor VIII. Classic hemophilia is the most common inherited coagulation disorder. It is seen in boys who inherit the defective gene on the X chromosome from their mother. The mother is usually heterozygous for the disorder and shows no symptoms. However, 25% of cases come from new X chromosome mutations. The defective gene may result from one of several different deletions or point mutations.

Without factor VIII, the intrinsic coagulation pathway is interrupted and extensive bleeding from small wounds or microvascular tears occurs. Bleeding is frequently into the joints and can cause significant pain and disability.

Other Types of Hemophilia

Other forms of hemophilia exist. These hemophilias result from the absence of different coagulation factors. Hemophilia B (also referred to as Christmas disease) is an X-linked disorder caused by a lack of factor IX. Hemophilia C is an autosomal disorder caused by a lack of factor XI. Von Willebrand disease is an autosomal-dominant disease resulting from an abnormality of vWF. This factor is released from endothelial cells and platelets and is essential for the formation of the platelet plug. With a reduction of vWF factor, factor VIII levels are also reduced.

Clinical Manifestations of Classic Hemophilia

- Prolonged bleeding and inability to form clots are the hallmark findings.
- Spontaneous or excessive bleeding after a minor wound.
- Joint swelling, pain, and degenerative changes.

Diagnostic Tools

- Laboratory studies show a normal bleeding time, but prolonged PTT.
- Measurement of factor VIII is reduced.
- Prenatal testing for the gene is possible.

Complications

- Intracranial hemorrhage may occur.
- Bleeding into the muscle, joints, and organs. Hemiarthrosis can lead to compartment syndrome and increase the risk for arthritis.
- Airway obstruction due to oropharyngeal bleeding.
- Infection with HIV was common before artificial production of factor VIII reduced the need for transfusions.

Treatment

- Factor VIII replacement. Factor VIII may be from frozen plasma concentrate donated from the father of the affected boy or may be produced by monoclonal antibody techniques. Multiple donor plasma extracts of Factor VIII are no longer used because of the risk of transmission of viral infections such as HIV and hepatitis B and C.
- DDAVP stimulates production of Factor VIII, but is only temporary.
- Analgesics to minimize pain during bleeding episodes.
- With bleeding, antifibrinolytics may be given to slow the fibrinolytic system and extend the effect of fibrin sheaths, thus slowing the effects of fibrin-degradation products.
- Minimize the risk for bleeding; safety to minimize injury, avoid aspirin or aspirin-containing products.

LIVER DISEASE AND VITAMIN K DEFICIENCY

The liver is the site of synthesis for many coagulation factors, several of which are vitamin K dependent. Disease of the liver or inadequate plasma levels of vitamin K will interrupt the coagulation pathways. Vitamin K is a fat-soluble vitamin absorbed in the diet by means of bile. Because bile is produced in the liver, a healthy liver and a clear bile duct are required for successful coagulation. Vitamin K is also synthesized by bacteria in the gut. Newborns are vitamin K deficient because of a lack of vitamin K–producing bacteria in the intestine and immature liver function.

Clinical Manifestations

- Bleeding characterized by petechia (small hemorrhage spots on the skin) and purpura (purplish discoloration of the skin).

Treatment

- Vitamin K is administered intramuscularly to the neonate and orally in children or adults.

DISSEMINATED INTRAVASCULAR COAGULATION

Disseminated intravascular coagulation (DIC) is a unique condition characterized by the formation of multiple blood clots throughout the microvasculature. Eventually, the components of the blood clotting cascade and the platelets are used up, and hemorrhages begin to occur at all bodily orifices, at sites of injury or venous puncture, and throughout many organ systems.

DIC is never a primary condition. Instead, it occurs as a complication of major clinical incidents or trauma such as shock, widespread infection, major burn, myocardial infarct, or obstetric complication. Hypoxemia and acidemia develop, damaging the endothelial cells of the vasculature. Multiple endothelial cell injuries initiate extensive activation of the platelets and the intrinsic coagulation pathway, leading to microthrombi throughout the vascular system. Tissue damage, occurring as the precipitating event or after hypoxia and acidemia, causes the production of thromboplastin, which activates the extrinsic coagulation pathway. Clotting is extensive, with fibrin strands firming and holding the emboli.

As the coagulation cascades proceed, fibrinolytic processes (breaking down of fibrin strands) are accelerated. These processes result in the release of anticoagulation enzymes into the circulation. Eventually, clotting factors and platelets are used up and hemorrhage and oozing of blood into mucous membranes occur. The loop is completed with bleeding and clotting occurring simultaneously.

Clinical Manifestations

- Hemorrhage from puncture sites, wounds, and mucous membranes in a patient with shock, obstetric complications, sepsis (widespread infection), or cancer. If bleeding is under the skin, vascular lesions will be apparent such as petechiae, ecchymosis, and purpura.
- Altered consciousness indicates a cerebral thrombus.
- Abdominal distention indicates a GI bleed.
- Cyanosis and tachypnea (increased respiratory rate) caused by poor tissue perfusion and oxygenation are common. Mottling of the skin indicates tissue ischemia.
- Hematuria (blood in urine) caused by hemorrhage or oliguria (decreased urine output) caused by poor renal perfusion.
- Decreased sensation in extremities.
- Extremities cool to touch.
- Hemoptysis.
- Pain which is described as swelling or sharp.
- Fatigue.
- Hypotension.

Diagnostic Tools

- Blood tests demonstrate accelerated clotting and decreased platelets.
- Fibrin degradation products are elevated. Platelets and plasma fibrinogen levels are reduced.

Complications

- The many clots cause obstruction to blood flow in all organs of the body. Widespread organ failure may occur. Mortality is greater than 50%.

Treatment

Treatment is difficult because of the combination of hemorrhage and clotting. Prevention of DIC and early identification of the condition is essential. Treatment is geared toward:

- Removal of the precipitating event.
- Heparin therapy may be initiated if organ failure caused by hypoxia is imminent. Heparin is not suggested when DIC is caused by sepsis or if central nervous system bleeding occurs.
- Low-molecular-weight heparin to minimize new thrombi formation.
- Fluid replacement is important to maintain organ perfusion as high as possible.
- Plasma containing factor VIII, red cells, and platelets may be administered.
- Antithrombin drugs such as activated protein C and antithrombin concentrations to restore anticoagulation pathways.

PEDIATRIC CONSIDERATIONS

- Newborn values of red blood cells, white blood cells, hemoglobin, and hematocrit are elevated compared with those of older infants, children, and some adults. High values begin to decrease within 2 weeks of birth, reaching a plateau after approximately 6 months. Levels reach adult values at approximately 18 years of age. Bleeding time, especially PT, is prolonged in infants because of a natural deficiency in vitamin K. At birth, infants in the United States are given injections of vitamin K to reduce the risk of bleeding.
- Dactylitis, also known as hand-foot syndrome, is a possible complication of sickle cell disease in children less than 2 years of age. Severe pain and swelling of the hands and feet are classical findings and are managed with nonprescription analgesics and hydration.

GERIATRIC CONSIDERATIONS

- The elderly are most prone to suffer from a dietary deficiency of vitamin B_{12}, as a result of poor diet. Any elderly person demonstrating fatigue, rapid heart rate, and mental and physical sluggishness should be evaluated for vitamin B_{12} deficiency.

- Although mononucleosis is usually seen in young adults or children, the elderly may contract the disease. When infected, the elderly may be difficult to diagnose because of the absence of the classic triad of symptoms. Jaundice may be present.

- Chronic lymphocytic leukemia (CLL) primarily affects older adults. Because progression is slow, treatment is typically not initiated until weight loss, fever, night sweats, and lymph node enlargement develop.

- Elderly patients with Hodgkin lymphoma have a poorer response to therapy than do young patients. This is largely because of the increased morbidity associated with aggressive chemotherapy. A more advanced stage of disease at the time of diagnosis may also be involved. Concurrent disease in the elderly (lung, cardiac, and renal) may affect the response to chemotherapy and radiation.

- Anemia in the older adult is a significant problem and greatly increases the risk for falls and infection. It also increases mortality and morbidity.

SELECTED BIBLIOGRAPHY

Adams, R. (2007). Sickle cell trait can take a sudden deadly turn. *American Nurse Today*, 2(11), 19–20.

Bielefeldt, S., & DeWitt, J. (2009). The rules of transfusion: Best practices for blood product administration. *American Nurse Today*, 4(2), 27–30.

Chamberlain, B. (2008). Are you prepared for malaria? *American Nurse Today*, 3(6), 10–12.

Chang, Y. C., Huang, H. P., Hsu, J. D., Yang, S. F., & Wang, C. J. (2005). *Hibiscus* anthocyanins rich extract-induced apoptotic cell death in human promyelocytic leukemia cells. *Toxicology* and *Applied Pharmacology*, 205, 201–212.

Copstead, L. C., & Banasik, J. L. (2010). *Pathophysiology* (4th ed.). St. Louis, MO: Saunders Elsevier.

Coyer, S. N., & Lash, A. A. (2008). Pathophysiology of anemia and nursing care implications. *MEDSURG Nursing*, 17(2), 77–83, 91.

Enserink, M. (2005). Mosquito-killing fungi may join the battle against malaria. *Science*, 308, 1531, 1533.

Freedman, D. O. (2008). Clinical practice: Malaria prevention in short-term travelers. *New England Journal of Medicine*, 359, 603–612.

Gunder, L. M. (2008, December). What you can learn from RBC analysis. The *Clinical Advisor*, 19–20, 22–23.

Guyton, A. C., & Hall, J. E. (2006). *Textbook of medical physiology* (11th ed.). Philadelphia, PA: W.B. Saunders.

Huether, S. E., & McCance, K. L. (2008). *Understanding pathophysiology* (4th ed.). St. Louis, MO: Mosby Elsevier.

Klein, H., Spahn, D., & Carson, J. (2007). Red blood cell transfusion in clinical practice. *The Lancet*, 370(9585), 415–426.

Kyle, R. A., & Rajkumar, S. V. (2004). Multiple myeloma. *New England Journal of Medicine*, 351, 1860–1873.

Lash, A. A., & Coyer, S. M. (2008). Anemia in older adults. *MEDSURG Nursing*, 17(5), 298–304.

Lew, V. L., & Bookchin, R. M. (2005). Ion transport pathology in the mechanism of sickle cell dehydration. *Physiological Reviews*, 85, 179–200.

National Newborn Screening and Genetics Resources Center. (August 15). *National newborn screening status report update*. Austin, TX: Author.

Osborne, K. S., Wraa, C. E., & Watson, A. B. (2010). *Medical-surgical nursing: Preparation for practice*. Upper Saddle River, NJ: Pearson.

Pack-Mabien, A., & Haynes, J. (2009). A primary care provider's guide to preventive and acute care management of adults and children with sickle cell disease. *Journal of the American Academy of Nurse Practitioners*, 21(5), 250–257.

Pagana, K. D. (2009). What does the absolute neutrophil count tell you? *American Nurse Today*, 4(2), 12–13.

Porth, C. M., & Matfin, G. (2009). *Pathophysiology: Concepts of altered health states* (8th ed.). Philadelphia: Lippincott Williams & Wilkins.

Re, D., Thomas, R. K., Behringer, K., & Diehl, V. (2005). From Hodgkin's disease to Hodgkin's lymphoma: Biologic insights and therapeutic potential. *Blood*, 105, 4553–4560.

Reyes, F., Lepage, E., Ganem, G., Molina, T. J., Brice, P., Coiffier, B. et al. (2005). ACVBP versus CHOP plus radiotherapy for localized aggressive lymphoma. *New England Journal of Medicine*, 352, 1197–1205.

Rosenthal, P. J. (2008). Artesunate for the treatment of severe falciparum malaria. *New England Journal of Medicine*, 358, 1829–1836.

Somjee, S. S., Warrier, R. P., Thomson, J. L., Ory-Ascani, J., & Hempe, J. M. (2005). Advanced glycation end-products in sickle cell anemia. *British Journal of Haematology*, 128, 112–118.

Stuart, M. J., & Nagel, R. L. (2004). Sickle-cell disease. *Lancet*, 364, 1343–1360.

Tabloski, P. A. (2010). *Gerontological nursing* (2nd ed.). Upper Saddle River, NJ: Pearson.

Thibodeau, G. A., & Patton, K. T. (2010). *The human body in health and disease* (5th ed.). St. Louis: Mosby Elsevier.

Van Leeuwen, A. M., & Poelhuis-Leth, D. J. (2009). *Davis's comprehensive handbook of laboratory and diagnostic tests with nursing implications* (3rd ed.). Philadelphia: F. A. Davis.

Werler, M. M. (1993). Periconceptual folic acid exposure and the risk of occurrent neural tube defects. *Journal of the American Medical Association*, 269, 1257–1261.

The Cardiovascular System

The final death reports for 2006 (National Vital Statistics Reports, 2009) indicate that the leading cause of death in the United States continues to be related to cardiovascular disease. According to the American Heart Association (2009), cardiovascular disease includes hypertension, coronary heart disease (myocardial infarction and angina), heart failure, stroke, and congenital heart disease. It is critical that health care providers and lay persons learn the concepts of cardiovascular disease, prevention, and health maintenance.

The cardiovascular system begins with the heart, a muscular pump that beats rhythmically and repeatedly 60 to 100 times a minute. Each beat causes blood to surge from the heart and travel throughout the body in a closed network of arteries, arterioles, and capillaries and return to the heart through venules and veins. The purpose of the cardiovascular system is to pick up oxygen in the lungs and nutrients absorbed across the gut and deliver them to all cells of the body. At the same time, the cardiovascular system removes the metabolic waste products produced by each cell and delivers them to the lungs or the kidneys to be excreted.

● Physiologic Concepts

ANATOMY OF THE HEART

The heart is a four-chambered, muscular organ that lies in the chest cavity, under the protection of the ribs, slightly to the left of the sternum. The heart sits within a loose, fluid-filled sac, called the **pericardium**. The four chambers of the heart include the left and right atria and the left and right ventricles.

The atria sit next to each other above the ventricles. The atria and ventricles are separated from each other by one-way valves. The right and left sides of the heart are separated by a wall of tissue called the septum. There is normally no mixing of blood between the two atria, except during fetal life, and there is never mixing of blood between the two ventricles in a healthy heart. Connective tissue surrounds all chambers. The heart is extensively innervated.

TWO CIRCULATIONS OF THE CARDIOVASCULAR SYSTEM

The left side of the heart pumps oxygenated blood through the **systemic circulation**, which reaches all cells of the body except those involved with gas exchange in the lungs. Blood leaves the heart via the aorta through a one-way valve. The right side of the heart pumps deoxygenated blood through the **pulmonary circulation**, which delivers blood only to the lungs to be oxygenated. Blood leaves the right side of the heart through the pulmonary artery, which has a one-way valve.

Systemic Circulation

Blood enters the left atrium from the pulmonary vein. The pulmonary vein is the only vein in the body that carries oxygenated blood. Blood in the left atrium flows into the left ventricle through the atrioventricular (AV) valve located at the juncture of the left atrium and ventricle. This valve is called the *mitral* valve. All cardiac valves open when pressure in the chamber or vessel above them is greater than the pressure in the chamber or vessel below.

Blood from the left ventricle outflows into a large, muscular artery, called the aorta, through the *aortic valve*. Blood in the aorta is delivered throughout the systemic circulation, through arteries, arterioles, and capillaries, which then rejoin to form veins. The veins from the lower part of the body return the blood to the largest vein, the inferior vena cava. The veins from the upper body return blood to the superior vena cava. The venae cavae empty into the right atrium.

Pulmonary Circulation

Blood in the right atrium moves into the right ventricle through another AV valve, called the *tricuspid valve*. Blood leaves the right ventricle and travels through a fourth valve, the *pulmonary valve*, into the pulmonary artery. The pulmonary artery is the only artery in the body that carries unoxygenated blood. The pulmonary artery branches into left and right pulmonary arteries, which travel to the left and right lungs, respectively. In the lungs, the pulmonary arteries branch many times into arterioles and then capillaries. Each capillary perfuses past an alveolus, the unit of respiration. All capillaries reform to become venules, and the venules become veins. The veins join to form the pulmonary veins.

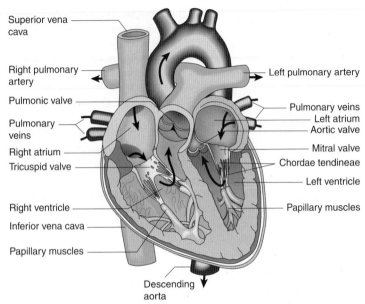

Superior vena cava
Right pulmonary artery
Pulmonic valve
Pulmonary veins
Right atrium
Tricuspid valve
Right ventricle
Inferior vena cava
Papillary muscles

Left pulmonary artery
Pulmonary veins
Left atrium
Aortic valve
Mitral valve
Chordae tendineae
Left ventricle
Papillary muscles

Descending aorta

FIGURE 13-1 Anatomy of the heart. (From Porth, C. & Matfin, G [2009]. *Pathophysiology, concepts of altered health states* [8th ed.]. Philadelphia: Lippincott Williams & Wilkins.)

Blood flows in the pulmonary veins back to the left atrium, completing the blood flow cycle. The heart and the systemic and pulmonary circulations are shown in Figure 13-1.

Functions of the Systemic and Pulmonary Circulations

As blood passes each cell of the body in the systemic circulation, carbon dioxide and other cellular waste products are added to the blood, while oxygen and nutrients are delivered from the blood to the cells. In the pulmonary circuit, the opposite occurs: carbon dioxide is eliminated from the blood and oxygen is added. By continual cycling of the blood through the pulmonary and systemic circulations, oxygen supply and waste removal are ensured for all cells.

Coronary Artery Blood Flow

Two large arteries, called the left and right coronary arteries, branch off the aorta as soon as it leaves the left ventricle and supply blood to the heart. The left coronary artery quickly branches into the left anterior descending artery and the circumflex artery. Table 13-1 summarizes the portions of the heart supplied by the coronary arteries.

TABLE 13-1 Coronary Arteries	
Coronary Artery	**Portion of the Heart Supplied**
Left anterior descending (LAD)	Anterior portion of septum
	Anterior muscle mass of left ventricle (LV)
Left circumflex	Lateral wall of left ventricle (LV)
Right coronary artery	Posterior portion of heart
	Posterior intraventricular septum
	Electrical sites of the heart: sinoatrial (SA) node and atrioventricular (AV) node

CARDIAC MUSCLE

Cardiac muscle is composed of highly specialized muscle fibers. Not only do these fibers contract in response to action potentials produced from neural stimulation, but many cardiac muscle fibers are capable of spontaneously firing action potentials that can initiate their own contractions. Excitation–contraction of cardiac muscle is described in the next several sections, beginning with a description of the cardiac muscle fibers and finishing with an outline of how an action potential leads to the contraction and beating of the heart.

Cardiac Muscle Fibers

As described fully in Chapter 10, cardiac muscle fibers are made up of bands of protein filaments, called myofilaments, lying in series with each other. Each band is called a sarcomere. A cardiac sarcomere is shown in Figure 13-2. Sarcomeres in cardiac muscle are fused together at their borders to form areas called intercalated disks. These are areas of low resistance across which electrical currents can pass.

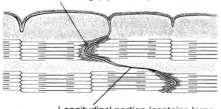

Transverse portion (myofibrillar junctions, desmosomes, and gap junctions)

Longitudinal portion (contains large gap junctions)

FIGURE 13-2 A sarcomere.

Myofilaments

Each cardiac sarcomere is made up of thick and thin filaments. Thick filaments consist of the contractile protein **myosin**. Thin filaments include the second contractile protein, **actin**, and two regulatory proteins, **tropomyosin** and **troponin**. Cross-bridges extend from the myosin filaments to the actin filaments. In the *absence* of calcium ion, tropomyosin is attached to each actin molecule in such a way that tropomyosin covers the binding site for myosin on actin, and thus inhibits cross-bridge connection. The troponin complex, which includes troponin-I, -T, and -C, is attached to the tropomyosin filament. When calcium *is* available, troponin-C binds the tropomyosin filament in such a way that the myosin cross-bridges are now exposed and able to bind actin.

At this point, energy stored from a previous myosin-based reaction, in which adenosine triphosphate (ATP) was split into adenosine diphosphate (ADP) and a phosphate molecule, is released and is used to swing the cross-bridges. This causes the myosin and actin filaments to slide past each other and muscle contraction to occur. Because all cardiac muscle cells are connected to each other at the intercalated disks, depolarization of one group of cardiac muscle cells spreads to neighboring cells and all cells contract as a unit. Each contraction represents a heartbeat.

Cardiac Muscle Depolarization and Action Potential Firing

An action potential in a cardiac muscle cell is triggered as a result of a depolarizing current reaching it from a neighboring muscle cell. Although in some ways similar to a skeletal muscle action potential, the cardiac action potential is unique due to its plateau phase and long duration.

Just like a skeletal muscle cell, a cardiac muscle cell fires an action potential when the inside of the cell becomes significantly more positively charged than the outside. As in skeletal muscle, this occurs when voltage-sensitive sodium channels open in the cell membrane, resulting in an in-rush of positively charged sodium ions. This is called Phase 0 of the cardiac action potential and is characterized by a rapid change in the membrane potential, from about -80 mV intracellularly to a positive intracellular value of approximately 20 to 25 mV (Fig. 13-3). Very quickly, closure of the sodium channels occurs, marking the end of Phase 0. Next begins Phase 1, a **repolarizing phase**. During Phase 1, potassium channels close in the cell membrane and positively charged potassium ions accumulate in the cell, preventing the return of the membrane potential toward its resting (negative) value. Closure of the potassium channels immediately following the onset of the action potential does not happen in skeletal muscle; in cardiac muscle, it contributes to the slowing of repolarization. Prolongation continues during the next

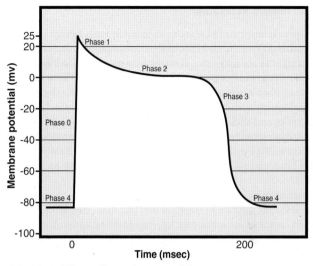

FIGURE 13-3 The cardiac action potential.

phase, Phase 2, as calcium ions begin to enter the cell through calcium channels present in the cell membrane. This increase in intracellular calcium triggers the opening of other, **slow calcium channels** located in the membrane of the sarcoplasmic reticulum, a storage compartment for intracellular calcium. This process, called "calcium stimulated calcium release," results in a further rise in intracellular calcium levels, reaching levels that effectively move the troponin off the tropomyosin molecule and thus trigger the muscle cell to contract. The slow inward movement of calcium also prolongs cellular depolarization. Phase 3 is the final repolarization phase, and it occurs when the influx of calcium decreases and the outflow of potassium ions through "delayed rectifier channels" begins, finally bringing the membrane potential back to its negative resting value. Intracellular levels of calcium decrease, by means of calcium moving out of membrane channels as well as via active transport of calcium back into the sarcoplasmic reticulum storage sites. As calcium falls, the cell relaxes and the heart enters diastole. The cell remains in Phase 4, the resting potential phase, until it is again stimulated to undergo an action potential. Prolongation of the action potential is significant because it makes it impossible to fire a second action potential before the first is completed, ensuring that cardiac cells will not undergo summation and tetany of contractions: If cardiac cells underwent tetany, the heart would stop pumping out blood because it would not be able to relax and fill with blood between beats.

Cardiac Muscle Relaxation

Adenosine diphosphate (ADP) releases from the cross-bridge after it swings, and another ATP molecule binds to the myosin protein, causing the myosin cross-bridges to separate from actin. As long as calcium ion is still available intracellularly to bind troponin, this new ATP will be split, and its energy will be released when a new cross-bridge connection forms, thereby repeating the cycle and ensuring that the muscle will continue to contract. Many cross-bridge cycles and sliding of the filaments occur during one action potential. The contraction ultimately stops when intracellular calcium levels fall. Without calcium, tropomyosin again blocks the site on actin to which the cross-bridges bind, and no further connection between myosin and actin can be made.

In skeletal muscle, there is always enough calcium released with each action potential to fully saturate all troponin sites and thus cause all cross-bridges to swing. In cardiac muscle, however, less than maximal amounts of calcium are usually released with a single action potential. This means that under certain circumstances, cardiac contractile strength may be increased if necessary.

The Pacemaker

Most cardiac muscle cells have the capacity to fire action potentials independently. However, certain cells are more permeable to sodium ions at rest than others, and therefore start off more positively charged than other cells. These slightly depolarized cells reach action potential threshold and fire sooner than other cells. The fast-firing cells pass their excitation easily to other cells through the connections between each cell. The fastest depolarizing cells of the heart control the rate, or pace, of contraction. The cells that normally depolarize fastest make up the SA node. The SA node, located in the wall of the right atrium, is the primary pacemaker of the heart.

Spread of Electrical Depolarization through the Myocardium

From the SA node, depolarization spreads rapidly through both atria and soon reaches the AV node, which is located in the lower right atrium near the juncture of the atria and ventricles. When the depolarization reaches the AV node, the electrical signal is delayed shortly before it is passed to the ventricles. During this delay, the atria reach action potential threshold and begin to contract, pumping their last bit of blood into the ventricles. While contraction of the atria is occurring, the electrical depolarization spreads through the AV node down specialized muscle fibers to an area of the ventricles called the bundle of His. Depolarization then spreads rapidly through the left and right bundle branches of the interventricular septum, and from there, down an extensive, wide-reaching group of specialized conducting fibers called Purkinje fibers. In a normal heart, the apex of the ventricle depolarizes first, after which the wave of depolarization spreads up toward the atria. This wave allows for the efficient ejection of blood from the ventricle.

THE CARDIAC CYCLE

Until the ventricles contract, the AV valves are open and blood flows from the atria into the relaxed, low-pressure ventricles. The aortic and pulmonary valves are closed because pressures are greater in the aortic and pulmonary arteries than in the relaxed ventricles. This allows blood to accumulate in the ventricles. This period of ventricular relaxation is called **diastole**. Blood volume in the ventricle immediately before ventricular contraction is called **end-diastolic volume**. When the ventricles contract, pressure inside the ventricles becomes greater than in the atria, and the AV valves snap shut. For a brief period of time, pressure in the aorta and pulmonary arteries is still higher than in the ventricles, so the aortic and pulmonary valves remain closed. With increasing pressure in the ventricles, the aortic and pulmonary valves burst open and blood flows out of the ventricles at high speed and pressure. This period of ventricular contraction is called **systole**.

With the end of systole, the ventricles relax again. As pressure in the relaxing ventricles falls below that in the aortic and pulmonary arteries, the aortic and pulmonary valves snap shut. Blood entering the atria from the venae cavae and pulmonary veins causes pressure to rebuild in the atria, opening the AV valves. The cycle of filling and emptying begins again.

ARTERIAL PRESSURES

The pulmonary artery and aorta are muscular vessels that expand with the surge of blood they receive from the ventricles. They hold this blood before releasing it into the rest of the vascular system, not in big pulses followed by ebbs of flow, but in a steady stream. Pressure generated in the arteries at the peak of ventricular contraction is much greater than pressure in the arteries when the ventricles are relaxed. Both of these pressures are frequently measured. **Systolic pressure** is the arterial blood pressure generated during ventricular contraction. **Diastolic pressure** is the arterial blood pressure generated when the ventricles are relaxed.

HEART SOUNDS

Heart sounds are produced when the AV valves (mitral and tricuspid valves) and the pulmonary and aortic valves snap shut. At least two (and sometimes four) heart sounds can be heard.

The first heart sound (S_1) is heard when the AV valves snap shut during ventricular contraction. This sound is somewhat prolonged and low in pitch, and occurs with the onset of systole when pressure in the ventricles becomes greater than that in the atria. The second heart sound (S_2) is shorter and occurs when outlet valves from the ventricles, the pulmonary and aortic valves, snap shut. This happens during diastole, when the ventricles relax and pressures in the pulmonary artery and aorta—which have just received the surging blood—are greater than pressures in the right and left ventricles. Third (S_3) and fourth heart sounds (S_4) are sometimes heard and are related to the sound of blood reverberating in the ventricles during rapid filling (S_3) or entering a ventricle that is stiff (S_4), for example, in conditions such as ventricular hypertrophy. S_3 heart sounds are considered to be benign in children and young adults; however, after about age 35, it may indicate systolic dysfunction and should be thoroughly assessed.

CARDIAC OUTPUT

Repeated contractions of the myocardium are the heartbeats. Each beat pumps blood out of the heart. The amount of blood pumped per beat is the **stroke volume**. Cardiac output (CO), the volume of blood pumped per minute, depends on the product of the heart rate (HR; in beats per minute) and the stroke volume (SV; in milliliters of blood pumped per beat) as shown in the following equation:

$$CO \text{ (mL/min)} = HR \text{ (beats/min)} \times SV \text{ (mL/beat)} \tag{13-1}$$

Cardiac output of an adult male ranges from 4.5 to 8 L/min. Increased cardiac output is possible with increased heart rate or stroke volume.

The cardiac index is often calculated clinically and offers input on heart performance in an individual. The cardiac index is found by dividing the measured cardiac output by the body surface area of the individual.

Cardiac output can increase or decrease as a result of forces acting intrinsically or extrinsically to the heart; that is, with or without external input. Intrinsic control of cardiac output is determined by the length of the cardiac muscle fibers. Extrinsic control refers to the effect of neural stimulation on the heart.

Intrinsic Control of Cardiac Output

The length of cardiac muscle fibers affects the tension they can produce because of the anatomic arrangement of muscle contractile proteins. In the resting heart, the muscle fibers are stretched to a degree less than that required to produce maximum tension. When cardiac muscle fibers are stretched, more myosin cross-bridges can reach their actin-binding sites, causing an increase in cross-bridge swinging and an increase in cardiac tension and cardiac contractility. This results in an increase in stroke volume and cardiac output (Equation 13-1). Increased stretch of the myofibrils occurs when there is increased filling of the heart; therefore, the tension that is produced by the heart is proportional to the volume of blood in the heart immediately before ventricular contraction: the end-diastolic volume (also referred to as preload). Because of this response, the heart has reserve capacity to pump more forcefully when the volume of blood flow is increased—for example, with exercise and volume loading.

Because an increase in venous return will increase end-diastolic volume, the length–tension relationship of the heart ensures that *under most conditions*, increased blood flow into the heart will be matched by increased blood pumped out. This serves to return the end-diastolic volume back toward normal, making this response typically of short duration. This intrinsic response of the heart to its own muscle fiber stretch is called **Starling's law of the heart**, after Frank Starling, the physiologist who first described it. The length–tension relationship of a normal heart under nonstimulated control conditions is shown in the lower curve of Figure 13-4. Note that, unlike in the skeletal muscle length–tension curve, the normal heart does not fall off the curve at higher fiber length.

The words "under most conditions" in the preceding paragraph refer to the fact that in a damaged heart, overstretch of the ventricle will not improve contractility, and the heart will not be able to pump out the extra blood. Therefore, a damaged heart continues to overfill and eventually becomes overstretched. This situation is characteristic of heart failure, which is described later.

A second reason why the stretch of cardiac muscle fibers determines cardiac output is that with increased venous return, the wall of the right atrium is stretched. This stretch causes an increased firing rate of the SA node and an increased heart rate of up to 20%. This increase in heart rate, coupled with an

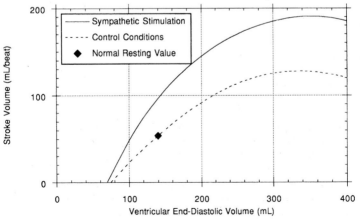

FIGURE 13-4 Length–tension curve: Starling law of the heart.

increase in stroke volume as a result of extra filling, can dramatically increase cardiac output. However, as mentioned earlier, because an increase in end-diastolic volume increases stroke volume, the intrinsic response to excess volume is usually temporary.

Extrinsic Control of Cardiac Output

Heart rate and stroke volume are affected by the sympathetic and parasympathetic nervous systems and by circulating hormones.

Sympathetic nerves travel in the thoracic spinal nerve tracts to the SA node and release the neurotransmitter norepinephrine. Norepinephrine binds to specific receptors called β_1 adrenergic receptors, present on the cells of the SA node. When this happens, activation of a second messenger system causes increased firing rate of the node, leading to an increase in heart rate. The heart rate is decreased if the activation of the sympathetic nerves and the release of norepinephrine are reduced. An increase or decrease in the heart rate is called a positive or negative **chronotropic** effect.

Sympathetic nerves also innervate cells throughout the myocardium, causing an increase in the force of each contraction (i.e., the contractility) at any given muscle fiber length. This causes an increase in stroke volume and is called a positive **inotropic** effect, as shown by the upper curve in Figure 13-4.

Parasympathetic nerves travel to the SA node and throughout the heart through the vagus nerve. Parasympathetic nerves release the neurotransmitter acetylcholine, which slows the rate of depolarization of the SA node and leads to a decrease in heart rate—a negative chronotropic effect. Parasympathetic stimulation to other sites in the myocardium appears to reduce contractility and therefore stroke volume, producing a negative inotropic effect.

Hormonal control of cardiac output mainly involves the adrenal medulla, an extension of the sympathetic nervous system. With sympathetic stimulation, the adrenal medulla releases norepinephrine and epinephrine into the circulation. These hormones travel to the heart and produce positive chronotropic and inotropic responses.

ARTERIES AND VEINS

All blood vessels except the capillaries are composed of three layers: the tunica adventitia, the tunica media, and the tunica intima.

The *tunica adventitia* is the outermost layer of the blood vessel, away from the lumen of the tube. It is primarily connective tissue and provides the vessels with physical support.

The *tunica media* is the middle layer of the vessel and is composed of vascular smooth muscle. This layer always has some basal tone, or tension, which can be increased or decreased. An increase in tension of the tunica media results in constriction of the vessel and a narrowing of its lumen, leading to an increase in the resistance to blood flow through the vessel. Relaxation of the smooth muscle causes dilation of the vessel and decreased resistance to flow. Increases or decreases in the radius of the vessels occur through neural, hormonal, and local mediators of blood flow. Because of their capacity to change their resistance through contraction or relaxation of the smooth muscle, the arterioles in particular are called the **resistance vessels** of the circulatory system.

The third layer of the blood vessels is the *tunica intima*, the innermost layer. This single-cell layer is made up of endothelial cells and is surrounded by a basement membrane.

SPECIAL CHARACTERISTICS OF VEINS

The veins, although composed of the tunicae adventitia, media, and intima, have much less smooth muscle than the arteries and arterioles. They are thin vessels that can easily expand to accommodate large volumes of blood and are easily collapsed. Because of their capacity to hold large volumes of blood, the veins are called the **capacitance vessels** of the circulatory system. This reservoir of venous blood can be called on in times of need when blood volume or pressure is low.

One-way valves are located periodically in the veins. These one-way valves allow blood to proceed toward the heart, but not back the other way. Blood is returned to the heart through the veins as a result of the pressure gradient that exists between the veins and the heart. Surrounding skeletal muscles contribute to returning venous blood to the heart by contracting and thus squeezing the veins. The valves prevent the blood squeezed up toward the heart from falling back down when the muscles relax. If one stands for a long period of time, the muscles relax and the valves do not close entirely, allowing blood to pool in the feet and ankles.

CAPILLARIES

The smallest of the blood vessels are the capillaries, with a diameter between 4 and 9 μm, barely large enough for a red blood cell to flow through. The capillaries are composed only of endothelial cells. Lipid-soluble substances, such as oxygen and carbon dioxide, pass out of the capillaries into the interstitial space by diffusing across the endothelial cells. Substances that are not lipid soluble, such as small ions and glucose, may move between the endothelial cells through intercellular clefts or pores to reach the interstitial space. Because the diameter of the capillary pores is much smaller than the diameter of the plasma proteins and red blood cells, and because neither is lipid soluble, proteins and red cells are prohibited from moving out of the vascular system into the interstitial space.

Precapillary Sphincter

Immediately proximal to the capillaries are the meta-arterioles, which deliver blood to the capillaries through a precapillary sphincter. The precapillary sphincter is a smooth muscle fiber encircling the entrance to the capillary. This fiber is not innervated by nerves, but responds to hormonal and local mediators of blood flow.

Bulk Flow Across the Capillary

Bulk flow is the movement of a fluid as a result of a pressure gradient from high to low. In the vascular system, fluid moves back and forth between the capillaries and the interstitial fluid. Interstitial fluid is a plasmalike filtrate surrounding all cells. It can store fluid in times of high plasma volume, or resupply the vascular system in times of plasma loss.

There are four forces affecting the bulk flow of fluid across a capillary into the interstitial space. They include capillary pressure, interstitial hydrostatic pressure, plasma colloid osmotic pressure, and interstitial fluid colloid osmotic pressure.

Capillary hydrostatic pressure is the remainder of the mean arterial pressure generated by the heart. For most capillaries, this pressure averages approximately 18 mm Hg over the length of the capillary (Fig. 13-5), with pressure at the arteriolar end (28 mm Hg) significantly greater than the pressure at the venous end (10 mm Hg). Capillary pressure is a reflection of mean blood pres-

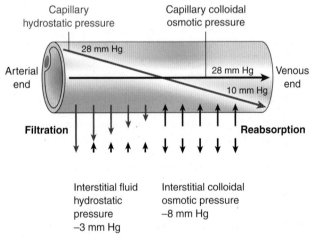

FIGURE 13-5 Forces of filtration and reabsorption across a capillary.(From Porth, C. & Matfin, G. [2009]. *Pathophysiology, concepts of altered health states* [8th ed.]. Philadelphia: Lippincott Williams & Wilkins.)

sure. Therefore, if blood pressure increases, capillary pressure increases. If blood pressure decreases, capillary pressure decreases. Capillary pressure favors filtration of plasma out of the capillary into the interstitial space.

Interstitial hydrostatic pressure is the pressure exerted by fluid in the interstitial space. Interstitial hydrostatic pressure is primarily caused by water. If positive, it opposes filtration of plasma out of the capillary; if negative, it draws fluid out of the capillary. Recent research suggests that the pressure is negative in most tissues, averaging approximately 3 mm Hg. In some tissues, it may be positive and oppose filtration.

Plasma (capillary) colloid osmotic pressure refers to osmotic pressure exerted by plasma proteins. Plasma colloid pressure opposes filtration of plasma out of the capillary. This pressure develops when water is pushed out of the capillary by the hydrostatic pressure and the proteins are too large and too charged to follow. The concentration of protein left behind increases, causing an increase in osmotic pressure. This pressure serves to draw water back into the capillary. Plasma colloid osmotic pressure in most capillaries averages approximately 28 mm Hg.

Interstitial fluid colloid osmotic pressure is normally a small force. Few proteins escape across the capillary into the interstitial compartment. Those that do are rapidly taken up into vessels of the lymph system. The lymph vessels return the proteins to the bloodstream by delivering them into the vena cava and the right atrium. Interstitial fluid colloid osmotic pressure averages approximately 8 mm Hg.

Adding up the forces, filtration (18 + 3 + 8 mm Hg = 29 mm Hg) nearly balances reabsorption (28 mm Hg) and little net movement of fluid across the capillary occurs (see Fig. 13-5). Extra fluid in the interstitial space is reabsorbed by the lymph flow.

BLOOD FLOW

Blood travels in the vascular system by bulk flow, the movement of a fluid through a tube based on the pressure difference between one end of the tube and the other. The pressure of the blood as it leaves the heart (P1) minus the pressure in a downstream vessel (P2), divided by the resistance offered by the blood vessels (R), determines the blood flow (F) through the vascular system, as expressed in the following equation:

$$F = (P1 - P2)/R \qquad (13\text{-}2)$$

Blood Pressure

Pressure at the beginning of the aorta is generated by the left ventricle. This pressure varies between approximately 120 mm Hg during systole and 80 mm Hg during diastole. Because diastole lasts longer than systole, the average, or mean, blood pressure equals approximately 40% of systolic pressure plus 60%

of diastolic pressure. The systolic pressure represents the maximum pressure on the aorta and major vessels and the diastolic pressure reflects the minimum pressure on the arteries. The difference in the systolic and diastolic pressure is referred to as **pulse pressure**.

As blood moves through the large and small arteries, some pressure is lost. Much more is lost as blood traverses the arterioles and capillaries. By the time blood flow reaches the capillary, blood pressure at the arteriole end of the capillary has decreased to approximately 35 mm Hg for most capillary beds. With movement through the capillary, this pressure decreases to 10 mm Hg at the venous end, resulting in a mean blood pressure in the capillary of approximately 18 mm Hg. By the time the blood reaches the vena cava, the pressure is zero.

Thus, the pressure gradient affecting flow is large between the aorta and the vena cava (90 to 0 mm Hg). This is the force that drives the blood through the systemic circulation.

Resistance

Resistance to flow through a vessel depends on the length and radius of the vessel, and on the viscosity of the fluid. In the body, the length of the blood vessels is essentially fixed. Although potentially variable, blood viscosity is also fixed. Therefore, when discussing resistance to blood flow in the vascular system, one usually considers only the radius of the blood vessels. Because of the dynamics of flow through a tube, a small decrease in the radius causes an enormous increase in resistance to flow. This is true both for blood flowing through a blood vessel and for water flowing through a hose or a pipe.

The smaller the vessel, the greater the effect narrowing that vessel has on blood flow. Varying the radius of the large arteries does not significantly affect blood flow. Likewise, because veins are so distensible, they offer little resistance to flow. Instead, resistance to blood flow is determined by the radius of the arterioles, thus making the arterioles the resistance vessels of the cardiovascular system.

Narrowing an arteriole decreases blood flow downstream into the capillaries and veins fed by that arteriole, backing up the blood upstream. Because blood pressure depends on blood flow, narrowing the arterioles decreases blood pressure downstream and increases blood pressure upstream.

In contrast, if the arterioles are dilated, flow increases, resulting in increased downstream pressure and decreased pressure upstream. With the dilation, force is decreased. Control of arteriole diameter is an intricate balance between local effects and nervous and hormonal stimulation.

Capillary Resistance to Blood Flow

The capillaries offer a great deal of resistance to blood flow because they are so narrow. However, because they have no smooth muscle, their diameter cannot be varied, so changes in capillary diameter cannot cause an increase or decrease in blood flow. The meta-arterioles immediately preceding the capillaries do change in diameter and affect capillary blood flow. Because of the extensive surface area covered by all the capillaries, blood flow through them is slow, allowing ample time for the diffusion of oxygen and carbon dioxide to occur.

Total Peripheral Resistance

Resistance in the systemic vascular system is referred to as total peripheral resistance (TPR). It is impossible to measure resistance directly. Resistance in the cardiovascular system is calculated by measuring flow and pressure. The resistance equals pressure divided by flow. Resistance to flow in the pulmonary vascular system is much less than in the systemic system. The amount of force that the ventricle must generate to overcome vascular resistance is referred to as afterload.

CONTROL OF MEAN ARTERIAL BLOOD PRESSURE

From the previous discussion, it should be apparent that in the vascular system it is difficult to discuss blood flow without referring to blood pressure. The variable regulated by the body, and usually measured clinically, is the systemic arterial blood pressure (BP). Equation 13-3 is used to describe the variables controlling systemic mean arterial blood pressure:

$$BP = CO \times TPR \qquad (13\text{-}3)$$

where, for the cardiovascular system,

- BP is the mean arterial blood pressure,
- CO is the cardiac output (which equals $HR \times SV$). Note: CO replaces F from Equation 13-2.
- TPR is the total peripheral resistance.
- Blood pressure control depends on sensors that continually measure blood pressure and send the information to the brain. The brain integrates all incoming information and responds by sending efferent (outgoing) stimulation to the heart and vasculature through the autonomic nerves. Various hormones and locally released chemical mediators add to the control of blood pressure.

Sensors

Blood pressure is continually monitored by sensors called baroreceptors (pressure receptors). There are baroreceptors in the carotid artery (in the neck) and in the aortic arch where the aorta leaves the heart; these sensors are called the carotid and aortic baroreceptors, respectively. There are baroreceptors located in the arterioles supplying the kidney nephrons. Receptors in both atria and in the pulmonary artery also respond to changes in pressure. Because the atrial and pulmonary artery receptors are in low-pressure areas of the vasculature, they are called low-pressure receptors.

All baroreceptors act as stretch receptors that respond to changes in blood pressure. Their stretch increases with increased blood pressure. This stretch increase causes afferent neurons receiving information from the receptors to increase their rate of firing. These neurons travel to the brain and innervate its cardiovascular center. A decrease in blood pressure decreases the stretch of the baroreceptors, which reduces the firing of the afferent nerves innervating the cardiovascular center.

Chemoreceptors located in the carotid bodies and the aorta, respond to changes in oxygen, carbon dioxide, and hydrogen ion concentration in arterial blood. Low blood pressure, decreased oxygen, or accumulation of metabolic end products stimulates the sympathetic nervous system causing the chemoreceptors and baroreceptors to respond and signal the brain. When blood pressure drops, the parasympathetic nervous system is inhibited and the sympathetic system is stimulated to increase heart rate. Chemoreceptors cause vasoconstriction and play a vital role in ventilation (see Chapter 14).

Integrating Center for the Control of Blood Pressure

The cardiovascular center in the brain is part of the reticular formation and is located in the lower medulla and pons. This center is the site of neural control for blood pressure regulation. If a change in blood pressure has occurred, the cardiovascular center activates the autonomic nervous system, leading to changes in sympathetic and parasympathetic stimulation to the heart and sympathetic stimulation to the entire vascular system. Resistance of the vasculature is altered and blood flow and blood pressure are affected.

Efferent Neural Innervation of the Vascular System

Sympathetic nerves stimulate heart rate and contractility by binding to β_1 receptors in the heart. Parasympathetic nerves decrease heart rate by binding to cholinergic receptors. In addition, sympathetic nerves traveling in the thoracic and upper lumbar spinal tracts influence blood pressure by exerting control over virtually the entire peripheral vascular system (except the capillaries) through innervation of the tunica media (the smooth muscle).

At most blood vessels, sympathetic nerves release norepinephrine, which binds to specific receptors on the smooth muscle cells, called alpha (α) receptors. Stimulation of the α receptors causes the smooth muscle to contract, constricting the vessel, which increases TPR and therefore increases blood pressure.

Blood vessels supplying skeletal muscle have a different type of receptor, called beta2 ($\beta2$) receptors, which, when stimulated by norepinephrine, cause the vessels to relax. It appears that this sympathetic vasodilatory response plays a significant role only in the anticipatory response to exercise, perhaps serving to prime the skeletal muscle with oxygen and nutrient support before exercise onset.

Skeletal muscle blood vessels also possess receptors for acetylcholine. These receptors are called muscarinic receptors and do not appear to be innervated by parasympathetic neurons. However, they respond to acetylcholine released by certain sympathetic cholinergic neurons. These neurons also supply the vascular smooth muscle in skeletal muscle and cause relaxation of the vessels, thus increasing blood flow through these vessels.

Hormonal Control of the Vascular System

There are several hormones that control the resistance of the vascular system. These hormones are released directly in response to changes in blood pressure, in response to neural stimulation, or both.

Norepinephrine and Epinephrine

The catecholamines, norepinephrine and epinephrine, are released from the adrenal medulla in response to activation of the sympathetic nervous system. Both substances act like norepinephrine released from nerve terminals and bind to α receptors to cause vasoconstriction, or to β_2 receptors to cause vasodilation of arterioles supplying skeletal muscles. Norepinephrine and epinephrine from the adrenal medulla also bind to β_1 receptors and increase heart rate.

Renin–Angiotensin System

Renin is produced and stored by the kidney. When renal baroreceptors sense a change in blood pressure the release of renin is increased or decreased. Renin release is also stimulated by sympathetic nerves to the kidney. If blood pressure is high, release of the hormone renin is decreased. When blood pressure drops, renin is released and acts as an enzyme to convert the protein angiotensinogen to angiotensin I.

Angiotensin I is a 10–amino acid protein, which is immediately split by angiotensin-converting enzyme (ACE) into the 8–amino acid peptide, angiotensin II. ACE is present in the blood vessels of the lungs and is the same enzyme that breaks down (and inactivates) the vasodilator hormone bradykinin. Blocking the action of ACE blocks the production of angiotensin II and the breakdown of bradykinin.

Angiotensin II is a powerful vasoconstrictor that primarily causes constriction of the small arterioles. This causes an increase in resistance to blood flow and an increase in blood pressure. The increase in blood pressure then acts in a negative feedback manner to reduce the stimulus for further renin release. Angiotensin II also circulates to the adrenal gland and causes cells of the adrenal cortex to synthesize another hormone, aldosterone.

Aldosterone.

Aldosterone circulates to the kidney and causes cells of the distal tubule to increase sodium reabsorption. Under many circumstances, reabsorption of water follows that of sodium, leading to an increase in plasma volume. An increase in plasma volume increases stroke volume, and hence cardiac output. It also causes increased blood pressure.

Renin–Angiotensin–Aldosterone Feedback Cycle.

It should be emphasized that the stimuli causing the release of renin—decreased blood pressure and decreased plasma sodium concentration—are reversed by the actions of angiotensin II and aldosterone. This is an excellent example of a negative feedback cycle.

Antidiuretic Hormone.

Antidiuretic hormone (ADH), also called **vasopressin**, is released from the posterior pituitary in response to increased plasma osmolality (decreased water concentration) or decreased blood pressure.

ADH is a potent vasoconstrictor with the potential to increase blood pressure by increasing the resistance to blood flow. Under most circumstances, except perhaps during severe hemorrhage, levels of circulating ADH are too low to affect the arterioles. However, ADH controls the reabsorption of water across the collecting ducts of the kidney back into the bloodstream. This effect influences blood pressure by increasing plasma volume and therefore cardiac output. Without ADH, water does not follow sodium reabsorption in the kidney and severe dehydration may occur. Reabsorption of water in response to ADH reduces the stimuli (increased plasma osmolality and decreased blood pressure) for ADH release.

Atrial Natriuretic Peptide.

Atrial natriuretic peptide (ANP) is a hormone released from cells of the right atrium in response to an increase in blood volume. ANP acts on the kidney to increase the excretion of sodium ion (natriuresis). Because water will follow sodium in the urine, ANP serves to decrease blood volume and blood pressure.

Summary of Blood Pressure Control

With a decrease in blood pressure, baroreceptor information is transmitted to the cardiovascular center in the brain. This causes the stimulation of sympathetic output to the heart and vascular system, increasing heart rate and TPR. Parasympathetic output is decreased, also increasing heart rate. Renin release increases, causing increased angiotensin II, which directly increases TPR and aldosterone synthesis. Increased aldosterone increases sodium reabsorption and, in the presence of ADH, water reabsorption. Increased plasma volume, stroke volume, and cardiac output result. Capillary pressure decreases directly with blood pressure and indirectly from sympathetic constriction of the arteriole

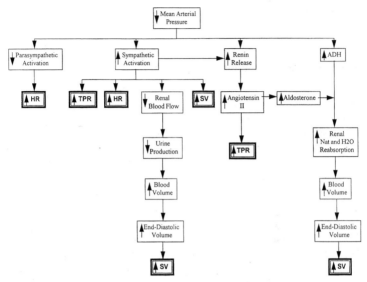

FIGURE 13-6 Flow diagram: reflex response to a fall in blood pressure.

feeding the capillary. This serves to decrease filtration of fluid out of the capillary. All of these responses serve to increase blood pressure toward normal, by increasing heart rate, stroke volume, and TPR (Fig. 13-6).

In contrast, if blood pressure increases, baroreceptor responses cause a decrease in sympathetic stimulation to the heart and vascular smooth muscle, and heart rate and TPR decrease. Increased parasympathetic stimulation to the heart contributes to the decrease in heart rate. There is a decrease in renin and ADH release, reducing TPR and plasma volume. ANP release increases. All these responses serve to decrease blood pressure toward normal.

Although hormonal and neural mechanisms can quickly regulate blood pressure, the effect is short-term. The kidneys are responsible for long-term blood pressure control by regulating extracellular fluid volume (ECF). For example, in response to ECF from increased water and sodium retention, the kidney responds by increasing the excretion of water and sodium. Autoregulation of blood flow also impacts how fluid volume affects blood pressure.

AUTOREGULATION OF BLOOD FLOW

In general, blood pressure is controlled through neural and hormonal influences. However, individual tissues have mechanisms that regulate their own blood flow. This is accomplished by local vasodilation or vasoconstriction of meta-arterioles and precapillary sphincters. This local control of blood flow is called **autoregulation**, and is the means by which some organs can maintain constant blood flow over a wide range of blood pressure, from approximately 70 to 180 mm Hg.

Theories of Autoregulation

Several theories are proposed to explain local control of blood flow. The most widely accepted is that chemical mediators are released by metabolizing cells that bind to meta-arterioles or precapillary sphincters, causing them to open or shut to blood flow.

Chemical mediators that control local blood flow include adenosine (a metabolite of ATP), carbon dioxide, histamine, lactic acid, potassium ions, and hydrogen ions. All of these substances except histamine are by-products of metabolism; as cell metabolism increases, so do their concentrations. This serves to match increased metabolic activity with increased blood flow. Mast cells present throughout the interstitial space release histamine in response to immune stimulation or local injury. Adenosine appears to particularly regulate local blood flow in the heart.

An alternative theory concerning local control suggests that the meta-arterioles and capillary sphincters sense an oxygen or nutrient deficit that causes them to relax, thereby increasing blood flow to the surrounding cells.

Other Chemical Mediators Influencing Blood Flow

Various other chemicals are released by the blood vessels or by mediators of inflammation or healing, which affect blood flow to an area.

Nitric Oxide

Endothelial cells of the small arteries and arterioles respond to the binding of various vasoactive substances such as acetylcholine with the production of the vasodilator nitric oxide (previously called endothelial-derived relaxing factor). Nitric oxide diffuses through endothelial cells to underlying smooth muscle cells, causing endothelial-dependent relaxation of the smooth muscle and inhibition of platelet aggregation. Nitric oxide release also occurs with increased blood flow through a vessel, allowing local dilation of the microvasculature to be matched by dilation of the small arteries and arterioles. Drugs that boost nitric oxide synthesis or prevent its breakdown are used to improve blood flow in a variety of clinical situations.

Endothelin

Endothelial cells also release endothelin, a 21–amino acid peptide that acts as a potent constrictor of vascular smooth muscle. Endothelin release is stimulated by angiotensin II, ADH, thrombin, cytokines, reactive oxygen species, and shearing forces acting on the vascular endothelium. Its release is inhibited by prostacyclin and nitric oxide. Deleterious effects of overproduction of endothelin on vascular smooth muscle include prolonged vasoconstriction, vascular hypertrophy, cell proliferation, and fibrosis. In addition, by binding to receptors on endothelial cells that are different from the ones on vascular smooth muscle, endothelin increases capillary permeability and contributes to inflammation. Endothelin has a long half-life (length of presence in the circulation or interstitial fluid), so even small changes in its production or clearance have significant impact on the vascular system. Overproduction of endothelin is implicated in numerous pathologies, including pulmonary hypertension, myocardial hypertrophy, and heart failure. Drugs to block endothelin receptors are being tested in a variety of clinical situations.

Serotonin

Serotonin (5-hydroxytryptamine) is primarily released by platelets drawn to an area of injury or inflammation. Effects of serotonin may be vasodilatory or vasoconstricting, depending on the site of release. Serotonin's ability to vasoconstrict and decrease blood flow appears to be one mechanism whereby platelets control or reduce bleeding.

Bradykinin

Bradykinin, like all members of the kinin family, is a small polypeptide that acts as a potent vasodilator of arterioles and as a mediator to increase capillary permeability. Bradykinin is produced in the plasma or interstitial fluid by enzymatic splitting of a serum globulin in response to vascular or tissue injury or inflammation. The half-life of bradykinin is short. Normally, it is broken down rapidly by circulating ACE or another enzyme, carboxypeptidase.

The effects of bradykinin are increased local blood flow, increased capillary permeability, and decreased vascular resistance. These effects allow delivery of mediators of the inflammatory and immune systems to a site of injury. Blockage of ACE by various pharmaceutical agents prolongs the half-life of bradykinin and its effects.

Prostaglandins

There are many different types of prostaglandins. Some cause dilation of the vascular system and some cause constriction. Prostaglandins are derived from the metabolism of arachidonic acid by cyclooxygenase (COX) enzymes one (COX1) and two (COX2). Arachidonic acid is present in all cell membranes and is released with tissue injury. Prostaglandins work to control local blood flow. They may circulate to affect distant cells.

One main group of prostaglandins, those of the E series, cause local vasodilation and increased blood flow, which makes them important mediators of inflammation. Prostaglandins of the I series, especially PGI_2, called prostacyclin, also are vasodilatory. PGI_2 inhibits platelet aggregation and blood clotting. Thromboxane A_2 is an important prostaglandin that causes vasoconstriction and blood clotting.

Prostaglandin synthesis is inhibited by drugs that block the function of the COX enzymes, including aspirin and nonsteroidal anti-inflammatory drugs (NSAIDs), and by specific COX enzyme inhibitors. Low concentration of aspirin particularly appears to cause a long-lasting block in production of thromboxane A_2. Glucocorticoids, including endogenously released cortisol and dexamethasome provided therapeutically, block prostaglandin synthesis at an early stage after membrane injury, prior to the formation of arachidonic acid, and are potent anti-inflammatory agents.

THE LYMPH SYSTEM

The lymph system consists of closed-end vessels that course through almost the entire interstitial fluid space. Lymph fluid is derived from interstitial fluid and is therefore very similar in composition to plasma.

Lymph Flow

The lymph system consists of small capillaries that drain into larger lymph vessels. Like blood vessels, these larger vessels are composed of smooth muscle and endothelial cells. Lymph from the lower body flows up the thoracic duct and empties into the left jugular and subclavian veins. Lymph flow from the left arm, shoulder, and left side of the head travels through the thoracic duct and then into the left jugular and subclavian arteries. Lymph flow from the right arm and right side of the neck and head empties into the right jugular and subclavian veins. The lymphatic system is illustrated in Figure 13-7.

Movement of lymph results from contraction of the smooth muscle lining the lymph vessels in response to its stretch, and the pumping action of the surrounding skeletal muscles. Valves present in lymph vessels prevent backflow.

Role of the Lymph System

The lymph system has three essential roles in the body, all of which depend on the greater permeability of lymph capillaries compared to blood capillaries.

First, lymph capillaries retrieve any proteins that escape from the capillaries into the interstitial fluid. These proteins move easily into lymph vessels and are then returned to the blood circulation via the thoracic duct. This is essential because it allows interstitial colloid osmotic pressure to remain low. If proteins were allowed to accumulate in the interstitial space, interstitial colloid osmotic pressure would increase. This would result in increased forces favoring filtration into the interstitial fluid, which would soon cause massive interstitial edema. Death of the individual could occur from circulatory collapse.

The second essential role played by the lymph system involves the absorption of fats from the small intestine. In the small intestine, fats and fat-soluble vitamins are absorbed into small lymph vessels called lacteals, and are then delivered to the general circulation. Fat and the fat-soluble vitamins are required for life.

LYMPHATIC SYSTEM

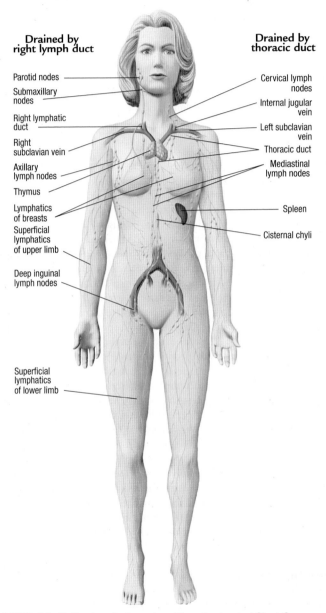

Drained by
right lymph duct

Drained by
thoracic duct

Parotid nodes

Submaxillary
nodes

Right lymphatic
duct

Right
subclavian vein

Axillary
lymph nodes

Thymus

Lymphatics
of breasts

Superficial
lymphatics
of upper limb

Deep inguinal
lymph nodes

Superficial
lymphatics
of lower limb

Cervical lymph
nodes

Internal jugular
vein

Left subclavian
vein

Thoracic duct

Mediastinal
lymph nodes

Spleen

Cisternal chyli

FIGURE 13-7 The lymphatic system. (From Anatomical Chart Company [2010]. *Atlas of pathophysiology* [3rd ed.]. Philadelphia: Lippincott Williams & Wilkins.)

The third essential role played by the lymph system involves immune function. Because of the high permeability of the lymph capillaries, bacteria and other microorganisms enter the lymph system from infected areas and are transported to and through lymph nodes, where they become trapped and removed from the circulation. Lymph nodes are an intertwining meshwork of vessels filled with tissue macrophages and T and B cells; bringing bacteria and other cellular debris to the lymph nodes allows the immune and inflammatory cells an opportunity to protect the host from widespread infection. Lymph nodes are spaced intermittently along the lymph vessels.

FETAL CIRCULATION

There are several major differences between fetal circulation and the circulation of infants, children, and adults. While in utero, a fetus does not receive oxygen through its own lungs. Rather, maternal oxygen is delivered across the placenta into the umbilical vein. The umbilical vein delivers oxygen-rich blood to the right side of the fetal heart through the vena cava. Because of the maternal source of oxygen, the fetal lungs and *most* of the blood vessels supplying them are collapsed, causing high resistance to blood flow through the fetal lungs, especially when compared to flow through the fetal systemic circulation, which offers low resistance because of the wide-open vessels of the placenta (Fig. 13.8).

There are also structural differences that characterize fetal circulation. In the fetus, there are two connections (shunts) that exist to take advantage of the maternal oxygen source and the high resistance of the pulmonary circulation. The first of these connections is an opening between the right atrium and the left atrium, called the **foramen ovale**. Because resistance is so high in the pulmonary circuit leaving the right ventricle, fetal blood travels in the direction of lower resistance: from right atrium to left through the foramen ovale. Because blood entering the vena cava in the fetus has already been oxygenated by passage through the placenta, this right to left shunting is an efficient adaptation. Well-oxygenated blood is delivered to the systemic (left side) circulation without the need to send blood through the collapsed, nonfunctioning pulmonary system.

The second shunting system between the right and left sides of circulation in the fetus is a vascular connection between the pulmonary artery and the aorta. This connection, called the **ductus arteriosus**, allows oxygenated blood leaving the right side of the heart to bypass the fetal lungs and flow directly into the low resistance of the systemic circulation. It should be noted that the fetal lungs do receive a small amount of blood flow through the pulmonary artery, allowing for their continued growth and development.

NEWBORN CIRCULATION

With birth, the situation changes dramatically and suddenly. The newborn is no longer supplied with oxygen from the placenta because the low-resistance vessels of the placenta are no longer connected to the fetus. At birth, the newborn

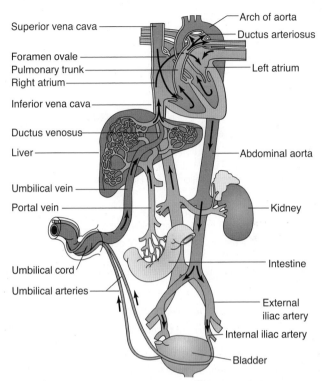

FIGURE 13-8 Fetal circulation. (From Porth, C. & Matfin, G [2009]. *Pathophysiology, concepts of altered health states* [8th ed.]. Philadelphia: Lippincott Williams & Wilkins.)

separates from the placenta, fluid in the lungs is squeezed out, and the newborn takes a deep breath, opening up the lungs and the blood vessels flowing through them. Immediately at birth, resistance of the pulmonary circulation falls while resistance of the systemic circulation increases. Blood flow no longer shunts right to left through the foramen ovale or the ductus arteriosus because those directions now offer higher resistance to flow. These shunt passages normally begin to close within a few hours after birth.

TESTS OF CARDIOVASCULAR FUNCTIONING

The Electrocardiogram

The electrocardiogram (ECG) is the measurement of the electrical currents of the heart. Contraction of the atria and ventricles results from action potentials occurring simultaneously in all muscle cells of the atria, followed by all muscle cells of the ventricles. Electrodes placed in specific locations on the body can

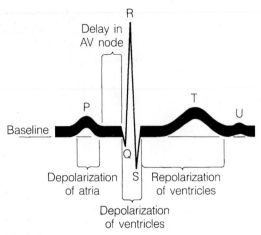

F I G U R E 1 3 - 9 The electrocardiogram (ECG) depiction.

detect these action potential currents. The currents can then be graphically displayed and interpreted.

Currents Measured by the Electrocardiogram

There are three currents produced in the normal ECG, as shown in Figure 13-9.

- The P wave corresponds to atrial depolarization.
- The QRS complex (beginning of Q wave to end of S wave) corresponds to depolarization of the ventricles.
- The T wave corresponds to repolarization of the ventricles.

Repolarization of the atria occurs during the QRS complex and is nondistinguishable. The U wave is an inconsistent finding that may represent slow repolarization of the papillary muscles involved in opening and closing the AV valves. Normal sinus rhythm is the expected rhythm of the heart, driven by the SA node and passed along the normal, intact conduction system.

Patterns of the Electrocardiogram

Several patterns in the normal ECG stand out. First, the pattern of the three waves repeats itself with each beat. A timescale is usually shown on the recording, allowing one to determine the heart rate by counting any one of the waves over time. The P wave or the QRS complex can be counted.

Second, the QRS complex always follows the P wave in a normal beating pattern because the atria undergo an action potential and contract first. Their action potential subsequently spreads to the ventricles. The time between the end of the P wave and the beginning of the QRS complex reflects the time during which the action potential is delayed at the AV node.

Third, the size of the atrial depolarization, as measured by the height of the P wave, is less than the depolarization of the ventricles, as measured by the height of the QRS complex. This reflects the much greater muscle mass of the ventricles compared to the atria. The ventricular depolarization is a rapid spike, as shown by the narrow displacement of the QRS complex, indicating that conduction throughout the ventricle is rapid, and that the entire ventricle contracts as one quick-firing unit. Increased horizontal spread of the QRS complex occurs with prolonged conduction of the electrical impulse through the ventricles, indicating ventricular hypertrophy. A bizarre QRS complex may indicate cardiac cell death.

Measurement of Cardiac Enzymes

When cardiac muscle cells die during a myocardial infarct (MI), they release their intracellular contents. Specific proteins and enzymes normally present only inside cardiac cells can be measured in the blood. This allows one to accurately diagnose the existence and frequently the extent of myocardial cell death. Because different enzyme levels are elevated at different times after infarction, the timing of the infarct can be determined.

Proteins released after injury to the myocardial cells include myoglobin, normally found only in skeletal and cardiac muscle cells, and the cardiac-specific contractile proteins, troponin T, C, and I. Highly sensitive bedside laboratory kits, capable of measuring the presence of very low amounts of serum troponin T and I within a short time of a suspected infarct, have the capacity to revolutionize early detection of an MI. Because troponin T elevates early and stays elevated for up to two weeks, it is useful for diagnosing cardiac events that may have occurred in the past 14 days. C-reactive protein is also released in the presence of myocardial injury. Myocardial creatine kinase (CK-MB) is an enzyme that is released with cardiac cell death. Lactic acid dehydrogenase (LDH), and serum glutamic oxaloacetic transaminase (SGOT) may also be elevated after myocardial injury, but are no longer considered the best indicators. The plasma concentration of each of these enzymes and proteins varies depending on the time since injury and the extent of the cell damage. Table 13-2 summarizes the most definitive serum markers of myocardial ischemia.

Stress Testing

Cardiac stress testing involves having an individual exercise up to his or her maximal capacity while observers monitor physical symptoms and the ECG. In a simple exercise stress test, the patient is asked to either walk on a treadmill or ride an exercise bike. The pattern of the ECG is observed for alterations in rhythm, the presence of AV blocks, and evidence of ST-segment changes indicative of hypoxia. Onset of physical symptoms, such as chest pain and extreme shortness of breath, is monitored.

TABLE 13-2 Serum Markers of Myocardial Ischemia

Marker	Initial Elevation after Injury	Peak Elevation after Injury	Return to Baseline
Myoglobin	1–3 hours	6–7 hours	24 hours
Troponin I	3–12 hours	24 hours	5–10 days
Troponin T	3–12 hours	12 hours–2 days	5–14 days
CK-MB	3–12 hours	24 hours	48–72 hours
C-reactive Protein	24 hours	2–3 days	2 weeks

Nuclear Stress Testing

Sometimes, an intravenous infusion of a radiolabeled isotope that has specific cardiac affinity is given during the exercise to monitor myocardial perfusion. An isotope commonly used is radioactive thallium-201, which can be substituted for potassium by cells and is infused during the peak portion of the exercise test. Other tracer isotopes include technetium 99m, sestamibi, and Tc 99m tetrofosmin. After a short delay, a nuclear scan of the heart is performed. Areas of the heart that have been perfused by blood will be labeled with the thallium. Areas of the heart that are poorly or not perfused by blood during the exercise test will be identified as cold spots, that is, without radiolabel. If the ischemia is temporary, the cold spots will disappear over time. Often patients are tested twice, once while at rest and once during exercise, and comparisons are made. If an individual is unable to exercise, dipyridamole or adenosine may be given to mimic the effect of physical activity on coronary blood flow.

In the majority of perfusion imaging studies single photon emission computed tomography (SPECT) is now being utilized. This allows better visualization of myocardial tissue from three different axes.

Echocardiography

Echocardiography involves ultrasound waves directed at the chest wall that are analyzed by a computer as they bounce back from the chest. The computer generates an image that is used to calculate the size and movement of the heart chambers, the performance of the valves, and the flow of blood through the heart. This test is highly sensitive and noninvasive and provides a visual image of the beating heart.

Because ultrasound waves cannot travel through air, transthoracic echocardiography may not be indicated for the patient with chronic lung disease or when mechanical ventilation is being used. The ultrasound waves are also impeded by bone, heavily calcified structures, and adipose tissue. In these cases, **transesophageal echocardiography** (TEF) may be indicated. Using conscious sedation, the transducer is guided down the esophagus to view the posterior heart structures and great vessels. TEF is useful for diagnosing endocarditis, valvular disorders, thrombi, tumors, aortic dissection, and congenital defects. The use of TEF during surgical repair of valvular disorders has been found to greatly improve outcomes. Since TEF is an invasive procedure it is reserved for situations in which transthoracic echocardiography would not be adequate for accurate diagnosis.

Cardiac Catheterization

In cardiac catheterization, also called **coronary angiogram**, a flexible tube (catheter) is inserted through a peripheral vein (femoral or brachial) into the right side of the heart, or through a peripheral artery (femoral or brachial) into the left side of the heart. Through the catheter, the chambers of the heart can be visualized and chamber pressures and oxygen content measured. A radiolabeled dye may be injected through the catheter, and the ability of the dye to move through the heart chambers and vessels may be monitored using x-ray techniques. Valve movement can be observed. Because cardiac catheterization is invasive, complications are possible, including tearing of the vessel wall. After the procedure, patients must lie still for 4 to 6 hours until leg vessels seal.

Computed Tomography Scan

The computed tomography (CT) scan is a combination of an x-ray scan of the heart coupled with multiple CT that produces highly detailed images of the arteries of the heart. Patients are given a radiolabeled dye to highlight the blood vessels, and then are exposed to a series of x-rays that create images of the heart in slices. These slices are reassembled by a computer to provide an image that can detail arterial narrowing, including that due to arterial calcium and fatty deposits. Risks include radiation exposure.

In a slightly different technique, called PET/CT scan, **positron emission tomography** (PET) is used in addition to the CT to provide even more detailed information than available by CT alone. Because a PET scan is expensive and not available at all facilities, it typically is used after specific vessels are identified by CT scan as being of concern.

A relatively new procedure for visualizing structures of the heart, great vessels, and the coronary arteries is the **multislice helical computed tomography**. Using 16-slice helican scanners, ECG gating, and iodinated contrast, the volume of the heart, the coronary arteries, and the proximal great vessels can be scanned in less than 25 seconds. Other advantages include:

- Spatial resolution is high enough to visualize branches in the coronary arteries, atherosclerotic plaques, and noncalcified plaques.
- Low-radiation scan.
- Visualization of the coronary artery lumen sufficient to measure the degree of luminal narrowing due to stenosis.

Magnetic Resonance Imaging

Magnetic resonance imaging (MRI) utilizes a powerful magnet that sets the nuclei of atoms in the heart cells vibrating at specific, recognized frequencies. The signals are analyzed by a computer to produce a detailed 3D image. MRI is noninvasive and very sensitive, but cannot be used on patients with pacemakers or metal implants such as stents. They also cannot identify calcium deposits in the coronary arteries.

Multiple-Gated Acquisition Scan (MUGA)

A radioactive substance is attached to red blood cells and then injected into the patient. The heart is scanned with a gamma camera that detects the tagged red blood cells. The MUGA scan shows the motion of the heart and measures the ejection fraction (amount of blood ejected from ventricle with each heart beat).

● Pathophysiologic Concepts

THROMBUS

A thrombus is a blood clot that can develop anywhere in the vascular system, causing the narrowing of a vessel. With a decrease in vessel diameter, blood flow can be occluded (reduced or totally blocked). A thrombus can develop from any injury to the vessel wall because endothelial cell injury draws platelets and other mediators of inflammation to the area. Many of these substances stimulate clotting and activation of the coagulation cascade. Thrombus formation can occur when blood flow through a vessel is sluggish, which is why most thrombi develop in the low-pressure venous side of the circulation, where platelets and clotting factors can accumulate and adhere to vessel walls. Similarly, when blood flow is irregular or erratic—for instance, during periods of irregular heartbeat or cardiac arrest—thrombus formation is enhanced. Endothelial damage, venous stasis, and hypercoagulability, commonly referred to as Virchow triad, summarize the etiology of venous thrombus formation.

EMBOLUS

An embolus is a substance that travels in the bloodstream from a primary site to a secondary site, becomes trapped in the vessels at the secondary site, and causes blood flow obstruction. Most emboli are blood clots (thromboemboli) that have broken off from their primary site (usually deep leg veins). Other sources of emboli include fat released during the break of a long bone or produced in response to any physical trauma, and amniotic fluid, which may enter maternal circulation during the intense pressure gradients generated by labor contractions. Air and displaced tumor cells may also act as emboli to obstruct flow.

Usually emboli are trapped in the first capillary network they encounter. For instance, emboli traveling from deep leg veins are delivered in the venous system to the vena cava and the right side of the heart. From there, they enter the pulmonary artery and arterioles, encounter pulmonary capillaries, and become trapped. Arterial thromboemboli usually develop in the heart, following a myocardial infarction or an episode of dysrhythmia. Thromboemboli from the heart can become trapped in the coronary vessels or any of the organs downstream, including the brain, kidneys, and lower extremities.

ANEURYSM

An aneurysm is a dilation of the arterial wall caused by a congenital or developed weakness in the wall. Weakness in the wall may develop as a result of an infection, from trauma, or, more commonly, from lesions produced by atherosclerosis. Aneurysms may burst with increased pressure, leading to massive internal hemorrhage.

ACUTE CORONARY SYNDROME

A term now being broadly used to encompass several cardiac events until a specific diagnosis is confirmed is acute coronary syndrome (ACS). ACS includes unstable angina, non-ST segment elevation myocardial infarction (MI), ST segment elevation MI, and any other manifestations which are the result of sudden myocardial ischemia. Fibrous plaque formation or thrombosis can cause occlusion of a coronary artery thus decreasing or totally occluding blood flow to the myocardium. Unstable and myocardial infarction will be discussed later in the chapter.

ALTERATIONS IN CAPILLARY FORCES OF FILTRATION OR REABSORPTION

Occasionally, forces favoring filtration from the capillary into the interstitial fluid are greater than forces favoring reabsorption of fluid into the capillary from the interstitial space. The result is net filtration. Net filtration across the capillary results in interstitial edema.

The opposite occurs when forces favoring reabsorption of fluid from the interstitial space into the capillary are greater than those favoring filtration. This results in net reabsorption, which leads to increased plasma volume, stroke volume, and cardiac output. Blood pressure may be increased significantly.

Causes of Increased Capillary Filtration

Causes of increased capillary filtration include increased capillary pressure, caused by high blood pressure, and increased capillary leakage, caused by injury or inflammation. An increase in protein concentration in the interstitial fluid caused by increased capillary breakdown or decreased lymph flow to the area would also cause net filtration, leading to edema and swelling of the interstitial space. Similarly, decreased production or increased loss of plasma proteins would reduce the reabsorption of fluid back into the capillary. This can occur with liver disease or loss of protein in the urine.

Causes of Increased Capillary Reabsorption

Causes of increased reabsorption of fluid from the interstitial space include decreased blood pressure in the capillary due to a decrease in systemic pressure or constriction of the arteriole or precapillary sphincter. Increased plasma colloid osmotic pressure also draws fluid back into the capillary. Plasma colloid osmotic pressure increases with dehydration, leading to a return of fluid from the interstitium to the plasma, which helps return plasma volume toward normal. Finally, increased interstitial fluid pressure increases reabsorption by opposing further accumulation of fluid.

STENOSIS

Stenosis is a narrowing of any vessel or opening. In the cardiovascular system, stenosis of the heart valves may occur. Stenosis of any valve usually occurs as a result of a congenital defect or an inflammatory process (e.g., after rheumatic fever). Stenosis results in increased pressure above the stenotic area and decreased blood flow below the area.

Results of Cardiac Valve Stenosis

Stenosis of a cardiac valve results in the chamber upstream of the stenosis pumping more forcefully to expel its blood through the narrowed orifice. After years of this extra work, cardiac muscle can hypertrophy (increase in size). If the chamber cannot pump forcefully enough to overcome the stenosis, blood flow out of the chamber will be reduced. Because of the chamber hypertrophy and the extra work it must do to pump through the narrowed orifice, the chamber increases its oxygen consumption and energy demands. The coronary arteries supplying the muscle may be unable to supply adequate oxygen to meet this demand.

As it becomes increasingly difficult for the upstream chamber to empty against the narrowed orifice, blood may accumulate in the chamber and stretch its muscle fibers. If this is significant or prolonged, a decrease in muscle contractility can result.

Examples of Cardiac Valve Stenosis

Any cardiac valve may become stenosed.

- Mitral stenosis is narrowing of the valve between the left atrium and left ventricle.

- Aortic stenosis is narrowing of the valve between the left ventricle and the aorta.
- Tricuspid stenosis is narrowing of the valve between the right atrium and the right ventricle.
- Pulmonary stenosis is narrowing of the valve between the right ventricle and the pulmonary artery.

VALVE INCOMPETENCE

An incompetent valve is one that does not close completely, allowing blood to move in both directions through that valve when the heart contracts (valve regurgitation). Any of the cardiac valves may be incompetent. Each chamber may hypertrophy. Stenosis and regurgitation result in turbulent blood flow, which can be auscultated as a **murmur** in the heart.

CARDIAC SHUNTS

In the cardiovascular system, a shunt is a connection between the pulmonary vascular system and the systemic vascular system. During fetal life, shunts between the right and left sides of the heart and between the aorta and pulmonary artery are normal. After birth, any shunting across the heart or between the pulmonary and systemic circulations is abnormal.

The direction in which blood flows through a shunt is determined by resistance to flow in each direction. Blood will flow in the direction of least resistance.

Right-to-Left Shunt

A right-to-left shunt is the flow of blood from the right side of the heart to the left, or from the pulmonary artery to the systemic circulation. After birth, right heart and pulmonary artery blood is poorly oxygenated. Therefore, a right-to-left shunt delivers poorly oxygenated blood to the systemic circulation. A right-to-left shunt is called a **cyanotic shunt** because delivery of poorly oxygenated blood to the systemic circulation causes cyanosis (bluish tinge to the skin). This is caused by deoxygenation of hemoglobin, as described in Chapter 14.

Fatigue results because cells of the muscles, brain, and other organs are not receiving adequate delivery of oxygen and nutrients. Respiratory rate increases as the body tries to compensate for the reduced oxygenation of the blood. Individuals with a cyanotic shunt may develop clubbing of the tips of the fingers, related to poor tissue perfusion.

Left-to-Right Shunt

A left-to-right shunt is the flow of blood from the left side of the heart to the right side, or from the aorta to the pulmonary circulation. Left heart blood is well oxygenated. Therefore, a left-to-right shunt overdelivers well-oxygenated blood directly into the right side of the heart, or it immediately returns the blood to the pulmonary artery and lungs. Blood going to the lungs from the left side of the heart recirculates to the left atrium and left ventricle. Because the blood is well oxygenated, this shunt is **acyanotic**.

A left-to-right shunt can be life-threatening because of the risk of hypertrophy of pulmonary vasculature as blood is continually recirculated through the lungs. Right-heart failure may develop if there is a high volume of blood entering the right side of the heart from the left side of the heart. In addition, left-heart failure may develop because of continual recycling of blood back into the left side of the heart from the lungs.

ALTERATIONS IN THE ELECTROCARDIOGRAM

Many conditions result in ECG alterations. Alterations in the ECG are associated with increased or decreased rate of contraction or changes in the force of contraction. Normal ranges for an ECG include:

- P–R interval (from the beginning of the P wave to the beginning of the QRS) 0.12 to 0.20 seconds.
- QRS complex (from beginning of QRS to end of S) 0.06 to 0.10 seconds.
- QT interval (from beginning of QRS to end of T wave) < 0.38 seconds.

Ectopic Pacemaker

An ectopic pacemaker is a site in the heart capable of automaticity that takes over control of the heart rate from the SA node. An ectopic pacemaker may occur if the SA node begins to depolarize very slowly, or if conduction of the signal from the SA node to the AV node is blocked. Usually, cells in the AV node or conducting cells of Purkinje fibers assume the pacemaker role.

If the SA node no longer controls the heart rate, an ECG will usually demonstrate a reduced heart rate and ventricular depolarization that does not follow atrial depolarization.

Sinus Arrest

Sinus arrest occurs when the SA node stops depolarizing and firing action potentials. This leads to an ectopic site taking control of the heart rate.

Atrial Dysrhythmias

Atrial dysrhythmias disrupt normal contraction of the atria. They may include ectopic pacemakers or irritation of the SA node.

Atrioventricular Blocks

Blocks of action potential spreading from the AV node may occur anywhere in the conducting system of Purkinje fibers or the bundle of His. A block may cause an extra long delay between the P wave and the QRS complex, or may totally uncouple the P wave from the QRS.

Blocks in Ventricular Conducting Branches

Conduction of the electrical signal from the AV node into and throughout the ventricle proceeds first through transitional fibers that join to form the bundle of His. The bundle of His enters the ventricles and immediately separates into left and right bundle branches. These branches supply the entire heart and terminate as very fine Purkinje fibers. Interruption of the signal anywhere in any of the conducting passages results in the entire ventricle taking longer to depolarize, spreading out the QRS complex. If some areas of the myocardium are completely blocked from receiving the excitation, the ventricular beat will be abnormal and inefficient. Cardiac output will decrease.

Ventricular Dysrhythmias

Ventricular dysrhythmia is an alteration in ventricular beating rate. A ventricular dysrhythmia can directly affect cardiac output; therefore, it is usually a more serious problem than an atrial dysrhythmia. Although an increase in heart rate can increase cardiac output, cardiac output also depends on stroke volume. An abnormally high heart rate can cause a significant decrease in stroke volume because if the heart rate increases too much, filling time for the ventricle will be inadequate. Table 13-3 summarizes some of the more common dysrhythmias and some ECG changes are shown in Figure 13-10.

TABLE 13-3 Common Cardiac Dysrhythmias	
Dysrhythmia	**Characteristics**
Sinus bradycardia	• Heart rate < 60 bpm • May occur in consistently conditioned athlete
Sinus tachycardia	• Heart rate > 100 bpm
Sinus arrhythmia	• Rhythm varies with respirations • Common in children and young adults
Sinus arrest	• P waves present and irregular • Rhythm is regular except when pause occurs
Premature atrial contraction (PAC)	• Early firing of action potential in the atria • Heart rate 60–100 bpm • Irregular rhythm due to premature beats

table continues on page 524

TABLE 13-3 Common Cardiac Dysrhythmias *(continued)*	
Dysrhythmia	**Characteristics**
Atrial flutter	• Atrial rate of 160–350 bpm • P waves are replaced with flutter waves • Regular rhythm • May result in hemodynamic instability
Atrial fibrillation	• Atrial rate > 350 bpm • No P waves • Irregular rhythm • Exercise may cause hemodynamic instability
First degree atrioventricular block	• P–R interval > 0.20 seconds
Second degree atrioventricular block	• Progressively lengthening P–R interval until a ventricular beat is dropped
Third degree atrioventricular block	• No relationship between P wave and QRS • Atrial rate 60–100 bpm • Ventricular or nodal rate 20–60 bpm
Bundle branch block	• QRS complex > 0.12 seconds
Premature ventricular contraction (PVC)	• Broad, premature QRS due to ectopic site in ventricle • Decreased stroke volume
Ventricular tachycardia	• QRS > 0.12 seconds, bizarre • Ventricular rate 100–250 bpm • Rhythm essentially regular • Significantly decreased stroke volume
Ventricular fibrillation	• Quivering ventricle • No cardiac output or BP • Results in death without intervention

● Conditions of Disease or Injury

ATHEROSCLEROSIS

Atherosclerosis, the most common type of arteriosclerosis or hardening of the arteries, is a condition of the large and small arteries characterized by accumulation of fatty deposits, platelets, neutrophils, monocytes, and macrophages throughout the tunica intima (endothelial cell layer) and eventually into the

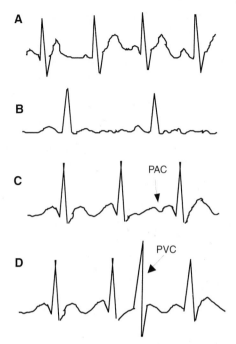

FIGURE 13-10 Electrocardiogram (ECG) depiction of a normal tracing (**A**); sinus bradycardia (**B**); premature atrial contraction (**C**); and premature ventricular contraction (**D**).

tunica media (smooth muscle layer). Arteries most often affected include the coronaries, the aorta, and the cerebral arteries.

The development of atherosclerosis begins with dysfunction of the endothelial cells lining the lumen of the artery. This may occur following injury to the endothelial cells, or from other stimuli. Injury to the endothelial cells increases their permeability to various plasma components, including fatty acids and triglycerides, allowing these substances access to the inside of the artery. Oxidation of fatty acids produces oxygen free radicals that further damage the vessel. Injury to the endothelial cells also initiates inflammatory and immune reactions, including the attraction of white blood cells (WBCs), especially neutrophils and monocytes, and platelets to the area. The white cells release potent proinflammatory cytokines that further aggravate the situation, drawing even more white cells and platelets to the area, stimulating clotting, activating T and B cells, and releasing chemicals that act as chemoattractants to perpetuate the cycle of inflammation, clotting, and fibrosis. Once drawn to the area of injury, the WBCs are caught there by activation of endothelial **adhesion factors** that act like Velcro to make the endothelium especially sticky to white cells. Once attached to the endothelial layer, the monocytes and neutrophils begin to emigrate between the endothelial cells, into the interstitial space. In the interstitium, the monocytes mature into macrophages and, along with the neutrophils, continue to release cytokines, which further the inflammatory cycle. The proinflammatory cytokines also stimulate smooth muscle cell proliferation, causing smooth muscle cells to grow into the tunica intima. Additional plasma cholesterol and fats gain access to the tunicae intima and media as permeability of the endothelial layer increases. An early indication of damage is the presence of a fatty streak in the artery. With continued injury and inflammation, platelet aggregation increases and a blood clot (thrombus) begins to form. Scar tissue replaces some of the vascular wall, changing the structure of the wall. The end results are cholesterol and fat buildup, scar tissue deposits, platelet-derived clots, and smooth muscle cell proliferation.

Even without direct injury to the endothelial cells, changes in the endothelial adhesion factors may occur, resulting in the accumulation of white cells and the release of inflammatory mediators and clot-forming substances. Why some individuals have especially active adhesion factors is unclear. It is likely that both genetic and environmental factors are involved.

Regardless of the precipitating event, atherosclerosis leads to a decrease in the diameter of the artery and an increase in its stiffness. The atherosclerotic area of an artery is called a **plaque**. The development of a plaque is shown in Figure 13-11.

Causes of Atherosclerosis

There are several hypotheses as to what first initiates dysfunction of the endothelial cells, thereby activating this cascade. It is likely that different initiating events are involved to different degrees in different people. Five hypotheses are presented.

High Serum Cholesterol

The first hypothesis suggests that high serum cholesterol and high levels of circulating triglycerides can cause development of atherosclerosis. Fatty deposits, called atheromas, are found throughout and inside the tunica media in persons with atherosclerosis.

Cholesterol and triglycerides are carried in the blood encased in fat-carrying proteins called **lipoproteins**. High-density lipoprotein (HDL) carries fat away from cells to be degraded and is known to be protective against atherosclerosis. Low-density lipoprotein (LDL) and very-low-density lipoprotein (VLDL) carry fat to the cells of the body, including the endothelial cells of the arteries. Especially at risk of atherosclerosis are persons who carry a defect in a specific apolipoprotein E protein normally involved in efficient hepatic uptake of lipoprotein particles, stimulation of cholesterol efflux from macrophages in the atherosclerotic lesion, and the regulation of immune and inflammatory responses. In the arterial wall, oxidation of cholesterol and triglycerides leads to inflammation and production of free radicals known to damage delicate endothelial cells.

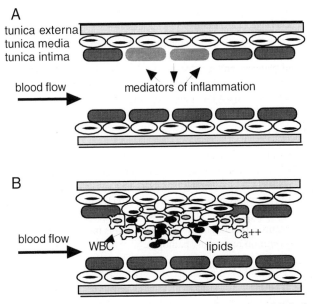

FIGURE 13-11 The formation of an atherosclerotic plaque with dysfunction of the endothelial cell (**A**) followed by white blood cell (WBC) migration and deposits of fat (foam) cells and calcium (**B**).

According to this hypothesis, the oxidative-modification hypothesis of atherosclerosis, the initial oxidation of LDL in the subendothelial layer of the arteries turns on various inflammatory reactions, which ultimately attract monocytes and neutrophils to the area. These WBCs become anchored to the endothelial layer by the adhesion molecules, and release additional inflammatory mediators that attract more white cells to the area and further stimulate LDL oxidation. Eventually, the monocytes move into the wall of the artery, where they mature into macrophages and internalize the LDL as fatty **foam cells**. Oxidized LDL is cytotoxic to vascular cells, further promoting inflammatory responses. According to this hypothesis, the higher the circulating level of LDL, the more frequently damage occurs.

Patients with diabetes mellitus often exhibit atherosclerosis caused by high cholesterol. Diabetes mellitus is a major risk factor for atherosclerosis. Persons with diabetes have high plasma cholesterol and triglycerides. Poor circulation to most organs causes hypoxia and tissue injury, also stimulating inflammatory reactions that contribute to atherosclerosis.

High Blood Pressure

The second hypothesis proposed for development of atherosclerosis is based on the finding that chronically high blood pressure produces shear forces that scrape away at the endothelial layer of the arteries and arterioles, initiating their injury. Shear forces especially occur in sites of arterial bifurcation (splitting) or bending, a trait characteristic of the coronary arteries, aorta, and cerebral arteries. With shearing of the endothelial layer, damage can occur repeatedly, leading to a cycle of inflammation, accumulation, and adhesion of WBCs and platelets, and clot formation. Any thrombus that develops can be sheared off the artery, leading to a thromboembolus downstream, or may grow large enough to obstruct blood flow. It may also weaken the artery, causing it to burst under the maintained high blood pressure.

Infection

A third hypothesis to explain how atherosclerosis develops suggests that some endothelial cells become infected by a circulating microorganism. Infection directly produces cell-damaging free radicals; it also initiates the cycle of inflammation, a process associated with free radicals and adhesion factor activation. WBCs and platelets arrive in the area and cause clots and scarring. A specific organism that has been implicated in this theory is *Chlamydia pneumoniae*, a common respiratory pathogen.

High Blood Iron Levels

A fourth hypothesis concerned with atherosclerosis of the coronary arteries is that high serum iron levels damage the coronary arteries or magnify damage from other insults. Iron is rapidly oxidized and capable of producing artery-damaging free radicals. This theory is suggested by some to explain the high incidence of coronary artery disease (CAD) in men compared with premenopausal women, who typically have lower levels of iron.

High Blood Homocysteine Levels

A fifth hypothesis suggests that persons with elevated plasma homocysteine levels have increased vascular disease. Homocysteine is an amino acid formed by the metabolism of methionine. Research suggests that hyperhomocysteinemia is associated with endothelial dysfunction, specifically manifested by a decreased availability of endothelium-derived nitric oxide, a local vasodilator. Hyperhomocysteinemia also increases susceptibility to arterial thrombosis and accelerates the development of atherosclerosis in apolipoprotein E–deficient mice. Homocysteine may also increase oxidation of LDL. Nutritional deficiencies in folic acid and the B vitamins are associated with elevated homocysteine.

Summary of Causes Inducing Atherosclerosis

Atherosclerosis occurs as a result of dysfunction of the endothelial cells lining the arteries, an occurrence that turns on inflammatory reactions and, in many cases, free radical production. Damage may occur from physical injury, such as hypertension, or chemical injury, such as elevated LDL, infection, heavy metal exposure, or chemical insult. Risk factors for the development of atherosclerosis may include smoking, glucose intolerance, elevated cholesterol, obesity, sedentary lifestyle, ineffective stress management, age, gender, and heredity.

Clinical Manifestations

Clinical manifestations of atherosclerosis usually occur late in the course of the disease and are the result of inadequate perfusion secondary to vessel obstruction.

- Intermittent claudication, an aching, cramping feeling in the lower extremities, occurs, especially during or after exercise. Intermittent claudication is caused by poor blood flow through atherosclerotic vessels supplying the lower limbs. When oxygen demand of the leg muscles increases, the limited flow cannot supply the extra oxygen required, and pain from muscle ischemia develops. As atherosclerosis worsens, intermittent pain can progress to pain during rest because even normal demands for oxygen cannot be met.
- Cold sensitivity occurs with inadequate blood flow to the extremities.
- Skin color changes occur as blood flow decreases to an area. With ischemia, the area becomes pale. This is followed by local autoregulatory responses, resulting in hyperemia (increased blood flow) to the area, causing the skin to flush red.
- Reduced arterial pulses may be felt downstream from an atherosclerotic lesion. If blood flow is inadequate to support metabolic needs, cell necrosis and gangrene may develop.
- Angina, stable or unstable, occurs with atherosclerosis of the coronary arteries.

Diagnostic Tools

- Elevated cholesterol and triglyceride levels may indicate a risk factor for atherosclerosis. Cholesterol levels higher than 180 mg/dL of blood are considered elevated, and the individual is considered especially at risk of CAD.
- Nuclear magnetic resonance (NMR) spectroscopy lipoprofiles are being recommended for high-risk individuals. This test quantifies different lipoproteins by subclass, identifies the amount of cholesterol carried by each LDL particle, and indicates the size of the particle. The tool has been helpful in early identification of high-risk individuals.
- A noninvasive technique called reactive hyperemia peripheral arterial tonometry (RH-PAT) is being evaluated for the potential to identify individuals with early-stage atherosclerosis. Return of digital blood volume is measured following a brief period of imposed ischemia. A sluggish return of blood in the extremities is postulated to indicate similar endothelial dysfunction at the level of the coronary arteries.

- Imaging of the arteries may allow visualization of atherosclerotic lesions. Identifying or monitoring atherosclerosis may be done using coronary or carotid artery CT, ultrasound, or MRI.

Complications

- Hypertension may develop from long-standing atherosclerosis, just as hypertension and high shear forces can cause atherosclerosis. With thrombus formation, scar tissue, and smooth muscle cell proliferation, the lumen of the artery is reduced and the resistance to flow through the artery increases. The left ventricle must pump more forcefully to produce enough pressure to drive blood through the atherosclerotic vascular system, which can result in increased systolic and diastolic blood pressures.

- A thrombus may dislodge by breaking off from an atherosclerotic plaque. This may lead to obstruction of blood flow downstream, causing a stroke if the blood vessels of the brain are occluded or a myocardial infarction if the blood vessels of the heart are affected.

- Development of an aneurysm, a weakening of the artery, may result from atherosclerosis. The aneurysm may burst, causing a stroke if it is located in the cerebral vasculature.

- Vasospasm may develop in atherosclerotic vessels. Normal endothelial cells act to block various vasoactive substances from directly binding to and acting on smooth muscle cells of the tunica media. If the endothelial layer is not intact, certain peptides such as serotonin and acetylcholine can diffuse directly to the underlying smooth muscle layer, causing the smooth muscle cells to constrict. This response may be involved in coronary artery spasm, or in the spasm of cerebral arteries known as a transient ischemic attack. Damage to the endothelial layer may also be a cause of male erectile dysfunction, since vasodilation of the penile arteries is required for an erection to develop.

- Myocardial infarction or sudden cardiac death may occur due to compromised myocardial perfusion.

Treatment

- Diet modification can lower LDL and improve HDL levels. High-fiber foods (fruits, vegetables, whole grains), fatty fish (omega 3 fatty acids), soy products (isoflavones), and garlic have been shown to lower LDL cholesterol.

- Drug therapy is frequently used to lower total cholesterol and triglyceride levels and improve HDL. Drugs known as statins are especially effective, although contraindications to their use exist and side effects may be serious. Fibrate therapy in conjunction with statins has been effective in reducing triglyceride levels.

- Aspirin or anticlotting drugs reduce risk of thrombus formation.

- A well-planned exercise program may reduce LDL, increase HDL concentrations, and lower body weight. Exercise may also stimulate development of collateral vessels around occluded sites.
- Good control of plasma glucose level is essential in diabetic patients.
- Cessation of smoking is essential for patients with atherosclerosis because of the damaging effects of smoke-related compounds on the endothelial cell wall.
- Antihypertensive medications will decrease shearing of the endothelial wall.
- Nitric oxide or nitroglycerin may be administered to patients experiencing vasospasm to relax the vessel wall.
- Antimicrobial therapy may offer protection against infectious injury to the endothelial layer.
- Blood donation by a man three times a year should reduce his iron levels to those seen in menstruating women, thereby reducing oxidative injury.

HYPERTENSION

Approximately 1 billion people worldwide are affected by hypertension, which is the most prevalent risk factor for cardiovascular disease. Hypertension is abnormally high blood pressure measured on at least three different occasions from a person who has been at rest at least for 5 minutes. Normal blood pressure varies with age, thus any diagnosis of hypertension must be age specific and based on serial readings. The 7th Joint National Committee on Prevention, Detection, Evaluation, and Treatment of High Blood Pressure has published revised guidelines on optimal and hypertensive values of systolic and diastolic pressures. In general, optimal pressures are considered less than 120 mm Hg systolic and 80 mm Hg diastolic, while pressures considered hypertensive are higher than 140 mm Hg systolic, and higher than 90 mm Hg diastolic. A state of "prehypertension" includes blood pressures between 120 and 139 mm Hg systolic and 80 and 89 mm Hg diastolic. For those with especially significant cardiovascular risk factors, including a strong family history of myocardial infarct or stroke, or a personal history of diabetes, even these prehypertensive values are too high.

Causes of Hypertension

Because blood pressure depends on heart rate, stroke volume, and TPR, an uncompensated increase in any of these variables can cause hypertension.

Increased heart rate may occur with abnormal sympathetic or hormonal stimulation to the SA node. Chronically increased heart rate frequently accompanies conditions of hyperthyroidism. However, increased heart rate is usually compensated for by decreases in stroke volume or TPR, and thus does not cause hypertension.

Chronically increased stroke volume may occur if there is a prolonged increase in plasma volume, since increased plasma volume is reflected as an increase in end-diastolic volume, and hence increased stroke volume and blood pressure. Increased end-diastolic volume is referred to as an increase in the **preload** of the heart. Increased preload is usually associated with an increased systolic blood pressure reading.

A prolonged increase in plasma volume may occur as a result of renal mishandling of salt and water, or it may result from excess salt consumption. Epidemiologic, migration, and genetic studies in humans and animals provide compelling evidence of a relationship between high salt intake and elevated blood pressure. From an evolutionary perspective, humans are adapted to ingest and excrete less than 1 g of salt per day, which is at least 10 times less than the average salt consumption in industrialized countries.

Besides excess dietary intake of salt, abnormally increased renin or aldosterone levels or decreased blood flow to the kidneys also may alter renal handling of salt and water.

Chronically increased TPR may occur with increased sympathetic or hormonal stimulation to the arterioles, or with an overresponsiveness of the arterioles to normal stimulation, both of which would cause a narrowing of the vessels. With increased TPR, the heart has to pump more forcefully, and therefore exert more pressure, to drive the blood through the narrow vessels. This is referred to as an increase in the **afterload** of the heart, and is usually associated with an increased diastolic pressure reading. With a prolonged increase in afterload, the left ventricle may begin to hypertrophy (increase in size). As a result, the ventricle's own oxygen demands increase further, causing it to pump even more forcefully to meet those demands.

Each of the possible causes of hypertension mentioned may result from increased sympathetic nervous system activity. For many people, increased sympathetic nerve stimulation, or perhaps overresponsiveness of the body to normal sympathetic stimulation, may contribute to the development of hypertension. This may result from a prolonged stress response, which is known to involve sympathetic activation, or from a genetic excess of receptors for norepinephrine in the heart or vascular smooth muscle. Other genetic influences may be racially determined. For instance, there is evidence that African Americans, who generally report more frequent and more severe hypertension, demonstrate an alteration in sodium–calcium pumping such that calcium accumulates in the smooth muscle cells, increasing muscle contraction and resistance. Other risk factors include obesity, excessive alcohol intake, low potassium intake, smoking, stress, sedentary lifestyle, family history, and advancing age.

Types of Hypertension

Hypertension is often classified as either primary or secondary, based on whether a cause can be identified. Most cases of hypertension have no known cause and are called primary or essential hypertension. When a clear cause of hypertension can be identified, it is called secondary hypertension.

Secondary Hypertension

An example of secondary hypertension is renal vascular hypertension, which develops as a result of renal artery stenosis. This condition may be congenital or a result of atherosclerosis. Renal artery stenosis reduces blood flow to the kidney, leading to activation of renal baroreceptors, stimulation of renin release, and production of angiotensin II. Angiotensin II increases blood pressure directly by increasing TPR, and indirectly by increasing aldosterone synthesis and sodium reabsorption. If repair of the stenosis is possible or the affected kidney is removed, blood pressure returns to normal.

Other causes of secondary hypertension include pheochromocytoma, an epinephrine-secreting tumor of the adrenal gland, which causes increased heart rate and stroke volume, and Cushing disease, which causes increased stroke volume from salt retention and increased TPR as a result of hypersensitivity of the sympathetic nervous system. Primary aldosteronism (increased aldosterone with no known cause), diabetes mellitus, coarctation of the aorta, brain tumor, head injury, thyroid or parathyroid dysfunction, cocaine, oral contraceptives, and other medications may also cause secondary hypertension.

Hypertension in Pregnancy

Hypertension in a pregnant woman carries risk to both the mother and fetus. Four categories of hypertension in pregnancy have been identified by the National Institutes of Health Working Group on High Blood Pressure in Pregnancy: gestational hypertension, chronic hypertension, preeclampsia–eclampsia, and preeclampsia superimposed on chronic hypertension.

Gestational hypertension is a type of secondary hypertension because, by definition, the elevation in blood pressure (>140 mm Hg systolic; >90 mm Hg diastolic) occurs after 20 weeks' gestation in a previously nonhypertensive woman, and reverses within 12 weeks postpartum. Gestational hypertension appears to result in part from a combination of increased cardiac output and increased TPR. If hypertension persists beyond 12 weeks postpartum, or was present before 20 weeks' gestation, it is categorized as chronic hypertension.

With preeclampsia, high blood pressure is accompanied by proteinuria (urinary excretion of at least 0.3 g protein in 24 hours). Preeclampsia typically develops after 20 weeks' gestation and is associated with decreased placental blood flow and the release of chemical mediators that cause dysfunction of vascular endothelial cells throughout the body. It is a very serious disorder, as is preeclampsia superimposed on chronic hypertension.

Clinical Manifestations

Hypertension has been referred to as the "silent killer" because symptoms may not be present until significant damage has occurred. Most clinical manifestations occur after years of hypertension, and include:

- Waking headache, sometimes with nausea and vomiting, caused by increased intracranial blood pressure.
- Epistaxis.
- Bruits.
- Blurred vision caused by hypertensive damage to the retina.
- Confusion.
- Fatigue.
- Dizziness or unsteadiness in the gait caused by central nervous system damage.
- Nocturia caused by increased renal blood flow and glomerular filtration.
- Dependent edema and swelling caused by increased capillary pressure.

Diagnostic Tools

- Diagnostic measurement of blood pressure using a sigmoid cuff manometer will show elevated systolic and diastolic pressures in an individual before any symptoms of the disease are present.
- Proteinuria is present in women with preeclampsia.
- Following a diagnosis of hypertension, further testing is indicated to determine if any target organ damage has occurred. Tests may include blood urea nitrogen, creatinine, chest x-ray, urinalysis, and complete eye exam.

Complications

See page C10 for illustrations of common complications.

- Stroke may result from a high-pressure hemorrhage in the brain or from an embolus broken off a noncerebral vessel exposed to high pressure. Strokes may occur with long-standing hypertension if arteries supplying the brain become hypertrophied and thickened, thereby reducing blood flow to areas of the brain that depend on them. The cerebral arteries that are atherosclerotic may become weak, increasing the likelihood of an aneurysm.
- A myocardial infarct (MI) may occur if the atherosclerotic coronary arteries cannot supply adequate oxygen to the myocardium or if a thrombus develops that blocks flow through a vessel. With chronic hypertension and the development of ventricular hypertrophy, the oxygen demands of the myocardium may not be met, and cardiac ischemia leading to an infarct may

occur. Likewise, ventricular hypertrophy may cause changes in the timing of electrical conductance through the ventricle, leading to dysrhythmia, cardiac hypoxia, and an increased risk of clot formation. Hypertrophy may also result in heart failure.

- Renal failure may occur with progressive high-pressure damage to the renal capillaries, the glomeruli. With glomerular injury, blood flow to the functional units of the kidney, the nephrons, is impaired, and these can become hypoxic and die. With damage to the glomerular membranes, proteins will be lost in the urine, decreasing the plasma colloid osmotic pressure and contributing to edema, which is often seen with long-standing hypertension.

- Encephalopathy (brain damage) may occur, especially with malignant (swiftly progressing, dangerous) hypertension. The dramatically high pressure seen in this condition causes increased cerebral capillary pressure and drives fluid into the interstitial space throughout the central nervous system. Surrounding neurons collapse, and coma and death may result.

- Retinopathy due to vascular damage.

- Metabolic syndrome (see Chapter 16).

- Seizures may develop in women with preeclampsia. The infant may be born small for his or her gestational age because of poor placental perfusion, and may suffer hypoxia and acidosis if the mother develops a seizure before or during the birth process.

Treatment

To treat hypertension, one can lower heart rate, stroke volume, or TPR. Pharmacologic and nonpharmacologic interventions may help an individual reduce his or her blood pressure.

- Weight loss appears to reduce blood pressure in some people, perhaps by reducing the workload of the heart, and therefore heart rate and stroke volume.

- Exercise, especially coupled with weight loss, reduces blood pressure by reducing resting heart rate and possibly TPR. Exercise increases HDL levels, which may reduce the development of atherosclerosis-associated hypertension.

- Relaxation techniques may reduce heart rate and TPR by interrupting the sympathetic stress response.

- Quitting smoking is important in reducing the long-term effects of hypertension because cigarette smoke is known to reduce blood flow to various organs and can increase the work of the heart.

- Diuretics act by several different mechanisms to reduce cardiac output by causing the kidney to increase its excretion of salt and water. Some diuretics (thiazides) also decrease TPR.

- Calcium channel blockers decrease cardiac or arterial smooth muscle contraction by interfering with the calcium influx needed for contraction. Some calcium channel blockers are more specific for cardiac muscle slow calcium channels; some are more specific for vascular smooth muscle calcium channels. Calcium channel blockers vary in their ability to preferentially reduce heart rate, stroke volume, and TPR.

- Angiotensin II–converting enzyme inhibitors (ACE inhibitors) act to decrease angiotensin II by blocking the enzyme needed to convert angiotensin I to angiotensin II. This decreases blood pressure directly by decreasing TPR, and indirectly by decreasing aldosterone secretion, thereby increasing loss of sodium in the urine and reducing plasma volume and cardiac output. Converting enzyme inhibitors also lower blood pressure by prolonging the effects of the vasodilator bradykinin, which is normally broken down by converting enzyme. *ACE inhibitors are contraindicated in pregnancy.*

- Angiotensin receptor blockers (ARBs) bind to angiotension I receptors, thus preventing the effects of angiotensin II. The result is decreased blood pressure, decreased vascular resistance, and smooth muscle contraction. Similar to ACE inhibitors, ARBs have not been as effective in black patients although in combination with thiazide diuretics, antihypertensive effects have been potentiated.

- Beta-receptor antagonists (β-blockers), especially selective β_1-blockers, act on the beta receptors of the heart to decrease heart rate and cardiac output.

- Alpha-receptor antagonists (α-blockers) block the vascular smooth muscle receptors that normally respond to sympathetic stimulation with vasoconstriction. This reduces TPR.

- Direct arteriolar vasodilators may be used to decrease TPR.

- Some individuals may benefit from a sodium-restricted diet. A healthy diet of fruits, vegetables, whole grains, low-fat milk products, low saturated fat, and low cholesterol foods with limited alcohol intake is also encouraged.

- Gestational hypertension and preeclampsia–eclampsia are reversed upon delivery of the infant.

RAYNAUD DISEASE

Raynaud disease is a primary vascular disease characterized by a temporary spasm of the small arteries and arterioles, usually in the fingers or, less frequently, the toes. Spasm of the blood vessels leads to tissue hypoxia. Spasms may be initiated by an abnormal epithelium. Usually, there is no lasting damage with an episode of spasm. However, if the spasms are extensive or very frequent, tissue injury and scarring can occur. The cause of Raynaud disease is unknown, but is usually seen in young women in response to cold exposure. Other triggers may include excessive alcohol or caffeine intake, smoking, cocaine, and amphetamines.

Raynaud phenomenon is a secondary disease that can occur following repeated exposure to vibration, such as would be experienced by a jackhammer operator. It might also develop in an individual who has suffered damage from previous cold exposure, or in an individual suffering from a systemic disease such as lupus erythematosus or scleroderma.

Clinical Manifestations

- Pallor (whiteness) due to vasospasms followed by cyanosis (bluish tinge) of the digits due to hypoxia, and then rubor (redness) as the local mechanisms of vasodilatation take over and arterial blood flow returns.
- Affected area will be cool due to arterial constriction and diminished blood flow.
- Numbness of the digits, then tingling and pain as the episode ends.

Diagnostic Tools

- A good physical examination and history will assist diagnosis.
- Cold stimulation challenge.
- Nail-fold capillaroscopy to determine the presence of deformed capillaries and distinguish between primary and secondary Raynaud disease.
- Antinuclear antibody (ANA) titer may be done to rule out an autoimmune disorder as the underlying cause.

Complications

- Gangrene may occur if episodes are extensive.
- Late onset of Raynaud disease may be an early indication of autoimmune disease.

Treatment

- Avoid unnecessary exposure to the cold and vibrations.
- Calcium channel blockers or alpha-adrenergic blockers.
- Biofeedback and relaxation techniques to manage stress.
- Treat underlying disease if present.

VARICOSE VEINS

Varicose veins are tortuous (twisted) distended veins occurring where blood has pooled, often in the legs. Since blood flow in the veins is driven by contraction of surrounding skeletal muscles that squeeze blood back to the heart, long episodes of standing without muscle contraction can lead to pooling of blood in the legs. Varicose veins may also develop if valves that normally prevent backflow of blood become incompetent, thereby delivering even more blood to the next backstream valve. If this valve becomes incompetent as well, blood will continue to fill up the veins below. The pressure from the blood causes the vein to distend and become weak. As elasticity is lost veins will become twisted and lumpy. Increased hydrostatic pressure pushes plasma into the interstitial spaces resulting in edema.

Valve incompetence (weakness) can be a hereditary predisposition, or it may occur following trauma to the valves. Obesity may contribute to the risk of developing varicose veins because of the associated sedentary lifestyle and the increased volume of blood pressing on the valves. Similarly, pregnant women are at increased risk of developing varicose veins because of their increased blood volume and body weight.

Clinical Manifestations

- Bulging, distended veins, showing prominent bluish streaks and pools in the legs.
- Pain may be present.

Diagnostic Tools

- Physical examination and family history will assist diagnosis.
- Doppler ultrasound to assess blood flow.
- Angiography to assess valve function.
- Manual compression test.

Complications

- A blood clot may develop, since the risk of clotting increases when blood pools or is sluggish in its flow.
- Chronic venous insufficiency may occur if blood pooled in the vascular system is enough to significantly reduce cardiac output. Edema in the feet and ankles will be apparent. Leg ulcers may eventually develop.
- Phlebitis.

Treatment

- Weight reduction.
- Elevation of the legs to assist blood flow return to the heart.
- Avoidance of tight-fitting clothes at the top of the legs or waist, which can restrict blood flow.
- Elastic support hose for the lower legs to compress the veins, assisting blood flow return to the heart.
- Walking and exercise to increase muscle strength and contraction of the leg muscles to increase blood flow return to the heart.

- Sclerotherapy, the injection of a sclerosing agent into a collapsed superficial vein, will cause fibrosis of the vein.
- Surgical stripping of the veins or cauterization may be performed.
- Radiofrequency vein ablation.

ANGINA PECTORIS

Angina pectoris is severe pain originating from the heart that occurs in response to an inadequate oxygen supply to the myocardial cells. The pain of angina may radiate down the left arm, to the back, to the jaw, or into the abdominal area.

When the workload of any tissue increases, oxygen demand goes up. If the oxygen demand increases in healthy hearts, the coronary arteries dilate and bring more blood flow and oxygen to the muscle. However, if the coronary arteries are stiffened or narrowed with atherosclerosis and cannot dilate in response to an increased demand for oxygen, myocardial ischemia (inadequate blood supply) occurs, and the myocardial cells begin to use anaerobic glycolysis to meet their energy requirements. This form of energy production is very inefficient and results in the production of lactic acid. Lactic acid decreases myocardial pH and causes the pain associated with angina pectoris. If the energy demands of the cardiac cells are lessened, the oxygen supply becomes adequate and the muscle cells revert to oxidative phosphorylation for energy production. This process does not produce lactic acid. With removal of the accumulated lactic acid, the pain of angina goes away. Angina pectoris is therefore a short-lived experience.

Types of Angina

There are three types of angina: stable, Prinzmetal (variant), and unstable.

Stable angina, also called classic angina, occurs when atherosclerotic coronary arteries cannot dilate to increase flow when oxygen demand is increased. Increased work of the heart can accompany physical exercise such as sports participation or climbing stairs. Exposure to the cold, especially in conjunction with work such as snow shoveling, increases the metabolic demands of the heart and is a strong stimulator of classic angina. Mental stress, such as that caused by anger or by mental tasks such as mathematics, may trigger classic angina. The pain of stable angina typically goes away when the individual stops the activity.

Prinzmetal angina occurs without any obvious increase in the workload of the heart, and in fact frequently occurs during rest or sleep. In Prinzmetal (variant) angina, a coronary artery undergoes a spasm, causing cardiac ischemia to occur downstream. Sometimes the site of spasm is related to atherosclerosis. At other times, the coronary arteries do not appear to be sclerotic. It is possible that even if no visible lesions are apparent on the artery, subtle damage to the endothelial layer may be present. This allows vasoactive peptides direct access to the smooth muscle layer, causing its contraction. Dysrhythmias are common with variant angina.

Unstable angina is a combination of classic and variant angina, and is seen in an individual with worsening CAD. It usually accompanies an increased workload of the heart. It appears to result from coronary atherosclerosis, characterized by a growing, spasm-prone thrombus. Spasm occurs in response to vasoactive peptides released from platelets drawn to the area of damage. The most potent constrictors released by the platelets are thromboxane, serotonin, and platelet-derived growth factors. As the thrombus continues to grow, episodes of unstable angina increase in frequency and severity, and the individual is at increased risk of suffering irreversible damage. Unstable angina is included along with myocardial infarction under the heading **acute coronary syndrome** and requires a thorough clinical workup, sometimes including hospitalization.

Clinical Manifestations

- Constricting or squeezing pain in the pericardial or substernal area of the chest, possibly radiating to the arms, jaw, or thorax.
- In stable and unstable angina, pain is typically relieved by rest. Prinzmetal angina is unrelieved by rest but usually disappears in about 5 minutes.

Diagnostic Tools

- Alteration in the ST segment of the ECG may occur.
- Areas of reduced blood flow may be observed using radioactive imaging during an induced angina episode as part of an exercise stress test.
- Cardiac enzymes and proteins may be measured to rule out MI.

Treatment

- Prevention: Aspirin is sometimes prescribed to prevent anginal symptoms. Also, individuals prone to angina are encouraged to avoid stressors known to precipitate attacks of classic angina, such as working in the cold. They are strongly encouraged not to smoke.
- Invasive techniques such as percutaneous transluminal **coronary angioplasty** (PTCA) and **coronary artery bypass** surgery reduce episodes of classic angina. With PTCA, the atherosclerotic lesion is dilated by a catheter inserted through the skin into the femoral or brachial artery and fed into the heart. Once in the affected coronary vessel, a balloon in the catheter is inflated. This cracks the plaque and stretches the artery. With bypass surgery, the diseased piece of a coronary artery is tied off, and an artery or vein taken from elsewhere in the body is connected to nondamaged areas. Flow is reinstated through this new vessel. The vessels most frequently transplanted are the saphenous vein and the internal mammary artery. Initial

response to PTCA appears good, but vessels frequently (20% to 40% of the time) become sclerotic again within a few months. Placing artificial tubes, or stents, into the artery to keep it open improves outcome. Drug-coated stents may reduce the rate of stent restenosis. Coronary bypass relieves the pain of angina, but does not appear to affect long-term mortality.

- Since the cause of angina is insufficient oxygen to meet the energy demands of the heart, once angina does occur, treatment is geared at reducing energy demands:

  - **Rest** allows the heart to pump out less blood (decreased stroke volume) at a slower rate (decreased heart rate). This reduces the work of the heart, and therefore its oxygen requirements. Sitting is the preferable posture for rest, since lying down increases blood return to the heart, leading to increased end-diastolic volume, stroke volume, and cardiac output.

  - **Nitroglycerin** and other nitrates act as potent dilators of the venous system, decreasing venous return of blood to the heart. A decreased venous return decreases end-diastolic volume, allowing the heart to decrease stroke volume. Nitrates dilate the arterial system as well, reducing the afterload against which the heart must pump, and increasing coronary blood flow. Dilation of a coronary artery undergoing spasm also may occur with nitrates. These effects reduce the inequalities of oxygen demand versus supply, and nitroglycerin given sublingually (under the tongue) usually reverses angina.

  - **Beta-adrenergic blockers** reduce angina by reducing heart rate and contractility of the heart, thereby reducing its oxygen demands. Calcium channel blockers also reduce the afterload against which the heart must pump by dilating the arteries and arterioles downstream and are particularly effective in reducing the spasm of variant angina. Calcium channel blockers should not be used in patients at risk of heart failure.

  - **Oxygen therapy** eases demands on the heart.

MYOCARDIAL INFARCTION

Myocardial infarction (MI) is the death of myocardial cells that occurs following prolonged oxygen deprivation. It is the culminating lethal response to unrelieved myocardial ischemia. Myocardial cells begin to die after about 20 minutes of oxygen deprivation. After this period, the ability of the cells to produce ATP aerobically is exhausted, and the cells fail to meet their energy demands.

Without ATP, the sodium–potassium pump quits, and the cells fill with sodium ions and water, eventually causing them to lyse (burst). With lysis, cells release intracellular potassium stores and intracellular enzymes, which injure neighboring cells. Intracellular proteins gain access to the general circulation and the interstitial space, contributing to interstitial edema and swelling around the myocardial cells. With cell death, inflammatory reactions are initiated. At the site of inflammation, platelets accumulate and release clotting factors. Mast cell degranulation occurs, resulting in the release of histamine and various prostaglandins. Some are vasoconstrictive and some stimulate clotting (thromboxane).

Effect of an MI on Cardiac Depolarization, Cardiac Contractility, and Blood Pressure

With the release of potassium ion and the various intracellular enzymes, and with the accumulation of lactic acid, the electrical conduction pathways of the heart are altered. This can result in interruption of atrial or ventricular depolarization, or in initiation of a dysrhythmia.

With the death of muscle cells and changes in the heart's electrical patterns, the heart begins to pump in a less-coordinated manner, causing contractility to decrease. Stroke volume falls, causing a fall in systemic blood pressure.

Reflex Responses to a Fall in Blood Pressure

Decreased blood pressure triggers the baroreceptor responses, leading to activation of the sympathetic nervous system and the renin–angiotensin system, and increasing the release of ADH. Stress hormones (ACTH and cortisol) are also released, which increases glucose production. Activity of the parasympathetic nervous system decreases.

With increased sympathetic and decreased parasympathetic nervous stimulation to the SA node, heart rate increases. Likewise, sympathetic and angiotensin stimulation of the arterioles causes an increase in TPR. Blood flow to the kidneys is reduced, reducing urine production and contributing to the stimulation of the renin–angiotensin system. Constriction of the arterioles causes a decrease in capillary pressure, reducing the capillary forces favoring filtration. Net reabsorption of interstitial fluid occurs, increasing the plasma volume and increasing venous return. Aldosterone synthesis stimulates sodium reabsorption which, in the presence of ADH, increases plasma volume further. Sympathetic simulation to the sweat glands and skin causes the individual to sweat and feel cool and clammy to the touch.

In summary, more blood (increased preload) is delivered to the heart, which is pumping at a faster rate against a narrowed arterial vasculature (increased afterload). The net result of activation of all the reflexes, which occur because of reduced cardiac contractility and fall in blood pressure, is to *increase the workload of the already damaged heart*. Oxygen demands of the heart increase. This can be disastrous because the initial problem causing the myocardial infarct was insufficient oxygen supply to heart cells. As the reflexes further increase the demands on the damaged heart, more and more cardiac cells become hypoxic. When oxygen demands of more cells cannot be met, zones of injured and ischemic cells increase around the central necrotic (dead) zone.

These injured and ischemic cells are at risk of dying. The pumping ability of the heart falls further, and hypoxia of all tissues and organs, including surviving areas of the heart, occurs. Finally, as blood is erratically or ineffectually pumped, it begins to move sluggishly through the vessels of the heart. This, along with accumulation of platelets and other clotting factors, increases the risk of blood clot development.

Causes of Myocardial Infarct

Myocardial infarct is usually the outcome of a long-standing CAD. For example, a common cause of an MI is the rupture and dislodgement of an atherosclerotic plaque from one of the coronary arteries, and the subsequent obstruction of blood flow that occurs as it is trapped downstream. An MI might also occur if a thrombotic lesion adhering to a damaged artery becomes large enough to totally obstruct flow downstream, or if a heart chamber becomes so hypertrophied that it is unable to meet its oxygen demands, for example, in a patient with long-standing hypertension.

Risk factors for developing CAD and/or MI (CAD/MI) include a positive family history, hypertension, hypercholesterolemia, obesity, smoking, and diabetes. Particular genotype patterns may also place individuals at risk of CAD/MI. For example, recent studies of a few families with high rates of CAD/MI have identified mutations in a gene known as *MEF2A*, which codes for one of the transcription factors known as myocyte enhancer factor–2. In its normal expression, this protein is involved in the early stages of vasculogenesis (formation of new blood vessels); mutations may compromise its ability to perform this function, resulting in increased susceptibility to heart disease. Hormonal factors may also contribute to CAD/MI. Although previously thought to be protective against CAD/MI, recent results from the Women's Health Initiative suggest that estrogen, given either alone or with progesterone to postmenopausal women, may increase the risk of heart attack. Cortisol, associated with the acute response to stress, is also associated with an increased risk of MI. Some evidence suggests that African Americans have poorer outcomes following an MI due late diagnosis, in addition to known risk factors including chronically high stress. Use of cocaine and amphetamines have also been shown to increase the risk of MI.

Clinical Manifestations

Although some individuals do not show any obvious signs of an MI (a silent heart attack), significant clinical manifestations usually occur:

- Abrupt (usually) onset of pain, often described as severe and crushing in nature. The pain may be compared to that of "an elephant sitting on my chest." The pain may radiate anywhere on the upper body, but most often radiates to the left arm, neck, or jaw. Nitrates and rest might relieve ischemia outside the necrotic zone by decreasing the workload of the heart but will not relieve the pain of infarct completely.

- Nausea and vomiting, probably related to intense pain, are common.
- Feelings of weakness related to decreased blood flow to the skeletal muscles occur. Studies have shown that, for women, lethargy or fatigue may be the key or only symptom present with infarct.
- Other symptoms commonly experienced by women include abdominal pain, indigestion, clammy skin, or light-headedness.
- The skin becomes cool, clammy, and pale due to sympathetic vasoconstriction.
- Urine output decreases related to decreased renal blood flow and increased aldosterone and ADH.
- Tachycardia develops, due to increased cardiac sympathetic stimulation and anxiety.
- A mental state of great anxiety and a feeling of doom often develop, perhaps related to release of stress hormones and ADH (vasopressin).

The European Society of Cardiology, American College of Cardiology Foundation, American Heart Association, and the World Health Foundation developed a universal definition of myocardial infarction and created a classification system for six types of MI. The criteria for Type 1 and Type 2, which are the most common, include a rise and/or fall in cardiac biomakers (one must be above 99th percentile of upper reference limit) plus at least one of the following:

- Manifestation of ischemia.
- ECG change consistent with ischemia.
- Pathologic Q waves in the ECG.
- New loss of viable myocardium or new regional wall motion abnormality identified with imaging.

Diagnostic Tools

- A good history and physical examination, including family history of heart disease, are important, especially for diagnosing an MI in a patient who might otherwise be considered at low risk, such as a premenopausal woman.
- Blood pressure may be decreased or normal depending on extent of myocardial damage and success of the baroreceptor reflexes. Heart rate is usually increased. A fourth heart sound may be heard.
- The ECG may show acute changes with elevation in the ST segment and T wave inversion. Within 1 or 2 days of the infarct, deepening of the Q wave occurs. Although the ST and T wave changes will disappear over time, the Q wave changes remain and can be used to detect a past infarct.
- Systemic signs of inflammation occur, including fever and elevated number of leukocytes. Sedimentation rate and C-reactive protein may be elevated

due to inflammation. These signs begin about 24 hours after the infarct and continue for up to 2 weeks.

- Cardiac enzyme levels (creatinine phosphokinase, SGOT, and lactic dehydrogenase) in the serum increase as a result of myocardial cell death. The increases occur in a characteristic pattern, beginning immediately after an infarct and continuing for about a week.

- Troponin T and troponin I levels become detectable in the blood within 15 to 20 minutes. Myoglobin is detected within 1 hour, peaking within 4 to 6 hours of the infarct. Table 13-2 summarizes changes in common cardiac enzymes.

- Elevated glucose due to catecholamine release.

- Echocardiogram, chest x-ray, nuclear imaging, and cardiac catheterization.

Complications

- Thromboemboli may develop as myocardial contractility falls. These emboli can block blood flow to other regions of the heart not previously damaged during the original infarct. They may also travel to other organs, blocking their blood flow and causing infarction in those organs.

- Congestive heart failure may occur when the failing heart cannot pump out all the blood it is receiving. Heart failure may develop soon after an infarct if the original infarct is very large, or may occur subsequent to activation of the baroreceptor reflexes. With activation of baroreceptor responses, there is increased blood returned to the damaged heart and constriction of the downstream arteries and arterioles. This causes blood to accumulate in the heart and leads to overstretch of the cardiac muscle cells. If the overstretch is severe enough, it can cause the contractility of the heart to decrease further as the muscle cells begin to fall down the length–tension curve.

- Dysrhythmia, the most common complication of an infarct, may develop due to alteration in electrolyte balance and decreased pH. Hypoxic areas of the heart may become irritable and initiate action potentials, also leading to dysrhythmia. The SA or AV nodes, or the transduction pathways (Purkinje fibers or the bundle of His), may be part of the necrotic or ischemic zones, thereby affecting signal initiation or passage. Fibrillation is the primary cause of death following a myocardial infarct outside the hospital setting.

- Cardiogenic shock (collapse of blood pressure) may occur with a prolonged, severe decrease in cardiac output. Cardiogenic shock may be fatal at the time of the infarct, or may cause death or disability days or weeks later as a result of subsequent pulmonary or renal failure following ischemia. Cardiogenic shock usually follows at least a 40% loss of myocardial muscle mass.

- Myocardial rupture may occur after a large infarct.

- Pericarditis, an inflammation of the heart, may occur, usually a few days after the infarct. Pericarditis occurs as part of the inflammatory reaction following cardiac cell injury and death. Some types of pericarditis may occur weeks after the infarct and may represent an immune hypersensitivity reaction to tissue necrosis.

- With healing after a myocardial infarct, scar tissue replaces dead myocardial cells. If this represents a large area of the myocardium, contractility of the heart may be permanently reduced. In some cases the scar tissue may be weak, leading to later myocardial rupture or development of an aneurysm.

Treatment

Prevention of heart disease is vital. Prevention involves:

- Reducing or eliminating modifiable risk factors. Since cardiovascular risk factors interact with each other, even moderate reductions in a few risk factors can be more effective than instituting a major reduction in any one risk factor. For example, a significant reduction in the risk of heart attack occurs with moderate levels of exercise (including walking), cessation of smoking, and moderate limitation of dietary fat. Cardiovascular risk management guidelines that integrate risk reductions should be used routinely.
- Individuals under stress, and especially those with a family history of heart disease, should be educated to reduce risks and to seek medical attention quickly if signs of an MI develop.

For a patient with acute coronary syndrome (ACS), the following treatment guidelines, using the acronym ABCDE, have been proposed:

- **A** for antiplatelet therapy, anticoagulation, ACE inhibition, and angiotensin receptor blockade
- **B** for beta-blockade and blood pressure control
- **C** for cholesterol treatment and cigarette smoking cessation
- **D** for diabetes management and diet
- **E** for exercise.

For a patient suffering a heart attack, the following treatments are added:

- Cessation of physical activity to reduce the workload of the heart helps to limit the area of damage.
- Cardiopulmonary resuscitation (CPR) may be required if the heart is in fibrillation or arrest. Electrical defibrillation to restore electrical rhythm within the first minutes of cardiac arrest is especially helpful in surviving an MI. Recent communitywide efforts that focus on intensive training of the public in the use of defibrillators have been shown to double the survival rate of cardiac arrest victims. Immediate care may also include lidocaine, atropine, epinephrine, transcutaneous pacing patches, or transvenous pacemaker.

- Immediate intravenous or intracoronary infusions of thrombolytic (clot-busting) drugs break up a causative embolus. Rapid use of these drugs (preferably within an hour of the infarct) is associated with a dramatically increased survival rate and a limited extent of further myocardial injury. Drugs to prevent new clot development, such as low-molecular-weight heparin or clopidogrel, are also required. Glycoprotein IIb/IIIa receptor blockers may reduce thrombus formation (not to be used in patients with a recent bleeding episode). Coronary angioplasty may be used to open coronary arteries instead of clot-busting drugs.

- Oxygen is provided to increase oxygenation of the blood, reducing demands on the heart and increasing systemic perfusion.

- Pain medications (usually morphine and meperidine [Demerol]) are used to make patients more comfortable, decrease mental stress and anxiety, and reduce the activity of the sympathetic nervous system, which raises heart rate and vascular resistance in response to acute pain. Morphine is also a vasodilator that works to decrease preload and afterload.

- Nitrates may be provided to decrease venous return and relax the arteries, decreasing preload and afterload and increasing coronary blood flow.

- Diuretics that increase blood flow may be provided. This preserves kidney function and prevents volume overload and development of congestive heart failure. Increased renal blood flow also reduces the release of renin.

- Positive inotropic agents (digitalis) may be used to increase the contractility of the heart.

- Coronary artery bypass may be considered if the infarct was due to a thrombotic occlusion.

After an MI, additional considerations include:

- Cardiac rehabilitation, involving a balance between rest and exercise and lifestyle modifications to reduce atherosclerotic risks and hypertension. Following the ABCDEs for ACS is essential. The family needs to be considered and involved.

- New research has shown that the heart contains stem cells that can regenerate cardiac muscle cells, and so is capable of repairing itself. These findings may offer hope to patients who have experienced an MI.

PERICARDITIS

Pericarditis is inflammation of the fluid-filled pericardial sac surrounding the heart. Pericarditis can occur with any cardiac trauma, including a myocardial infarct, blunt or penetrating trauma to the chest, infection (bacterial, fungal, or viral), or neoplasm. Radiation to the chest, uremia, autoimmune disease, certain drugs, aortic aneurysm, myxedema, kidney disease, rheumatic fever, and other systemic diseases may also cause pericarditis.

A noxious stimulus to the pericardial tissue stimulates the release of chemical mediators of inflammation into the surrounding areas initiating the inflammatory process. The release of histamine causes vessel dilation and increased vessel permeability, which results in protein leakage and edema formation. Phagocytosis causes an accumulation of exudates and necrotic tissue that is usually reabsorbed within a few days. This exudate may be purulent if a bacterial infection is present. Acute pericarditis usually resolves on its own in 2 to 6 weeks. Chronic pericarditis is diagnosed if the condition does not resolve. It is usually associated with other symptoms of heart disease or systemic inflammation.

Clinical Manifestations

- Sharp chest pain, usually with a rapid onset, that worsens when the individual breathes, coughs, or changes position. Pain is lessened when the individual sits up and leans forward.
- Difficulty breathing and a dry cough.
- Fever is usually present.

Diagnostic Tools

- A friction rub can be heard with a stethoscope due to the inflamed sac rubbing over the heart with each beat. Heart sounds may be muffled.
- Systemic signs of inflammation (fever, elevated sedimentation rate, and increased leukocyte count) may occur.
- Cardiography can indicate fluid accumulation in the pericardial sac.

Complications

- Pericardial effusion may develop due to fluid accumulation. If the accumulation is rapid, cardiac compression can occur.
- Cardiac tamponade, compression of the heart due to extensive buildup of fluid or blood in the pericardial sac, may occur if the pressure in the pericardial sac increases to a level equal to or greater than that of the diastolic pressure of the heart. This causes diastolic filling of the heart to cease, collapsing stroke volume and cardiac output.

Treatment

- Bed rest, with elevation of the head of the bed to improve breathing.
- Oxygen therapy.
- Nonsteroidal anti-inflammatories, corticosteroids, and diuretics.
- Antibacterial, antifungal, or antiviral therapy if an infectious cause is suspected.

- Drainage of the pericardial fluid (pericardiocentesis) or removal of the pericardium (pericardectomy) may be performed.

MYOCARDITIS

Myocarditis is inflammation of the heart not related to CAD or myocardial infarct. The inflammation may result in hypertrophy, fibrosis, and inflammatory changes, which affect the myocardium and the conduction system. Myocarditis most often is a result of a viral infection of the myocardium, but may be caused by a bacterial or fungal infection. Coxsackievirus is often implicated. Systemic disease such as lupus erythematosus may also cause the disorder.

Myocarditis results in weakening of the heart muscle and a decrease in cardiac contractility. The heart becomes flabby and dilated, with many foci of pinpoint hemorrhage developing in the endocardium, myocardium, and epicardial layers. Myocarditis is a major cause of heart transplantation in the United States.

Clinical Manifestations

- Chest pain.
- Fatigue and dyspnea.
- Tachycardia, S_3 and S_4 gallops, murmur, pericardial friction rub, dysrhythmias.

Diagnostic Tools

- Systemic signs of inflammation include elevated sedimentation rate and leukocytosis.
- Elevated levels of antiviral antibodies, frequently against the coxsackievirus, are seen.
- ECG shows diffuse ST-segment and T-wave abnormalities, conduction problems, supraventricular arrhythmias.
- Radionuclide scan indicates inflammatory and necrotic changes.
- Echocardiography and coronary artery catheterization show normal arteries and cardiac valves. Biopsy of the muscle shows inflammation.

Complications

- Heart failure.
- Arrhythmia leading to sudden death.
- Thromboembolism.

Treatment

- Treatment of infectious cause or systemic disease.
- Corticosteroids and immunosuppressants.

- Control of heart failure.
- Heart transplantation.

CARDIOMYOPATHY

Cardiomyopathy refers to any disease or injury of the heart not related to CAD, hypertension, or congenital malformations. Cardiomyopathy may occur following an infection of the heart, as a result of an autoimmune disease, or following the exposure of an individual to certain toxins, including alcohol and many anticancer drugs. Cardiomyopathy may also occur idiopathically.

Cardiomyopathies can be divided into four categories based on abnormal structure and function. With dilated cardiomyopathy, the ventricle stretches, leading to heart failure. With hypertrophic myopathy, cardiac muscle thickens, especially along the interventricular septum. This makes the ventricle stiff, resulting in reduced compliance and diastolic filling. Restrictive cardiomyopathy is the result of decreased ventricular compliance and endocardial fibrosis and thickening that causes restricted ventricular filling and can be irreversible in severe cases. Arrhythmogenic right ventricular cardiomyopathy (ARVC) involves replacement of the normal myocardial tissue with fibrous fatty tissue. It may also involve the left ventricle. There tends to be a high familial association and most often occurs in young adults.

Clinical Manifestations

- Dyspnea (difficulty breathing) and fatigue may occur if cardiac output is reduced.
- Dysrhythmia may occur as a result of atrial stretching.
- Palpitations and syncope.
- Weight gain, bloating, and edema.
- Emboli may develop as a result of sluggish coronary blood flow.
- Chest pain may be present.

Diagnostic Tools

- An ECG or echocardiogram will demonstrate a thickened myocardium.
- Chest x-ray shows an enlarged heart.
- Echocardiography reveals dilation, dysfunction, and/or hypertrophy of the left ventricle and a thickened asymmetrical intraventricular septum.
- Thallium scan to determine perfusion defects.
- Cardiac catheterization to determine filling pressures and myocardial perfusion.

Complications

- A myocardial infarct may occur if oxygen demand of the thickened ventricle cannot be met. Sudden death may also occur.
- Heart failure may occur in dilated cardiomyopathy if the heart cannot pump out as much blood as is entering.
- Emboli formation from pooled blood.

Treatment

- Salt restriction and diuretics are used for dilated cardiomyopathy to reduce end-diastolic volume. Other treatments for heart failure may be required.
- Anticoagulants are provided to prevent the formation of emboli. Examples include warfarin, heparin, and a new therapy, ximelagatran. Recent findings show that ximelagatran has fewer side effects than the older drugs, and monitoring may not need to be as stringent. Ximelagatran has few known food or drug interactions.
- β-blockers are provided for hypertrophic cardiomyopathy in order to decrease the heart rate, allowing increased diastolic filling time. They also reduce ventricular stiffness.
- Surgical resection of some areas of hypertrophied myocardium may be attempted (myotomy or myectomy).
- Calcium channel blockers are not used since they may further decrease contractility of the heart.
- Valve repair and cardiac transplant may be necessary.

HEART FAILURE

Heart failure occurs when the heart is unable to pump out enough blood to meet the oxygen and nutrient demands of the body. Heart failure can result from either diastolic or systolic dysfunction.

Diastolic heart failure may develop alone or in conjunction with systolic heart failure. It often follows prolonged hypertension. When the ventricle must pump continually against a very high afterload (increased resistance), muscle cells hypertrophy and become stiff. Stiffness of the muscle cells causes a reduction in ventricular compliance, leading to decreased ventricular filling, abnormal diastolic relaxation, and decreased stroke volume. Left ventricular end-diastolic volume (LVEDV) and left ventricular end-diastolic pressure (LVEDP) are elevated and reflected back into the pulmonary circulation, causing pulmonary hypertension. Because stroke volume and hence blood pressure fall, baroreceptor reflexes are activated.

Systolic dysfunction as a cause of heart failure results from injury to the ventricle, usually from a myocardial infarct. The damaged muscle is unable to contract forcefully, and again, stroke volume falls. Decreased stroke volume leads to a decrease in blood pressure, quickly followed by the initiation of reflex responses geared to reverse the trend. Because the damaged ventricle is unable to bring stroke volume back up, the reflexes continue. In particular, sympathetic stimulation of cardiac β_1-receptors becomes chronic. Research suggests that the chronically activated sympathetic response ultimately reduces calcium levels in, and release of calcium from, the myocardial cell's sarcoplasmic reticulum. Reduction in myocardial calcium causes defective excitation–contraction coupling, leading to diminished myocardial force production, dysrhythmia, and eventual contractile dysfunction and cardiac muscle cell remodeling.

Also worsening the path of heart failure is the effect the progressive increase in end-diastolic volume has on stretching the cardiac muscle cell well beyond its optimum length, causing less tension to be produced as the ventricle becomes more distended with blood. Heart failure becomes a worsening cycle: the more overfilled the ventricle becomes, the less blood it can pump out, leading to further accumulation of blood and additional stretch of the muscle fibers. As a result, stroke volume, cardiac output, and blood pressure all remain low. The body's reflex responses initiated in response to the fall in pressure continue unabated and significantly worsen the situation.

Reflexes Initiated During Heart Failure

Decreased blood pressure is sensed by the baroreceptors. Most reflex responses initiated by baroreceptor activation significantly advance heart failure progression as shown in Figure 13-12. This occurs because the reflex responses either further increase ventricular filling (preload) or further reduce stroke volume by increasing the afterload against which the ventricle must pump. Increased preload and afterload serve to increase the workload and oxygen demand of the heart. If the increased oxygen demand cannot be met, the muscle fibers become increasingly hypoxic and contractility worsens. The downward spiral of heart failure continues.

As each of these reflexes further fill and stretch the heart and/or increase afterload, blood pressure continues to be below normal, causing those same reflexes to be maintained and heightened. As described above, the chronically activated sympathetic response leads to diminished intracellular calcium release from the sarcoplasmic reticulum, and ultimately to contractile dysfunction. Heart failure continues unless the cycle of overfill, decreased stroke volume, and decreased blood pressure is broken.

One reflex response that is advantageous during heart failure is that which occurs from atrial overfilling. As blood is poorly pumped out of the ventricle, it soon begins to accumulate in the atria. Expansion of the atria leads to stretching of atrial baroreceptors and the release of the hormone ANP. ANP works on the kidney to increase the excretion of sodium ion (natriuresis). Since, under most circumstances, water excretion follows sodium excretion, production

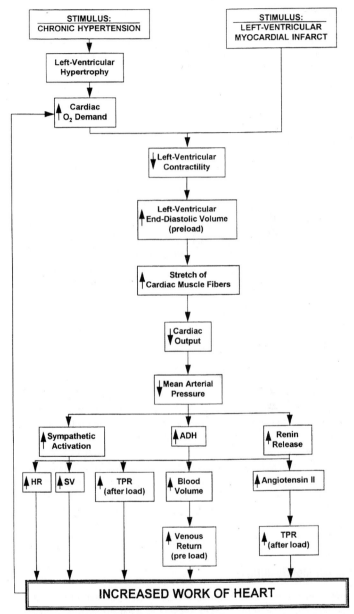

FIGURE 13-12 Flow diagram of heart failure.

of ANP is one mechanism by which the body is able to rid itself of excess fluid volume. ANP also relaxes vascular smooth muscle, causing vasodilation. A second natriuretic peptide, called B-type natriuretic peptide (BNP), is released in the form of a precursor peptide, pro-BNP, from an overstretched ventricle. Once in the circulation, pro-BNP is converted to BNP. Similar to ANP, BNP is natriuretic and vasodilatory. Serum levels of both of these hormones, especially BNP, are significantly correlated with heart failure severity and are excellent markers of disease progression.

Causes of Heart Failure

Heart failure may result from noncardiac causes such as long-standing systemic or pulmonary hypertension or, less commonly, disorders such as kidney failure or water intoxication, which increase plasma volume to such a degree that the ventricular fibers are stretched beyond their optimum length.

Cardiac causes of heart failure include myocardial infarct, cardiac myopathy, valvular defects, and congenital malformation. Pathways leading to heart failure following myocardial infarct and chronic hypertension are highlighted in Figure 13-12. As shown in the figure, if increased oxygen demand of a hypertrophied ventricle cannot be met by increased blood flow (usually because of coronary atherosclerosis), ventricular contractility will fall. In this case, diastolic dysfunction and systolic dysfunction are both present.

Progression of Heart Failure

Heart failure can begin on either the left or right side of the heart. For instance, long-standing systemic hypertension would cause the left ventricle to hypertrophy and fail. Long-standing pulmonary hypertension would cause the right ventricle to hypertrophy and fail. The site of a myocardial infarct would determine which side of the heart is first affected following a heart attack.

Because a failing left ventricle would cause blood to back up in the left atrium, and then to the pulmonary circuit, right ventricle, and right atrium, it is apparent that left heart failure can eventually lead to right heart failure. In fact, the main cause of right heart failure is left heart failure. As blood is poorly pumped out of the right side of the heart, it begins to pool in the peripheral venous system. The end result is a further reduction in circulating blood volume and blood pressure, and a worsening cycle of heart failure.

Clinical Manifestations

Clinical manifestations of heart failure are often separated into forward and backward effects, with the right or left side of the heart as the starting point. Forward effects are considered downstream from the failing myocardium. Backward effects are considered upstream from the failing myocardium.

Forward Effects of Left Heart Failure

- Decreased systemic blood pressure
- Fatigue
- Increased heart rate
- Decreased urine output
- Plasma volume expansion

Backward Effects of Left Heart Failure

- Increased pulmonary congestion, especially when lying down
- Dyspnea (difficult breathing)
- Right heart failure if the condition worsens

Forward Effects of Right Heart Failure

- Decreased pulmonary blood flow
- Decreased blood oxygenation
- Fatigue
- Decreased systemic blood pressure (due to decreased left heart filling), and all the signs of left heart failure

Backward Effects of Right Heart Failure

- Increased venous pooling of blood, edema of the ankles and feet
- Jugular venous distension
- Hepatomegaly and splenomegaly

Diagnostic Tools

- A third heart sound may be present.
- Radiologic identification of pulmonary congestion and ventricular enlargement may indicate heart failure.
- MRI or ultrasound identification of ventricular enlargement may indicate heart failure.
- Measurement of ventricular end-diastolic pressure with a catheter inserted into the pulmonary artery (reflecting left ventricular pressure) or into the vena cava (reflecting right ventricular pressure) can diagnose heart failure. Left ventricular pressure usually reflects left ventricular volume.
- Echocardiography can demonstrate abnormal dilation of the cardiac chambers and abnormalities in contractility.
- Measurement of serum BNP (and to a lesser extent, ANP) provides information on disease severity and progression. Normal levels vary with age (baseline increases with age) and gender (increased levels in women compared to men), so a patient's age and sex need to be considered when evaluating results.

Treatment

- Health-promotion behaviors such as smoking cessation, limited alcohol consumption, regular physical activity, sodium-restricted diet, and medication compliance to manage hypertension and metabolic syndrome.
- Best-practice guidelines released by the American Heart Association have identified the use of β-blockers and ACE inhibitors as the most effective therapies for heart failure unless specific contraindications exist. β-blockers reduce heart rate, allowing for improved stroke volume. ACE inhibitors reduce afterload (TPR) and plasma volume (preload). ARBs may be used in place of ACE inhibitors.
- Diuretics are administered to decrease plasma volume, thereby decreasing venous return and removing some of the stretch on the cardiac muscle fibers.
- Oxygen therapy may be used to reduce the demands of the heart.
- Nitrates may be administered to reduce afterload and preload.
- Clinical trials of nitric oxide boosting drugs (BiDil) for some patients with heart failure, in particular African Americans, suggest that such drugs both improve patients' quality of life and prolong survival.
- Aldosterone blockers (epleronone) have been approved for the treatment of congestive heart failure following a heart attack.
- Digoxin (digitalis) may be administered to increase contractility. Digoxin acts directly on the cardiac muscle fibers to increase the strength of each contraction regardless of the length of the muscle fibers. This increases cardiac output, relieving the ventricle of volume and lessening the stretch of the chamber. Digitalis is used less for the treatment of heart failure now than in the past.
- Implantable cardioverter defibrillators (ICD). Although there is a risk for another heart failure event with the use of ICDs, evidence supports a decreased risk when accompanied with β-blockers and ACE inhibitors.
- Cardiac resynchronization therapy with or without a defibrillator.
- Compassionate end-of-life care and hospice when heart failure becomes refractory.

RHEUMATIC FEVER

Rheumatic fever is a serious inflammatory disease that may occur in an individual 1 to 4 weeks following an untreated throat infection by the group A beta-hemolytic *Streptococcus* bacteria. The acute condition is characterized by fever and inflammation of the joints, heart, nervous system, and skin. In some cases, it can permanently affect the structure and function of the heart, especially the heart valves. Rheumatic fever is a relatively rare illness, however, affecting only 3% of those with untreated streptococcal infections. Rheumatic fever is preventable with prompt antibiotic therapy.

Rheumatic fever can occur at any age, but mainly affects children between the ages of 5 and 15. It is likely that individuals who develop the disease, and those who experience repeated infections, have a genetic tendency to do so.

Rheumatic Heart Disease

Approximately 10% of individuals who acquire rheumatic fever develop rheumatic heart disease. Rheumatic heart disease is the major cause of acquired cardiac valve disease. Damage to the heart with rheumatic fever occurs as a result of a robust host immune response that, although produced against the streptococcal antigens, cross-reacts against self-antigens expressed on the heart valves. This immune response involves both humoral (B cell) and cell-mediated (T cell) immunity. The attack against self-antigens is likely related to an antigenic similarity between cardiac valves and antigens of the group A beta-hemolytic streptococcus, and/or to an error in the presentation of host antigens to the immune cells. Immune attack can occur against any of the four cardiac valves, but is usually seen against the mitral and aortic valves.

The course of rheumatic heart disease can be separated into acute and chronic stages. In the acute stage, the valves become swollen and red as the inflammatory reaction begins. Lesions may develop on the valve leaflets. As the acute inflammation subsides, scar tissue develops. Scar tissue may deform the valves and, in some cases, cause the leaflets to fuse together, narrowing the orifice. A chronic stage of the disease may follow, characterized by repeated inflammation and continued scarring.

Associated Effects of Rheumatic Fever

Besides affecting the heart, rheumatic fever has other systemic effects. These include migratory (moving) joint inflammation and pain, occurrence of skin nodules, and occasionally a rash. The central nervous system is affected, causing behavioral changes, awkwardness in walking and speech, and a type of movement called chorea, characterized by spontaneous, jerky motions. These nervous system manifestations usually regress over the course of a few weeks or months.

Clinical Manifestations

- Throat culture is positive for group A beta-hemolytic streptococcus. History of the infection usually includes headache, fever, swollen lymph nodes along the jaw, and stomach pain or nausea.
- Migratory polyarthritis occurs, with inflammation of the joints (swelling, redness, pain, heat). The large joints of the elbows, knees, ankles, and wrists are often affected.
- Subcutaneous hard nodules develop over the muscles of affected joints. These nodules are painless and transitory.
- Erythema marginatum (a transitory rash) is seen, especially on trunk, inner arms, and thighs.

- Chorea (rapid, jerky movements) may occur, accompanied by clumsiness in movement.
- Behavioral changes may become apparent.

Diagnostic Tools

- Antistreptolysin O titer is increased in individuals after a streptococcal infection.
- Signs of inflammation during the acute phase of rheumatic heart disease include fever, arthralgia (joint pain), elevated sedimentation rate, and increased number of leukocytes.
- Elevated C-reactive protein is measurable in the serum. This protein is released by the liver as part of the immune system response to the streptococcal bacteria.
- An Aschoff body, a fibrous area of tissue necrosis, may be present on the heart.

Complications

- A heart murmur may develop in an individual without a previous murmur, or a worsening of a previous murmur may occur, if rheumatic heart disease develops.
- Cardiomegaly (increased size of the heart), pericarditis, or congestive heart failure in a previously well individual may also occur.

Treatment

- The most important method available for reducing the harmful effects of rheumatic fever and rheumatic heart disease is to promptly identify the occurrence of a beta-hemolytic streptococcal infection and provide a full course of antibiotic therapy.
- If rheumatic fever develops, interventions to limit the disease include administration of antibiotics and anti-inflammatory drugs. Restriction of activities to reduce cardiac demand is also suggested.
- To prevent recurrence of rheumatic fever in susceptible individuals, prophylactic antibiotics (usually penicillin) are administered for at least 5 years after the most recent occurrence. Education on the signs and symptoms of a streptococcal infection, and the need for prompt treatment, should be provided to the entire family.

VALVULAR DISORDERS

The two main types of valvular disorders are stenosis and regurgitation. Stenosis is a narrowing that prevents full opening of the valve. A regurgitant valve is unable to completely close, thus allowing the backflow of blood. Regurgitation may also be referred to as insufficient or incompetent. Table 13-4 summarizes

TABLE 13-4   Valvular Disorders

	Description	Clinical Manifestations
Mitral valve stenosis	• Narrowing in the opening of the valve between the left atrium and left ventricle • May be due to scar tissue following cardiac infection or congenital defect • Blood will pool in the left atrium and back up into the lung and eventually into the right heart if the atria is not able to generate enough force to push the blood through the stenosed valve • If cardiac output is decreased, right heart failure may occur • If systemic blood pressure drops, baroreceptor reflexes will stimulate sympathetic and hormonal responses to increase plasma volume and TPR	• Absent or severe depending on level of stenosis • Pulmonary congestion with dyspnea and pulmonary hypertension • Dizziness and fatigue due to decreased left ventricular output • Tachycardia due to sympathetic stimulation
Aortic valve stenosis	• Narrowing in the opening of the valve between the left ventricle and the aorta • Result of rheumatic fever or congenital defect • Left ventricle must pump hard to overcome stenotic valve resulting in hypertrophy and decreased compliance • Blood backs up in ventricle, then atria, then pulmonary system and right heart	• Absent or severe depending on level of stenosis • Pulmonary congestion with dyspnea and pulmonary hypertension from blood backing up in the pulmonary vascular system • Dizziness and fatigue due to decreased cardiac output and decreased stroke volume • Tachycardia due to sympathetic stimulation

table continues on page 560

TABLE 13-4 Valvular Disorders *(continued)*

	Description	Clinical Manifestations
Pulmonary valve stenosis	• Narrowing in the opening between the right ventricle and pulmonary vein • Typically due to congenital defect • Right ventricle must pump more forcefully resulting in hypertrophy • Blood backs up in right atrium causing dilation of vena cava and blood accumulation in systemic veins • Decreased blood flow to lungs and left heart if severe resulting in decreased BP	• Absent or severe depending on level of stenosis • Weakness and fatigue due to poorly oxygenated blood from decreased pulmonary blood flow • Venous distention and swelling of ankles and feet
Mitral valve regurgitation	• Blood returns to left atrium from left ventricle, especially with ventricular contraction • Due to failure of mitral valve to completely snap shut with ventricular systole • Caused by bacterial heart infection or valve rupture from coronary artery disease • Decreased ventricular stroke volume and cardiac output resulting in decreased BP and baroreceptor reflex activation • Chronic ventricular dilation and filling can lead to hypertrophy	• Absent or severe depending on degree of valve incompetence • Pulmonary congestion, dyspnea, pulmonary hypertension • Dizziness and fatigue due to decreased stroke volume and decreased cardiac output • Tachycardia due to sympathetic stimulation
Aortic valve regurgitation	• Blood returns to left ventricle from aorta during diastole	• Wide pulse pressure (difference between systolic and diastolic pressures)

Description	Clinical Manifestations
• Due to cardiac infection • Decreased diastolic pressure in aorta leading to increase in pulse pressure • Increased left ventricular diastolic volume due to blood entering from left atrium and aorta • Increased stroke volume and cardiac output	• Hyperkinetic (very strong) peripheral and carotid pulsations • Symptoms of heart failure may develop

the valvular disorders based on location and structural dysfunction. Diagnostic tools, complications, and treatment for all types of valvular disorders are included below.

Diagnostic Tools

- Auscultation of a murmur.
- Echocardiography may be used to diagnose abnormal valve structure and motion.

Complications

- Mitral valve stenosis: left atrial hypertrophy may cause atrial dysrhythmia or right heart failure.
- Aortic valve stenosis: left ventricular hypertrophy may develop, leading to congestive heart failure.
- Pulmonary valve stenosis: right heart hypertrophy and subsequent right heart failure may occur.
- Mitral valve regurgitation: left ventricular and left atrial hypertrophy may develop, leading to congestive heart failure.
- Aotic valve regurgitation: left ventricular hypertrophy that may lead to congestive heart failure.

Treatment

- Treatment for congestive heart failure may be required.
- Valve replacement or surgical correction of the stenosis may be attempted.

Mitral Valve Prolapse

Mitral valve prolapse (MVP), also referred to as systolic-click-murmur syndrome, floppy mitral valve syndrome, or Barlow syndrome, is the most common cardiac valve disease in the United States. The mitral valve leaflets bulge into the left atrium causing regurgitation during systole. MVP occurs more frequently in females and tends to be genetically inherited as a dominant gene. Other possible causes include endocarditis, myocarditis, connective tissue disorder, and it may just be idiopathic.

The vast majority of people with MVP are asymptomatic or only mildly symptomatic. The pain associated with MVP is due to stretching of the chordae tendineae and papillary muscle during the prolapse. Feelings of impending doom and anxiety may also be present.

CONGENITAL HEART DEFECTS

Congenital heart defects involve abnormal shunting between the left and right sides of the heart or between the aorta and pulmonary artery. The direction of blood flow in the shunt depends on the relative resistance of the pulmonary and systemic circulations.

Usually, pulmonary vascular resistance falls and systemic vascular resistance increases following birth. If a shunt is present under these conditions, the direction will be left to right. Well-oxygenated blood will flow from the left side of the heart into the right side or into the pulmonary circulation, resulting in overfilling of the pulmonary circuit and, since the blood is immediately delivered again into the left atrium, overfilling of the left side of the heart. Overfilling may lead to pulmonary congestion and left heart failure. If blood is delivered directly to the right side of the heart from the left through an opening in the septal wall, right heart failure may develop.

In a premature infant, resistance to flow in the pulmonary circulation may be greater than resistance in the systemic circulation due to immature development of the lungs, resulting in a right-to-left shunt. In a right-to-left shunt, poorly oxygenated blood is delivered into the systemic blood supply, causing cyanosis. A shunting pathway that causes cyanosis is called a cyanotic defect.

Types of Congenital Heart Defects

Congenital heart defects may involve the atria, the ventricles, any of the valves, or the great arteries.

Atrial Septal Defect

An atrial septal defect (ASD) is an abnormal opening between the left and right atria. It is a congenital disorder that occurs when the foramen ovale fails to close after birth, or when another opening between the left and right atria is present due to improper closure of the wall between the two atria during gestation.

Ventricular Septal Defect

A ventricular septal defect (VSD) is an abnormal opening between the left and right ventricles that occurs when the wall between the ventricles fails to close properly during gestation. VSD is the most common cardiac congenital defect. The size of the defect determines the severity of the symptoms.

Patent Ductus Arteriosus

Patent ductus arteriosus (PDA) occurs when the ductus arteriosus, the connection between the pulmonary artery and the aorta, remains open after birth. Normally, the ductus closes soon after birth as a result of increased oxygenation in the pulmonary circulation. If the ductus does not close, blood will shunt between the two main arteries. The direction of blood flow will depend on the relative resistance to flow of the pulmonary and systemic circulation.

Transposition of the Great Vessels

Transposition of the great vessels is a congenital heart defect in which the openings of the aorta and pulmonary artery are switched; that is, the aorta originates in the right ventricle and the pulmonary artery originates in the left ventricle. This reversal results in separation of the left and right heart circulations.

Blood flows in the pulmonary vein to the left atrium. From there it flows to the left ventricle and back through the pulmonary artery to the lungs, to cycle again to the left atrium. This blood is oxygenated, but does not supply the systemic circulation.

At the same time, blood flows in the vena cava to the right atrium, to the right ventricle, through the aorta to the systemic circulation, and back again to the vena cava. This blood is not oxygenated. Obvious signs of cyanosis will be apparent.

Transposition of the great vessels is incompatible with life unless, as is frequently the case, a septal defect or a PDA maintains communication between the two circulations. If no communication is present, surgical opening of the atrial septum is required until major surgery to redirect blood flow can be performed.

Coarctation of the Aorta

Coarctation of the aorta is a congenital defect that results in the narrowing of the aorta as it leaves the left ventricle. The narrowing can be proximal or distal to the ductus arteriosus.

Aortic coarctation that occurs proximal to the ductus arteriosus is called preductal coarctation. If the coarctation is severe, the major source of systemic blood flow will be pulmonary artery blood flowing through the ductus arteriosus. In order to keep infants with preductal coarctation alive until the stenosis can be surgically repaired, the ductus must remain open. This is accomplished by administering prostaglandin E intravenously or into the duct. Preductal coarctation is a cyanotic defect.

Postductal coarctation occurs if the narrowing is distal to the ductus arteriosus. In this case, the duct usually closes. However, blood leaves the aorta via subclavian arteries, which branch off before the coarctation, and travels to the upper body. The result is an obvious disparity in the upper and lower body pulses, depending on the degree of coarctation. Systemic signs of poor blood flow will be apparent. Collateral vessels that deliver blood to the systemic circulation frequently develop around the coarctation.

Tetralogy of Fallot

Tetralogy of Fallot is a congenital heart defect characterized by four presenting abnormalities: VSD, pulmonary artery stenosis, right ventricular hypertrophy, and a shifting of the position of the aorta so that it opens into the right ventricle (an overriding aorta). Tetralogy of Fallot is a cyanotic defect.

Clinical Manifestations

- With a right-to-left shunt, cyanosis, fatigue, and weakness occur. Knee-to-chest or squatting behavior may be observed. Clubbing of the digits may develop.
- With a left-to-right shunt, pulmonary congestion and dyspnea may occur. Left heart failure may develop.

Diagnostic Tools

- With an ASD, a splitting of the second heart sound is frequently heard because closure of the pulmonary valve may be prolonged.
- With a VSD, a systolic murmur is usually present.
- Postductal coarctation causes disparity in upper and lower body pulses and blood pressure.
- Doppler echocardiography to show cardiovascular structures and blood flow direction and velocity.
- MDCT has a fast scan time, excellent resolution, and is more cost effective than MRI.

Treatment

- Some defects may be small, require no treatment, or close spontaneously.
- Surgical correction of the defect is often required.
- Treatment for congestive heart failure may be necessary.
- Prostaglandin E is administered to maintain patency of the ductus arteriosus in preductal coarctation.
- Administration of the prostaglandin inhibitor indomethacin will initiate closure of the ductus in patent ductus arteriosus.

SHOCK

Shock is the collapse of systemic arterial blood pressure. With a severe fall in blood pressure, blood flow does not adequately meet the energy demands of tissues and organs. In addition, the body responds by diverting blood away from most tissues and organs to ensure that vital organs—that is, the brain, heart, and lungs—receive blood. The tissues and organs that are deemed expendable are severely jeopardized, especially the kidneys, the gut, and the skin. If the individual survives the shock episode, renal failure, gastric ulcers, intestinal infarction, and a sloughing of the skin often follow.

The Baroreceptor Response to Shock

With the beginning of shock, baroreceptor reflexes are activated and the body tries to compensate for the drastically reduced blood pressure. If the cause of shock continues, compensation will become inadequate and deterioration of all organs, including the lungs, heart, and brain, will progress. As the heart and lungs deteriorate, a deadly cycle is initiated. Oxygenation and cardiac output progressively fall, and shock worsens, soon becoming irreversible. Irreversible shock results in death of the individual.

Causes of Shock

Blood pressure depends on the product of the cardiac output (heart rate × stroke volume) and TPR. Therefore, anything that causes heart rate, stroke volume, or TPR to plummet can cause shock. There are six major causes of shock.

Cardiogenic shock can occur following collapse of the cardiac output, which often results from a myocardial infarct, fibrillation, or congestive heart failure.

Hypovolemic shock can occur if there is a loss of circulating blood volume, causing a severe drop in cardiac output and blood pressure. Hemorrhage and dehydration can cause hypovolemic shock.

Anaphylactic shock can occur following a widespread allergic response associated with mast cell degranulation and the release of inflammatory mediators, such as histamine and prostaglandin. These inflammatory mediators cause widespread systemic vasodilatation and edema, which cause TPR and blood pressure to fall dramatically.

Septic shock can occur following a massive systemic infection and the subsequent release of vasoactive mediators of inflammation. These substances initiate widespread vasodilation and edema, causing TPR and blood pressure to collapse. Septic shock may occur with a blood-borne bacterial infection or result from the release of gut contents, for example, with gastrointestinal perforation or a burst appendix. Some bacteria seem to be superantigens capable of rapidly stimulating septic shock.

Neurogenic shock occurs following sudden loss of vascular tone throughout the body. Neurogenic shock may result from an injury to the cardiovascular center of the brain, a spinal cord injury, or deep general anesthesia. It may also occur as a result of a burst of parasympathetic stimulation to the heart that slows the heart rate, with a corresponding decrease in sympathetic stimulation to the blood vessels. This type of occurrence may explain sudden fainting during a severe emotional disturbance.

Burn shock occurs following a severe burn involving a substantial amount of total body surface area. Burn shock is an interesting combination of shock due to the systemic release of the vasodilatory mediators of inflammation causing a fall in TPR, and a collapse of the blood volume as plasma leaks across suddenly porous capillary membranes.

Clinical Manifestations

Specific manifestations will depend on the cause of shock, but all, except neurogenic shock, will include the following:

- Cool, clammy skin.
- Pallor.
- Increased heart and respiratory rate.
- Dramatically decreased blood pressure.

Individuals with neurogenic shock will have a normal or slow heart rate, and will be warm and dry to the touch.

Diagnostic Tools

- A measured severe decrease in blood pressure.
- Decreased or absent urine output.

Complications

- Tissue hypoxia, cell death, and multi-organ failure following a prolonged decrease in blood flow.
- Adult respiratory distress syndrome from hypoxic destruction of the alveolar–capillary interface.
- Most patients who die of shock do so because of disseminated intravascular coagulation resulting from extensive tissue hypoxia and subsequent tissue death that leads to massive stimulation of the coagulation cascade.

Treatment

- The cause of shock must be identified and reversed if possible.
- Plasma volume replacement is essential, except with cardiogenic shock. What is used for replacement depends on the cause of shock.
- Supplemental oxygen or artificial ventilation may be required.
- Vasopressor agents are given in order to return blood pressure toward normal.

PEDIATRIC CONSIDERATIONS

- An infant with a right-to-left shunt may assume a knee-to-chest position, which increases flow through the pulmonary system and results in improved blood oxygenation. In older children, this maneuver is performed by squatting.

- Increasing incidence of obesity in children and adolescents require careful screening for those with significant risk factors (elevated cholesterol, family history, overweight).

- Autopsy studies of children who have died in accidents have shown that fatty streaks on the arteries may occur in children 10 years of age or younger. Even though these early indications of atherosclerosis may be asymptomatic, they may be predictive of later coronary disease. Children with risk factors for atherosclerosis, including high body mass index, elevated systolic and diastolic pressures, and elevated cholesterol, show a larger percentage of fatty streaks than do children with few risk factors. Smoking in the teen years also increases incidence of fatty streaks.

GERIATRIC CONSIDERATIONS

- Aging increases the risk for varicose veins and chronic venous insufficiency due to increased vein stretching and dilation.

- The older adult may not experience the typical sensation of pain associated with MI. Manifestations may include acute confusion or delirium, pale skin, and weakness.

- Pulmonary thromboembolism (PTE) is a major cause of morbidity and mortality in the older adult. Along with being difficult to diagnose in any individual, frailty and co-morbidities in the older adult increase the risk.

SELECTED BIBLIOGRAPHY

American Heart Association. (2009). Heart disease and stroke statistics. Retrieved August 11, 2009 from http://www.americanheart.org/downloadable/heart/123783441267009 Heart%20and%20Stroke%20Update.pdf.

Anderson, K. M. (2008). Clinical uses of brain natriuretic peptide in diagnosing and managing heart failure. *Journal of the American Academy of Nurse Practitioners*, 20(6), 305–310.

Armbrister, K. A. (2008). Self-management: Improving heart failure outcomes. *The Nurse Practitioner*, 33(11), 20–28.

Atlas of Pathophysiology (3rd ed.). (2010). Philadelphia, PA: Lippincott Williams & Wilkins.

Attina, T., Camidge, R., Newby, D. E., & Webb, D. J. (2005). Endothelin antagonism in pulmonary hypertension, heart failure, and beyond. *Heart*, 91, 825–831.

Barclay, L. (2009). BMI may be a poor marker for hypercholesterolemia in children, adolescents. *Archives of Pediatric and Adolescent Medicine*, 163, 716–722.

Berra, K., & Miller, N. H. (2009). Inhibiting the renin–angiotensin system. *Journal of the American Academy of Nurse Practitioners*, 21(1), 67–75.

Birkeland, J. A., Sejersted, O. M., Taraldsen, T., & Sjaastad, I. (2005). E–C coupling in normal and failing hearts. *Scandinavian Cardiovascular Journal*, 39, 13–23.

Bonetti, P. O., Pumper, G. M., Higano, S. T., Holmes Jr., D. R., Kuvin, J. T., & Lerman, A. (2004). Noninvasive identification of patients with early coronary atherosclerosis by assessment of digital reactive hyperemia. *Journal of the American College of Cardiology*, 44, 2137–2141.

Buczkowski, G., Munschauer, C., & Vasquez, M. A. (2009). Chronic venous insufficiency. *Clinician Reviews*, 19(3), 18–24.

Capik, L. (2008). A double dose of risk: Heart disease and metabolic syndrome in South Asians. *Advance for Nurse Practitioners*, 16(7), 65–68.

Copstead, L. C., & Banasik, J. L. (2010). *Pathophysiology* (4th ed.). St. Louis, MO: Saunders Elsevier.

Cottrell, D. B., Mack, K. (2008). Atrial fibrillation: An emergency nurses's rapid response. *Journal of Emergency Nursing*, 34(3), 207–210.

Coughlin, R. M. (2008). Attacking anterior-wall myocardial infarction in time. *American Nurse Today*, 3(1), 26–30.

Dembrow, M. (2009). Specialists call for tighter BP control. *The Clinical Advisor*, February, 29–30, 32, 34.

DeSimone, M. E., & Crowe, A. (2009). Nonpharmacological approaches in the management of hypertension. *Journal of the American Academy of Nurse Practitioners*, 21, 189–196.

Dibra, A., Kastrati, A., Mehilli, J., Pache, J. Schuhlen, H., von Beckerath, N., et al. (2005). Paclitaxel-eluting or sirolimus-eluting stents to prevent restenosis in diabetic patients. *New England Journal of Medicine*, 353, 663–670.

Dogar, M., Caboral, M. F., & Mitchell, J. E. (2009). Chronic heart failure: When to consider device therapy. *Consultant*, 49(5), 305–310.

Eliopoulos, C. (2010). *Gerontological nursing* (7th ed.). Philadelphia, PA: Lippincott Williams & Wilkins.

Flannery, M., & Flanagan, A. (2008). Beyond the donor shortage: Mechanical help for the failing heart. *American Nurse Today*, 3(2), 35–37.

Furlow, B. (2008). Pediatric heart malformations. *Radiologic Technology*, 80(2), 131CI–145CI.

Greer, D. M. (2008). Coronary CT angiography. *Advance for Nurse Practitioners*, 16(8), 31–34.

Hayman, L. L., & Stuart-Shor, E. M. (2009). The heart of the matter: Reducing CVD risk. *The Nurse Practitioner*, 34(5), 30–35.

Held, M. L., & Sturtz, M. (2009). Managing acute decompensated heart failure. *American Nurse Today*, 4(2), 18–22.

Hughes, S. (2009). On the road to better dyslipidemia outcomes. *The Nurse Practitioner*, 34(2), 14–21.

Jurewitz, D. L., & Lee, M. S. (2008). Shifting the paradigm for ACS management: Pathways in achieving improved outcomes. *Advances in Primary Care Medicine*, December, 3–8.

Mascotti, L. (2008). Diagnosis and treatment of acute pulmonary thromboembolism in the elderly: Clinical practice and implications for nurses. *Journal of Emergency Nursing*, 34(4), 330–339.

Mason, C., Watson, K., & Codario, R. (2009). Focus on hypertriglyceridemia: Improving patient outcomes. [Supplement]. *Journal of the American Academy of Nurse Practitioners*, 19(2), 3–14.

Meneton, P., Jeunemaitre, X., de Wardener, H. E., & Macgregor, G. A. (2005). Links between dietary salt intake, renal salt handling, blood pressure, and cardiovascular diseases. *Physiological Reviews*, 85, 679–715.

Moore, T. D., Witte, A. P., Chilton, R. (2009). Silent myocardial ischemia: Diagnosis, treatment, and prognosis. *Consultant*, 82–85, 89–90.

Naples, R., Ellison, E., & Brady, W. J. (2009). Cranial computed tomography in the resuscitated patient with cardiac arrest. *American Journal of Emergency Medicine*, 27, 63–67.

Narayan, S. M., Bayer, J. D., Lalani, G., Trayanova, N. A. (2008). Action potential dynamics explain arrhythmic vulnerability in human heart failure. *Journal of the American College of Cardiology*, 52(22), 1782–1792.

National Vital Statistics Report. (2009). Vol 57 #14, available at http://www.cdc.gov/nchs/data/nvsr/nvsr57/nvsr57_14.pdf. Retrieved August 11, 2009.

Ohtsuka, S., Hyodo, K., Jin, W., Takeda, T., Maruhashi, A., & Yamaguchi, I. (2005). Overview of clinical intravenous coronary angiography both in Japan and at ESRF. *Nuclear Instruments and Methods in Physics Research*, 548, 78–83.

Osborn, K. S., Wraa, C. E., & Watson, A. B. (2010). *Medical-surgical nursing: Preparation for practice*. Boston, MA: Pearson.

Overbaugh, K. J. (2009). Acute coronary syndrome. *American Journal of Neurology*, 109(5), 42–52.

Pearson, T. A., Mensah, G. A., Alexander, R. W., Anderson, J. L., Cannon, R. O. III, Criqui, M., et al. (2003). Markers of inflammation and cardiovascular disease. A statement for healthcare professionals from the Centers for Disease Control and Prevention and the American Heart Association. *Circulation*, 107, 499–511.

Pierson, C. A., Epstein, B. J., Roberts, M. E. (2008). The importance of managing cardiovascular risk in the treatment of hypertension: The role of ACE inhibitors and ARBs. *Journal of the American Academy of Nurse Practitioners*, 20(11), 529–538.

Pietrasik, G., Goldenberg, I., Mcnitt, S., Polonsky, B., Moss, A. J., & Zareba, W. (2009). Efficacy of medical therapy for the reduction of heart failure events in patients with implanted cardioverter defibrillators. *Journal of Cardiovascular Electrophysiology*, 20(4), 395–400.

Porth, C.M., Matfin, G. (2009). *Pathophysiology: Concepts of altered health states* (8th ed.). Philadelphia, PA: Lippincott Williams & Wilkins.

Rankin, F. M., & Cohen, J. D. (2008). Managing the patient with hypertriglyceridemia: A practical approach for nurse practitioners. [Supplement]. *Journal of the American Academy of Nurse Practitioners*, 20(12), 3–14.

Reaven, G. M. (2005). Hemostatic abnormalities associated with obesity and the metabolic syndrome. *Journal of Thrombosis and Haemostasis*, 3, 1074–1075.

Redderson, L. A., Keen, C., Nasir, L., & Berry, D. (2008). Diastolic heart failure: State of the science on best treatment practices. *Journal of the American Academy of Nurse Practitioners*, 20(10), 506–514.

Richie, R. (2008, October). Updating the latest in hypertension therapy. *The Clinical Advisor*, 48, 50, 53–55, 59.

Rosenfeld, A. G. (2006). State of the health: Building science to improve women's cardiovascular health. *American Journal of Critical Care*, 15(6), 556–567.

Shahady, E. J. (2008). Non-HDL cholesterol: When—and how—to treat. *Consultant*, 48(10), 745–752.

Shirley, S., Davis, L. L., & Carlson, B. W. (2008). The relationship between body mass index/body composition and survival in patients with heart failure. *Journal of the American Academy of Nurse Practitioners*, 20(6), 326–332.

Strimike, C. L. (2006). B-type natriuretic peptide: An emerging cardiac risk marker. *American Journal for Nurse Practitioners*, 10, 27–34.

Taylor, A., Shaw, L. J., Fayad, Z., O'Leary, D., Brown, B. G., Nissen, S., et al. (2005). Tracking atherosclerosis regression: A clinical tool in preventive cardiology. *Atherosclerosis*, 180, 1–10.

Thornton-Miller, D. A. (2008). NMR lipoprofiles: Moving beyond cholesterol. *The Nurse Practitioner*, 33(11), 30–33.

Thygesen, K., Alpert, J. S., & White, H. D. (2007). Joint ESC/ACCF/AHA/WHF task force for the redefinition of myocardial infarction. Universal definition of myocardial infarction. *Journal of American College of Cardiology*, 50(22), 2173–2195.

U.S. Department of Health and Human Services. (2004). *The seventh report of the Joint National Committee on Prevention, Detection, Evaluation, and Treatment of High Blood Pressure (JNC 7).* Washington, DC: National Institutes of Health, National Heart, Lung, and Blood Institute.

Wehrens, X. H. T., Lehnart, S. E., & Marks, A. R. (2004). Intracellular calcium release and cardiac disease. *Annual Review of Physiology*, 67, 69–98.

Weng, L., Kavaslar, N., Ustaszewska, A., Doelle, H., Schackwitz, W., Hébert, S., et al. (2005). Lack of *MEF2A* mutations in coronary artery disease. *Journal of Clinical Investigation*, 115, 1016–1020.

Women's Health Initiative Steering Committee. (2005). Effects of conjugated equine estrogen in postmenopausal women with hysterectomy. The Women's Health Initiative Randomized Controlled Trial. *Journal of the American Medical Association*, 291, 1701–1712.

Wright, W. L. (2008). Hypertension update: Getting patients to goal with newer agents. *Advance for Nurse Practitioners*, 16(12), 37–42.

14

The Respiratory System

The respiratory system is responsible for the exchange of oxygen and carbon dioxide between the air and the blood. Oxygen is required by all cells so that the life-sustaining energy source, adenosine triphosphate (ATP), can be produced. Carbon dioxide is produced by metabolically active cells and forms an acid that must be removed from the body. For gas exchange to be performed, the cardiovascular and respiratory systems must work together. The cardiovascular system is responsible for perfusion of blood through the lungs. The respiratory system performs two separate functions: ventilation and respiration.

● Physiologic Concepts

ALVEOLUS

The functional unit of the lungs is the alveolus (plural, alveoli). There are more than a million alveoli in each lung. Alveoli are small, air-filled sacs across which oxygen and carbon dioxide and other gases diffuse. The large number of small alveoli ensures that the total area available for the diffusion of gas in each lung is enormous. If the airflow into an alveolus is blocked, it collapses and is unavailable for gas exchange. If airflow into several alveoli is blocked, exchange of gases may be impaired to the extent that the person becomes hypoxic or unconscious or dies.

VENTILATION

The movement of air from the atmosphere into and out of the lungs is called ventilation. Ventilation occurs by bulk flow. Bulk flow is the movement of a gas or a fluid from high to low pressure.

Factors that Affect Ventilation

Ventilation is determined by the variables in the following equation:

$$F = P/R$$

where F is the bulk flow of air, P is the difference in pressure between the atmosphere and the alveoli, and R is the resistance offered by the conducting airways.

Pressure

Alveolar pressure varies with each inspiration and drives the flow of air. With the onset of inspiration, the thoracic cavity expands. As the thoracic cavity expands, the lungs also expand. According to the Boyle law, if the volume of an air-filled chamber increases, the pressure of the air in the chamber decreases. Therefore, as the lungs expand, pressure in the alveoli decreases to below atmospheric pressure, and air rushes into the lungs from the atmosphere (from high pressure to low pressure). At the end of inspiration, the thoracic cavity relaxes, causing pressures in the alveoli, which are filled with the air of inspiration, to be higher than in the atmosphere. Air then flows out of the lungs and down the pressure gradient.

Bronchial Resistance

Resistance of the airways is usually low. Resistance is increased when the smooth muscle of the bronchiolar tubes constricts. Constriction of the bronchi results in a decrease in airflow into the lungs. Resistance is inversely proportional to the radius of a vessel to the fourth power. This means that if the radius of a bronchiolar tube decreases by one-half, the resistance to airflow in that tube increases by 16 (i.e., 2^4). Therefore, *when the air passages constrict even slightly, resistance to airflow goes up significantly.*

Bronchiolar resistance is determined by parasympathetic and sympathetic nervous system innervation of the smooth muscle of the bronchi and local chemical mediators.

Parasympathetic nerves are carried to the bronchial smooth muscle by way of the vagus nerve and cause contraction or narrowing of the airways, increasing resistance and reducing airflow. Parasympathetic nerves release the neurotransmitter acetylcholine (ACh). ACh acts by binding to cholinergic receptors on the smooth muscle of the bronchi.

Sympathetic innervation of the bronchial smooth muscle occurs by way of nerve fibers from the upper thoracic and cervical ganglia and causes relaxation of the bronchi. This reduces resistance and increases airflow. Sympathetic nerves release the neurotransmitter norepinephrine. Norepinephrine acts by binding to β_2 adrenergic receptors on the smooth muscle of the bronchi.

Nervous Control of Respiration

Ventilation is controlled by the respiratory center in the lower brainstem areas of the medulla and pons. In the medulla, there are inspiratory and expiratory neurons that fire at opposite times in a preset pattern of rate and rhythm. Respiratory neurons drive ventilation by exciting motor neurons that innervate the main muscle of inspiration (the **diaphragm**) and the accessory muscles (the intercostal muscles).

Central Chemoreceptors

Central chemoreceptors in the brain respond to changes in the hydrogen ion concentration of the cerebral spinal fluid. Increased hydrogen ion concentration increases the firing rate of the chemoreceptors, while decreased hydrogen ion concentration decreases the firing rate of the chemoreceptors. Information from the central chemoreceptors is delivered to the respiratory center in the brain, which in response increases or decreases the breathing pattern. Hydrogen ion concentration usually reflects carbon dioxide concentration. Therefore, when carbon dioxide levels rise, hydrogen ion levels rise, and the firing rate of inspiratory neurons is increased, causing an increase in respiratory rate. This is an example of negative feedback, because with an increase in the rate of breathing, the excess carbon dioxide and hydrogen ion will be blown off. With low carbon dioxide and low hydrogen ion levels, the firing rate of the inspiratory neurons returns toward baseline, and respiration slows.

Peripheral Chemoreceptors

Peripheral chemoreceptors exist in the carotid and the aortic arteries, and monitor oxygen concentration in arterial blood. These receptors, called the carotid and the aortic bodies, send their impulses to the respiratory center of the medulla and pons primarily to increase the rate of ventilation when oxygen is low. They are less sensitive than the central chemoreceptors. The peripheral chemoreceptors also respond with an increase in firing rate to increased hydrogen ion dissolved in the blood. This is important because under certain circumstances free hydrogen ion increases without causing a change in carbon dioxide concentration (e.g., during conditions of metabolic acidosis caused by prolonged diarrhea or diabetes mellitus). Free hydrogen ion is relatively impermeable across the blood–brain barrier, so it is unable to activate the central chemoreceptors directly.

Motor Neurons Driving Respiration

The major motor neuron controlling respiration is the phrenic nerve. When activated by the central inspiratory neurons, the phrenic nerve causes the diaphragm muscle to contract and the chest to expand. As the chest expands, air begins to flow from the atmosphere into the lungs. Airflow into the lungs is called **inspiration**. As inspiration continues, firing of the central inspiratory neurons slows and firing of the expiratory neurons increases, causing cessation of motor neuron activity and relaxation of the diaphragm. Chest expansion reverses and air flows out of the lungs. Airflow out of the lungs is referred to as **expiration** and is a passive process.

RESPIRATION

Respiration refers to the diffusion of gases between an alveolus and the capillary that perfuses it. Respiration occurs by diffusion, which involves the movement of a gas down its concentration gradient.

Factors that Affect Respiration

The rate of diffusion of a gas (e.g., oxygen and carbon dioxide) is determined with the following equation:

$$D = \frac{[(X_a - X_c)] \times SA \times T}{d \times k}$$

where D is the rate of diffusion, X_a is the concentration of gas in the alveolus, X_c is the concentration of gas in the capillary, SA is the surface area available for diffusion, T is the temperature of the solution, d is the distance across which diffusion must occur, and k is a physical constant that takes into account non-variable characteristics of the gas such as its molecular weight and its specific solubility coefficient.

Concentration of Oxygen and Carbon Dioxide in the Alveolus and the Capillary

Alveolar oxygen concentration reflects atmospheric oxygen, whereas pulmonary capillary oxygen concentration reflects the oxygen concentration of systemic venous blood. Because systemic venous blood is blood returning from the peripheral circulation, where much of the oxygen has been used by the cells of the body, it has a low oxygen concentration. The atmosphere is typically well supplied with oxygen. Therefore, oxygen is normally in higher concentration in the alveolus than it is in the pulmonary capillary. Values for oxygen concentration are directly proportional to the partial pressure of the gas and are usually expressed in millimeters of mercury (mm Hg).

At sea level, the partial pressure of oxygen is approximately 100 mm Hg in the alveolus and 40 mm Hg in the pulmonary capillary. Because alveolar oxygen concentration in the alveolus is greater than in the capillary, oxygen diffuses down its concentration gradient from the alveolus into the capillary. This is how deoxygenated blood is replenished with oxygen by respiration.

Carbon dioxide normally diffuses in the opposite direction. It is in low concentration in the atmosphere and thus in low concentration in the alveolus

(40 mm Hg). Pulmonary capillary blood reflects systemic venous blood. Because carbon dioxide is a waste product of metabolizing cells, the concentration of carbon dioxide in the capillary is high (46 mm Hg). Therefore, in the lungs, carbon dioxide diffuses down its concentration gradient, from the blood into the alveolus, where it will be expired.

Under some circumstances, concentration gradients of oxygen and carbon dioxide between the blood and the alveolus may be increased or decreased; magnified concentration gradients affect the diffusion rate of the gas. For example, during exercise, oxygen concentration in the blood entering the pulmonary capillaries may be less than 40 mm Hg because the exercising muscles have increased their oxygen usage. Carbon dioxide concentration would be greater in blood flowing to the lungs from exercising tissue because its metabolic production would be increased. In this situation, diffusion rates for both gases would be increased, allowing more oxygen to diffuse into the blood and more carbon dioxide to diffuse out of the blood.

Surface Area

Surface area (SA) refers to the expanse of alveolar and capillary membranes available for gas diffusion. Surface area is normally high in the lungs. Some diseases, including emphysema, tuberculosis (TB), and lung cancer, can decrease the surface area available for diffusion, thus reducing the diffusion rates of oxygen and carbon dioxide.

Distance for Diffusion

The distance (d) across which oxygen and carbon dioxide must diffuse is normally quite small. Alveolar and capillary membranes are close to each other, separated only by a thin layer of interstitial fluid (Fig. 14-1).

Certain conditions, including pneumonia, can increase the distance of diffusion by causing edema and swelling of the interstitial space. This decreases the diffusion rate of the gases (Fig. 14-2). Interstitial fibrosis (scarring) can also

HOW PULMONARY EDEMA DEVELOPS

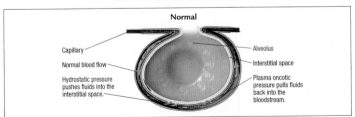

FIGURE 14-1 Normal alveolus–capillary distance allows for efficient diffusion of oxygen and carbon dioxide between the capillary and alveolus. (From Anatomical Chart Company [2010]. *Atlas of pathophysiology* [3rd ed.]. Philadelphia: Lippincott Williams & Wilkins.)

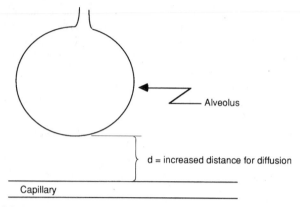

FIGURE 14-2 With interstitial edema, the alveolus–capillary distance is increased, resulting in reduced diffusion of oxygen and carbon dioxide between the capillary and the alveolus.

increase the distance between the alveoli and the capillaries and therefore slow diffusion.

Temperature

A decrease in temperature (T) would decrease the diffusion rate of oxygen and carbon dioxide. An increase in T would increase the diffusion rate of both gases. An increase in temperature may play a role in meeting the increased metabolic demands during fever.

Permeability Coefficient

Carbon dioxide and, to a lesser extent, oxygen have high permeability. Because the variable k in the equation is fixed for each gas, k does not play an active role in determining respiration.

Oxygen Carrying in the Blood

Oxygen is carried in the blood in dissolved form and bound to hemoglobin. The amount of oxygen dissolved in the blood depends on the partial pressure of oxygen in the air entering the alveoli and the solubility of oxygen. Normally the dissolved amount carried is small (only approximately 3 mL/L). Instead, most oxygen (98%) is carried bound to hemoglobin.

Hemoglobin is a protein molecule composed of four subunits, each combining a globulin molecule with a molecule of iron. Each iron molecule has a binding site for oxygen. Dissolved oxygen combines with hemoglobin until all four sites are saturated. At normal arterial oxygen concentration of 100 mm Hg,

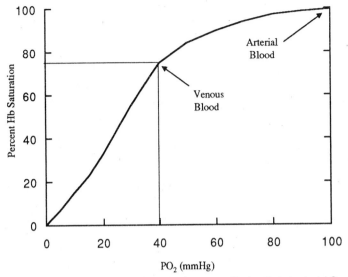

FIGURE 14-3 Oxygen–hemoglobin saturation curve. Notice that at arterial O₂ levels (PO₂), nearly 100% of hemoglobin is saturated. Even at PO₂ of 60 mm Hg, 90% of Hb is saturated. In venous blood (PO₂ 40), 75% of Hb is saturated with blood.

nearly 100% of hemoglobin molecules are saturated with oxygen. Even in the venous blood, with a reduced oxygen concentration of 40 mm Hg, hemoglobin is still at least 75% saturated with oxygen (Fig. 14-3). The ability of hemoglobin to bind oxygen is reduced by increased hydrogen ion concentration, increased temperature, and increased amount of a substance produced by red blood cells during glycolysis, 2,3-diphosphoglycerate (DPG). A reduced affinity for oxygen means that hemoglobin releases oxygen to the tissues more readily. Increases in hydrogen ion, temperature, and DPG occur during periods of increased metabolism; therefore, decreased hemoglobin affinity releases more oxygen to a cell and allows it to meet its elevated metabolic demands.

PERFUSION

For the respiratory system, perfusion refers to the movement of blood in the pulmonary vascular system, past the alveolar capillaries. Perfusion, like blood flow and ventilation, occurs by bulk flow. In the lungs, perfusion and ventilation usually are well matched. This ensures that there is adequate oxygen available in each alveolus to replenish the blood flowing past it and adequate blood flow to support each alveolus.

CIRCULATIONS THAT PROVIDE BLOOD FLOW TO THE LUNGS

Two separate blood circulations supply blood flow to the lungs from the heart: the pulmonary circulation and the bronchial circulation.

Pulmonary Circulation

The pulmonary circulation consists of deoxygenated blood traveling in the pulmonary artery from the right side of the heart. This blood perfuses the respiratory portions of the lungs and participates in the exchange of oxygen and carbon dioxide across the capillaries and alveoli. After picking up oxygen and releasing carbon dioxide, the blood returns to the heart by way of the pulmonary vein. Pressure and resistance to flow in the pulmonary circulation are usually low, with a mean pulmonary pressure of approximately 12 mm Hg compared with a mean systemic pressure of approximately 90 mm Hg. The pulmonary circulation is compliant and can accommodate large variations in blood volume. Therefore, the pulmonary circulation can act as a reservoir for blood that can be called upon in times of decreased systemic blood volume or pressure.

Bronchial Circulation

The bronchial circulation carries blood from the left side of the heart to the lungs through the thoracic aorta. The bronchial circulation accounts for approximately 8% to 9% of the total cardiac output. Blood in the bronchial circulation is well oxygenated and supplies oxygen to the structures of the lungs not involved in the exchange of gases, including the connective tissue and the large and small bronchi. Blood returns to the left side of the heart through the pulmonary vein. Returning bronchial blood is deoxygenated because it has been used by metabolically active cells of the lungs but has not been involved in gas exchange. The deoxygenated blood mixes with the well-oxygenated blood coming from the pulmonary circulation also back to the left side of the heart, and slightly reduces the overall oxygen concentration of that blood.

VENTILATION:PERFUSION RATIO

Ventilation refers to air moving into and out of the lungs. Perfusion is the blood passing through the pulmonary circulation to be oxygenated. The ventilation:perfusion ratio, V/Q, is the ratio of airflow into the lungs divided by the pulmonary blood flow. In this expression, V is the volume of air moved with each breath, expressed as milliliters per minute (mL/min), and Q is the rate of blood flow in the pulmonary circulation, also expressed as mL/min. Normally, perfusion is slightly greater than ventilation and the V/Q ratio is approximately 0.8. Therefore, the alveoli receiving oxygen are well perfused by blood, allowing optimal conditions for gas exchange.

ELASTICITY

Elasticity of the respiratory system refers to the degree to which the lungs resist inflation or stretching. The alveoli and other lung tissue normally resist stretching and recoil after the force causing the stretch or expansion is removed. This situation is partially caused by the surface tension of each alveolus and partially by the presence of elastic fibers throughout the lungs, which tend to recoil after stretch. Conditions such as emphysema reduce the elastic recoil of the lungs, resulting in chronic overinflation.

The reciprocal of elasticity of the lungs is termed **lung compliance**. Compliance refers to the ease of inflation or stretching of the lungs. Lung compliance is reduced by fibrosis, infection, or adult respiratory distress syndrome (ARDS).

PLEURAL PRESSURE

The lungs are surrounded by a thin membrane called the pleura. The outer layer of the pleural membrane is attached to the wall of the thoracic cavity. The inner layer of the pleura is attached to the lungs. With expansion of the thoracic cavity during inspiration, the outer layer is pulled out; this force is transmitted to the inner layer, which expands the lungs. In between the inner and outer layers of the pleura is the pleural space. This space is filled with a few milliliters of fluid that surround and lubricate the lungs. The pleural fluid is at negative pressure and opposes the elastic recoil (collapse) of the lungs. This negative pressure helps keep the lungs expanded.

SURFACE TENSION

Surface tension refers to the tendency of water molecules to pull toward each other and to collapse a sphere. Because each alveolus is lined with a thin water layer, the surface tension within each alveolus could be high, making it extremely difficult to expand an alveolus. With each breath, a certain pressure must be exerted to overcome the surface tension of the water layer. The amount of pressure needed to expand the alveolus is described by Laplace law in the following equation:

$$P = 2T/r$$

where P is the pressure needed to expand the alveolus, T is the surface tension of the water molecules, and r is the radius of the alveolus. As shown in this equation, the smaller the alveolus, the greater the pressure required to expand it. An inability to overcome the surface tension of an alveolus could lead to alveolar collapse. Normally, however, the surface tension of an alveolus is kept low by the presence of surfactant.

SURFACTANT

Certain cells inside the alveolus, called **type II alveolar cells**, produce an important substance called **surfactant** that helps reduce the surface tension of the alveolus, making it easier to inflate. Surfactant is a phospholipid that acts like a detergent to intersperse between water molecules in the alveolus, thereby weakening the bonds between them. This reduces surface tension and the tendency of the sphere to collapse.

When surfactant is present, a small alveolus actually requires less pressure to inflate than a large one because the surfactant is packed tightly together, greatly reducing the surface tension of the alveolus. This serves to compensate for the effect of small radius in Laplace law.

TESTS OF PULMONARY FUNCTIONING
Lung Volumes

Spirometry is the measurement of the volume of air moving into and out of the lungs and is measured as an individual inhales and exhales into a closed chamber. It is used to determine lung volumes, including tidal, inspiratory reserve, expiratory reserve, and residual volumes, and, calculated from these, vital capacity (Fig. 14-4). The average values presented in the figure for each of these volumes are for an adult male. Values for adult females are approximately 20% to 25% less.

Tidal Volume

The amount of air entering or leaving the lungs during a single breath is the tidal volume. The amount of air inspired at rest (inspiratory volume) usually equals the amount expired (expiratory volume). Tidal volume averages approximately 500 mL at rest.

Inspiratory Reserve Volume

The amount of air above the normal inspiration that can be maximally inspired with each breath is the inspiratory reserve volume. It averages approximately 3000 mL.

Expiratory Reserve Volume

The maximum amount of air that can be exhaled beyond normal exhalation is the expiratory reserve volume. This value averages approximately 1000 mL.

Residual Volume

The air remaining in the lungs after maximum exhalation is the residual volume. The normal value is approximately 1000 mL.

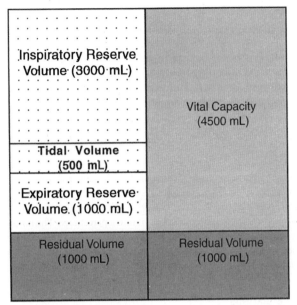

FIGURE 14-4 Approximate lung volumes per breath for a 70-kg male. Average lung volumes are proportional to body mass index.

Vital Capacity

The maximum amount of air that an individual can inspire and expire during a single breath is the vital capacity. It is the sum of the normal tidal volume and the inspiratory reserve volume and the expiratory reserve volume. It is measured by having an individual take a maximum breath and then exhale as much as possible into the measurement chamber. In restrictive pulmonary disorders (e.g., resulting from neuromuscular disease, fibrosis, or loss of surfactant-producing cells), vital capacity is reduced.

A common test of pulmonary function is to plot the volume of air an individual can expire in the first second of expiration, called the **forced expiratory volume in one second** (FEV_1). A healthy individual can expire approximately 80% of vital capacity as fast as possible in the first second (FEV_1/vital capacity). In obstructive pulmonary diseases such as asthma and emphysema, expiration is particularly affected, and the amount of air an individual can forcefully expire in the first second is reduced. In patients who have restrictive airway disease, expiration is usually normal. Therefore, whereas overall vital capacity is reduced in those who have restrictive airway disease, FEV_1 is normal.

Anatomic Dead Space

The amount of air in each breath that is measured as part of the tidal volume but does not actually participate in gas exchange is the anatomic dead space. This air fills the conducting passages of the nose, mouth, pharynx, larynx, trachea, bronchi, and the bronchioles. With rapid, shallow respirations, a greater percentage of each breath is wasted simply moving air in and out of the anatomic dead space compared with that seen with slow, deeper breathing.

Pulse Oximetry

Pulse oximetry is a noninvasive method that uses infrared technology to measure the percentage of hemoglobin that is saturated with oxygen. A transducer placed on an extremity detects light absorption by hemoglobin during pulsatile arterial waves and a computer translates it into a percentage. The normal range for oxygen saturation (SPO_2) is 95% to 100%. Inaccurate readings may be caused by excessive movement, nail polish, and conditions that alter perfusion such as shock or hypovolemia.

Arterial Blood Gas

Arterial blood gases (ABGs) offer information about pH and the amount of oxygen, carbon dioxide, and bicarbonate in the blood. Normal values are:

- pH   7.35 to 7.45
- PaO_2 80 to 100 mm Hg
- $PaCO_2$ 35 to 45 mm Hg
- HCO_3^- 22 to 26 mEq/L

Capnography

Measurement of the amount of exhaled carbon dioxide may be done by treated paper which changes color in the presence of acid or via spectography. This test is useful in determining the effectiveness of ventilation and may actually help identify impending respiratory depression.

Radiographs

A chest x-ray offers information about structural abnormalities of the lung. For example, atelectasis, consolidation, densities, hyperinflation, edema, or collapsed areas offer valuable information for the diagnosis of respiratory problems.

● Pathophysiologic Concepts

ATELECTASIS

The collapse of either a lung or an alveolus is called atelectasis. Collapsed alveoli are airless, and therefore do not participate in gas exchange. This results in a reduction in the surface area available for diffusion, and respiration is decreased. Newborns may be born with alveoli collapsed at birth. This condition is called **primary atelectasis**. The collapse of previously expanded alveoli is called **secondary atelectasis**. The two main types of atelectasis are compression atelectasis and absorption atelectasis.

Compression Atelectasis

Compression atelectasis occurs when a source outside the alveolus exerts enough pressure on the alveolus to collapse it. This occurs if the chest wall is punctured or opened because atmospheric pressure is greater than the pressure holding the lungs expanded (pleural pressure), and with exposure to atmospheric pressure the lungs will collapse. Compression atelectasis can also occur if there is pressure exerted on the lungs or alveoli from a growing tumor, abdominal distention, or edema and swelling of the interstitial space around an alveolus.

Absorption Atelectasis

Absence of air in the alveolus results in absorption atelectasis. If flow of air into an alveolus is blocked, the air currently inside eventually diffuses out and the alveolus collapses. Blockage usually occurs after mucus buildup and obstruction of airflow through a bronchus supplying a given group of alveoli. Any situation that results in mucus accumulation, such as cystic fibrosis, pneumonia, or chronic bronchitis, increases the risk of absorption atelectasis. Surgery is also a risk factor for absorption atelectasis because of the mucus-producing effects of anesthesia as well as a resultant hesitancy to cough up accumulated mucus after surgery. This is especially true if the surgery was in the abdominal or thoracic area, where pain associated with coughing is intense. Prolonged bed rest after surgery increases the risk of developing absorption atelectasis, because lying down causes a pooling of mucus secretions in dependent areas of the lung, decreasing ventilation to those areas. Mucus accumulation increases the risk of pneumonia because mucus can act as a breeding ground for growth of microorganisms.

Absorption atelectasis can also be caused by anything that reduces the production or concentration of surfactant. Without surfactant, surface tension in the alveolus is high, increasing the likelihood of alveolar collapse. Premature birth is associated with a reduction in surfactant and a high incidence of absorption atelectasis. Near drowning may dilute out surfactant and thus may be associated with absorption atelectasis as well.

Damage to the type II alveolar cells that produce surfactant can also lead to absorption atelectasis. These cells are destroyed by the breakdown of the alveolar wall that occurs during some forms of respiratory disease, as well as by high oxygen therapy for a period longer than 24 hours. With loss of these cells, surfactant production is reduced.

HYPOXEMIA

The condition of reduced oxygen concentration in arterial blood is called hypoxemia. There are many causes of hypoxemia. Hypoxemia can occur if there is decreased oxygen in the air (hypoxia) or if hypoventilation occurs because of decreased lung compliance or atelectasis. Hypoxemia related to hypoperfusion (decreased blood flow past the alveoli) can occur from pulmonary hypertension, a pulmonary embolus, or a myocardial infarct. Hypoxemia may also occur if there is a problem with diffusion of oxygen across the alveolus into the capillary. This may happen with destruction of the alveolar–capillary interface or with edema of the alveolar–capillary interstitial space.

Because oxygen is carried in the red blood cell bound to hemoglobin, any decrease in hemoglobin concentration or carrying capacity can result in hypoxemia. Hemoglobin concentration is reduced in certain types of anemia. Binding sites for oxygen on the hemoglobin molecule may be occupied by other gases (e.g., carbon monoxide) that would also decrease the oxygen-carrying capacity of hemoglobin.

CYANOSIS

Bluish discoloration of the blood that occurs if large amounts of hemoglobin in the blood are not completely bound with oxygen molecules is called cyanosis. There are four sites on hemoglobin where oxygen may bind. Hemoglobin fully bound with oxygen at all four sites is called saturated. Desaturated or deoxygenated hemoglobin is not fully bound with oxygen.

If the hemoglobin concentration in the blood is normal, but the availability of oxygen to bind to hemoglobin is reduced, the hemoglobin molecules will be deoxygenated. Normally there is approximately 15 g of hemoglobin per 100 mL of blood. In arterial blood, more than 98%, or 14.7 g per l00 mL of blood, will be saturated with oxygen. Venous blood normally has an oxygen saturation of 75%; this comes to 11.3 g of hemoglobin per 100 mL of blood saturated with oxygen and about 4 g per 100 mL of unsaturated blood. If arterial hemoglobin oxygen saturation falls below 70%, resulting in *5 g or more of unsaturated hemoglobin per 100 mL of blood*, cyanosis will be apparent.

In hypoxemia caused by low hemoglobin concentration, such as with microcytic hypochromic anemia, cyanosis will not develop because there will not be greater than 5 g of deoxygenated hemoglobin per 100 mL of blood. Cyanosis will not occur with carbon monoxide poisoning because the hemoglobin-binding sites will still be saturated, although with the carbon monoxide molecule rather than oxygen. In both of these situations, hypoxemia would be present in the absence of cyanosis.

ALTERATIONS IN VENTILATION:PERFUSION RATIO

A decrease in ventilation may occur when the delivery of air to some alveoli is obstructed, for example, with mucus or by foreign-body aspiration. With decreased ventilation (V), the ventilation:perfusion ratio is decreased, because the blood flow (Q) will pass by underventilated alveoli. This mismatch in ventilation and perfusion is not beneficial for gas exchange, and is an example of a right-to-left shunt of blood. A right-to-left shunt, described in Chapter 13, is characterized by delivery of deoxygenated blood to the systemic circulation. A decrease in the ventilation:perfusion ratio, however, will not last long in the lungs because of the pulmonary arteriolar response when exposed to low oxygen.

Pulmonary arterioles vasoconstrict in response to low oxygen concentration in underventilated alveoli. This serves to decrease blood flow to those alveoli, returning the ventilation:perfusion ratio back toward 1.0. This response is called **hypoxic vasoconstriction**. Hypoxic vasoconstriction is effective only if the extent of underventilated alveoli is limited. In conditions such as chronic bronchitis, alveolar obstruction is so widespread that a normal ventilation:perfusion ratio cannot be maintained. Hypoxic vasoconstriction of the pulmonary arterioles can lead to pulmonary hypertension as described later.

Under some circumstances, it is possible for ventilation of an alveolus to be adequate but capillary perfusion to be compromised. The result is a decrease in Q and an increase in the ventilation:perfusion ratio. This situation could occur as a result of a pulmonary embolus. A myocardial infarct would also cause decreased perfusion of the alveoli.

PULMONARY HYPERTENSION

Elevated blood pressure in the pulmonary vascular system is called pulmonary hypertension. It is a common condition in serious respiratory or cardiovascular disease. It is a progressive condition characterized by elevated pulmonary artery pressure and increased pulmonary vascular resistance. Although a definitive diagnosis is based on findings from cardiac catheterization, echocardiography is a valuable way to assess for, and monitor the progression of pulmonary hypertension.

Causes of Pulmonary Hypertension

The pulmonary circulation is usually a low-pressure, low-resistance circulation. Anything that causes (1) a prolonged increase in pulmonary blood flow, (2) an increase in pulmonary resistance to flow, or (3) an impediment in pulmonary vascular outflow can result in pulmonary hypertension.

Increased Pulmonary Blood Flow

If excessive blood volume is delivered to the lungs, increased pulmonary blood flow occurs. For example, with a left-to-right shunt, blood from the left side of the heart goes back to the lungs rather than to the systemic circulation, thus overloading the lungs.

Increased Pulmonary Resistance to Flow

Anything that obstructs the passage of blood into or through the lungs causes increased pulmonary resistance to flow. This includes pulmonary fibrosis (scarring) and the changes in the structure of the lungs that accompany chronic obstructive pulmonary disease (COPD). Long-term pulmonary hypoxic vaso-constriction is also a significant cause of increased pulmonary resistance and hypertension. Hypoxic vasoconstriction of the pulmonary arterioles occurs when the pulmonary circulation is exposed to low oxygen, causing the vascular smooth muscle of the pulmonary arterioles to constrict. This can be useful because it allows the ventilation:perfusion ratio to return toward 1.0. However, if the condition is chronic or extensive, hypertrophy of the arterioles and increased pulmonary resistance can result.

Impediment to Outflow

This condition occurs with left-heart failure, as blood backs up in the left side of the heart, opposing continued flow out of the lungs. Other causes of impediment to outflow are mitral or aortic stenosis or incompetence, which also interfere with blood leaving the heart.

Consequences of Pulmonary Hypertension

Pulmonary hypertension can make it more difficult for the right side of the heart to pump. A type of heart failure called **cor pulmonale** can result. Cor pulmonale is right-sided heart failure caused by chronic lung disease. Pulmonary hypertension can also result in pulmonary edema because the capillary hydrostatic force favoring filtration is increased. Edema of the pulmonary interstitial space leads to a decreased diffusion rate of oxygen from the alveolus to the capillary because of increased distance for diffusion.

BRONCHIECTASIS

Bronchiectasis is abnormal dilation of a bronchus or bronchi. Bronchiectasis occurs from long-standing pulmonary obstruction of the lower airways by tumors, chronic infections, mucus accumulation as seen in cystic fibrosis, and exposure to toxins. The bronchi fill with mucus, resulting in atelectasis and development of abnormal connections between the bronchi. Ventilation of the alveoli is impaired.

COUGH

In 2006, the American College of Chest Physicians' updated the guidelines for the diagnosis and management of cough and reclassified it as a symptom rather than a defense mechanism. As one of the most common reasons for visiting health care providers in the United States, chronic cough interferes with the quality of life (i.e., sleep deprivation, urinary incontinence). Based on the new guidelines, idiopathic cough is any unexplained cough, and cough due to postnasal drip is referred to as upper airway cough syndrome.

Irritating substances stimulate receptors in the tracheobronchial wall sending afferent impulses through the vagus nerve to the medullary center where the cough response is initiated. Allergens, postnasal drip, smoking, heart failure, esophageal reflux, and some medications, such as angiotensin converting enzyme (ACE) inhibitors, are possible stimulants that initiate the cough response.

CENTRAL NERVOUS SYSTEM DEPRESSION

Central nervous system depression is a depressed respiratory drive resulting from alteration in function of the respiratory centers of the brain. Central nervous system depression can occur with hypoxemia or chronic elevation of carbon dioxide concentration, both of which occur when there is decreased pulmonary ventilation or perfusion. The respiratory center of the medulla and pons, which normally drives respiration, requires adequate oxygenation to function. Although the normal stimulus to breathe is the carbon dioxide concentration of the cerebral spinal fluid (as reflected in hydrogen ion concentration), high carbon dioxide levels can depress the respiratory center enough to cause a cessation of breathing.

● Conditions of Disease or Injury

UPPER RESPIRATORY TRACT INFECTIONS

Infections caused by any microorganism of the non–gas-exchanging upper structures of the respiratory tract, including the nasal passages, the pharynx, and the larynx, are known as upper respiratory tract infections. Upper respiratory tract infections include the common cold, otitis media, sinusitis, pharyngitis or sore throat, laryngitis, and uncomplicated influenza. Most upper respiratory tract infections are caused by viruses, although bacteria may also be involved either initially or secondary to a viral infection. All types of infections activate the immune and the inflammatory responses, leading to swelling and edema of the infected tissue. The inflammatory reaction leads to increased mucus production, contributing to the symptoms seen with upper respiratory tract infections, including congestion, excess sputum, and nasal discharge. Headache, low-grade fever, and malaise may also occur as a result of the inflammatory reaction.

Respiratory Defenses against Infection

Although the upper respiratory tract is directly exposed to the environment, infections are uncommon and seldom progress to lower respiratory tract infections involving the lower airways and alveoli. Protective mechanisms abound throughout the respiratory tract to prevent infection. The **cough reflex** expels foreign bodies and microorganisms, and removes accumulated mucus. The **mucociliary blanket** consists of cells, located upwards from the level of the bronchi, which make mucus, and cilia cells that line the mucus-producing cells. The mucus-producing cells trap foreign particles, and the cilia beat rhythmically to propel the mucus and any trapped particles up the respiratory tree to the nasopharynx, where they can be expelled as sputum, blown out the nose, or swallowed. This complex is sometimes referred to as the mucociliary escalator system. The cilia are delicate structures that can be paralyzed or injured by a variety of noxious stimuli, including cigarette smoke, as described later.

If microorganisms evade these defense mechanisms and colonize the upper respiratory tract, a third important line of defense, the **immune system**, is in position to prevent their passage to the lower respiratory tract. This response is mediated by lymphocytes, but also involves other white blood cells such as macrophages and neutrophils brought to the area by the inflammatory process. If there is a breakdown of a defense mechanism of the respiratory system or if the microorganism is especially virulent, a lower respiratory tract infection can result.

Effects of Cigarette Smoking on Respiratory Defenses

Cigarette smoke is known to alter the effectiveness of some respiratory defense mechanisms. Products of cigarette smoke stimulate mucus production while paralyzing the cilia. This leads to the accumulation of thick mucus and any trapped particles or microorganisms in the airways, decreasing the movement of air and increasing the risk of microbial growth. A smoker's cough is an attempt to expel this thick mucus out of the respiratory tract. Lower respiratory tract infections are more common in smokers and in those exposed to second-hand smoke, especially infants and children.

Clinical Manifestations

Clinical indications of upper respiratory tract infections depend on the infection site as well as the microorganism responsible for the infection. All clinical manifestations result from the inflammatory processes and any direct damage the microorganism inflicts. Clinical manifestations include:

- Cough.
- Sneezing and nasal congestion.
- Mucus production and drainage from the nose and down the throat.

- Headache.
- Sore throat.
- Earache.
- Facial pain and pressure.
- Low-grade fever.
- Malaise (physical discomfort).

Diagnostic Tools

- A good history and physical examination will assist diagnosis.
- Complete blood cell count and sputum culture to rule out bacterial infection.

Complications

- Sinusitis and acute otitis media may develop.
- Lower respiratory tract infections, including pneumonia and bronchitis, may follow an upper respiratory infection.

Treatment

- Rest to reduce the body's metabolic demands.
- Extra hydration helps liquefy the thick mucus, making it easier to move it out of the respiratory tract. This is important because mucus accumulation offers a breeding ground for secondary bacterial infection.
- Decongestants, antihistamines, and cough suppressants may provide some symptom relief.
- Some studies suggest zinc lozenges or increased vitamin C consumption may reduce the severity or likelihood of certain viral infections.
- Antibiotics are required if the infection is bacterial either initially or secondary to a viral infection.

LOWER RESPIRATORY TRACT INFECTIONS

Pneumonia

Pneumonia, an acute infection of the lung tissue by a microorganism, is a lower respiratory tract infection. Most pneumonias are bacterial in origin, occurring as a primary condition or secondary to a previous viral infection. Pneumonia is classified as **community acquired** (CAP) when it occurs outside a health care facility or in someone other than a health care provider. It is more prevalent in smokers and has a much higher incidence in the winter months. Pneumonia diagnosed at least 48 hours after being admitted to a health care facility is referred to as **hospital-acquired (or nosocomial) pneumonia** and has a mortality rate of up to 50%. Almost 90% is bacterial in nature.

The most common cause of bacterial pneumonia is the gram-positive bacterium *Streptococcus pneumoniae*, which is responsible for pneumococcal pneumonia. The bacteria *Staphylococcus aureus* and group A beta-hemolytic streptococci are also frequent causes of pneumonia, as is *Pseudomonas aeruginosa*. Other pneumonias are caused directly by viruses, such as that seen occasionally with influenza. Young children especially are susceptible to viral pneumonia, usually from infection with respiratory syncytial virus (RSV), parainfluenza, adenovirus, or rhinovirus. Mycoplasmal pneumonia, a relatively common pneumonia, is caused by a microorganism that is, in some respects, between a virus and a bacterium. Individuals who have acquired immunodeficiency syndrome (AIDS) frequently develop an otherwise rare pneumonia called *Pneumocystis carinii* pneumonia. Individuals exposed to aerosols of previously standing water, for instance, from air-conditioning units or dirty humidifiers, may develop *Legionella* pneumonia. Finally, individuals who aspirate stomach contents after vomiting or who aspirate water in an experience of near-drowning may develop aspiration pneumonia. For these individuals, the aspirated material itself rather than a microorganism may cause pneumonia by stimulating an inflammatory reaction. Subsequent bacterial infection may also develop.

The risks of developing the pneumonias described above are greater for the young, the old, or for anyone immunocompromised or weakened by another disease or disability. Risk of death after pneumonia is also stratified based on age (over 50 or young, especially the newborn) and the presence of coexisting illness such as congestive heart failure, neoplastic disease, or renal disease.

Much of the damage to the lung tissue after successful colonization of the lungs by a microorganism is the result of the usually vigorous immune and inflammatory reaction mounted by the host. In addition, toxins released by the bacteria causing bacterial pneumonia can directly damage cells of the lower respiratory system, including the surfactant-producing type II alveolar cells. Bacterial pneumonia results in the most striking immune and inflammatory response, the course of which has been well described for pneumococcal pneumonia.

Stages of Bacterial Pneumonia

For pneumococcal pneumonia, four stages of disease have been described. These four stages are similar for the other types of pneumonia.

Stage 1, called hyperemia, refers to the initial inflammatory response occurring in the area of lung infection. It is characterized by increased blood flow and increased capillary permeability at the site of infection. It occurs as a result of inflammatory mediators released from mast cells after immune cell activation and tissue injury. These components include histamine and prostaglandin. Mast cell degranulation also activates the complement pathway. Complement acts with histamine and prostaglandin to vasodilate the pulmonary vascular smooth muscle, leading to increased blood flow to the area and increased capillary permeability. This results in movement of plasma exudate into the interstitial space, causing swelling and edema between the capillary and the alveolus. Fluid buildup between the capillary and the alveolus increases the distance over which oxygen and carbon dioxide must diffuse, thereby decreasing the rate of gas diffusion. Because oxygen is less soluble than carbon dioxide, its movement into the blood is most affected, often leading to a decrease in hemoglobin oxygen saturation. During this first stage of pneumonia, infection spreads to neighboring tissue as a result of increased blood flow and breakdown of neighboring alveolar and capillary membranes as the inflammatory processes continue.

Stage 2 is called red hepatization. It occurs when the alveoli fill with red blood cells, exudate, and fibrin, produced by the host as part of the inflammatory reaction.

Stage 3, called gray hepatization, occurs as white blood cells colonize the infected part of the lung. Then, fibrin deposits accumulate throughout the area of injury and phagocytosis of cell debris occurs.

Stage 4, called the resolution stage, occurs when the inflammatory and immune responses wane; cell debris, fibrin, and bacteria are digested; and macrophages, the cleanup cells of the inflammatory reaction, dominate.

Clinical Manifestations

Symptoms are similar for all types of pneumonia but are usually most pronounced for those of bacterial origin.

- Significantly increased respiratory rate. Normal and abnormal respiratory rates vary with age, with young infants and children having more rapid normal rates of breathing than older children and adults.
- Grunting, intercostal and substernal retractions, and nasal flaring may be experienced by infants in an attempt to improve airflow.
- Fever and chills from the inflammatory processes and a cough that is often productive, purulent, and present throughout the day.
- Chest pain as a result of pleural irritation. The pain may be diffuse or referred to the abdominal area.
- Sputum that is rust colored (for *S. pneumoniae*), pink (for *S. aureus*), or greenish with a particular odor (for *P. aeruginosa*).
- Crackles, a poplike sound when the airways open suddenly, are indicative of lower airway infection.
- Wheezing, the high-pitched sound heard when air rushes through a narrow orifice, signifies obstruction to airflow.
- Fatigue, from both inflammatory reactions and hypoxia, if the infection is serious.
- Pleural pain from inflammation and edema.

- The subjective response of dyspnea is common. Dyspnea is a feeling of air hunger or a reported difficulty in breathing, which can be attributed in part to decreased gas exchange.
- Hemoptysis, the coughing up of blood, may occur as a result of direct toxin injury to the capillaries or as a result of the inflammatory reaction and subsequent capillary breakdown.

Diagnostic Tools

- White blood cell count generally increases (unless the patient is immunodeficient). This is especially true for bacterial pneumonia.
- Edema of the interstitial space is often apparent on chest radiograph (x-ray).
- ABGs may be abnormal.
- Sputum culture and gram stain.

Complications

- Cyanosis with accompanying hypoxia may develop.
- Ventilation may be reduced because of mucus accumulation, which may lead to absorption atelectasis.
- Respiratory failure and death may occur in extreme cases and may be related to either exhaustion or sepsis (spread of the infection in the blood).

Treatment

The causative agent as determined by a pretreatment sputum sample determines the treatment for pneumonia. Such treatment includes:

- Antibiotics, especially for a bacterial pneumonia. Other pneumonias may be treated with antibiotics to reduce the risk that a bacterial infection will develop secondary to the original infection.
- Analgesics.
- Rest and well-balanced diet.
- Hydration to help loosen secretions.
- Humidified oxygen.
- Deep-breathing techniques to increase ventilation of alveoli and to reduce the risk of atelectasis.
- Other drugs specific for the type of microorganism identified in a sputum culture.

TUBERCULOSIS

TB is another example of a lower respiratory tract infection. It is caused by the microorganism *Mycobacterium tuberculosis*, which usually infects by inhalation of droplets, person to person, and colonizes the respiratory bronchioles or alveoli. It can also enter the body through the gastrointestinal tract, by means of ingestion of contaminated unpasteurized milk, or, occasionally, through a skin lesion. Although TB typically affects the lungs, any organ in the body can be involved.

After nearly 30 years of decline, starting in the mid-1980s, the number of cases of TB diagnosed in the United States began to increase. Reasons for this included increasing numbers of immigrants from areas where TB is endemic, increased poverty and homelessness in this country, and the advent of HIV/AIDS and a surge of immunocompromised persons. Although this increase has begun to taper off, the U.S. Center for Disease Control and Prevention noted that despite a low TB rate reported in 2004 (4.9 cases per 100,000 population), the rate of decline for 2003 and 2004 were the smallest since 1993.

If a significant amount of the *Mycobacterium* bypasses the defense mechanisms of the respiratory system and successfully implants in the lower respiratory tract, the host mounts a vigorous immune and inflammatory response. Because of this vigorous response, which is primarily T-cell mediated, only approximately 5% of people exposed to the bacillus develop active TB. Only those individuals who develop an active tuberculin infection are contagious to others and only during the time of active infection.

Racial and Ethnic Implications

TB rates greater than the U.S. average were observed in certain racial/ethnic populations in 2006. Hispanics, African Americans, and Asians living in the United States have a disproportionately higher incidence than whites. In 2006, the TB rate for foreign-born individuals was 9.5 times higher than in individuals born in the United States. To address the high rate of TB among foreign-born persons living in the United States, custom and immigration efforts are directed to improve the screening of overseas immigrants and refugees, strengthen the current notification system about the arrival of those suspected of having TB, ensure completion of treatment among TB patients who cross the border, test recent arrivals from high-incidence countries for latent infection, and treat to completion. March 24 of each year is being celebrated as World TB Day.

Risk Factors for Tuberculosis Exposure and Infection

Those most at risk of exposure to the bacillus are those living in close quarters with someone who has an active infection. This includes homeless individuals living in shelters where TB is present, as well as family members of infected individuals. Children and the elderly may be especially susceptible. Immigrants to the United States from developing nations frequently arrive with active or latent infection. Substance abusers, incarcerated individuals, and the chronically ill are also at a greater risk.

Also at risk of exposure to and development of TB are health care workers caring for the infected, and those individuals using the same health care clinics or hospital units as people who have active infection. Of those exposed to the bacillus, individuals who have inadequate immune systems, including the undernourished, the elderly and the young, individuals receiving immunosuppressant drugs, and those infected with the human immunodeficiency virus (HIV), are most likely to become infected. The virulence of the strain also affects transmission, with certain highly infective strains identified. TB control is hindered by the emergence of multidrug resistance and the synergistic effect of HIV/AIDS. A significant number of TB cases in Africa have been linked to HIV infection.

Immune Response to Tuberculosis

Because the TB bacillus is difficult to destroy once colonization of the lower respiratory tract occurs, the goal of the immune response is to surround and seal off the bacilli, rather than to kill them. The cell-mediated response involves T cells as well as macrophages. Macrophages encircle the bacilli, after which T cells and fibrous tissue wall off the bacilli and macrophage complex. This complex of bacilli, macrophages, T cells, and scar tissue is called a **tubercle**. The tubercle eventually becomes calcified and is called Ghon complex, which can be seen on chest radiograph. Before engulfment of the bacteria is complete, the material liquefies. At this time, viable microorganisms can gain access to the tracheobronchial system and spread airborne to infect others. Even when adequately walled off, the bacillus may survive within the tubercle. It is believed that because of this viability, approximately 5% to 10% of individuals who do not initially develop TB may have a clinical demonstration of the disease at some other time in their lives, perhaps when they have become immunocompromised by age, other infection, or the need for anti-inflammatory medications. In fact, many if not most cases of active TB occur in individuals whose primary infection occurred decades earlier.

Among those infected, damage to the lung is caused by the bacilli as well as by a vigorous immune and inflammatory reaction. Interstitial edema and permanent scarring of the alveoli increase the distance for diffusion of oxygen and carbon dioxide, decreasing gas exchange. Also, the deposition of scar tissue and production of tubercles decrease surface area available for gas diffusion, decreasing diffusion capacity. If the disease is extensive, abnormalities in the ventilation:perfusion ratio occur that can lead to hypoxic vasoconstriction of pulmonary arterioles and pulmonary hypertension. Decreased lung compliance occurs with scar tissue.

Multidrug-Resistant Tuberculosis

A recent worldwide and serious complication of TB is the development of tuberculin bacilli that are resistant to many drug combinations. Resistance develops when individuals do not complete the course of their therapy, and mutations of the bacillus make it nonresponsive to the antibiotics that were used for a short time. The tuberculin bacillus mutates rapidly and often. Drug-resistant TB can also occur if an individual cannot mount an effective immune response, for instance, as seen in AIDS patients or in the malnourished. In these cases, antibiotic therapy is only partially effective. Health care workers or others who are exposed to these strains of bacillus may also develop drug-resistant TB, which can result in years of morbidity and frequently even in death. Those who have multidrug-resistant TB will need to undergo more toxic and expensive treatments that are more likely to fail.

Clinical Manifestations

Clinical indications of TB may be absent with initial infection and may never be present if active infection does not occur. If active TB develops, an individual usually demonstrates the following:

- Fevers, especially in the afternoon.
- Malaise.
- Chills.
- Shortness of breath.
- Night sweats.
- Loss of appetite and weight loss.
- A productive, purulent cough accompanied by chest pain is common with active infection. Hemoptysis may also be present.

Diagnostic Tools

- A positive skin test for TB demonstrates cell-mediated immunity and gives evidence only of previous exposure of the lower respiratory tract to the bacillus. It is however not an evidence to show that active TB ever developed. Individuals who have received the bacilli Calmette–Guérin (BCG) vaccine may have a false–positive result, but they may not have immunity to TB.
- The QuantiFERON®-TB test is a new-generation blood test that is not affected by the BCG vaccination and does not affect future testing.
- Active TB is diagnosed by collection of a sputum sample followed by microscopic examination for the presence of acid-fast bacilli or culturing of the cells followed by identification and drug susceptibility testing of the isolates. Microscopy suffers from low sensitivity, especially in extrapulmonary TB and conditions of low bacillus count, which are common among HIV-infected individuals. Sputum culture of an actively infected individual will reveal the bacillus but takes a significantly longer time to complete.
- Drug-resistance testing is traditionally performed using conventional methods in either solid or liquid media. More recently, molecular techniques

based on PCR in conjunction with electrophoresis, sequencing, or hybridization are being used to detect gene mutations associated with the development of drug resistance. These molecular techniques have been used to complement smear results and clinical diagnosis.

- Chest radiograph demonstrates current or previous tubercle formation.

Complications

- Severe disease may lead to pneumothorax, hemorrhage, pleural effusion, pneumonia, overwhelming sepsis, respiratory failure, and death.
- Multidrug-resistant TB may develop. Passage to others of the drug-resistant strain may occur.
- Liver damage due to drug therapy.

Treatment

- Treatment of individuals who have active TB is lengthy because the bacillus is resistant to most antibiotics and rapidly mutates when exposed to antibiotics to which it is sensitive. Currently, treatment of individuals who have an active infection includes a combination of four drugs and lasts at least 9 months or longer. If the person does not respond to those drugs, other drugs will be tried and different protocols will be followed. Baseline data should include complete blood cell count, eye exam (vision and color blindness), and HIV test.
- Individuals who develop a positive TB skin test after having been previously negative, even if they show no symptoms of active disease, are usually put on a 6- to 9-month antibiotic regimen to support their immune response and to increase the likelihood that the bacillus will be eradicated completely.
- Vitamin B6 may be prescribed to minimize neuropathy associated with drug therapy.
- If drug-resistant TB develops, more toxic drugs will be administered. The patient may be kept in the hospital or under some type of forced quarantine if compliance with the medical therapy is unlikely or impossible.

A new antibiotic (PA-824) is currently in clinical trials, which has the potential to shorten treatment time.

PNEUMOCONIOSIS

Pneumoconiosis, or **occupational lung disease**, is defined as a restrictive pulmonary disease that results from occupational inhalation of dust, usually from stone, coal plants, or artificial fibers. Pneumoconiosis usually only develops after many years of dust inhalation.

Dust that reaches the lower respiratory tract stimulates an immune and inflammatory reaction resulting in the accumulation of dust-filled macrophages and the development of diffuse pulmonary fibrosis. Pulmonary fibrosis increases the distance across which diffusion of gases must occur, resulting in a decrease in gas exchange. Fibrosis also limits chest compliance and reduces ventilation. Additional influences such as cigarette smoking, which incapacitates the mucociliary escalator system, promote the likelihood of dust reaching the lower respiratory system and increasing its damage.

Examples of diseases from dust inhalation include black lung disease, seen in coal miners; silicosis, which occurs in stone workers, including masons and potters; and brown-lung disease, seen in those exposed to cotton dust. Asbestos exposure also leads to fibrosis and may cause lung cancer.

Clinical Manifestations

- Dyspnea.
- A generally nonproductive cough unless chronic bronchitis develops.
- Dry crackles.
- Interstitial fibrosis.
- A severe restriction of inspiratory volume due to shrinkage of the lung from fibrosis.
- Cyanosis may develop from decreased ventilation coupled with decreased diffusion rate.
- Clubbing.
- Sputum which is black in color.

Diagnostic Tools

- A complete history and physical examination.
- Chest x-ray.

Complications

- Pulmonary hypertension leading to cor pulmonale may develop from severe fibrosis and decreased alveolar ventilation.
- Pneumonias may repeatedly occur as restrictive disease contributes to atelectasis and poor gas exchange.

Treatment

- A reduction of further exposure and avoidance of additive influences such as smoking.
- Prevention and treatment of pneumonia with antibiotic therapy is also important.
- Palliative care.

PNEUMOTHORAX

Pneumothorax is the collapse of all or part of a lung that occurs when air or another gas enters the pleural space surrounding the lungs. Accumulation of air causes separation of the visceral and parietal pleura resulting in the loss of negative pressure which is necessary to keep the lungs inflated. There are different types of pneumothorax: open, spontaneous, and tension.

Open and Spontaneous Pneumothorax

An **open** pneumothorax occurs when the chest wall has been opened and air is allowed into the pleural space from the atmosphere. Atmospheric pressure is greater than pleural pressure and collapses the lungs. Causes of open pneumothorax include stab and gunshot wounds, rib fractures, and penetrating and non-penetrating trauma to the chest wall. With chest trauma, a **hemothorax** may also occur. A hemothorax occurs when blood is lost into the thoracic cavity.

A **spontaneous** pneumothorax occurs when the chest wall is intact, but the lungs spontaneously develop a leak (primary) or are injured and begin to leak air into the pleural space (secondary). Air entering the pleural space from the lungs can cause the underlying alveoli to collapse. A spontaneous pneumothorax may be the result of a ruptured bulla or bleb in the patient with emphysema.

Tension Pneumothorax

It is also possible to have a **tension** pneumothorax in which there is one-way movement of air from the lung into the pleural space through a small hole in the lung structure. In this case, air leaves the lung and enters the pleural space during inspiration. However, air cannot move back into the lungs with expiration because the small hole collapses as the lungs deflate. It is also possible for air to enter the pleural cavity from damage to the tracheobronchial tree. Any tension pneumothorax is a life-threatening situation as it results in increased pressure in the pleural space. As pleural pressure increases, widespread compression atelectasis can occur. Displacement of the heart and great vessels in the thoracic cavity may also occur, resulting in severe alterations of cardiovascular function.

Clinical Manifestations

- Acute onset of pain in the thoracic area resulting from pleural trauma.
- Diminished or absent breath sounds and decreased respiratory movement over the area of the collapsed lung.
- Rapid, shallow breathing (tachypnea) and dyspnea are common.
- If the pneumothorax is extensive, or if it is a tension pneumothorax and air is accumulating in the pleural space, the heart and large blood vessels may be displaced toward the other lung, which would give the chest the appearance of asymmetry. Tracheal deviation may also be apparent.

Diagnostic Tools

- Blood gases and hemoglobin saturation will indicate hypoxia.
- Radiographs can identify a collapsed lung.
- If the pneumothorax is small, a CT scan may be necessary.

Complications

- A tension pneumothorax may collapse blood vessels, leading to reduced cardiac filling and causing a fall in blood pressure. The other lung may also be affected.
- A pneumothorax may lead to hypoxia and severe dyspnea. Death may occur.

Treatment

- A tension pneumothorax is a life-threatening condition because the buildup of air in the pleural space can eventually collapse the underlying lungs and blood vessels. It must be treated immediately with insertion of a chest tube or a large-bore needle into the pleural space with subsequent suction of the air out of the space.
- A small spontaneous pneumothorax or a pneumothorax resulting secondarily to chest trauma is treated by insertion of a chest tube connected to a drainage tube that is kept in place until the pleural injury is healed. Any penetrating wound should be covered or closed.

RESPIRATORY FAILURE

Inadequate exchange of gas that results in hypoxia, hypercapnia (increased arterial carbon dioxide concentration), and acidosis is called respiratory failure. It frequently develops when breathing becomes so difficult that exhaustion sets in and the individual no longer has enough energy to breathe. Respiratory failure becomes a vicious cycle; the more difficult it is to breathe, the less the alveoli themselves are oxygenated, leading to death of the surfactant-producing cells, and an increased resistance to expansion. This means that the work of breathing is even harder, and the cycle continues and worsens. Respiratory failure can develop after a variety of respiratory diseases, including widespread pneumonia, sepsis, and infection with certain viruses such as Hantavirus.

Clinical Manifestations

- Cyanosis.
- Severe dyspnea.
- Hypoxemia.
- Tachycardia, tachypnea, agitation, confusion, disorientation.

Diagnostic Tools

- Respiratory failure is defined clinically as a partial pressure of oxygen in arterial blood of ≤50 mm Hg, and a partial pressure of carbon dioxide in arterial blood of ≧50 mm Hg, with a pH ≤7.25.

Complications

- Poor oxygenation of other organs may lead to multiorgan failure.
- Individuals in respiratory failure are at a high risk of dying.

Treatment

- Oxygen support, including intubation and artificial ventilation. In general, the sooner a person is put on ventilatory support, the better the prognosis.
- Noninvasive positive pressure ventilation (NPPV).

ADULT RESPIRATORY DISTRESS SYNDROME (ARDS)

ARDS is a disease characterized by widespread breakdown of the alveolar and/or pulmonary capillary membranes. ARDS occurs after a major pulmonary, cardiovascular, or system-wide insult. It may also occur following excessive fluid resuscitation, blood transfusions, or blunt chest trauma. See page C11 for illustrations.

Causes of Adult Respiratory Distress Syndrome

ARDS can occur as a result of direct injury to the capillaries of the lungs or to the alveoli. However, because the capillary and the alveolus are so intimately connected, extensive destruction of one typically leads to destruction of the other. This destruction occurs because of the release of lytic enzymes when cells die; it also occurs with activation of the inflammatory reaction subsequent to cell injury and death. Examples of conditions that affect the capillaries and/or the alveoli and can lead to ARDS are presented in the following sections.

Capillary Destruction

If the initial breakdown is of the capillary membrane, movement of plasma and red blood cells into the interstitial space occurs. This increases the distance across which oxygen and carbon dioxide must diffuse, decreasing the rate of gas exchange. Fluid accumulating in the interstitial space moves into the alveoli, diluting surfactant and increasing surface tension. The exertion of pressure needed to inflate the alveoli is vastly increased. Increased surface tension coupled with edema and swelling of the interstitial space leads to widespread compression atelectasis, resulting in a loss of lung compliance, significantly decreased ventilation, and hypoxia. Causes of pulmonary capillary breakdown include septicemia, pancreatitis, venoms, and uremia. Pneumonia, smoke inhalation, trauma, and near drowning can also destroy the capillary membrane and initiate ARDS.

Alveolar Destruction

When the alveoli are the initial damage site, the surface area available for gas exchange is reduced, and, again, the rate of gas exchange is decreased. Causes of alveolar damage include pneumonia, aspiration, and smoke inhalation. Oxygen toxicity, which occurs after 24 to 36 hours of high-oxygen treatment, can also be a cause of alveolar membrane damage through the production of oxygen free radicals and by damaging the surfactant-producing cells.

Without oxygen, vascular and pulmonary tissues become hypoxic, leading to further cell injury and death. Once the alveoli and capillaries are damaged, inflammatory reactions, including macrophage and neutrophil infiltration and the release of various cytokines, are initiated that lead to swelling and edema of the interstitial space and damage to the neighboring capillaries and alveoli. Within 24 hours of ARDS onset, hyaline membranes form within the alveoli. These are white fibrin deposits that progressively accumulate and further decrease gas exchange. Eventually, fibrosis obliterates the alveoli. Ventilation, respiration, and perfusion are all compromised. Mortality associated with ARDS can be as high as 50% and is usually the result of multiple-organ failure.

Clinical Manifestations

- Significant dyspnea.
- Decreased lung compliance.
- Inspiratory crackles.
- Diffuse alveolar infiltrates on chest radiograph.
- Rapid shallow breathing initially, resulting in respiratory alkalosis as carbon dioxide is blown off. Dyspnea and hypoxemia lead to a metabolic acidosis which results in hypoventilation and resulting respiratory acidosis. Respiratory acidosis causes further hypoxemia (unresponsive to O_2 therapy) which eventually results in hypotension, decreased cardiac output, and death.

Diagnostic Tools

- Arterial blood–gas analysis demonstrates reduced arterial oxygen concentration despite oxygen therapy. Oxygen therapy is ineffective in ARDS, regardless of the amount of oxygen supplied, because diffusion of the gas is limited owing to fibrin accumulation, edema, and capillary and alveolar breakdown.
- Chest radiograph.

Complications

- Respiratory failure may develop as the disease progresses and the individual has to work harder to overcome decreased compliance of the lungs. Eventually, exhaustion sets in and ventilation slows. This results in respiratory acidosis as carbon dioxide accumulates in the blood. Respiratory slowing and a fall in arterial pH are indications of impending respiratory failure and possible death.
- Pneumonia may develop after ARDS because of fluid accumulation in the lungs and poor lung expansion.
- Renal failure and gastrointestinal stress ulcer can occur as a result of hypoxia.
- Disseminated intravascular coagulation may develop because of the large amount of tissue that can be destroyed during ARDS.

Treatment

Initially, treatment of ARDS is geared toward prevention, because ARDS is never a primary disease but always occurs after a major body catastrophe. When present, ARDS is treated as follows:

- Diuretics to decrease fluid load and cardiostimulatory drugs to increase cardiac contractility and stroke volume are used. These interventions serve to reduce fluid buildup in the lungs and to reduce the likelihood of right-heart failure.
- Oxygen therapy and mechanical ventilation are often initiated.
- Anti-inflammatory drugs to reduce the damaging effects of inflammation are occasionally used, although their effectiveness is questionable.
- Vasopressor medications are indicated if fluid resuscitation has not been effective in preventing shock. Vasopressors are given to prevent tissue hypoxia and hypotension and to increase cardiac output to minimize the risk for renal failure.

SEVERE ACUTE RESPIRATORY SYNDROME (SARS)

SARS was first recognized as a global threat by the World Health Organization in mid-March 2003. The SARS coronavirus (SARS-CoV) is the etiological agent and is believed to be an animal virus that crossed the species barrier to humans. The natural reservoir of SARS-CoV has not been identified, but a number of wildlife species, including the Himalayan masked palm civet (*Paguma larvata*), the Chinese ferret badger (*Melogale moschata*), and the raccoon dog (*Nyctereutes procyonoides*), are suspect. The most probable sources of human infection with the SARS-CoV are either from these or other animal reservoirs or from exposure in laboratories where the virus is used or stored for diagnostic and research purposes.

Clinical Manifestations

- During the first week, patients develop influenza-like prodromal symptoms such as fever, malaise, myalgia, headache, and lymphopenia.
- Dry cough, dyspnea, and large-volume diarrhea may be present in the first to second weeks.
- Sore throat.
- Rash.
- Dizziness.
- Confusion.
- Transmission occurs during the second week.
- Severe cases develop rapidly progressing respiratory distress and oxygen desaturation, with about 20% requiring intensive care.

Diagnostic Tools

A detailed history and chest radiograph are recommended along with the following tests.

Laboratory Tests

- Diagnosis requires reverse transcription-polymerase chain reaction (RT-PCR) positive for the SARS-CoV, using a validated method from at least two different clinical specimens (e.g., nasopharyngeal and stool) or from the same clinical specimen collected on two or more occasions during the course of the illness (e.g., sequential nasopharyngeal aspirates). Two different assays or repeat RT-PCR are required, using a new RNA extract from the original clinical sample on each occasion of testing.
- Seroconversion by ELISA. Negative antibody test on acute serum (collected prior to the development of antibody) followed by positive antibody test on convalescent phase serum tested in parallel.

Virus Isolation

- Isolation in cell culture from any clinical specimen and identification of the SARS-CoV using a validated method such as RT-PCR.

Laboratory Findings

- Proliferation of the cytokine interferon-gamma has been identified after SARS-CoV infection. It is hypothesized that this cytokine might be involved in immunopathologic damage in SARS patients.
- Lymphopenia, thrombocytopenia, and elevated lactate dehydrogenase and creatine kinase levels. Age, male sex, high lactate dehydrogenase level, high

creatine kinase level, and high initial absolute neutrophil count are significant predictive factors for intensive care unit admission and death.
- Hyponatremia, hypokalemia, hypomagnesemia, and hypocalcemia have been reported.

Complications

- Respiratory failure and death may occur.
- Those who survive may experience compromised pulmonary function for months after.
- For pregnant women who develop SARS, there is an increase in fetal loss in early pregnancy and maternal mortality in later pregnancy.

Treatment

- The anti-inflammatory agent dexamethasone and intravenous immunoglobulin are given. Dexamethasone inhibits cytokine production and delayed chemokine-recruited inflammation, while the immunoglobulin appears to modulate cytokine overaction and inhibit lymphocyte or macrophage activation.
- Antivirals may be prescribed.
- Antibiotics if superimposed bacterial infection is present.

INFLUENZA

Influenza is a contagious viral disease transmitted by small-particle aerosols. Transmission may occur through coughing, sneezing, or by direct contact between respiratory droplets and the nose or mouth. After being deposited in the lower respiratory tract, the virus attaches to the epithelial cells and causes an infection. The two types of influenza are type A and type B. Because of antigenic mutations in the virus from year to year, annual influenza vaccinations are necessary. The disease is typically self-limiting although the risk of complications is higher in older adults and those with chronic illnesses.

Clinical Manifestations

- Abrupt onset of fever, chills, and myalgia.
- Headache, fatigue, nonproductive cough.
- Sore throat and nasal congestion.

Diagnostic Tools

- Rapid flu test.
- Other viral tests may be done to rule out other diseases.

Complications

- Pneumonia.

Treatment

- If antivirals are begun within two days of the onset of clinical manifestations, the clinical course may be shorter and less severe.
- Symptomatic treatment including fluids, rest, acetaminophen, or aspirin.
- No alcohol or tobacco.

RESPIRATORY DISTRESS SYNDROME OF THE NEWBORN

Respiratory distress syndrome (RDS) of the newborn, also called **hyaline membrane disease**, can be attributed to an immature pulmonary system and decreased surfactant. It is a condition of pulmonary hypoxia and injury resulting from widespread primary atelectasis. Primary atelectasis refers to the state of substantial alveolar collapse seen in a newborn. With alveolar collapse, ventilation is decreased. Hypoxia develops, leading to pulmonary injury and a subsequent inflammatory reaction with the accumulation of white blood cells and the release of various cytokines. The inflammatory reaction leads to edema and swelling of the interstitial space, further reducing gas exchange between capillaries and any functioning alveoli. Inflammation also results in the production of hyaline membranes, which are white fibrin accumulations lining the alveoli. Fibrin deposits further decrease gas exchange and reduce lung compliance. With a decrease in lung compliance, the work of breathing is increased.

Decreased alveolar ventilation results in a decreased ventilation: perfusion ratio and pulmonary arteriolar vasoconstriction. Pulmonary vasoconstriction can lead to an increase in right-heart volume and pressure, resulting in a shunting of blood from the right atrium through the still-patent foramen ovale of the newborn, and directly to the left atrium. Likewise, high pulmonary resistance can result in deoxygenated blood bypassing the lungs and being delivered directly to the left side of the body via the ductus arteriosus. Both of these blood flow routes are considered right-to-left shunts, in that they bypass the lungs and so deliver poorly oxygenated blood to the systemic circulation. These examples of shunting worsen the condition of hypoxia, leading to significant cyanosis.

With each attempt to ventilate the collapsed alveoli, the infant must exert a large amount of energy. Such energy expenditure results in a correspondingly large oxygen demand, contributing to the evident cyanosis. With increased oxygen demand, the infant is caught in a positive-feedback cycle as shown in Figure 14-5.

At first the infant demonstrates rapid, shallow breathing in an attempt to meet this high oxygen demand, causing initial blood gases to indicate respiratory alkalosis as carbon dioxide is blown off. However, the infant soon tires

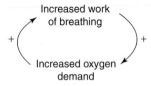

FIGURE 14-5 When the work of breathing is increased, oxygen demand increases, which further increases the work of breathing.

from the extraordinarily difficult alveolar and lung expansion and is unable to keep up the respiratory effort. When this occurs, respiratory effort slows and blood gases reflect respiratory acidosis (buildup of carbon dioxide) and the onset of respiratory failure.

Risk Factors for Respiratory Distress Syndrome

The primary risk factor for the development of RDS of the newborn is prematurity. Between 5% and 10% of premature infants suffer from this syndrome. The more premature the infant, the more likely that RDS will develop. The mechanism whereby prematurity is associated with RDS is threefold.

Most significantly, the type II alveolar cells that produce surfactant do not mature until between 28 and 32 weeks of gestation. Therefore, any infant born before surfactant is present in the alveoli encounters high alveolar surface tension with each breath. This contributes significantly to the primary atelectasis seen in RDS and results in decreased alveolar ventilation and hypoxia. Second, alveoli of premature infants are small and unfolded. By Laplace law, this factor also contributes to the increased pressure that must be exerted to overcome their surface tension. Third, premature infants have weak, immature chest muscles, making it almost impossible for an infant without surfactant to successfully expand his alveoli, breath after breath for hours.

Infants born to insulin-dependent diabetic mothers are also at risk for developing RDS. It appears that insulin provided by injection interferes with the development of type II alveolar cells. Other categories of risk include preterm males, white infants, infants exposed to cold stress or asphyxia during delivery, and infants born via cesarean section. Because cortisol accelerates surfactant production and vaginal delivery tends to increase the newborn's cortisol production, infants born via cesarean section are not afforded this benefit.

Clinical Manifestations

The following clinical manifestations are usually present at birth:

- Increased respiratory rate.
- Central cyanosis.
- Duskiness of the skin caused by hypoxia.

- Intercostal or chest retractions with each breath.
- Nasal flaring with each breath.
- Many infants survive RDS, and in these cases the symptoms lessen and resolve, usually within 3 days.

Diagnostic Tools

- Diagnosis is usually made from the clinical appearance of the infant at birth coupled with the pregnancy history.
- ABGs may be drawn to assist in diagnosis and management.
- Chest radiograph typically shows diffuse granular densities within hours of birth.

Complications

- Some infants who survive RDS go on to develop bronchopulmonary dysplasia (BPD), which is a chronic respiratory disease characterized by alveolar scarring, inflammation of the alveoli and the capillaries, and pulmonary hypertension. Effects of BPD may continue for years.
- Patent ductus arteriosus may develop due to increased pulmonary effort that increases resistance to pulmonary blood flow.
- Signs of dyspnea and hypoxia may continue and proceed to infant exhaustion, respiratory failure, and death, usually within 3 days.

Treatment

- Prevention is the first treatment of RDS. This includes behavioral and pharmacologic attempts to delay or stop labor and accurate dating of pregnancy to minimize delivery of premature infants by cesarean section.
- Delay of parturition (delivery of an infant) for even 24 to 48 hours has been shown to reduce the incidence and severity of RDS. This is because the stress of labor increases maternal and fetal cortisol release from the adrenal cortex. Naturally occurring increases in cortisol have been shown to stimulate the type II alveolar cells to produce surfactant.
- Maternal injections of corticosteroids at least 24 hours before a premature infant is delivered can significantly reduce the incidence of RDS. Concerns exist, however, about the long-term effects of exposing newborns to high levels of steroids.
- If an infant is born with RDS, treatment is supportive and consists of oxygen therapy, maintenance of a quiet, warm environment to decrease oxygen requirements, nutritional support, and repeated evaluation of blood gases and acid–base status.
- Continuous positive airway pressure through nasal prongs.

- A major treatment advance has been the development of artificial surfactant. Surfactant can be delivered directly into the lower respiratory tract of infants demonstrating signs of RDS and has been shown to be successful in reducing clinical manifestations of the disease. This treatment, combined with maternal corticosteroid injections, offers the best hope for reducing the morbidity and mortality caused by RDS.
- Diabetic women are closely monitored throughout pregnancy.
- Mechanical ventilation may be employed to treat RDS. However, it is associated with increased risk of developing BPD.

SUDDEN INFANT DEATH SYNDROME

Characterized by the unexpected and the unexplained death of a previously healthy infant, sudden infant death syndrome (SIDS) typically occurs when the infant is between 1 week and 1 year of age. The highest incidence of SIDS is between 2 and 4 months of age, and occurs primarily during the night. African Americans and Native Americans have a higher rate of SIDS than Hispanics, Asians, or whites.

At risk of developing SIDS are premature infants, infants born small for gestational age, and those born in multiple-birth pregnancies. Males are at slightly increased risk. In some cases, there is also a history of an upper respiratory tract infection during the week before death. Also at increased risk of developing SIDS are siblings of a child who has died of SIDS, and infants who have already experienced an episode of prolonged apnea, a near-miss occurrence of SIDS.

The incidence of SIDS has declined in recent years. This decline appears to be because of an understanding of behavioral risk factors as well as more restrictive diagnostic criteria. SIDS, however, remains the major cause of death in otherwise healthy infants during the first year of life.

Causes of Sudden Infant Death Syndrome

The cause of SIDS is unknown. Some evidence suggests that an immature central nervous system fails to respond appropriately to increasing levels of carbon dioxide. Normally, increasing carbon dioxide is a stimulation to breathe, until high levels eventually depress ventilation. Healthy infants show occasional periods of apnea, during which carbon dioxide levels rise, stimulating the infant to breathe. Infants who experience SIDS or who experience near-miss episodes of SIDS appear not to respond to rising carbon dioxide with a stimulation of ventilation. Instead, they may show only a depression of ventilation in response to carbon dioxide. In these infants, apnea would occur, carbon dioxide levels would rise, and instead of stimulating breathing, the apneic episode would continue. Eventually, the high carbon dioxide levels completely suppress ventilation and the child dies.

Another phenomenon that may be involved in the development of SIDS in some infants is a prolongation of the cardiac QT interval (time before ventricular repolarization). It is suggested that this may lead to a fatal arrhythmia. Both respiratory and cardiac causes of SIDS are believed to have developmental as well as genetic influences.

Other Causes of Unexpected Infant Death

The major behavioral intervention that has resulted in a significant reduction in the occurrence of SIDS has to do with the positioning of infants during sleep periods. It appears that many infants who were assumed to have died of SIDS in the past actually suffocated while lying on mattresses or pillows that were too soft. When an infant lies face down, it has an increased risk of suffocation caused by its inability to move its head and face freely out of a confining position. This is especially true if the infant is weak because of prematurity or if the bed is too soft. In addition, if a baby's face is pressed into a small, soft depression on a mattress or pillow, it exhales into that depression and then rebreathes the same air. The carbon dioxide concentration in this pocket of rebreathed air increases, leading to central nervous system depression and cessation of breathing. Thus, it is recommended that infants should be propped on their back, not placed face down, and never left unattended on a water bed, soft mattress, pillow, or fur rug.

Other areas that are being explored include maternal smoking, secondhand smoke, and gastroesophageal reflux disease. Another cause of infant death that is occasionally diagnosed as SIDS is child abuse. Injuries to the infant brainstem can occur with even moderate shaking, leading to respiratory depression and death. This condition is known as shaken-baby syndrome.

Clinical Manifestations

- Death by suffocation or heart failure caused by respiratory arrest.
- Symptoms of near-miss apneic episodes are cyanosis and, upon revival, gasping for air.

Treatment

- Treatment of SIDS is aimed at prevention. Infants at high risk (as defined by having suffered a near-miss episode or having had a sibling who experienced SIDS) may wear monitors to signal apneic episodes.
- If a cardiac tendency to dysrhythmia is documented, antiarrhythmic drugs or monitors may be used.
- Prevention of other causes of infant death include careful placement of an infant to avoid face-down positions and vigilant prevention of child abuse.

CYSTIC FIBROSIS

Cystic fibrosis is a hereditary disease characterized by alterations of exocrine gland function throughout the body. It results in production of large amounts of thick mucus and increased concentration of sodium and chloride in the sweat. Cystic fibrosis is a relatively common genetic disease, affecting mostly whites (1 in 3200 born in the United States). It is much less common in other races, although it does happen. Cystic fibrosis occurs as a result of a mutation in the 230 kb gene, a gene located in the middle of chromosome 7. This gene normally produces a protein called the cystic fibrosis transmembrane regulator (CFTR) protein, which functions as a chloride channel in epithelial cell membranes, thus affecting the flow of chloride through virtually all cells of the body. Without this protein, phenylalanine is absent and secretions dry out and become thick and obstructive. Cystic fibrosis is typically inherited as an autosomal-recessive disease. Only individuals who carry two copies of the defective gene, one from each parent, will have the disease. Over 1000 mutations in this gene have been described, although the most common mutation is one that results in defective processing of the protein. Carriers of one cystic fibrosis gene and one normal gene are heterozygotic for the trait and do not demonstrate the disease.

Effects of Cystic Fibrosis

When the CFTR protein is absent, copious amounts of mucus and heavily concentrated sweat are produced. Phenylalanine deficit leads to dehydration, which leads to increased viscosity of mucous gland secretions and eventually results in glandular duct obstruction. The main body systems affected by the mucus accumulation are the pulmonary and the gastrointestinal systems. Other organs are also victims of the excess mucus, including the liver and the reproductive organs. Sweat glands oversecrete sodium chloride, and sweat accumulates on the skin.

Pulmonary Effects of Cystic Fibrosis

In the lungs, the thick mucus increases the risk of repeated pneumonias and chronic bronchitis. It also blocks alveolar ventilation, leading to absorption atelectasis. In addition, an exaggerated and extended inflammatory response to pathogens, characterized by neutrophil-dominated airway inflammation, is chronically present. This leads to edema of the capillary and alveolar interface that accelerates progression of disease. Bronchial scarring and fibrosis progressively destroy the bronchial passages. Lung compliance is reduced and ventilation impaired.

Gastrointestinal Effects of Cystic Fibrosis

In the gastrointestinal tract, thick mucus accumulates, blocking digestion and absorption of nutrients. The pancreatic duct becomes clogged, thereby preventing the pancreatic digestive enzymes from reaching the small intestine and further compromising digestion and absorption of nutrients. A common complication is failure to thrive which is defined as a downward deviation in weight in an infant or a child from a previously recorded maximum crossing one or two percentile lines and persisting for longer than 1 month. Poor nutritional status contributes to the frequency and severity of pulmonary infections. Frequently, the pancreas is destroyed, resulting in decreased insulin secretion and diabetes.

Clinical Manifestations

- A protuberant abdomen may be apparent soon after birth, resulting from an inability to pass meconium in the first stool.
- Salty taste when kissed, caused by salt buildup from sweat on the skin.
- Repeated occurrences of respiratory tract infections throughout infancy and early childhood.
- Thick, sticky secretions.
- Bulky, greasy stools.
- Dehydration.
- Chronic rhinitis (or nasal drainage), and chronic cough and sputum production.
- Failure to thrive because nutrients are poorly absorbed.

Diagnostic Tools

- In the United States, 50% of patients with cystic fibrosis are diagnosed by 6 months of age, and 90% are diagnosed by 8 years. While early diagnosis may improve weight gain and early growth of infants via improved nutritional management, whether early diagnosis affects long-term outcome is unclear.
- Testing for excess chloride in a sample of sweat; a positive result and presence of an obstructive pulmonary disease is indicative of disease. A concentration of sweat chloride greater than 60 mmol/L on repeated analysis is diagnostic.
- Genetic testing can be used to confirm the diagnosis. Testing for CFTR.
- Abnormal pancreatic enzymes support the diagnosis.
- Measurement of transepithelial potential differences in nasal membrane.
- Cystic fibrosis may be diagnosed prenatally by amniocentesis in couples who are known heterozygotes for the disease. Even eggs fertilized in vitro can be identified as being heterozygotic or homozygotic for the cystic fibrosis gene at the eight-cell stage. The option to implant the embryo or abort the fetus is available.

Complications

- Most individuals who have cystic fibrosis become progressively worse, and many die in their 20s or 30s, usually of bacterial pneumonia. Pulmonary hypertension can also develop as a result of decreased ventilation-perfusion, leading to cor pulmonale.

- Frequent respiratory infections are present throughout life.
- Nearly 98% of men with cystic fibrosis are infertile. Aspermia is present secondary to atrophied or absent vas deferens or seminal vesicles. Spermatogenesis and sexual functioning are normal, however, and men have successfully become fathers with assisted technology. Female reproductive function is normal, although cervical mucus may be especially thick.
- Nasal polyps, pneumothroax, cholecystitis, rectal prolapse, bowel obstruction.

Treatment

- Prevention of bacterial lung infection is a primary aim of treatment. The use of improved antibiotic treatment strategies both for prophylaxis and in response to acute infection is the main reason for the increased life span currently seen. Lung injury and scarring are reduced.
- Drugs that block inflammation are being tested as a mechanism to reduce pulmonary damage, including drugs that reduce the production of proinflammatory cytokines or increase anti-inflammatory cytokine levels. Other drugs have been developed that target specific components of neutrophils or block enzymes that accumulate at sites of neutrophil degradation. These enzymes are largely responsible for the damage to associated airway tissues. Clinical trials are underway to test the efficacy of such drugs, including recombinant human DNase (dornase alpha). Early studies suggest that cystic fibrosis patients have improved lung function and minimal pulmonary exacerbations following use of DNase. DNase appears to facilitate expectoration of mucus and more effective clearance of neutrophils and by-products from the lungs.
- Daily chest physiotherapy is essential to assist the individual in clearing the respiratory passages of mucus accumulations. Techniques include chest percussion and postural drainage, and frequent rest periods are advised to decrease energy demands.
- Bronchodilators and mucus-thinning medications.
- Increased nutrient intake is important to maintain a well-functioning immune system and to minimize growth deficiencies. Dietary education and digestive enzyme supplements can improve nutritional balance and growth.
- Double lung or heart–lung transplantation is a treatment option for some patients with end-stage lung disease. Survival is poorer than for other types of organ transplantation, however, with a 3-year survival of about 60%. Better results are seen in adults than in children.
- There is ongoing genetic research aimed at correcting cystic fibrosis at the gene level. Experimental techniques include introducing the gene for transmembrane regulator protein into the lungs of an individual with cystic fibrosis, via exposure of the person to a genetically engineered virus that has

been designed to carry that gene in its own DNA. It is intended that the virus, typically an attenuated cold virus, when delivered into the lower respiratory tract will incorporate its DNA into the host's respiratory cell DNA. This is the normal pattern of viral infection in the lungs. However, in this case, the virus would also be incorporating the genetically altered DNA into the host's genome, replacing the host's missing gene. Preliminary results of these initial trials have been unsuccessful, although hope is that in the future their success will be a standard for cure.

- Additional studies are underway to investigate the use of supplements, including the following:
  - Glutathione, a naturally occurring antioxidant that protects the lungs from germs and pollutants. Patients with cystic fibrosis appear to have low levels of pulmonary glutathione. Glutathione administered by inhalation or as an oral supplement may reduce oxidative stress in patients, thereby reducing cell damage and lung inflammation.
  - Cucumin, the component of the spice turmeric that gives it a bright yellow color and strong taste. In animal studies, cucumin appeared to stimulate the function of the cystic fibrosis transmembrane conductance regulator. Phase 1 clinical trials are underway to test if similar effects will be manifested in humans.

ASTHMA

Asthma is a progressive respiratory disease characterized by inflammation of the respiratory tract and spasm of airway bronchiolar smooth muscle. This results in excess mucus production and accumulation, obstruction to airflow, and a decrease in ventilation of the alveoli. See page C12 for illustrations.

Asthma occurs in individuals who aggressively respond to various airway irritants. Risk factors for this type of hyperresponsiveness include a family history of asthma or allergy, suggesting a genetic tendency. Repeated or intense exposure to some irritating stimuli, perhaps at a key developmental time, may also increase risk of this disease. Although most cases of asthma are diagnosed in childhood, adults may develop asthma without a previous history of the disease. According to the Center for Disease Control (2007), in 2005 childhood asthma was more prevalent in boys while adult-onset asthma was more prevalent in females. Stimulation of adult-onset asthma often appears related to a worsening of previous allergies. Repeated upper respiratory infections may also trigger adult-onset asthma, as can occupational exposure to dusts and irritants.

Inflammatory Reaction in Asthma

The pathophysiology of asthma involves a hyperresponsiveness of the airways after exposure to one or more irritating stimuli. Known stimuli for inducing an asthmatic reaction include viral infections; an allergic response to dust, pollen, mites, or pet dander; exercise; cold exposure; and gastrointestinal reflux. With airway irritability and hyperresponsiveness, both an **inflammatory reaction** and **bronchoconstriction** result. Although bronchoconstriction and a feeling that the air passages are closing may be the first symptom of an asthmatic attack, it is the delayed inflammatory reaction that makes asthma such a serious disease.

The primary mediators of inflammation in an asthmatic reaction are the eosinophils, a type of white blood cell. Eosinophils concentrate in the area and release chemicals that stimulate mast-cell degranulation. They also draw other white blood cells to the area, including basophils and neutrophils; stimulate the production of mucus; and increase swelling and edema of the tissues. The inflammatory response begins with the initial stimulus, but it may take as long as 12 hours to become apparent.

More acutely felt is the effect of the chemical histamine on the bronchiolar smooth muscle. Histamine is released with IgE-mediated mast-cell degranulation and quickly causes bronchiolar smooth muscle constriction and spasm. Histamine also stimulates mucus production and increased capillary permeability, further contributing to the more delayed congestion and swelling of the interstitial spaces.

Individuals who develop asthma may have either an overabundance of eosinophils or perhaps an over-responsiveness of the mast cells to stimuli initiating degranulation. IgE antibody, responsible for allergic attacks, may overreact in response to foreign antigens, turning on the inflammatory cascade. Regardless of the source of the hypersensitivity, the final result is bronchospasm, mucus production and accumulation, edema, and obstruction to airflow. Viral infection, allergy, and reflux appear to trigger a hypersensitivity response by means of irritating the airways. Exercise might also act as an irritant because large volumes of air are moved rapidly in and out of the lungs. This air has not been adequately humidified, warmed, or cleared of particulates and can trigger an attack.

Psychological Stimuli for Asthma

Psychological stimuli may worsen an asthmatic attack. Because parasympathetic stimulation constricts bronchiolar smooth muscle, anything that increases parasympathetic activity could worsen the symptoms of asthma. The parasympathetic system is activated with the emotions of anxiety and sometimes fear. An individual having an attack may experience worsening of symptoms as his anxiety peaks. In contrast, sympathetic innervation of bronchiolar smooth muscle leads to dilation of the bronchi. Typically, sympathetic stimulation is associated with conditions of fright and flight, during which increased ventilation is an important component of escape. Many of the therapeutic interventions traditionally used to treat asthma have relied on blocking parasympathetic or stimulating sympathetic responses.

Clinical Manifestations

- Significant dyspnea and tightness in the chest.
- Coughing, especially at night.
- Rapid, shallow breathing.
- Audible wheezing can be heard on auscultation of the lungs. Typically wheezing is heard only on expiration, unless the patient's condition is severe.
- An increase in the work of breathing, exemplified by chest retractions and, with a worsening of condition, nasal flaring.
- Hyperresonant lung fields and diminished breath sounds.
- Tachycardia.
- Anxiety, related to the inability to get enough air.
- Air trapping because of the obstruction to airflow, especially seen during expiration in patients who have asthma. This is demonstrated as prolonged expiration time.
- Between asthmatic attacks, a person is usually asymptomatic. However, changes in lung function tests may be apparent even between attacks in patients who have persistent asthma.

Diagnostic Tools

- Asthma is diagnosed by spirometry, a technique that measures and identifies reductions in vital capacity and reduced peak expiratory flow rates. During an asthmatic attack, maximum expiratory volume and maximum rate of expiration are reduced.
- To evaluate asthma symptoms at home, peak flowmeters are available. With a peak flowmeter, maximum forced expiratory flow rate (FEV), also called peak flow, is measured during an attack and during times between asthmatic episodes. (Note: since personal flowmeters do not actually measure exhalation over just 1 second, FEV will give slightly different values than the more exact FEV_1 measurements.) By comparing his or her personal best FEV with that produced during an exacerbation, an individual or a family member can recognize mild versus moderate or severe worsening of symptoms. Appropriate therapeutic or emergency interventions can then be initiated.
- Individuals who have asthma typically show a significant diurnal pattern, with peak flowmeter readings significantly poorer in the early hours after midnight than in late afternoon. This may be related to exacerbation of symptoms by exposure to the cool air of night, or related to diurnal changes in hormones such as cortisol, known to affect inflammatory reactions.
- The saturation of hemoglobin with oxygen (oxygen saturation) may be measured to determine how well the blood is being oxygenated in a person showing asthmatic symptoms. This technique involves placing a sensor over

the finger and obtaining the information concerning the color of the blood flowing beneath it. Unsaturated hemoglobin is darker in color than saturated. This tool is easily used in the clinical setting and provides a rapid indication of a patient's ability to move air.

- Blood–gas analysis may demonstrate a decrease in arterial oxygen concentration and at first respiratory alkalosis as carbon dioxide is blown off in rapid breathing. If the condition persists and worsens, respiratory acidosis may develop as a result of status asthmaticus, as described in the following section.

Complications

- **Status asthmaticus**, a life-threatening condition of prolonged bronchiolar spasm that cannot be reversed with medication, may develop in some individuals. In this case, the work of breathing is greatly increased. When the work of breathing increases, oxygen demand also increases. Because individuals in an asthmatic attack are not meeting a normal oxygen demand, they certainly cannot meet the high-oxygen demands needed to inspire and expire against prolonged bronchiolar spasm, bronchiolar swelling, and thick mucus.
- Pneumothorax from the enormous pressures exerted to ventilate.
- As the individual becomes exhausted with effort, respiratory acidosis, respiratory failure, and death can occur.

Treatment

The goals of treatment are to (1) control the disease, (2) maintain control, and (3) minimize risk and impairment associated with asthma. According to the National Asthma Education and Prevention Program (2007), medications should be individualized using a stepwise approach based on each patient's age and responsiveness to therapy. Self-monitoring and routine follow-up with a consistent health care provider are essential.

- The first step in treatment involves evaluating a patient's severity of asthma. Staging is currently separated into four levels, depending on the frequency of symptoms and the frequency with which medications are needed to provide relief. Stages of asthma include (1) intermittent, (2) mild, (3) persistent moderate, and (4) severe. Treatment is based on staging.
- For all stages of asthma, prevention of exposure to known allergens is vital. This involves identifying triggers and allergy-proofing the home—including removal of pets as necessary—avoidance of cigarette and wood-burning smoke, and the use of air conditioners to minimize the opening of windows, especially during high-pollen seasons.
- Monitoring peak flow rate frequently, especially during times of increased asthma incidence, such as the cold season (winter) or the pollen season

(spring), is key for early recognition of exacerbations, reduction of symptoms, and prevention of hospitalization. This is true even for mild intermittent asthma. If a significant decrease in peak flow rate is observed, adding pharmacologic intervention immediately instead of waiting until an attack is full blown can block its progression.

- An important advance in prevention and treatment of an asthmatic attack has been the use of oral or inhaled corticosteroids early in the course of an attack or as preventive therapy. Corticosteroids act as potent anti-inflammatory agents. Similarly, inhaled drugs that stabilize mast cells are used to prevent an asthmatic attack. The effects of these inhaled medications appear to be localized to the respiratory system, making their use safe and effective as treatments for asthma. Because asthma is a progressive disease, it is important to maintain treatment even between episodes of asthmatic attacks. Any individual, regardless of stage of disease, may require anti-inflammatory drugs. For those who have persistent, moderate, and severe asthma, low doses of inhaled steroids may be used daily to assist in stabilizing the patient.

- Bronchodilators that act by stimulating the beta-adrenergic receptors of the airways (beta agonists) are a mainstay of asthma therapy. These drugs are inhaled (or given as a liquid in young children) at the onset of an attack and between attacks as needed. Bronchodilators do not prevent the delayed inflammatory response and so are not effective alone during a moderate or severe exacerbation of asthma; too-frequent or sole reliance on them has led to a significant number of fatalities. Newly available long-acting beta-adrenergic agonists (LABAs) may reduce the need for frequent use of inhalers for some patients. For individuals $\geqq 12$ years of age, a combination of ICS and LABA may be more effective.

- Combined products containing low-dose inhaled corticosteroids and long-acting beta-2 agonists appear to improve adherence and reduce exacerbations.

- Beta-agonists may also be used before exercise in those who have exercise-induced asthma.

- Although potent in the prevention and treatment of asthma and allergies, corticosteroids do not affect leukotriene synthesis or release. Leukotrienes are a product of arachidonic acid metabolism and contribute to the inflammation process. The production of leukotrienes may be prevented by using a 5-lipoxygenase inhibitor (zileuton) or by blocking specific leukotriene receptors using a leukotriene receptor antagonist (LTRA) such as montelukast or zafirlukast. LTRA medications manifest both bronchodilator and anti-inflammatory properties and may be used to complement corticosteroids.

- Anticholinergic drugs may be given to decrease parasympathetic effects and to relax the bronchiolar smooth muscle. However, these drugs have a narrow therapeutic range of safety and so are used infrequently in general practice.

- Immunomodulators are now available to assist with long-term control. Given once a month by injection, it binds to the IgE on basophils and mast cells thus decreasing symptoms and exacerbations.
- Behavioral intervention, aimed at calming the person to reduce parasympathetic stimulation of the airways, is important. When a person who is crying stops, this also allows for a slowing and a warming of the airflow, thereby reducing stimulation to the airways.

ACUTE BRONCHITIS

Acute bronchitis is a sudden inflammation of the tracheobronchial tree caused by a chemical or microorganism. The most common cause is a viral infection although it can be caused by bacteria, fungi, or yeast. It may also result from the inhalation of irritants such as cigarette smoke or chemicals present in air pollution. It is characterized by excess mucus production.

Clinical Manifestations

- Cough, usually productive with thick mucus and purulent sputum.
- Dyspnea.
- Fever.
- Hoarseness.
- Crackles (discontinuous fine or coarse lung sounds), especially on inspiration. Wheezing and shortness of breath may also be present.
- Malaise.
- Chest pain occasionally may be present.

Diagnostic Tools

- Chest radiograph.

Complications

- Repeated episodes of acute bronchitis may result in the pathologic changes characteristic of chronic bronchitis.
- Pneumonia may develop in high-risk individuals.

Treatment

- Antibiotics for secondary or primary bacterial infections.
- Increased fluid intake and expectorants to loosen mucus.
- Rest to reduce oxygen demands.

CHRONIC BRONCHITIS

Chronic bronchitis is defined as an obstructive pulmonary disorder characterized by excessive mucus production in the lower respiratory tract and a resulting chronic cough. It must last for at least 3 consecutive months of the year for 2 consecutive years.

Excess mucus results from pathologic changes (hypertrophy and hyperplasia) of the mucus-producing cells of the bronchi. In addition, the cilia lining the bronchi become paralyzed or dysfunctional, and undergo metaplasia. These changes to the mucus-producing cells and the cilia cells derail the mucociliary escalator system and cause the accumulation of large amounts of thick mucus that cannot be easily removed from the respiratory tract. The mucus acts as a breeding ground for infection and becomes highly purulent. Inflammation sets in, resulting in edema and swelling of the tissues and changes in the pulmonary architecture. Ventilation, especially exhalation, is obstructed. Hypercapnia (increased carbon dioxide) develops, as exhalation is prolonged and difficult to accomplish through the mucus and inflammation. The decrease in ventilation causes a decrease in ventilation:perfusion ratio, with resulting pulmonary hypoxic vasoconstriction and pulmonary hypertension. Although the alveoli are normal, hypoxic vasoconstriction and poor ventilation result in decreased oxygen exchange and hypoxia.

The main risk factor for development of chronic bronchitis is cigarette smoking. Components of cigarette smoke stimulate changes in both the mucus-producing cells of the bronchi and the cilia. They also induce chronic inflammation, which is the distinguishing characteristic of chronic bronchitis.

Clinical Manifestations

- A productive, purulent cough, easily worsened by inspired irritants, cold weather, or an infection.
- Copious amounts of sputum production. Color may be gray, white, or yellow.
- Air hunger, accessory muscle use, and dyspnea.
- Wheezing, rhonchi, prolonged expiratory phase.
- Cyanosis.
- Pedal edema and jugular vein distention.

Diagnostic Tools

- Pulmonary function tests demonstrate a reduction in FEV_1 and vital capacity.
- Blood gases show decreased arterial oxygen and increased arterial carbon dioxide.
- Chest radiograph may document chronic bronchitis (hyperinflation) and fibrosis of the lung tissue.
- Sputum culture.

Complications

- Pulmonary hypertension, resulting from chronic pulmonary hypoxic vaso-constriction, can occur, leading to cor pulmonale.
- Clubbing of the end segment of the fingers, an indication of chronic hypoxic stress, may develop.
- Polycythemia (an increase in red blood cell concentration) occurs due to chronic hypoxia and the stimulation of erythropoietin secretion. This, coupled with cyanosis, gives the skin a bluish coloration.
- Lung cancer.

Treatment

- Education on decreasing further irritant exposure, especially cigarette smoke.
- Prophylactic antibiotic therapy, especially in the winter months, to reduce incidence of lower respiratory tract infections. This is important because any infectious process further increases the inflammatory outcomes of mucus production and swelling.
- Because many patients experience spasms of the respiratory tract with chronic bronchitis that are similar to spasms seen in chronic asthma, bronchodilators are frequently prescribed.
- Anti-inflammatory drugs reduce mucus production and relieve blockage.
- Expectorants and increased fluid intake loosen the mucus.
- Chest physiotherapy.
- Corticosteroids.
- Oxygen therapy may be required.
- Vaccination against pneumococcal pneumonia is highly advised.

EMPHYSEMA

Emphysema is a chronic obstructive disease characterized by loss of lung elasticity and a reduction in alveolar surface area due to the destruction of the alveolar walls and the enlargement of air spaces distal to the terminal bronchioles. Damage can be either restricted to the central part of the lobe, which results in the bronchiolar wall integrity being affected most, or it can be throughout the entire lung, which results in damage both to the bronchi and to the alveoli.

Loss of lung elasticity can affect both the alveoli and the bronchi. Elasticity is lost as a result of destruction of the elastin and collagen fibers found throughout the lung from products produced by activated alveolar macrophages. The exact cause of emphysema is unclear, but in over 80% of cases, the disease occurs after years of smoking. It appears that components of cigarette smoke directly change the structure of the elastic molecules. There may also be an effect on the elastic fibers related to repeated infectious ailments and the state of chronic inflammation that accompanies infection. As a result of the loss of elasticity, air passages and alveoli collapse, reducing ventilation. Airways collapse primarily on expiration because normal expiration occurs as a result of passive recoil after inspiration. Therefore, if there is no passive recoil, air is trapped in the lung and the airways collapse.

The walls between the alveoli, called the alveolar septa, can also be destroyed. This reduces the surface area of alveoli available for gas exchange and decreases the rate of diffusion.

Although the primary risk factor for emphysema is smoking, repeated exposure to secondhand smoke might also result in emphysema. In addition, there is a familial form of emphysema, related to a deficiency in an antiprotease, alpha-1 antitrypsin. This is a much less common cause of emphysema that occurs in individuals not necessarily exposed to cigarette smoke, although tobacco smoke exposure worsens the course of emphysema in those with this deficiency as well.

Clinical Manifestations

- Air trapping, resulting from the loss of lung elasticity and leading to expansion of the chest (increased anterior–posterior diameter).
- Diminished breath sounds on auscultation.
- Use of accessory muscles of respiration.
- Tachypnea (increased respiratory rate) caused by hypoxia and hypercapnia. Because of the effectiveness of increasing respiratory rate in this disease, most individuals who have emphysema do not show a significant alteration in ABGs until late in the course of the disease, when the respiratory rate cannot mask hypoxia or hypercapnia. Eventually, all blood–gas values deteriorate, and frank hypoxia, hypercapnia, and acidosis are present.
- Central nervous system depression, resulting from high carbon dioxide levels (carbon dioxide narcosis), can occur.
- Cachexia.
- One key difference between emphysema and chronic bronchitis is the lack of sputum production in emphysema.

Diagnostic Tools

- Abnormal pulmonary function tests, including decreased measured FEV_1, decreased vital capacity, and increased residual volume (air left in the respiratory tract after each breath) caused by loss of lung elasticity.
- As the disease progresses, blood–gas analysis will first demonstrate hypoxia. Late in the disease, carbon dioxide levels may also be elevated.

Complications

- Pulmonary hypertension from chronic pulmonary hypoxic vasoconstriction, leading to cor pulmonale, may occur.
- A reduction in quality of life is common in severely affected individuals.
- Respiratory failure.

Treatment

Relieving the symptoms and preventing a worsening of the condition is the objective in emphysema treatment. There is no cure. Treatments include:

- Encouraging the individual to stop smoking.
- Using breathing positions and patterns to reduce air trapping.
- Teaching the individual relaxation techniques and means of energy conservation.
- Oxygen therapy is needed for many patients who have emphysema, so that they can complete tasks of daily living. Oxygen therapy may slow the progression of the disease and lessen morbidity and mortality.
- Well-designed exercise therapy can improve symptoms.

CHRONIC OBSTRUCTIVE PULMONARY DISEASE

Individuals who have long-standing emphysema also usually have chronic bronchitis and demonstrate indications of both diseases. This condition is called COPD. Chronic asthma in association with either emphysema or chronic bronchitis may also result in COPD.

Clinical Manifestations

- Symptoms of both emphysema and chronic bronchitis are usually present.
- Dyspnea is constant.

Diagnostic Tools

- History and physical examination.
- Chest x-ray.

Complications

- Pulmonary hypertension leading to cor pulmonale.
- Pneumothorax.

Treatment

Treatment is focused on minimizing symptoms and exacerbations and maintaining quality of life.

- Long-acting beta-2 agonists (LABAs), rather than short-acting beta-2 agonists, have the potential to improve the mucociliary clearance and act as bronchodilators. A combination therapy consisting of LABA and an inhaled corticosteroid provides anti-inflammatory activity and improves mucociliary clearance.

- In general, COPD treatment is as described for chronic bronchitis and emphysema, with the exception that oxygen therapy must be closely monitored. Individuals who have COPD have chronic hypercapnia that causes the central chemoreceptors, which normally respond to carbon dioxide, to adapt. What keeps these individuals breathing is the low oxygen concentration of the arterial blood that continues to stimulate the less-sensitive peripheral chemoreceptors. These peripheral chemoreceptors only fire if the arterial partial pressure of oxygen decreases to less than 50 mm Hg. Therefore, if oxygen therapy were to result in a partial pressure of oxygen of greater than 50 mm Hg, this remaining drive to breathe would be extinguished. Individuals who have COPD typically have low oxygen levels and cannot be treated with high-oxygen therapy. This severely affects quality of life.

- Phosphodiesterase 4 (PDE4) inhibitors are a promising and potent drug class that controls the inflammatory process in patients with COPD by reducing the number of bronchial mucosal CD8+ T cells and CD68+ macrophages and neutrophils.

- Lifestyle changes such as smoking cessation, avoidance of aggravating stimuli, relaxation, positioning and physical activity (as tolerated).

- Routine vaccinations such as influenza and pneumococcal vaccine.

- Palliative care.

LUNG CANCER

Lung cancer is defined as a cancer of the epithelial lining of the respiratory tract (bronchogenic carcinoma). It can occur anywhere in the lung and is the leading cause of cancer death in adults. There are four general types of lung cancer: three non–small-cell carcinomas and one small-cell carcinoma. The non–small-cell carcinomas are squamous cell carcinoma, adenocarcinoma, and large-cell carcinoma.

Squamous cell carcinoma accounts for about 30% of lung cancers. This cancer is clearly associated with cigarette smoking and exposure to environmental toxins, such as asbestos and components of air pollution. Squamous cell tumors are usually located in the bronchi at the site where the bronchi enter the lungs, called the hila, and from there extend down into the bronchi. Because the bronchi are obstructed to some degree, absorption atelectasis and pneumonia, as well as decreased ventilatory capacity, can occur. This tumor grows relatively slowly and has the best prognosis for a 5-year survival if diagnosed prior to metastasis.

Adenocarcinoma is a type of lung cancer arising from the glands of the lung. It usually occurs in the periphery of lung tissue, including the terminal bronchioles and the alveoli. This type of cancer accounts for approximately 30% of lung cancers and is increasing among women. Adenocarcinomas are typically slow growing, but they metastasize early and have a poor 5-year survival rate.

Large-cell undifferentiated cancer is highly anaplastic and associated with rapid metastasis. These tumors account for approximately 10% to 15% of all lung cancers, often occurring peripherally and spreading centrally in the lung. They are highly correlated with cigarette smoking and can cause chest pain. This type of cancer has a poor prognosis for survival.

Small-cell carcinoma accounts for approximately 25% of all lung cancers. This type of tumor is also referred to as oat-cell carcinoma and usually occurs in the central areas of the lung. Small-cell carcinoma is an anaplastic, or embryonic, type of tumor, and therefore shows a high incidence of metastasis. It is often a site of ectopic tumor production and may cause early symptoms based on endocrine disturbances. Pulmonary manifestations that occur with this tumor also result from obstruction to airflow. This type of tumor is the most strongly associated with cigarette smoking, and has the worst prognosis.

Risk Factors for Lung Cancer

Although the incidence of lung cancer in the United States has begun to fall for men, it is holding steady or continues to rise among women. The reason for this is the clear fact that the primary risk factor for lung cancer in approximately 90% of cases is cigarette smoking, a behavior that peaked and then began its fall among men at least a decade or more before a similar change in behavior developed in women. Lung cancer is often associated with chronic bronchitis, because of the overlap in risk factors as well as excess mucus possibly causing abnormal epithelial cell changes. Air pollution and exposure to chemicals and dusts, including asbestos, also contribute to the disease. A familial susceptibility tends to exist.

Although there are more than 50 known carcinogens in tobacco smoke, it is still not exactly understood how cigarette smoking causes cancer. It is likely, however, that these carcinogens or other metabolites of cigarette smoke interfere with the functioning of key genes regulating epithelial cell growth and development. In particular, specific mutations in certain cancer suppressor genes have been shown to occur with prolonged exposure to tobacco smoke. Without properly functioning tumor suppressor genes, uncontrolled cell division can occur and cancer may develop.

Epithelial cells change progressively with the development of lung cancer, first showing subtle signs of metaplasia, then dysplasia, and finally neoplasia. These conditions preceding neoplasia are visible histologically in individuals who have chronic bronchitis and emphysema. The bronchial epithelial cells that appear to be most damaged by toxins are those at the bronchial bifurcations. It appears that mucus and toxins accumulate there, causing the most injury to these cells. The result is that the epithelial cells become thickened, the mucus-producing cells hypertrophy, and metaplasia and dysplasia occur. Alveolar cells may also be altered in structure and function.

Clinical Manifestations

- A persistent cough.
- Recurring lower respiratory tract infections.
- Wheezing, dyspnea.
- Hemoptysis (the coughing up of blood), atelectasis, or pneumonitis.
- Weight loss.
- Fatigue.
- Hoarseness.
- Pain or dysfunction in a distant organ reflecting metastasis may be the first clue of lung cancer.
- Other symptoms seen with each particular type of lung cancer may vary, as described previously.

Diagnostic Tools

- Chest x-ray followed by biopsy of suspicious lesions may diagnose the disease.

Complications

- Paraneoplastic syndromes such as Cushing syndrome, hypercalcemia, SIADH.
- Superior vena cava syndrome.
- Metastasis to thoracic structures, brain, liver, bone, adrenal glands.
- Prognosis is poor. The 5-year survival rate for all types of lung cancer is only 13%. Some types of lung cancer have an even worse prognosis. For instance, oat-cell carcinoma has a less than 5% survival rate 2 years after diagnosis.

Treatment

- Any combination of surgery, radiation, and chemotherapy.

PEDIATRIC CONSIDERATIONS

- Primary atelectasis of the alveoli results in poor oxygenation of the newborn and is associated with significant morbidity and mortality. The cause of alveolar collapse is usually inadequate production of surfactant, resulting in high surface tension in the alveoli. The infant must work hard with each breath to overcome the surface tension and expand the alveoli. This can lead to exhaustion and an ever-worsening exchange of gases.

- Infants and children exposed to cigarette smoke before or after birth experience increased rates of upper respiratory tract infections, lower respiratory tract infections such as pneumonia, and childhood asthma compared with infants and children of parents who do not smoke. Urinary output of nicotine metabolites is grossly elevated in children whose parents smoke compared with those whose parents do not. Several metabolites of nicotine are known carcinogens as well as pulmonary irritants.

- In children, **croup**, a viral infection of the larynx or trachea, and **epiglottitis**, a bacterial infection of the epiglottis, may occur. Like adults, children develop significant inflammation and swelling of the respiratory tract with infections. In fact, children may demonstrate more drastic clinical manifestations with upper airway infections because the upper airways are much narrower to begin with, resulting in a significant increase in resistance to airflow with even slight swelling and airway blockage. Symptoms of croup include a barking cough, hoarse voice, and stridor. Treatment for children who have mild-to-moderate croup may include a vaporizer, mist tent, or oxygen therapy. Those who have moderate-to-severe croup are likely to benefit from intramuscular or nebulized glucocorticoids. The inflammation seen with epiglottitis may result in total obstruction to airflow, significant anxiety, and death. Children typically sit forward and may drool. For children who have epiglottitis, hospitalization and perhaps intubation or tracheotomy may be required. Children who have epiglottitis should be kept as calm as possible (and so should their parents) to maintain airway patency until emergency support can be given.

- Streptococcal pharyngitis is more common in children. It is present in up to 36% of pediatric patients with a sore throat. The Center for Disease Control recommends a quick strep and antibiotic treatment for a positive result and for a positive follow-up culture if quick strep was negative.

- In the newborn period, pneumonia is most often caused by infection with group B streptococcal disease transmitted in utero. This disease can have a devastating effect, with an infant developing severe illness within hours of delivery. Treatment requires hospitalization, oxygen therapy, and intravenous antibiotics. This terrible disease may be reduced by prenatal screening of expectant mothers and treatment of women shown to be infected.

- SARS-CoV is seen less frequently in children and has a milder presentation. The reasons for this are unknown.

- Being exposed to cigarette smoke in utero or in early childhood is considered a risk factor for childhood asthma. Infection in infancy with RSV may also be a risk factor for childhood asthma. Children may outgrow asthma, although a tendency toward allergies often remains.

- The daily use of oral steroids may be necessary to control conditions of severe asthma, or they may be prescribed as a burst for 5 to 7 days to help return normal function more rapidly during an exacerbation in patients who have mild or moderate asthma. The chronic use of oral steroids for the long-term treatment of childhood asthma is associated with a reduction in growth potential and a thinning of the bones (osteoporosis).

GERIATRIC CONSIDERATIONS

- The most common cause of pneumonia in the elderly is pneumococcal pneumonia. The elderly are at the greatest risk of dying from pneumonia, usually related to preexisting disease, poor nutrition, and reduced immune responsiveness. Those in long-term care facilities are especially susceptible to outbreaks of pneumococcal pneumonia. The risk of acquiring pneumococcal pneumonia can be reduced or eliminated by immunization; it is recommended that those who are older than 65 years of age or who live in a long-term care facility be vaccinated. Reports indicate, however, that less than 30% of those over 65 have been vaccinated against pneumococcal pneumonia.

- The risk of aspiration pneumonia is greater for those with neurological disorders such as dementia, stroke, or Parkinson disease. A normal change associated with aging is a slower swallowing rate which further increases the risk of dysphagia and aspiration pneumonia for the older adult with a neurologic disorder.

- Geriatric patients may not demonstrate these typical signs of pneumonia. Instead, complaints of fatigue or disorientation, or both, may be made by the patient or the caregiver.

- Afebrile illness or concurrent bacterial sepsis/pneumonia has been seen among SARS-infected elderly (those over 60 years of age). Those among the elderly with coexisting conditions should be excluded from caring for SARS patients and handling SARS-CoV.

- The risk of aspiration coupled with inadequate oral care greatly increases the risk of aspiration pneumonia in the older adult.

SELECTED BIBLIOGRAPHY

Atlas of Pathophysiology (3rd ed.). (2010). Philadelphia, PA: Lippincott Williams & Wilkins.

Barclay, L. (2009). WHO issues guidelines for antiviral treatment of H1N1 and other influenza. *Medscape Medical News CME*. Available at http://cme.medscape.com/viewarticle/708032.

Bender, J. (2009). Evaluation of cough in adults: A review of evidence-based guidelines. *Advance for Nurse Practitioners*, 17(3), 42–44, 46–47.

Chalwin, R. P., Moran, J. L., & Graham, P. L. (2008). The role of extracorporeal membrane oxygenation for treatment of the adult respiratory distress syndrome: Review and quantitative analysis. *Anesthesia and Intensive Care*, 36(2), 152–161.

Copstead, L. C., & Banasik, J. L. (2010). *Pathophysiology* (4th ed.). St. Louis, MO: Saunders Elsevier.

Drummond, M. B., Dasenbrook, E. C., Pitz, M. W., Murphy, D. J., & Fan, E. (2008). Inhaled corticosteroids in patients with stable chronic obstructive pulmonary disease: A systemic review and meta-analysis. *Journal of American Medical Association*, 300(20), 2407–2416.

Egan, M. E., Pearson, M., Weiner, S. A., Rajendran, V., Rubin, D., et al. (2004). Cucumin, a major constituent of turmeric, corrects cystic fibrosis defects. *Science*, 304, 600–602.

Ellis, K. C. (2008). Keeping asthma at bay. *American Nurse Today*, 3(2), 20–26.

Fowler, S. B. (2008). Community-acquired pneumonia: Follow the guidelines to better outcomes. *American Nurse Today*, 3(9), 26–30.

Gahbauer, M. (2009). Chronic cough: Stepwise application in primary care practice of the ACCP guidelines for diagnosis and management of cough. *Journal of the American Academy of Nurse Practitioners*, 21(8), 409–416.

George, K. J. (2008). A systematic approach to care: Adult respiratory distress syndrome. *Journal of Trauma Nursing*, 15(1), 19–22.

Grey, V., Mohammed, S. R., Smountas, A. A., Bahlool, R., & Lands, L. C. (2003). Improved glutathione status in young adult patients with cystic fibrosis supplemented with whey protein. *Journal of Cystic Fibrosis*, 2, 195–198.

Guyton, A. C., & Hall, J. (2006). *Textbook of medical physiology* (11th ed.). Philadelphia, PA: W.B. Saunders.

Hallman, M. (2004). Lung surfactant, respiratory failure, and genes. *New England Journal of Medicine*, 350, 1278–1280.

Hayden, M. L., & Rachelefsky, G. (2008). Partners for better asthma control. *Advance for Nurse Practitioners*, 16(9), 45–48, 50–52, 54–56.

Heimer, K. A., Hart, A. M., Martin, L. G., & Rubio-Wallace, S. (2009). Examining the evidence for the use of vitamin C in the prophylaxis and treatment of the common cold. *Journal of the American Academy of Nurse Practitioners*, 21(5), 295–300.

Hutchison, R., & Rodiguez, L. (2008). Capnography and respiratory depression. *American Journal of Nursing*, 108(2), 35–39.

Jeffery, P. (2005). Phosphodiesterase 4-selective inhibition: Novel therapy for the inflammation of COPD. *Pulmonary Pharmacology and Therapeutics*, 18, 9–17.

Kuebler, K. K., Buchsel, P. C., & Balkstra, C. R. (2008). Differentiating chronic obstructive pulmonary disease from asthma. *Journal of the American Academy of Nurse Practitioners*, 20(9), 445–454.

Mathai, S. C., & Hassoun, P. M. (2009). The role of echocardiography in the diagnosis and assessment of pulmonary hypertension. *Advances in Pulmonary Hypertension*, 7(4), 379–382, 384–385.

McShane, H. (2005). Co-infection with HIV and TB: Double trouble. *International Journal of STD and AIDS*, 16, 95–101.

MMWR. (2005). Trends in tuberculosis—United States, 2004. *MMWR*, 54(10), 245–249.

National Asthma Education Prevention Program (2007). The Expert Panel Report-3. Guidelines for the diagnosis and management of asthma (EPR-3). Available at http://www.nhlbi.nih.gov/guidelines/asthma/asthgdln.htm.

O'Laughlen, M. C., Hollen, P., & Ting, S. (2009). An intervention to change clinician behavior: Conceptual framework for the multicolored simplified asthma guideline reminder (MSAGR). *Journal of the American Academy of Nurse Practitioners*, 21(8), 417–422.

Osborn, K. S., Wraa, C. E., & Watson, A. B. (2010). *Medical-surgical nursing: Preparation for practice. Boston, MA: Pearson.*

Palmer, J. L., & Metheny, N. A. (2008). Preventing aspiration in older adults with dysphagia. *American Journal of Nursing*, 108(2), 40–48.

Poole, P. J., Saini, R., Brodie, S. M., & Black, P. N. (2005). Comparison of the effects of nebulised and inhaled salbutamol on breathlessness in severe COPD. *Respiratory Medicine*, 99, 372–376.

Porth, C. M., & Matfin, G. (2009). *Pathophysiology: Concepts of altered health states* (8th ed.). Philadelphia, PA: Lippincott Williams & Wilkins.

Ratjen, F., Paul, K., van Koningsbruggen, S., Breitenstein, S., Rietschel, E., Nikolaizik, W., et al. (2005). DNA concentrations in BAL fluid of cystic fibrosis patients with early lung disease: Influence of treatment with dornase alpha. *Pediatric Pulmonology*, 39, 1–4.

Rogers, D. F. (2005). Mucociliary dysfunction in COPD: Effect of current pharmacotherapeutic options. *Pulmonary Pharmacology and Therapeutics*, 18, 1–8.

Rothman, R. E., Moran, G. J., Bradshaw, Y. S., Josephine, E. B., & Hirshon, J. M. (2007). Respiratory hygiene in the emergency department. *Journal of Emergency Nursing*, 33(2), 119–134.

Ruppert, R. (2007). Tuberculosis today: Fighting an ancient adversary. *American Nurse Today*, 2(11), 32–36.

Sarver, N., & Murphy, K. (2009). Management of asthma: New approaches to establishing control. *Journal of the American Academy of Nurse Practitioners*, 21(1), 54–65.

Schwartz, P. J., Stramba-Badiale, M., Segantini, A., et al. (1998). Prolongation of the QT interval and the sudden infant death syndrome. *New England Journal of Medicine*, 338, 1709–1714.

Severe acute respiratory syndrome (SARS). (2009, February). *Weekly Epidemiological Record*, 7, 54–55.

Shamputa, I.C., Rigouts, L., & Portaels, F. (2004). Molecular genetic methods for diagnosis and antibiotic resistance detection of mycobacteria from clinical specimens. *Acta Pathologica, Microbiologica et Immunologica Scandinavica*, 112, 728–752.

Snider, D. E., & Castro, K. G. (1998). The global threat of drug-resistant tuberculosis. *New England Journal of Medicine*, 338, 1689–1690.

Taylor, C., Allen, A., Sumner, S., & Vought, M. (2007). Are you prepared to deal with a high-risk respiratory illness? *Journal of Emergency Nursing*, 33(2), 110–118.

Taylor, J., Wentworth, D. E., Bernard, K. A., Masters, P. S., & Trimarchi, C. V. (2005). SARS coronaviruses and highly pathogenic influenza viruses: Safety and occupational health for laboratory workers [conference summary]. *Emerging Infectious Diseases* [serial on the Internet]. Available from http://www.cdc.gov/ncidod/EID/vol11no04/04-1304.htm.

Seemungal, T., Wilkinson, T., Hurst, J., Perera, W., Sapsford, R., & Wedzicha, J. (2008). Long-term erythromycin therapy is associated with decreased chronic obstructive pulmonary disease exacerbations. *American Journal of Respiratory and Critical Care Medicine*, 178, 1139–1147.

Umetsu, D. T. (2005). Revising the immunological theories of asthma and allergy. *Lancet*, 365, 98–100.

Valdez-Lowe, C., Ghareeb, S. A., & Artinian, N. T. (2009). Pulse oximetry in adults. *American Journal of Nursing*, 109(6), 52–60.

Visitainer, C., & Byars, D. (2008). How serious is that sore throat? *Clinician Reviews*, 18(12), 29–31.

Wagner, F. P., & Mathiason, M. A. (2008). Using centor criteria to diagnose streptococcal pharyngitis. *The Nurse Practitioner*, 33(9), 10–12.

Wingrove, B. R. (2009). Pediatric respiratory infections. *Clinician Reviews*, 19(2), 20–26.

World Health Organization. (2005). Global tuberculosis control: Surveillance, planning, financing. *WHO Report 2005* (WHO/HTM/TB/2005.349). Geneva: World Health Organization.

Wouters, E. F. M. (2004). Management of severe COPD. *Lancet*, 364, 883–895.

Yu, I. T. S., Li, Y. G., Wong, T. W., Tam, W., Chan, A. T., Lee, J. H. W., et al. (2004). Evidence of airborne transmission of the severe acute respiratory syndrome virus. *New England Journal of Medicine*, 350, 1731–1739.

Zimmerman, R. (2009). Treatment options for respiratory infections. *The Clinical Advisor*, February, 21–22, 25–26, 28.

Nutrition, Elimination, and Reproductive Function and Dysfunction

The Gastrointestinal System

The gastrointestinal (GI) tract is a hollow tube that extends from the mouth to the anus. The GI tract is responsible for the ingestion, propulsion, digestion, and absorption of nutrients necessary to sustain life and maintain optimal functioning of the body.

● Physiologic Concepts

ANATOMY

As shown in Figure 15-1, the GI tract begins with the oral cavity, and continues into the esophagus and stomach. Food is stored in the stomach until it is released into the small intestine. The small intestine is divided into three sections: the duodenum, the jejunum, and the ileum. Digestion and absorption of food occur primarily in the small intestine. From the small intestine, food is passed to the large intestine, which consists of the colon and rectum. Accessory organs include the liver, pancreas, gallbladder, and appendix.

The entire GI tract is composed of several tissue layers that include:

- the innermost mucosa (secreting) layer;
- a submucosa connective tissue layer;
- circular and longitudinal smooth muscle layers, called the muscularis externa; and

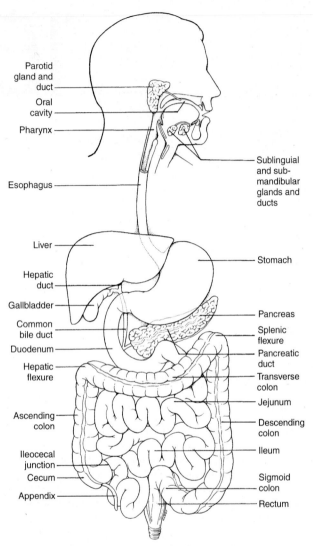

FIGURE 15-1 Digestive system. (From Chaffee, E.E. & Lytle, I.M. [1980]. *Basic physiology and anatomy*. [4th ed.]. Philadelphia: J.B. Lippincott.)

- an outermost serous membrane, called the peritoneum or serosal layer, which is composed of a layer of mesothelium and a layer of connective tissue (Fig. 15-2).

These layers are connected to one another physically and through neural connections.

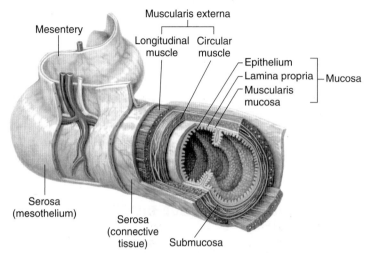

FIGURE 15-2 Transverse section of the digestive system. (From Porth, C. & Matfin, G [2009]. *Pathophysiology, concepts of altered health states.* [8th ed.]. Philadelphia: Lippincott Williams & Wilkins.)

Mucosa

The mucosa layer of the small intestine is the site of food absorption. The mucosa layer consists of a lining of epithelial cells, a thin connective tissue layer called the lamina propria, and an underlying layer called the muscularis mucosa. Food particles leave the gut and enter the internal environment of the body by moving across the epithelial cells.

Submucosa

The submucosa layer of the gut is a connective tissue matrix. It contains one of the two nerve networks of the gut, called the submucosal plexus, and a system of blood vessels and lymphatics. The submucosal plexus is primarily concerned with maintaining function within each very small section of the intestinal wall. For example, the submucosal plexus helps control *local* intestinal secretions, *local* absorption of foodstuffs, and *local* contraction of the muscularis mucosa.

Muscularis Externa

The muscularis externa contains a thick circular muscle layer, and a thinner, longitudinal muscle layer. Contraction of the circular smooth muscle causes mixing of the food in the gut. Contraction of the longitudinal layer shortens the tube. Extending all the way along the intestine, in between the circular and longitudinal smooth muscle layers, is the second neural network of the gut, called the myenteric plexus. The myenteric plexus controls muscle contractions along the entire gut, in contrast to the localized effects of the submucosal plexus.

Peritoneum or Serosal Layer

The outer layer of the GI tract is the largest serous membrane in the body and is composed of the visceral peritoneum and the parietal peritoneum. The visceral peritoneum lines the viscera such as the intestines and stomach. The parietal peritoneum is attached to the abdominal wall. The peritoneal cavity is a fluid-filled space between the visceral peritoneum and the parietal peritoneum which facilitates movement of the abdominal structures.

NEURAL REGULATION OF THE GUT: THE ENTERIC NERVOUS SYSTEM

The two neural networks of the gut, the submucosal plexus and the myenteric plexus, make up the self-contained nervous system of the gut, referred to as the enteric nervous system. The nerves of this system fire on their own without external stimuli. Because the smooth muscle cells of the gut are connected to each other via gap junctions, firing of the nerves in one area spreads to the entire length of the gut. The neurons in the two plexuses synapse on each other, as well as on the surrounding smooth muscle cells, the exocrine glands throughout the GI tract, and the epithelial cells. They can affect contraction of the smooth muscle, the production of mucus, and the release of digestive enzymes. The neurons of the enteric nervous system include both adrenergic and cholinergic nerves, as well as nerves that release a variety of other neurotransmitters, including nitric oxide, endorphin, and various intestinal peptides. Although the firing of the enteric nervous system can occur without external input, the plexuses also receive external stimuli that influence their rate of firing.

External Neural Input

Both the myenteric and the submucosal nerve plexuses are innervated by sympathetic and parasympathetic nerves. Sympathetic fibers originate in the spinal cord between the levels of T8 and L3 and innervate the plexuses throughout the gut. They inhibit firing of the plexus, slowing the basic rhythm. Sympathetic nerves release norepinephrine in the gut. Parasympathetic nerves travel in the vagus nerve to the esophagus, the stomach, the small intestine, and the upper half of the large intestine. Other parasympathetic fibers travel in sacral divisions and innervate the distal half of the large intestine. Parasympathetic nerves release acetylcholine and stimulate firing of both the plexuses, speeding peristalsis and increasing mixing. Innervation of this distal part of the large intestine is important for stimulating defecation.

Other External Input

In addition to external neural innervation, the cells of the enteric nervous system are affected by gut hormones as well as by a variety of irritants, including those present in some foods and in certain drugs. Toxins released by infectious agents and chemicals participating in the body's response to infection also increase the firing rate of the enteric nervous system.

THE MUSCULATURE OF THE GUT

As described previously, the GI tract is composed of an outer longitudinal layer and an inner circular layer of muscle. The longitudinal and the circular muscle layers are responsible for mixing and moving the food throughout the entire GI tract.

The longitudinal and circular smooth muscles show an inherent rate of spontaneous muscle-cell depolarization at each segment of the GI tract. These inherent depolarizations cause action potentials, resulting in muscle contractions. The contractions in each segment may vary in strength in response to internal or external nervous input, hormonal stimuli, and stretch. Although they vary in strength, gut contractions vary little in frequency. Gut contractions are slow, calcium-dependent contractions that occur over a wide range of muscle length. The contractions of the muscles at each gut segment determine the motility of that segment (i.e., the propulsion of food and secretions from one area to the next).

GUT MOTILITY

Esophageal Motility

Movement of food in the esophagus occurs by the process known as peristalsis. When food enters the esophagus, the smooth muscle is stretched; this initiates a peristaltic wave that proceeds along the length of the esophagus, propelling the food with it. When the peristaltic wave reaches the end of the esophagus, the smooth muscle at the opening into the stomach relaxes and food moves into the stomach. The end of the esophagus, called the lower esophageal sphincter (LES), is located in the abdominal cavity, below the level of the diaphragm. Because this area is not anatomically different than the rest of the esophagus, there has been a debate about whether or not the LES is a true sphincter; however, for the sake of this discussion, it will be considered a sphincter. When a peristaltic wave is not passing down the esophagus, the esophageal sphincter is relaxed and in the closed position, preventing reflux of stomach contents into the esophagus. Reflux is also prevented by the fact that the LES is in the abdominal rather than in the thoracic cavity; if this were not so, backflow of food from the high-pressure zone of the abdomen to the low-pressure thoracic area would easily occur. By having part of the esophagus in the abdominal cavity, the pressure difference is minimized.

Stomach Motility

When food enters the stomach, the stomach also responds with a peristaltic wave. As the wave of contraction reaches the lower end of the stomach, called the antrum, the wave picks up strength, which effectively mixes the food. This wave of contraction also causes the closure of the junction between the distal end of the stomach and the beginning of the duodenum, called the pyloric sphincter. This is a true sphincter and is normally relaxed when food is not entering the stomach.

Gastric peristaltic waves occur as a result of the depolarization of the smooth muscle cells of the stomach. Pacemaker cells in the smooth muscle of the stomach depolarize continually at an inherent rate; this is called the basic electrical rhythm of the stomach. Normally, the depolarizations associated with the basic electrical rhythm are too slight to cause the muscle of the stomach to reach threshold and therefore do not lead to contractions. With increased stretch of the stomach or with neural and hormonal stimulation, the smooth muscle does depolarize to threshold and the strength of gastric peristalsis increases.

As the peristaltic waves continue in the stomach, a small amount of material is forced through the pyloric sphincter into the duodenum. The more material in the stomach, the more rapid is the rate of emptying. Eventually, all of the stomach content empties into the small intestine.

Small Intestinal Motility

Once the food, now called chyme, enters the small intestine, it continues to be mixed as a result of smooth muscle contraction. In the small intestine, the contractions result in mostly stationary mixing, with slow forward propulsion down the gut. The slow propulsion occurs as a result of segmentation. Segmentation refers to the process by which slightly more frequent contractions in the upper intestine, compared with the lower, eventually propel the chyme through the length of the small intestine. The thorough mixing during segmentation ensures that the chyme is acted upon by digestive enzymes and that it comes into repeated contact with the intestinal wall to facilitate absorption.

Large Intestine Motility

The large intestine consists of the cecum, followed by the ascending, transverse, and descending colon; the sigmoid colon; and the rectum. The appendix is a blind pouch, growing off of the cecum. The rectum ends at the anus, the exit point from the body. Contraction of the large intestine occurs at a slow rate compared with that of the small intestine. This means that food entering the large intestine takes approximately a day to travel the entire length of the structure. A few times a day, usually after a meal, a wave of contraction, called a mass movement occurs. This is a powerful contraction that initiates the urge to defecate.

HORMONES OF THE GASTROINTESTINAL TRACT

Many GI hormones, including gastrin, secretin, cholecystokinin (CCK), glucagon-like peptide-1 (GLP-1), and glucose-dependent insulinotropic polypeptide (GIP), play important roles in the digestive function of the GI tract. Other hormones released from the stomach or intestine, including ghrelin and peptide YY (PYY), are involved in controlling appetite. These hormones and their roles are summarized in Table 15-1.

TABLE 15-1 Summary of Gastrointestinal Hormones		
Hormone	**Source**	**Function**
Gastrin	Stomach antrum due to distention and presence of protein from food	Stimulates secretion of histamine and gastric juices from gut lining
	Stimulated by gastrin-releasing peptide from nerves of submucosal plexus secondary to parasympathetic stimulation	Stimulates secretion of hydrochloric acid (HCl) from stomach's parietal cells
		Stimulates intestinal motility
		HCl activates pepsin
		Pepsin + gastric juices stop gastrin secretion
Secretin	Small intestine in response to HCl in chyme	Stimulates intestinal secretions of base
		Stimulates pancreatic release of bicarbonate to neutralize acid
		Slows passage of food from stomach into the small intestine to facilitate adequate digestion of food already in the small intestine
Cholecystokinin (CCK)	Small intestine as a result of fat and other food entering the intestine in chyme	Stimulates gallbladder contraction
		Causes release of pancreatic and intestinal digestive enzymes and of bile that facilitates digestion and absorption of food

table continues on page 640

TABLE 15-1 Summary of Gastrointestinal Hormones *(continued)*

Hormone	Source	Function
Glucagon-like pepetide-1 (GLP-1) and glucose-dependent insulinotropic polypeptide (GIP)	Upper small intestine in response to fatty acids, amino acids, and glucose in chyme	Slows stomach emptying to facilitate effective digestion of food already in the small intestine
		Increases insulin release from the pancreas— responsible for up to 60% of insulin released during a meal
		Deficit may be the underlying cause for glucose intolerance in type 2 diabetes
Ghrelin	Stomach	Modulates appetite Regulates energy balance by stimulating food intake and decreasing fat metabolism
		Signals CNS about food intake and body fat mass
		Stimulates growth-releasing hormone from hypothalamus
		Affects hypothalamic–pituitary–gonadal axis
Peptide YY (PYY)	Small intestine as a result of food entry from the stomach	Satiety hormone that inhibits further food intake
		Levels are proportionate to meal energy content and plasma levels peak about 1 hour postprandially

DIGESTION OF FOOD

Digestion of food begins in the mouth with the release of saliva, continues in the stomach, and is mostly accomplished in the small intestine. The process of digestion involves enzymes that are secreted in response to specific foodstuffs and that act to break down carbohydrates into simple sugars, fats into free fatty acids and monoglycerides, and proteins into amino acids. It is only in these simple forms that these nutrients can be absorbed across the gut and used by the body.

Protein and Carbohydrate Digestion

Protein digestion begins in the stomach with the enzyme pepsin and is completed in the small intestine by the action of the pancreatic enzymes trypsin and chymotrypsin. Carbohydrate digestion begins in the mouth with the activity of the enzyme salivary amylase and is completed in the small intestine by the enzyme pancreatic amylase.

Fat Digestion

Fat digestion occurs in the small intestine, primarily as a result of the activity of the pancreatic enzyme lipase. Fats are digested by the action of lipase into free fatty acids and monoglycerides. Lipase, however, is a water-soluble enzyme; because fats are insoluble in water, their digestion by lipase would be extremely slow if it were not for emulsification, the process by which large fat complexes are broken down into smaller droplets. Emulsification increases the surface area of the fats available for digestion by pancreatic lipase. By increasing the surface area, lipase is a much more effective agent for digestion. Emulsification occurs by the mechanical mixing of the food in the intestine and by the action of bile in the small intestine. The emulsification and digestion of fat is illustrated in Figure 15-3.

STEP 1: EMULSIFICATION OF FAT

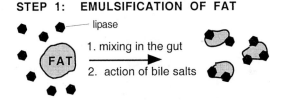

STEP 2: DIGESTION OF FAT

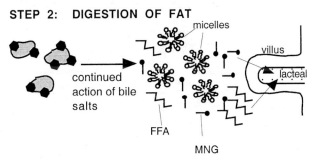

FIGURE 15-3 Emulsification (step 1) and digestion (step 2) of fat (free fatty acid [FFA]; monoglyceride [MNG]).

BILE

Bile is a substance produced in the liver and contains bile salts, water, cholesterol, electrolytes, and bilirubin, which is a breakdown product of hemoglobin. Although bile is continually released from the liver, it is usually stored and concentrated in the gallbladder. Bile then is released from the gallbladder and travels to the small intestine via the common bile duct, in response to the hormone CCK. In individuals who do not have a gallbladder, bile is released directly from the liver into the common bile duct in response to CCK.

Although bile contains no digestive enzymes, it does contain bile salts, the substance that serves to emulsify fats. Bile salts are phospholipids that act as detergents to break down (emulsify) fats into the small droplets. Once emulsified into droplets, lipase is then capable of digesting the fats into fatty acids and monoglycerides.

ABSORPTION OF FOOD

Although a small amount of lipid-soluble material may be absorbed across the stomach wall, most absorption of digested food occurs in the small intestine, across millions of fingerlike projections called villi (singular: villus). Each villus consists of epithelial cells of the mucosal layer, a capillary network, and a central lymph vessel called lacteal (Fig. 15-4). Nerve fibers of the intrinsic plexuses and smooth muscle cells are also present. The presence of villi on the mucosal surface of the intestine increases the surface area available for the absorption of

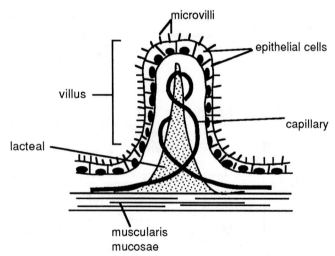

FIGURE 15-4 Villus showing a central lacteal, capillary network, microvilli, and the epithelial cells across which nutrients are absorbed.

food by at least 10-fold. Finally, each villus is topped by almost 1000 microvilli, adding even more to the enormous surface area available for the absorption of food. Certain digestive enzymes (brush border enzymes) are produced by cells of the villus as well.

Absorption of food occurs when digested food particles enter a villus from the lumen of the gut and move either into the capillary or into the lacteal, thereby gaining access to the general circulation. The movement of food particles into the epithelial cells and across the capillary or the lacteal may occur by simple or facilitated diffusion or by active transport, depending on the substance.

Absorption of Amino Acids

Amino acids and small di- or tri-peptides, the result of protein digestion, are actively transported into the epithelial cells of the villus, mostly via sodium co-transport. Once in the villus, they move into the capillary by facilitated diffusion. In the bloodstream, they are delivered to body cells, especially the muscle cells, where they are used for protein synthesis. The amino acids and small peptides not used for protein synthesis travel to the liver, where they are converted to carbohydrates or fats and are either used for energy or stored throughout the body.

Absorption of Simple Sugars

Most of the simple sugars that result from carbohydrate digestion, including glucose and galactose, are transported from the lumen of the intestine into the epithelial cells through sodium-coupled active transport. Once in the epithelial cell, these sugars then move through the basolateral membrane into the space between cells via facilitated diffusion and, from there, into the blood. Other sugars, for example fructose, move both into and out of the epithelial cells only by facilitated diffusion. Once in the blood, sugars are delivered to all body cells and are used for energy production. Sugars not used immediately for energy production can be stored as fat or glycogen in all cells, especially liver cells.

Absorption of Free Fatty Acids and Monoglycerides

Even after being digested, the absorption of free fatty acids and monoglycerides would be extremely slow if it were not for the continued action of the bile salts. Bile salts further break the emulsified fat droplets into even smaller droplets called micelles (see Fig. 15-3). The micelles contain fatty acids and monoglycerides, bile salts and other phospholipids, cholesterol, and several fat-soluble vitamins all combined together. The micelles stay in equilibrium with a *small amount* of free fatty acids and monoglycerides; these free fatty acids and monoglycerides are the substances actually absorbed into the circulation. As each molecule of free fatty acid or monoglyceride is absorbed, the micelles release replacements, thereby continuing the cycle of absorption. Without the micelles, the fat molecules would once again clump together and be unavailable for absorption.

Because the free fatty acids and monoglycerides are lipid soluble, they move by passive diffusion into the intestinal epithelial cells. In the cells, they are changed back into triglycerides, a process requiring energy. Then, triglycerides join in the epithelial cell with cholesterol and phospholipids. This complex is encased in a protein coat, exits the epithelial cell, and moves by passive diffusion into the lacteal in the center of the villi. The complex of the triglyceride, cholesterol, and phospholipid is similar to a micelle and is called a chylomicron. Chylomicrons are carried in the lymph to the thoracic duct and then enter the general circulation.

Triglycerides can be used directly as an energy source for most cells of the body, or the glycerol portion can be changed into glucose in the liver and used as an energy source. Excess triglycerides are stored in adipose tissue.

SECRETION OF MUCUS

Mucus is secreted along the entire length of the gut. Mucus is a thick substance that coats the wall of the gut and serves to protect it from being digested by the enzymes to which it is exposed. It also serves to lubricate food, allowing for easier passage. HCl, which is highly concentrated in the stomach and serves as an essential component of protein digestion, could severely compromise the gut wall integrity if mucus production were not adequate to provide protection. In addition, without the lubricating effects of mucus, stools would be hard.

RECIRCULATION OF BILE

After the bile salts deliver fatty acids and monoglycerides to the villi, some travel back into the chyme to pick up more molecules and repeat the process. Most of the remaining bile salts are eventually reabsorbed at the end of the small intestine and are recycled back to the liver via the portal vein to be used again. This process is called **enterohepatic circulation**.

ELIMINATION OF WASTE PRODUCTS

Absorption, primarily of water and electrolytes, continues to occur in the large intestine. Most absorption occurs in the upper half of the colon. Of the approximately 1000 mL of chyme that enters the large intestine each day, only 100 mL of fluid and virtually no electrolytes are excreted. Besides water, which makes up approximately 75% of feces, feces contain dead bacteria, some undigested fat and roughage, and a small amount of protein. Bilirubin byproducts give the feces its color.

The process of elimination, or defecation, occurs as a result of peristaltic contractions of the rectum. These contractions are produced in response to stimulation of the longitudinal and circular smooth muscles by the myenteric plexus. The myenteric plexus is stimulated by parasympathetic nerves traveling in sacral segments of the spinal cord. Mechanical stretching of the rectum with stool is also a strong stimulator of peristalsis. When a peristaltic wave is initiated, the internal anal sphincter, a smooth muscle, relaxes. If the external anal sphincter is also relaxed, defecation occurs. The external anal sphincter is a skeletal muscle and thus under voluntary control. In fact, relaxation of the internal sphincter causes reflex contraction of the external sphincter in all individuals except babies and some people who have spinal cord transection. Reflex contraction of the external sphincter effectively stops defecation. If the defecation reflex occurs at an acceptable time, the reflex contraction of the external sphincter can be consciously reversed to allow defecation.

HUNGER AND THE INGESTION OF FOOD

Hunger is controlled by an area of the brain in the lateral hypothalamus. Stimulation of this area causes a strong desire to seek out and to eat food. The lateral hypothalamus receives numerous inputs that can stimulate hunger. For instance, hunger can be stimulated by the occurrence of hunger contractions in the stomach. These contractions appear to increase in frequency and intensity the longer the stomach remains empty. The exact mechanism by which they occur is unclear.

Hunger is also stimulated by a fall in blood nutrients, such as amino acids, fats, and glucose, and by a rise in the hormones that accompany nutrient deficit (e.g., glucagons and ghrelin). A decrease in the level of hormones present when food is plentiful may also stimulate hunger (e.g., decreased insulin and PYY). Input to the hypothalamic hunger center can include input from other areas of the brain as well. For instance, higher brain centers can stimulate hunger in response to certain situations or experiences. Likewise, input from the emotional center of the brain, the limbic system, may also stimulate hunger, as may different smells activating from the olfactory center.

Conversely, the ventromedial nucleus of the hypothalamus appears to be the site where satiety, the opposite of a hunger drive, occurs. This center is influenced by the fullness of the stomach and blood levels of nutrients and hormones, and also in the opposite direction, as is required for hunger stimulation. Emotions and habits may also influence the satiety center.

TESTS OF GASTROINTESTINAL FUNCTIONING

Barium Contrast x-Ray Films: Upper and Lower Gastrointestinal Series

In these tests, a radiopaque solution is introduced into the upper or the lower GI tract, and then x-ray films are obtained to follow its progress. This technique is able to identify the positions and sizes of the GI structures and any obstructions that are present; however, its ability to identify ulcers, fissures, or early stage cancers is poor.

Endoscopy

Endoscopy is the process whereby a thin, rigid or flexible scope is passed into the GI tract to visualize the esophagus (*esophagoscopy*), stomach (*gastroscopy*), upper small intestine (*duodenoscopy*), large intestine (*colonoscopy*), or sigmoid colon (*sigmoidoscopy*). With this instrument, the walls of the GI tract can be visualized, allowing identification of ulcerations, blockages, and other irregularities. Special tools at the end of the scope allow tissue to be sampled for biopsy and culture.

Whether patients should have colonoscopy or sigmoidoscopy for screening of colon cancer depends on personal risk factors, including age, family history of GI or other cancers, and personal history of polyps or cancer. With colonoscopy, the practitioner can fully visualize the entire large intestine. Because many colon cancers develop in the sigmoid colon and because sigmoidoscopy is usually accomplished without general anesthesia, this procedure may be recommended for screening in low-risk populations.

Endoscopic Retrograde Cholangiopancreatography (ERCP)

The gallbladder and pancreas are accessory organs of the GI system and play a major role in the production and storage of bile salts that are necessary for the emulsification of fat. When a problem with either of these organs is suspected, an ERCP is performed. ERCP is similar to the endoscopy but the focus is on the pancreatic and bile ducts. Dye is injected and the ducts are visualized. Stone removal, biopsy, and sphincterotomy are possible with this procedure.

Ultrasound

Ultrasound is a procedure whereby sound waves are reflected from tissue to provide an image. It is a highly sensitive technique and can be used to visualize the structure of the abdominal organs to identify abnormalities, abscesses, stones, and other structures.

Computed Tomography

The process whereby a computer integrates images from several x-ray projections to provide a vivid cross-sectional image is called computed tomography (CT). CT is used to image all GI organs and to identify structural and other abnormalities.

Magnetic Resonance Imaging

Magnetic resonance imaging (MRI) is the process whereby shifts in the magnetic axis of atoms in response to externally applied electromagnetic fields are transformed by computer to produce a cross-sectional image of the structures of the GI tract. MRI is used extensively to identify structural abnormalities, alterations in blood flow, and vessel patency.

● Pathophysiologic Concepts

ANOREXIA

Defined as a loss of appetite or desire for food, anorexia often occurs as a symptom with other GI alterations, including nausea, vomiting, and diarrhea. It can also be present with conditions not associated with the GI tract, such as cancer or as a side effect of some medications.

Anorexia nervosa is a condition in which one chooses not to eat because of a morbid fear of being fat. The term anorexia nervosa is actually a misnomer because individuals who have this disorder still have a desire to eat and are still hungry; so by definition they are not truly anorectic.

NAUSEA

Nausea is a subjective, unpleasant sensation that often precedes vomiting. Nausea is caused by distention or irritation anywhere in the GI tract, but it can also be stimulated by higher brain centers. Interpretation of nausea occurs in the medulla, which is either adjacent to or part of the vomiting center.

VOMITING

Rapid emptying of stomach contents through the esophagus and into the mouth is referred to as vomiting. Vomiting is a complex reflex mediated through the vomiting center in the medulla oblongata of the brain. Afferent impulses travel to the vomiting center as both vagal and sympathetic afferents. Afferent impulses originate in the stomach or duodenum in response to excessive distention or irritation, or sometimes they originate in response to chemical stimulation by emetics (agents that cause vomiting), such as syrup of ipecac. Hypoxia and pain can also stimulate vomiting by means of activation of the vomiting center. Vomiting can also occur through direct stimulation of an area of the brain adjacent to the vomiting center in the brain. Certain drugs initiate vomiting by activating this center, called the chemoreceptor trigger zone, which lies in the floor of the fourth ventricle. Vomiting as a result of rapid motion change is believed to work through stimulation of this trigger zone. Activation of the chemoreceptor trigger zone can cause vomiting either directly or indirectly by its subsequent activation of the vomiting center. Input from higher brain centers in the cortex and increased intracranial pressure (ICP) can also stimulate vomiting, probably by directly stimulating the vomiting center. Projectile vomiting occurs when the vomiting center is directly stimulated, frequently by increased ICP.

When the vomiting reflex is initiated in the vomiting center, it is carried out by activation of several cranial nerves to the face and throat, and spinal motor neurons to the diaphragm and abdominal muscles. Excitation of these pathways results in the coordinated response of vomiting. Certain symptoms generally precede vomiting, including nausea, tachycardia, and sweating.

DIARRHEA

Diarrhea is an increase in fluidity and frequency of stools. It may be large or small volume and may or may not contain blood. Large-volume diarrhea can occur as a result of the presence of a nonabsorbable solute in the stool, called osmotic diarrhea, or as a result of irritation of the intestinal tract. The most common cause of large-volume diarrhea due to irritation is a viral or bacterial infection of the large intestine or the distal small intestine.

Irritation of the intestines by a pathogen affects the mucosal layer, leading to increased secretory products, including mucus. Microbial irritation also affects the muscular layer, leading to increased motility. Increased motility causes large amounts of water and electrolytes to be lost in the stool because the time available for reabsorption in the colon is reduced. An individual who has severe diarrhea can die from hypovolemic shock and electrolyte irregularities. Cholera toxin released from the cholera bacteria is an example of a substance that strongly stimulates motility and directly causes secretion of water and electrolytes into the large intestine, contributing to the devastating loss of these important plasma constituents. Other infectious agents can also cause diarrhea, either severe or mild. Infection with *Escherichia coli* O157, found in undercooked ground beef, causes a severe bloody diarrhea. Large-volume diarrhea can also be caused by psychological factors, such as fear or some types of stress, mediated through parasympathetic stimulation of the gut.

Small-volume diarrhea is characterized by frequent loss of small amounts of stool. Causes of this type of diarrhea include ulcerative colitis and Crohn disease. Both of these illnesses have physical and psychogenic components and are discussed later.

CONSTIPATION

Constipation is defined as small, difficult, or infrequent defecation. Because frequency of stool varies among individuals, part of this definition is subjective and should be interpreted as a relative decrease in the number of stools for that particular individual. In general, however, bowel movements fewer than once every 3 days are considered to indicate constipation.

Delayed peristalsis is the major underlying factor related to constipation. When peristalsis is slowed, the stool can become hard and compact and defecation can become difficult. This can occur when an individual is dehydrated or if a bowel movement is delayed, which allows more water to be absorbed out of the stool as it sits in the large intestine. Bulk or high-fiber diets keep stools moist by osmotically drawing water into the stool and by stimulating peristalsis of the colon by distention. Therefore, people who eat low-bulk diets or highly refined foods are at a greater risk for constipation. Exercise promotes defecation by physical stimulation of the GI tract. Therefore, individuals who lead sedentary lives are at a higher risk of suffering from constipation.

Fear of pain during defecation can be a psychological stimulus to withhold a bowel movement and can cause constipation. Other psychological inputs might also cause delay of defecation. Sympathetic stimulation of the GI tract decreases motility and can slow defecation. Sympathetic activity is increased in individuals who have long-term stress. Certain drugs such as antacids and opiates may also cause constipation.

Spinal cord trauma, multiple sclerosis, intestinal neoplasm, and hypothyroidism can result in constipation. A disease characterized by a dysfunctional myenteric plexus in the large intestine, called Hirschsprung disease (congenital megacolon), also causes constipation. This disease should be apparent soon after birth.

● Conditions of Disease or Injury

PERITONITIS

Inflammation of the peritoneum, a membrane that lines the abdominal cavity, is called peritonitis. Peritonitis usually occurs as a result of the passage of bacteria through the GI tract or abdominal organs into the peritoneal space as a result of perforation of the gut or rupture of an organ. GI surgery or a penetrating wound to the gut may also result in spillage into the peritoneal cavity. The severe infection that occurs with the movement of gut contents into the peritoneal cavity emphasizes the fact that the GI tract is really external to the body, rather than a part of the internal environment.

Clinical Manifestations

- Pain, especially over the inflamed area. Pain may change in location, being centrally located at first, and then becoming more site-specific as the inflammation worsens. Pain may be rebound in nature; that is, the person may complain of more pain when pressure on the abdomen is removed quickly. Rebound pain is related to the sudden wave of movement that occurs through the peritoneal fluid when pressure is released.
- Tachycardia due to hypovolemia as fluid moves into the peritoneum.

- Nausea and vomiting.
- Rigid abdomen indicative of widespread inflammation.
- General signs of inflammation such as fever, an increase in white blood cell count, and increased sedimentation rate.

Diagnostic Tools

- Abdominal paracentesis that reveals pus, bacteria, exudates, and/or blood.
- Abdominal and chest radiographs.
- Complete blood cell count revealing leukocytosis.

Complications

- Dehydration due to vascular fluid loss into the peritoneal cavity.
- Sepsis leading to multiorgan failure.
- Bowel obstruction.
- Respiratory compromise as the diaphragm is forced upward from increasing abdominal pressure.

Treatment

- Antibiotics.
- Nothing by mouth in an effort to slow peristalsis and minimize the risk of perforation.
- Nasogastric intubation.
- Fluid and electrolyte replacement.
- Analgesics.
- Surgery.

GASTROESOPHAGEAL REFLUX DISEASE

The condition of gastroesophageal reflux disease (GERD) is caused by the reflux of stomach contents into the esophagus. GERD is commonly called heartburn because of the pain that occurs when the acid, normally present only in the stomach, enters and burns or irritates the esophagus.

GERD is a significant problem in Western societies but relatively uncommon in Asian countries. Risk factors for GERD include male gender, increased body mass index (BMI), smoking, and regular alcohol intake. Epidemiologic studies have shown a negative relationship between *Helicobacter pylori* (*H. pylori*) infection and GERD, perhaps related to a reduced ability of the stomach to produce acid over time in patients with *H. pylori* or perhaps

Normal Gastroesophageal Junction

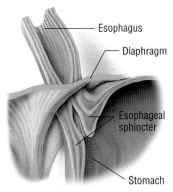

FIGURE 15-5 Normal gastroesophageal junction.

related to the proton-pump inhibitors used in the treatment of *H. pylori* as described later in this chapter.

Causes of GERD

GERD usually occurs after a meal and results from conditions that either weaken the tone of the esophageal sphincter or increase the pressure in the stomach compared with the esophagus. By either of these mechanisms, acidic stomach contents move into the esophagus.

The contents of the stomach are usually prevented from entering the esophagus by the esophageal sphincter (Fig. 15-1). This sphincter normally opens only when a peristaltic wave delivering a bolus of food moves down the esophagus. When this happens, the smooth muscle of the sphincter relaxes, and food enters the stomach (Fig. 15-5). It is important that the esophageal sphincter always remains closed except at this time, because many organs are crowded together in the abdominal cavity, causing abdominal pressure to be greater than thoracic pressure. Therefore, the tendency is for contents of the stomach to be pushed up into the esophagus. If one has a weakened or incompetent sphincter, it will not remain closed to stomach contents. Reflux will occur from the high-pressure zone (the stomach) to the low-pressure zone (the esophagus). A weakened sphincter can be a congenital defect or a result of damage to the esophagus. Repeated episodes of GERD may themselves worsen the condition by causing inflammation and scarring in the lower esophageal area (Fig. 15-6).

In some circumstances, even if the sphincter has normal tone, reflux will occur if there is an unusually high-pressure gradient at the sphincter. For example, if stomach contents are excessive, abdominal pressure may increase

GERD (Gastroesophageal Reflux Disease)

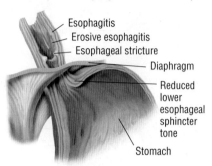

FIGURE 15-6 Gastroesophageal reflux disease (GERD): acid reflux occurs when gastric acid flows backwards into the esophagus, causing inflammation and erosion of esophageal tissue.

significantly. This may result from an extra large meal, pregnancy, or obesity. High abdominal pressures tend to push the esophageal sphincter into the thoracic cavity; this exaggerates the pressure gradient between the esophagus and the abdominal cavity. Lying down, especially after a large meal, lifting, bending, straining, certain foods, and some medications can also contribute to reflux.

A hiatal hernia may also cause reflux. A hiatal hernia is a protrusion of a part of the stomach through the opening in the diaphragm. If this occurs, high pressure in that part of the stomach results in stomach contents being pushed into the esophagus. Reflux of stomach contents irritates the esophagus because of the high acid content in the stomach. Although the esophagus also has mucus-producing cells, they are not as active or as prevalent as they are in the stomach.

Clinical Manifestations

- Burning pain in the epigastric area, called dyspepsia, may occur, and may radiate to shoulders, back, or neck.
- Belching and a sour taste may accompany the pain.
- Pain usually occurs within 30 to 60 minutes after a meal or during sleep, when the individual is lying down.
- Regurgitation, dysphagia, coughing.

Diagnostic Tools

- A good history identifies many individuals at risk of GERD.
- A pH probe, passed into the lower esophageal area may reveal an abnormally low pH (below 4.0) in individuals who have GERD. False positives and false negatives exist.

- Esophageal manometry to measure pressure of the LES.
- Barium swallows are *ineffective* in identifying GERD although they may be used to visualize a hiatal hernia.

Complications

- Barrett esophagitis is an irritation of the lining of the esophagus characterized by cell changes that can result from chronic reflux. It is a premalignant condition that may lead to esophageal carcinoma.
- Chronic irritation of the esophagus can cause chronic inflammation, spasm of the muscles, and scarring of the esophagus, all of which may lead to stricture development, thereby interfering with or blocking food passage.
- Vomiting and dysphagia (difficulty swallowing) with eating may occur.
- Pulmonary complications and reflux aspiration.

Treatment

- Identify and avoid aggravating factors.
- Abdominal pressure can be reduced by eating frequent small meals rather than large meals. If obesity is a problem, nutritional and exercise counseling are advised.
- Sitting up during and after eating, and sleeping with the head elevated, will reduce abdominal pressure on the esophageal sphincter.
- Drinking extra fluids will help wash refluxed material out of the esophagus.
- Histamine type-2 (H2) receptor antagonists and proton-pump inhibitors are used to reduce acid secretion by the stomach, in combination with the behavioral changes described above.
- Proton-pump inhibitor therapy is the treatment of choice in acute cases of GERD and as maintenance therapy for patients with documented esophageal erosion.
- Antireflux surgery may be considered if symptoms are resistant to treatment or are caused by hiatal hernia.
- Antacids may be used to neutralize the acidic content of the stomach.
- Medications that promote gastric motility may be used on a short-term basis to minimize the time gastric contents have to irritate the mucosa.
- Smoking cessation and elimination of alcohol intake.

PEPTIC ULCER

The term peptic ulcer refers to an erosion of the mucosal layer anywhere in the GI tract; however, it usually refers to erosions in the stomach or duodenum. Gastric ulcer refers only to an ulcer in the stomach.

Causes of Peptic Ulcer

There are two main causes of ulcers: (1) too little mucus production or (2) too much acid being produced in the stomach or delivered to the intestine. A variety of conditions may cause either or both of these disturbances.

Decreased Mucus Production as a Cause of Ulcer

Ulcers most commonly develop when the mucosal cells of the gut do not produce adequate mucus to protect against acid digestion. Causes of decreased mucus production can include anything that decreases blood flow to the gut, causing hypoxia of the mucosal layer and injury to or death of mucus-producing cells. This type of ulcer is called an ischemic ulcer. Decreased blood flow occurs with all types of shock. A particular type of ischemic ulcer that develops after a severe burn is called a Curling ulcer.

Decreased mucus production in the duodenum can also occur as a result of inhibition of mucus-producing glands, called Brunner glands, located there. Their activity is inhibited by sympathetic stimulation. Sympathetic stimulation is increased by chronic stress, thus making a connection between chronic stress and ulcer development.

The main cause of decreased mucus production is related to infection with *H. pylori* bacteria. *H. pylori* colonize the mucus-secreting cells of the stomach and duodenum, reducing their ability to produce mucus. Approximately 90% of patients who have duodenal ulcer and 70% of patients who have gastric ulcer show *H. pylori* infection. *H. pylori* infection is endemic in some countries. Infection appears to occur by means of ingestion of the microorganism.

The use of various drugs, especially nonsteroidal anti-inflammatory drugs (NSAIDs) is also associated with an increased risk of ulcer development. Aspirin, especially, causes irritation of the mucosal wall, as do the other NSAIDs and glucocorticosteroids. These drugs contribute to ulcer development by inhibiting protective prostaglandins both systemically and in the gut wall. Approximately 10% of patients taking NSAIDs develop an active ulcer while a much higher percentage develops less-serious erosions. Gastric or intestinal bleeding can occur from NSAIDs, with little early warning. The elderly are especially susceptible to GI injury from NSAIDs. Other drugs or foods associated with ulcer development include caffeine, alcohol, and nicotine. These drugs seem to injure the protective mucosal layer also.

Excess Acid as a Cause of Ulcer

Acid production in the stomach is necessary for activation of stomach digestive enzymes. Hydrochloric acid (HCl) is produced by the parietal cells in response to certain foods, drugs, hormones (including gastrin), histamine, and parasympathetic stimulation. Foods and drugs such as caffeine and alcohol stimulate the parietal cells to produce acid. Some individuals might be overreactive in their parietal response to these substances or other foods, or they may simply have a greater number of parietal cells than normal and therefore release excess acid. Aspirin is an acid, which may directly irritate or erode the lining of the stomach.

Because gastrin stimulates the production of acid, anything that increases the secretion of gastrin can lead to excess acid production. The main example of this condition is called Zollinger–Ellison syndrome, a disease characterized by tumors of the gastrin-secreting endocrine cells. Other causes of excess acid include excessive vagal stimulation to the parietal cells that is seen after severe brain injury or trauma. Ulcers that develop under these circumstances are called Cushing ulcers. Excess vagal stimulation during psychological stress may also cause excess HCl production.

Increased Delivery of Acid as a Cause of Duodenal Ulcer

Too rapid movement of stomach contents into the duodenum can overwhelm the protective mucus layer there. This occurs with irritation of the stomach by certain foods or microorganisms, as well as by excess gastrin secretion or abnormal distention.

Rapid movement of stomach contents into the intestine also occurs in the condition called dumping syndrome. Dumping syndrome happens when the ability of the stomach to hold and slowly release chyme into the duodenum is compromised. One cause of dumping syndrome is surgical removal of a large part of the stomach. Dumping syndrome not only results in rapid delivery of acid to the intestine, but it can cause cardiovascular hypotension. Hypotension occurs because the delivery of multiple food particles to the intestine all at once results in a large amount of water moving from the circulation into the gut by osmosis.

Clinical Manifestations

- Burning abdominal pain (dyspepsia) often occurs at night. The pain is usually located in the midline epigastric area, and is often rhythmic in nature.
- Pain that occurs when the stomach is empty (e.g., at night) often signifies a duodenal ulcer. This is most common.
- Pain that occurs immediately after or during eating suggests a gastric ulcer. Occasionally, the pain may be referred to the back or shoulder as well.
- The occurrence of pain often comes and goes; it sometimes occurs daily for several weeks and then disappears altogether until the next exacerbation.
- Weight loss is common with gastric ulcers. Weight gain may occur with duodenal ulcers because eating relieves the discomfort.
- Nausea, anorexia, pallor, epigastric tenderness, hyperactive bowel sounds.

Diagnostic Tools

- Ulcers are diagnosed primarily by history and endoscopy. With esophagogastroduodenoscopy not only can the gut lining be viewed for ulcers, but tissue samples can also be taken for biopsy and the presence or absence of *H. pylori* can be determined.

- *H. pylori* infection may also be diagnosed by blood tests for antibody and by breath tests that measure metabolic waste production by the microbe.
- Stool analysis for occult blood.

Complications

- An ulcer may in some instances go through all mucosal layers, causing perforation of the gut. Because gut contents are not sterile, this can lead to infection of the abdominal cavity. The pain of perforation is severe and radiating. It is unrelieved by eating or antacids.
- Obstruction of the lumen of the GI tract may occur as a result of repeated episodes of injury, inflammation, and scarring. Obstruction is most often at the pylorus, the narrow passageway between the stomach and the small intestine. Obstruction causes feelings of stomach and epigastric distention, heaviness, nausea, and vomiting.
- Hemorrhage may occur when the ulcer has eroded an artery or vein in the gut. This can result in hematemesis (vomiting of blood) or in melena (passage of upper GI blood in the stool). If bleeding is extensive and sudden, symptoms of shock may occur. If bleeding is slow and insidious, microcytic hypochromic anemia may develop.

Treatment

- Identify and instruct patients to avoid foods that cause excess HCl secretion; doing so improves the symptoms for some individuals.
- Educate patients that avoidance of alcohol and caffeine improves symptoms and increases healing of a pre-existing ulcer.
- Discontinue or reduce NSAID ingestion; this often relieves symptoms in mild cases.
- Strongly urge individuals who smoke to quit because tobacco both irritates the gut and delays healing.
- Antihistamines or proton-pump inhibitors to neutralize stomach acid and to relieve symptoms of an ulcer.
- Anticholinergics, prostaglandin analogs, and cytoprotectant medications.
- Individuals documented to have an ulcer caused by *H. pylori*—the majority of patients by far—are treated with the addition of an antibiotic to the standard antacid therapy previously used. Typically, patients are placed on one or two effective antibiotics plus bismuth or on a proton-pump inhibitor and antibiotics. Adding antibiotics to the acid-lowering strategies used previously can truly cure many patients of their ulcers rather than just temporarily improving their symptoms.

- Stress management, relaxation techniques, or sedatives can be used to relieve psychological influences.

MALABSORPTION

Failure of the small intestine to absorb certain foodstuffs is called malabsorption. Inability to absorb can be (1) of one type of amino acid, fat, sugar, or vitamin; (2) of all amino acids, fats, sugars; or (3) of all fat-soluble vitamins. Malabsorption of everything absorbed in one segment of the small intestine can also occur, with other small intestine segments being spared.

Causes of malabsorption include pancreatic digestive enzyme deficiency; microorganism infection; damage to the mucosal layer of the gut; or, for fats and fat-soluble vitamins, impairment of bile production or lymph function. Genetic deficiencies in specific enzymes may also occur. Lactose malabsorption can result from the inability to break down lactose into absorbable monosaccharides. Lactose malabsorption can result from a congenital deficiency in the enzyme lactase or a decrease in lactase after an intestinal disease. Crohn disease and bowel resection are common causes of malabsorption, as is sprue, a disease characterized by injury to the villi that apparently is caused by a hypersensitivity to gluten, a product of wheat, barley, rye, and oats.

Clinical Manifestations

Clinical manifestations of malabsorption depend on what is not being absorbed and whether other areas of the bowel can compensate. Specific symptoms are related to the dietary deficiency that occurs. Generalized symptoms usually include those related to the GI tract or to the loss of fat-soluble vitamins:
- Fat malabsorption results in steatorrhea (fat in the stool). Diarrhea, flatulence, bloating, and cramps often occur. Stools are bulky but of light weight, float, and are malodorous.
- Bile salt deficiency results in malabsorption of fat-soluble vitamins, causing the following:
  - Vitamin A deficiency—night blindness.
  - Vitamin D deficiency—bone demineralization and increased risk of fractures.
  - Vitamin K deficiency—poor coagulation with prolonged prothrombin time, easy bruising, and petechia (hemorrhagic spots on the skin).
  - Vitamin E deficiency—perhaps resulting in poor immune function.
  - Lactose malabsorption results in osmotic diarrhea and flatulence (gas).

Diagnostic Tools

- The presence of over 7 g of fat per day in the stool of an adult consuming a typical American diet is considered malabsorption. Weight loss or failure to gain weight in infancy or early childhood may indicate malabsorption.

Complications

- Failure to thrive may occur in severe cases, leading to malnutrition, infection, and even death.

Treatment

- Identification of the cause of malabsorption.
- Provision of needed nutrients through other food sources or supplements.

APPENDICITIS

Inflammation of the appendix, known as appendicitis, may occur (1) for no obvious reason, (2) after obstruction of the appendix with stool, or (3) from either the organ or its blood supply being twisted. Decreased blood supply may be the result of infection, strictures, neoplasms, or a foreign body. Irritation to the mucosa triggers the inflammatory process that obstructs the appendix. The obstruction prevents the mucus from flowing out thus increasing pressure in the appendix. As the pressure continues to increase, inflammation increases and results in a swollen, tender appendix, which can lead to gangrene of the organ as blood supply is compromised. The appendix may also burst; this typically happens between 36 and 48 hours after the onset of symptoms.

Clinical Manifestations

- Abrupt or gradual onset of diffuse pain in the epigastric or periumbilical area is common.
- Over the next few hours, the pain becomes more localized and may be described as a pinpoint tenderness in the lower right quadrant (McBurney's point).
- Rebound tenderness (pain that occurs when pressure is removed from the tender area) is a classic symptom of peritonitis and is common with appendicitis. Guarding of the abdomen occurs.
- Fever.
- Anorexia, nausea, and vomiting.

Diagnostic Tools

The diagnosis of appendicitis continues to be difficult for clinicians. In at least 20% of cases of appendicitis, the diagnosis is missed; in another 15% to 40% of cases, the appendix is normal in patients sent to surgery for suspected appendicitis. Diagnostic criteria for identifying appendicitis include:

- Elevated white cell count greater than 10,000/mL.
- Fever greater than 37.50°C (99.5°F).

- The presence of pain in the right lower quadrant.
- CT scanning is an excellent tool for the diagnosis of appendicitis, especially appendiceal CT used in the emergency department by radiologists trained in its use.
- Ultrasound may also be effective.
- Elevated C-reactive protein due to inflammatory process.

Complications

- Peritonitis can occur if the swollen appendix bursts. Peritonitis significantly increases the risk of postoperative complications.

Treatment

- Nothing by mouth.
- Parenteral fluids and electrolytes.
- Nasogastric intubation.
- Surgical removal of the appendix.
- If the appendix bursts before surgery, antibiotics are necessary to reduce the risk of peritonitis and sepsis.

CHOLECYSTITIS

Acute or chronic inflammation of the gallbladder is known as cholecystitis and is most often the result of a gallstone. Abnormal metabolism of cholesterol and bile salts can lead to the development of gallstones. The stone lodges in the cystic duct, inhibiting the release of bile, which causes the gallbladder to become distended and inflamed. Bacteria and diminished blood flow contribute to the inflammation.

Clinical Manifestations

- Acute right upper quadrant abdominal pain, usually after a high-fat meal. May radiate to the back, between the shoulders or to the chest.
- Colic, nausea, and vomiting.
- Chills, low-grade fever.
- Jaundice.

Diagnostic Tools

- Radiographs.
- CT or MRI.

- Percutaneous transhepatic cholangiography.
- Laboratory findings include: elevated alkaline phosphate, lactate dehydrogenase, aspirate aminotransferase, total bilirubin, serum amylase, icteric index, and white blood cell count.

Complications

- Perforation.
- Gangrene.
- Peritonitis.
- Fistula formation.
- Pancreatitis.

Treatment

- Surgical removal of gallstones and/or gallbladder.
- Lithotripsy.
- Vitamin K.
- Antibiotics.

INFLAMMATORY BOWEL DISEASE

Inflammatory bowel disease includes Crohn disease and ulcerative colitis. Both of these conditions appear to be autoimmune diseases of unknown cause, with widespread activation of proinflammatory cytokines contributing to the scarring and inflammation of the tissue. Both of them have strong genetic influences, are exacerbated by stress, and tend to occur more often in females. A constellation of factors must be present, which include:

- Genetic susceptibility.
- Abnormal immune response.
- Imbalance of pathogenic and beneficial bacteria in the intestine.
- Defects in the intestinal epithelium.

CROHN DISEASE

Crohn disease, also known as regional enteritis, is a chronic inflammatory disease of the bowel characterized by inflammation of all layers of the GI tract. It especially affects the submucosal layer and the small and large intestines. Regional lymph nodes and the mesentery may also be involved.

The inflammation of Crohn occurs as sharply outlined granulomatous lesions that appear in a skip pattern scattered throughout the affected area of the gut. Interspersed between areas of inflammation is normal gut tissue. With chronic inflammation, fibrosis and scarring occur and make the bowel stiff and inflexible. If the fibrosis occurs in the small intestine, it can significantly interfere with the absorption of nutrients. If the disease is primarily localized in the colon, water and electrolyte balances can be disturbed. Abnormal connections or fistulas sometimes develop between different parts of the digestive tract and between the GI tract and the vagina, bladder, or rectum. These fistulas can contribute to malabsorption and cause infection.

Clinical Manifestations

- Intermittent, usually nonbloody diarrhea. Steatorrhea.
- Colicky pain, usually in the right lower quadrant.
- Weight loss.
- Malabsorption.
- Fluid and electrolyte imbalances may result.
- Malaise.
- Low-grade fevers.

Diagnostic Tools

- Colonoscopy reveals irregular, scarred bowel.
- Small bowel radiograph shows irregular mucosa and ulceration.
- Barium enema reveals segments of strictures separated by normal bowel (string sign), fissures, and narrowed bowel.
- Biopsy.
- Laboratory findings include increased white blood cell count and erythrocyte sedimentation rate; decreased potassium, calcium, magnesium, and hemoglobin.

Complications

- Toxic megacolon, dilation of the colon resulting from interference with its neural or vascular integrity, may occur. This condition can be life threatening.
- Obstruction of the intestine caused by scarring may occur. Fistulas between the colon and other abdominal organs may occur.
- Systemic manifestations of Crohn disease include arthritis, skin lesions, and various blood disorders, including autoimmune anemia and hypercoagulability. Persons may demonstrate signs of depression.
- Children afflicted with Crohn disease may experience growth retardation, resulting from malabsorption as well as from the anti-inflammatory drugs used to treat the disease.

Treatment

- Anti-inflammatory drugs are used to interrupt the constant cycle of inflammation.
- Corticosteroids, immunosuppressants, aminosalicylates, antidiarrheals, antibiotics.
- Nutritional supplementation and diet education.
- Surgery involving gut resection may be required.
- Psychological support.
- Total parenteral nutrition, which involves food solutions being delivered intravenously, may be needed during exacerbations to allow the gut to heal.
- Given the role of proinflammatory cytokines in contributing to the course of Crohn disease, use of antibodies against one proinflammatory cytokine in particular, tumor necrosis factor alpha (TNF-α) is an effective treatment for many.

ULCERATIVE COLITIS

Ulcerative colitis is an inflammatory disease of the rectum and colon that primarily affects the mucosal layer of the large intestine. It is spread continuously throughout the affected area. There is no skip pattern. Ulcerative lesions in the crypts located in the base of the mucosal layer, called Lieberkuhn crypts, become inflamed, causing hemorrhage and abscess formation. Thickening of the wall of the bowel can occur.

Ulcerative colitis typically goes through stages of exacerbations and remissions. The disease can be mild, moderate, or fulminating. Bloody diarrhea mixed with mucus is characteristic of each stage, but it is intensified with increasing severity of the disease.

Clinical Manifestations

- Mild cases demonstrate small-volume, chronic, bloody diarrhea.
- With worsening cases, more and more of the colon is affected, resulting in increasing diarrhea, with loss of electrolytes.
- A hallmark sign is recurrent bloody diarrhea that typically contains pus and mucus.
- Foul-smelling stools.
- Fever.
- Weight loss.
- Abdominal pain increasing with severity of disease.

Diagnostic Tools

- Sigmoidoscopy reveals hemorrhagic mucosa with ulceration.
- Colonoscopy reveals strictures and pseudopolyps. Biopsy shows areas of inflammation.
- Blood analysis demonstrates anemia and low hemoglobin, white blood cell count, serum potassium, magnesium, and albumin.

Complications

- Toxic megacolon may develop.
- Perforation of the gut wall with peritonitis may occur.
- There is an increased risk of colon cancer with ulcerative colitis.
- Systemic manifestations of ulcerative colitis include arthritis, skin lesions, and various blood disorders, including autoimmune anemia and hypercoagulability.
- Nutritional deficits.
- Loss of muscle mass.
- Children afflicted with ulcerative colitis may experience growth retardation, resulting from malabsorption and diarrhea, as well as from the anti-inflammatory drugs used to treat the disease.

Treatment

- Anti-inflammatory drugs to inhibit prostaglandin production in the gut in an effort to decrease the inflammatory process.
- Corticosteroids or immunomodulators.
- Biologic modifiers.
- Nutritional supplementation.
- Bulk-free diet to decrease stool frequency.
- Psychological support.
- Surgical resection of the bowel may be necessary.

DIVERTICULAR DISEASE

Diverticular disease is characterized by one or multiple herniations of the mucosal layer of the colon through the muscular layers. Herniations of the mucosal layer are believed to occur when an individual frequently exerts high pressures inside the lumen of the colon while straining to pass a low-bulk stool. Although the exact cause is unknown, contributing factors may include diminished colonic motility, increased intraluminal pressure, low-fiber and low-bulk meals, and defects in colon wall strength.

Clinical Manifestations

Some individuals may be asymptomatic while others may have mild, severe, or chronic complaints. Clinical manifestations usually include the following:
- A change in bowel habits.
- Excess gas.
- Left lower abdominal pain.
- Low-grade fever to high fever, chills, hypotension, and shock.
- Nausea and vomiting.
- Microscopic to massive hemorrhage.
- Abdominal rigidity, pain, absent bowel sounds.
- Leukocytosis.

Diagnostic Tools

- A good history and physical examination assist diagnosis.
- An enema containing the contrast medium barium followed by x-ray may identify diverticula. Barium enemas should be avoided if risk of perforation is high.
- Laboratory findings: elevated white blood cell count and erythrocyte sedimentation rate.

Complications

- Diverticulitis, an inflammation or infection of the diverticula, may occur. The diverticula may become infected if bacteria-rich pieces of stool become trapped in the diverticula. Systemic signs of an infection, including fever and elevated white cell count, occur.
- Perforation of the gut from severe diverticulitis may occur. With perforation, pain (usually in the lower left quadrant), nausea, and vomiting occur. Fever and elevated white cell count are present.
- Rectal hemorrhage or obstruction.

Treatment

- Dietary modification to increase stool bulk.
- Exercise to increase the rate of stool passage.
- Diverticulitis is usually treated with antibiotics and the withholding of solid food until healing occurs. High-residue diet after pain subsides.

- Antispasmodics, analgesics.
- Colon resection with removal of involved segment. Temporary colostomy if needed.
- Possible blood transfusion.
- Perforation requires surgery and antibiotic therapy.

HIRSCHSPRUNG DISEASE

Hirschsprung disease, also called congenital megacolon, results from the congenital absence of autonomic ganglia innervating the myenteric plexus in the anorectal junction and some or most of the rectum and colon. In most cases, the absence of ganglia is restricted to the sigmoid (distal) colon, although in approximately 20% of cases, the disorder extends proximally as well. Involvement of the entire bowel is rare and fatal. Autonomic ganglia to the myenteric plexus normally stimulate motility and ensure the passage of stool. With Hirschsprung, stool accumulates in the bowel. The prevalence of Hirschsprung is about 1:5000 live births, with most cases (approximately 85%) occurring sporadically or without a clear autosomal dominant pattern. Nevertheless, there are at least nine genes involved in affecting susceptibility to the disorder. Nearly 1 in 3 afflicted children will have an additional congenital malformation. In adults, Hirschsprung disease may develop following damage to the myenteric plexus.

Clinical Manifestations

- Neonates
  - Failure to pass the first stool within 48 hours of birth carries a high suspicion of Hirschsprung.
  - Bile-stained or fecal vomitus.
  - Distended abdomen and/or vomiting.
  - Dehydration, failure to thrive.
- Children
  - Intractable constipation.
  - Protruding abdomen with palpable fecal mass.
- Adults (rare occurrence)
  - Abdominal distention.
  - Chronic, intermittent constipation.

Diagnostic Tools

- Rectal biopsy that demonstrates an absence of ganglion cells confirms diagnosis.

- Barium enema shows narrowed segment of distal colon.
- Rectal manometry to evaluate anal sphincter.
- Abdominal radiograph reveals colonic distention.

Complications

- Electrolyte disturbances and perforation of the bowel if distension is unrelieved.
- Fecal impaction.
- Nutritional deficits.

Treatment

- Surgical resection of the affected area.

ESOPHAGEAL CANCER

Esophageal cancer is relatively uncommon in the United States; in other countries, this is not true. Worldwide, the highest rate of esophageal squamous cell carcinoma is in North Central China. Esophageal cancer is primarily related to alcohol and tobacco use. In some countries, such as China, these standard risks are combined with exposure to polycyclic aromatic hydrocarbons and malnutrition. Injury to the esophagus from accidental exposure to caustic materials or from the repeated ingestion of extremely hot liquids (such as tea) also has been implicated. And finally, chronic GERD may stimulate development of Barrett esophagus and esophageal cancer. Prognosis for esophageal cancer has traditionally been poor, but it is improving with better diagnostic techniques that allow for earlier recognition and treatment. The most common sites for metastasis are the liver and the lungs.

Clinical Manifestations

- Dysphagia (difficulty swallowing) is the most common symptom.
- Anorexia and weight loss follow.
- Pain from bone metastases often is the first symptom that stimulates a person to seek care.

Diagnostic Tools

- Endoscopy followed by tissue biopsy is used to diagnose esophageal cancer.
- x-ray or other diagnostic tests may be used to identify the secondary tumors.
- Endoscopic ultrasonography.

Treatment

The goals of treatment are to control dysphagia and improve nutritional status.

- Surgical resection, radiation, and chemotherapy.
- Analgesics.

STOMACH CANCER

Stomach cancer has decreased in the United States; however, it is still the seventh leading cause of death in this country. There appears to be a genetic predisposition to stomach cancer and an increased risk associated with consumption of preserved and smoked meats. Stomach cancer has also been linked to *H. pylori* infection. It has been suggested that the decreasing rates of stomach cancer in the United States over the last several decades may be due to the frequent use of antibiotics and hence the eradication of *H. pylori*. Decreased use of nitrate preservatives with better refrigeration has also contributed to the decrease in occurrence of stomach cancer.

Clinical Manifestations

Stomach cancer is frequently asymptomatic until advanced. When symptoms are present they include the following:

- Vague abdominal discomfort.
- Indigestion.
- Weight loss.
- Anorexia.
- Fatigue.
- A palpable abdominal mass may be present.

Diagnostic Tools

- A careful history and the use of endoscopy followed by tissue biopsy enable diagnosis.

Treatment

- Partial or complete surgical resection of the stomach.
- Chemotherapy and/or radiation therapy may be used.

COLORECTAL CANCER

Colorectal or intestinal cancer is common in the United States. Most colorectal cancers are carcinomas and usually begin in the secretory glands of the mucosal layer. Most colorectal cancers begin in pre-existing polyps. The focus is now shifting from early detection to more comprehensive screening.

Risk factors for colorectal cancer include a high-fat and low-fiber diet, as well as high consumption of red meat and processed meats. Withholding stools may also allow toxins present in the stool to initiate or promote cancer. There is a genetic risk factor for colorectal cancer, and specific genes associated with colon cancer have been identified. The presence or history of polyps in the colon and rectum indicates an increased risk of cancer development. With regard to prevention, high intake of fruits and vegetables may protect against the development of colorectal cancer by increasing dietary bulk and by providing antioxidants that may protect cells from damage by carcinogens. Long-term (>10 years) use of aspirin and other NSAIDs significantly reduces the risk of colorectal cancer in a dose-dependent manner. However, risks associated with aspirin and NSAIDs, including GI bleeding, also increase with usage and dose. Finally, although still under investigation, there is evidence to suggest that colon cancer risk is lower in individuals taking statins for treatment of hyperlipidemia, although the mechanism by which this occurs is unclear.

Clinical Manifestations

- Changes in bowel habits resulting in diarrhea or constipation may occur.
- Occult or frank blood in the stool is a strong warning sign.
- Fatigue, weakness, exertional dyspnea, anorexia,
- Signs of obstruction or metastasis (pressure, pain in adjacent organs).

Diagnostic Tools

- Anemia may show up in a complete blood count (CBC), prompting further evaluation.
- A palpable mass may be felt by digital examination.
- Tests for occult blood in the stool may indicate cancer. Fecal immunochemical test or stool DNA testing.
- Early identification of polyps with digital examination, sigmoidoscopy, or colonoscopy (examination of the entire rectum and colon with a fiber-optic lens), and surgical removal of any visualized polyps may prevent cancer from developing.
- Double-contrast barium enema.

- Genetic markers for colon cancer may predict who is at greatest risk of developing the disease, thus allowing appropriate preventive measures to be initiated.
- Blood tests for specific antigens associated with colorectal cancer, especially carcinoembryonic antigen (CEA), can be useful in the early identification of a recurring colorectal cancer. CEA levels are poor screening tools for cancer for the general population because measurable levels of CEA are only present with advanced disease. In addition, false–positive results (prediction of cancer when it is not present) frequently occur.

Treatment

- Preventive measures are important and include dietary education on increasing roughage, fruits, vegetables, and grains to increase bulk, decrease fat, and provide protective antioxidants.
- Staging of the disease based on dissemination of tumor cells to regional lymph nodes is important in determining the prognosis and treatment of the disease. Identification of even micrometastases can influence outcome.
- If colorectal cancer is present, surgery is required with or without follow-up chemotherapy and/or radiation.

 PEDIATRIC CONSIDERATIONS

- Most people who develop anorexia nervosa are adolescent or postadolescent females, frequently perfectionists for whom being thin is a sign of success or athletes who may believe that their performance depends on a level of thinness only possible by the strict avoidance of food. Although less common, young men may also develop anorexia nervosa. In young men, the condition may be associated with depression or concerns about sexual orientation. Some male athletes who participate in sports with strict weight categories, such as wrestling, may also develop anorexia nervosa. Anyone who has anorexia nervosa needs intense and prolonged therapy to overcome the condition.
- Infants and children are especially susceptible to the severe effects of diarrhea and should be monitored closely for early signs of dehydration. In developing countries, diarrhea from infectious disease, especially cholera, is the number one cause of infant and early childhood death. Any child who has moderate or severe diarrhea should receive fluid replacement with osmotically balanced products.
- Rotavirus is a major cause of diarrhea in the United States, affecting about 3 million infants and young children annually.
- The peak age of incidence of appendicitis in children is between ages 10 and 12. In children, especially infants and toddlers, appendicitis is often misdiagnosed, with a perforation incidence greater than 90% in children less than 3 years of age.

GERIATRIC CONSIDERATIONS

- Slowed peristalsis, which is a normal part of the aging process, in combination with decreased physical activity can increase the risk for chronic constipation in the older adult.

- Colorectal cancer usually occurs in the elderly. Recommendations for digital examination and tests for occult blood in the stool usually begin after the age of 40, and visualization of the rectum and colon is recommended after the age of 50. Individuals who have a first-degree relative with colon cancer are advised to undergo colonoscopy before the age of 50.

SELECTED BIBLIOGRAPHY

Avunduk, C. (2008). *Manual of gastroenterology* (4th ed.). Philadelphia, PA: Lippincott Williams & Wilkins.

Garber, B. (2009). Peptic ulcer disease: What you need to know. *Clinician Review,* 19(2), 28–31.

Guyton, A. C., & Hall, J. (2006). *Textbook of medical physiology* (11th ed.). Philadelphia, PA: W.B. Saunders.

Hedden, A. Z. (2008). *E coli* O 157:H7 infection. *Advance for Nurse Practitioners,* 16(10), 69–72.

Holcomb, S. S. (2008). Colorectal cancer: New screening guideline. *The Nurse Practitioner,* 33(9), 13–15, 17–19.

Levin, B., Lieberman, D. A., McFarland, B., Smith, R. A., Brooks, D., Andrews, K. S., et al. (2008). Screening and surveillance for the early detection of colorectal cancer and adenomatous polyps, 2008: A joint guideline from the American Cancer Society, the US Multi-Society Task Force on Colorectal Cancer, and the American College of Radiology. *CA Cancer Journal of Clinicians,* 58, 130–160 or available at http://caonline.amcancersoc.org/cgi/content/full/58/3/130, accessed September 5, 2009.

Otto, B., Spranger, J., Benoit, S. C., Clegg, D. J., & Tschöp, M. H. (2005). The many faces of ghrelin: New perspectives for nutrition research? *British Journal of Nutrition,* 93, 765–771.

Peters, D. P. (2008). Colon cancer screening: Recommendations and barriers to patient participation. *The Nurse Practitioner,* 33(12), 14–20.

Porth, C. M., & Matfin, G. (2009). *Pathophysiology: Concepts of altered health states* (8th ed.). Philadelphia, PA: Lippincott Williams & Wilkins.

Pregerson, D. B. (2008). Colonoscopy: A guide to endoscopic screening and therapy. *Consultant,* 48(10), 763–766, 768–771.

Rizzo, M. (2008). Suboptimal vitamin D status common in patients with inflammatory bowel disease. *American Journal of Gastroenterology,* 103, 1451–1459.

Sandborn, W. J. (2005). New concepts in anti-tumor necrosis factor therapy for inflammatory bowel disease. *Review of Gastroenterological Disorders,* 5, 10–18.

Sherman, C. (2009). Colorectal cancer: Prevention vs. detection. *The Clinical Advisor,* 37–39, 43.

Zimmerman, P. G. (2008). Is it appendicitis? *American Journal of Nursing,* 108(9), 27–31.

Zitkus, B. S. (2009). Evaluation of the acute abdomen: Key issues in primary care settings. *Advance for Nurse Practitioners,* 17(2), 28–33.

16

The Pancreas and Diabetes Mellitus

The pancreas is a large, diffuse abdominal organ that functions as both an exocrine and an endocrine gland. Endocrine functions include the production and release of insulin, glucagon, and somatostatin. The secretion of digestive juices into the digestive tract is part of the exocrine function. In this chapter, both roles are presented, followed by a detailed description of diabetes mellitus, a condition in which the pancreatic hormone, insulin, is either ineffective or absent. Pancreatitis and pancreatic cancer are discussed briefly.

● Physiologic Concepts

EXOCRINE FUNCTIONS OF THE PANCREAS

The exocrine functions of the pancreas involve the synthesis and release of digestive enzymes and sodium bicarbonate from specialized cells of the pancreas called acini cells. The acini cells release their contents into the pancreatic duct. From the pancreatic duct, the enzymes and bicarbonate solution travel through the sphincter of Oddi into the first section of the small intestine, the duodenum. The pancreatic enzymes and bicarbonate solution both play important roles in the digestion and absorption of food in the small intestine.

Secretion of Pancreatic Enzymes

The secretion of the various pancreatic enzymes occurs primarily as a result of stimulation of the pancreas by cholecystokinin (CCK), a hormone released from the small intestine. The stimulus for the release of CCK is the presence of a mixture of food particles entering the duodenum from the stomach. This food mixture coming from the stomach is called **chyme.** The pancreatic enzymes are secreted as inactive proenzymes that are activated when they reach the duodenum. The activated enzymes include:

- trypsin, which is responsible for the digestion of proteins to amino acids
- amylase, which is responsible for the digestion of carbohydrates to simple sugars
- lipase, which is responsible for the digestion of fats to free fatty acids and monoglycerides

Secretion of Sodium Bicarbonate

Sodium bicarbonate is secreted from pancreatic ductal cells in response to a second small-intestine hormone, secretin. Secretin is released in response to the acidic chyme entering from the stomach. When delivered to the small intestine, sodium bicarbonate, which is a base, neutralizes acidic chyme. This function is essential because the digestive enzymes are inactivated in an acidic environment. Neutralization of the acid in the duodenum also protects this area against acid injury to the mucosal wall and subsequent development of ulcer.

ENDOCRINE FUNCTIONS OF THE PANCREAS

The endocrine functions of the pancreas involve the synthesis and release of the hormones insulin, glucagon, and somatostatin. These hormones are each produced by separate, specialized cells of the pancreas, called the **islets of Langerhans**.

Synthesis and Secretion of Insulin

The synthesis of insulin in the pancreas comes from the enzymatic cleavage of the molecule proinsulin, which itself is the cleavage product of an even larger preproinsulin molecule. Proinsulin is composed of an A peptide fragment connected to a B peptide fragment by a C peptide fragment and two disulfide bonds (Fig. 16-1). Enzymatic cleavage of the C peptide connections leaves the A and the B peptides connected to each other only through the two disulfide bonds. In this form, insulin circulates unbound in the plasma.

Insulin is released at a basal rate by the *beta cells* of the islets of Langerhans. A rise in blood glucose is the primary stimulus to increase insulin release above the baseline. Fasting blood glucose level is normally 80 to 90 mg/100 mL of blood. When blood glucose increases to more than 100 mg/100 mL of blood, insulin secretion from the pancreas increases rapidly and then returns to baseline in 2 to 3 hours. Insulin is the main hormone of the **absorptive stage** of digestion that occurs immediately after a meal. Insulin levels are low between meals.

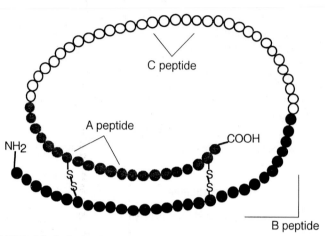

FIGURE 16-1 Proinsulin molecule.

Insulin circulates in the plasma and acts by binding to insulin receptors present in most cells of the body. Once bound, insulin works through a protein kinase messenger system to cause an increase in the number of glucose-transporter molecules present on the outside of the cell membrane. The glucose-transporter molecules, called glut-4 glucose transporters, are necessary for the facilitated diffusion of glucose into most cells. Once transported inside the cells, glucose can be used for immediate energy production through the Krebs cycle or it can be stored in the cell as glycogen, a glucose polymer, which is the storage form of glucose. When glucose is carried into the cell, it results in decreased blood levels of glucose, reducing further stimulation of insulin release. This cycle is an example of negative feedback, as shown in Figure 16-2.

Insulin release is also stimulated by amino acids and the digestive hormones (i.e., CCK, secretin, and glucose-dependent insulinotropic polypeptide [GIP]; see Chapter 15). The autonomic nervous system also stimulates insulin release by means of parasympathetic nerves to the pancreas. Both the release of GIP and the activation of the autonomic nervous system occur when one starts eating, resulting in a release of insulin at the beginning of a meal, even before glucose is absorbed. Sympathetic stimulation of the pancreas decreases insulin release.

Insulin is the major anabolic (building) hormone of the body and has a variety of other effects besides stimulating glucose transport. It also increases amino acid transport into cells, stimulates protein synthesis, and inhibits the breakdown of fat, protein, and glycogen stores. Insulin also inhibits **gluconeogenesis**, the synthesis of a new form of glucose, by the liver. In summary,

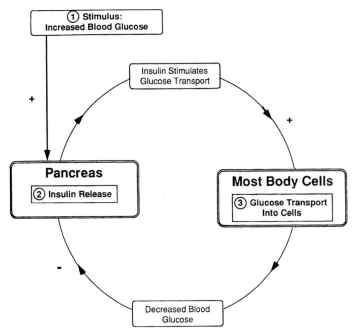

FIGURE 16-2 Feedback cycle demonstrating the effect of decreased blood glucose on insulin release.

insulin serves to provide glucose to our cells, build protein, and maintain low plasma glucose levels.

The Brain, Glucose, and Insulin

Unlike most other cells, brain cells do not require insulin for glucose entry. Also unlike other cells that may use free fatty acids or amino acids for energy, brain cells must use only glucose or glycogen to meet their energy demands and drive their cellular functions. In other words, brain cells are obligate users of glucose and glycogen. This means that gluconeogenesis by the liver is important; if glucose were not produced between meals by the liver, the brain would have no usable energy source during that time.

Secretion of Glucagon

Glucagon is a protein hormone released from the *alpha cells* of the islets of Langerhans in response to *low* blood glucose levels and increased plasma amino acids. Glucagon is primarily a hormone of the **postabsorptive stage** of digestion that occurs during fasting periods in between meals. Its functions are mainly catabolic (breaking down). In most respects, the functions of glucagon are opposite to that of insulin. For example, glucagon acts as an insulin antagonist by inhibiting glucose movement into cells. Glucagon also stimulates liver gluconeogenesis and causes the breakdown of stored glycogen to be used as an energy source instead of glucose. Glucagon stimulates the breakdown of fats and the release of free fatty acids into the bloodstream so they may be used as an energy source instead of glucose. These functions serve to increase blood glucose levels. The release of glucagon by the pancreas is stimulated by sympathetic nerves.

Secretion of Somatostatin

Somatostatin is secreted by *delta cells* of the islets of Langerhans. Somatostatin is also called growth hormone–inhibiting hormone and is released by the hypothalamus as well. Somatostatin from the hypothalamus inhibits the release of growth hormone from the anterior pituitary. Somatostatin from the pancreas appears to have a minimal effect on the release of growth hormone from the pituitary. It rather controls metabolism by inhibiting the secretion of insulin and glucagon. The exact function of somatostatin is otherwise unclear.

Counter-Regulatory Hormones

Glucose levels may also be affected by catecholamines, growth hormone, or glucocorticoid. These are known as counter-regulatory hormones and they facilitate glucose regulation when glucose intake is decreased or glucose stores are depleted. Table 16-1 includes a brief description of each.

TESTS OF PANCREATIC FUNCTION
Fasting Plasma Glucose

Plasma glucose levels provide instantaneous data about the glucose level at that moment. Measurement of plasma glucose above 126 mg/100 mL (corresponding to fasting blood glucose of 110 mg/100 mL) on more than one occasion is diagnostic of diabetes mellitus. Plasma glucose levels greater than 110 mg/100 mL indicate insulin resistance. Nonfasting plasma glucose level greater than 200 mg/100 mL with symptoms of polyurea, polydipsia, and polyphagia is also diagnostic of diabetes.

Urine Glucose Tests

Glucose in the urine may or may not be indicative of diabetes. Likewise, the absence of glucose in the urine cannot be used to discount diabetes. Under most conditions, however, glucose is not present in the urine of healthy, nonpregnant individuals and further assessment is necessary when it is present.

TABLE 16-1	Counter-Regulatory Hormones
Hormone	**Description**
Epinephrine	• Released from adrenal medulla during stressful periods
	• Causes glycogenolysis in the liver
	• Inhibits insulin release from beta cells
	• Increases breakdown of muscle glycogen stores which in turn frees up glucose to be used by other organs
	• Lipolytic effect on adipose cells which mobilizes fatty acids for energy use
	• Facilitates homeostasis during a hypoglycemic episode
Growth hormone	• Increases protein synthesis
	• Mobilizes fatty acids from adipose tissue
	• Decreases cellular uptake and use of insulin
	• Antagonizes effects of insulin
	• Decreases peripheral use of glucose
Glucocorticoid hormones	• Essential for survival during starvation
	• Stimulate gluconeogenesis by the liver
	• Moderately decrease tissue use of glucose

Glycosylated Hemoglobin

Throughout the 120-day life span of the red blood cell, hemoglobin slowly and irreversibly becomes glycosylated (glucose bound). Normally, approximately 4% to 6% of red blood cell hemoglobin is glycosylated. If there is chronic hyperglycemia, the level of glycosylated hemoglobin increases. Patients with poorly controlled diabetes show the highest level of glycosylated hemoglobin, which may be greater than 10%. The particular hemoglobin most often measured and reported is glycohemoglobin A1c (HbA1c). Measurement of HbA1c is important because it offers an indication of how well controlled the blood glucose has been over the previous 2 to 4 months.

1,5-Anhydroglucitol (1,5-AG)

A relatively new measurement offers hope for improving therapeutic management of glucose control. 1,5-AG offers information about glucose control over days to weeks as opposed to the 2 to 4 month period of HbA1C.

Serum Amylase and Lipase

Amylase is a pancreatic enzyme. Its increased concentration in the serum suggests pancreatic acinar damage and pancreatic destruction. Lipase is a digestive enzyme secreted solely by the pancreas and elevated serum levels indicate damage to pancreatic acinar cells.

● Pathophysiologic Concepts

HYPOGLYCEMIA

Hypoglycemia occurs when the blood glucose level falls below 50 mg/100 mL of blood. Hypoglycemia is caused by an imbalance between glucose production and utilization. It can be caused by fasting or, especially, fasting coupled with exercise, because exercise increases the usage of glucose by skeletal muscle. Most commonly, hypoglycemia is caused by an insulin overdose in an insulin-dependent diabetic.

The brain relies on glucose as its main energy source and because it cannot synthesize or store glucose, it is dependent on circulating blood glucose to maintain normal functioning. Hypoglycemia results in many symptoms of altered central nervous system (CNS) functioning, including confusion, irritability, seizure, and coma. Hypoglycemia can cause headache, as a result of alteration of cerebral blood flow, and changes in water balance. Systemically, hypoglycemia causes activation of the sympathetic nervous system, stimulating hunger, nervousness, sweating, and tachycardia. Anxiety levels increase due to the diabetic being shaky and agitated.

HYPERGLYCEMIA

Hyperglycemia is defined as a condition when plasma glucose level is higher than the normal (fasting range of 126 mg/100 mL of blood). Hyperglycemia is usually caused by insulin deficiency, as seen in type 1 diabetes, or as a result of decreased cellular responsiveness to insulin, as seen in type 2 diabetes (the types of diabetes are discussed in the following section). Hypercortisolemia, which occurs in Cushing syndrome and in response to chronic stress, can cause hyperglycemia by the stimulation of liver gluconeogenesis. Acute conditions of elevated thyroid hormone, prolactin, and growth hormone all increase blood glucose as well. Prolonged high levels of these hormones, especially growth hormone, are considered diabetogenic (producing diabetes) because they overstimulate insulin release by beta cells of the pancreas, leading to an eventual decrease in the cellular response to insulin. Sympathetic nervous stimulation and epinephrine released from the adrenal gland also raise plasma glucose levels, especially during periods of stress. The catecholamines epinephrine and norepinephrine inhibit insulin secretion, increase the breakdown of stored fats, and promote the use of glycogen for energy. By these mechanisms, the catecholamines make a variety of alternative energy sources available for the body to use instead of glucose, thereby raising plasma glucose levels and increasing its availability for use by the brain.

● Conditions of Disease or Injury

DIABETES MELLITUS

Diabetes is a Greek word that means "to siphon or pass through." Mellitus is a Latin word meaning honey or sweet. The disease diabetes mellitus is one in which an individual siphons large volumes of urine with a high glucose level. It is a disease of hyperglycemia characterized by the absolute lack of insulin or a relative lack of cellular insensitivity to insulin. Based on recent epidemiological evidence, the number of people afflicted with diabetes around the globe, currently nearly 200 million, is expected to increase to over 330 million by the year 2025. Reasons for the increase include longer life expectancy and higher population growth coupled with increased rates of obesity associated with urbanization and reliance on processed foods. In the United States, of the 18.2 million persons with diabetes (6.3% of the population), nearly one third are unaware that they have the disease. It is further projected that 57 million people in the United States have prediabetes.

Tests used to diagnose diabetes include the fasting plasma glucose (FPG) test and the oral glucose tolerance test (OGTT). The American Diabetes Association recommends the FPG test because it is faster, easier to perform, and less expensive than the OGTT. An FPG level between 100 and 125 mg/dL is indicative of prediabetes, and an FPG level of 126 mg/dL or more is considered as frank diabetes. For the OGTT, a person's blood glucose is measured after a fast and 2 hours after drinking a glucose-rich beverage. A 2-hour OGTT between 140 and 199 mg/dL indicates prediabetes; a level of 200 mg/dL or higher indicates diabetes. Providing a range of values indicative of prediabetes allows for earlier intervention in patients at risk of developing frank diabetes. Early intervention is extremely important because, at the time of diagnosis of type 2 diabetes, 20% of patients already have retinal damage, 8% have renal dysfunction, and 9% have neurologic symptoms. Even if the FPG is within normal limits, an OGTT should be conducted if the individual has risk factors for prediabetes. Box 16-1 includes risk factors identified by the American Diabetes Association.

Types of Diabetes Mellitus

In 2007, the American Diabetes Association updated the classification of diabetes and abnormal glucose tolerance to include five types of diabetes. The new criteria are based on the etiology of the disease rather than the presentation. The five types include type 1, type 2, gestational diabetes, other types of diabetes, and prediabetes (Table 16-2). Types 1, 2, and gestational diabetes are discussed in the following sections. Other specific types of diabetes include those due to pancreatic trauma, neoplasm, or diseases characterized by other endocrine disorders, for example, Cushing disease (see Chapter 9).

B O X 1 6 - 1 Risk Factors for Prediabetes and Diabetes in Asymptomatic Individuals

- Body mass index (BMI) $\geq$ 25 kg/m^2 in adults
- Sedentary lifestyle
- Blood pressure $\geq$ 140/90 mm Hg or currently taking antihypertensives
- First-degree relative with diabetes
- HDL < 36 mg/dL or triglycerides > 250 mg/dL
- Females with a history of polycystic ovarian syndrome, giving birth to an infant > 9 lb, or gestational diabetes mellitus
- Previous impaired fasting glucose (IFG) or impaired glucose tolerance (IGT) tests
- Clinical findings consistent with insulin resistance such as *Acanthosis nigricans* or skin tags
- African-American, American Indian, Asian American, Pacific Islander, or Hispanic
- History of cardiovascular disease or other factors specific to cardiovascular risk

TABLE 16-2 Diabetes Mellitus: A Classification Scheme

Type	Characteristics	Etiology	Treatment
Type 1	Absolute lack of insulin	Autoimmune	Insulin
Type 2	Insulin insensitivity and insulin-secreting deficiency	Obesity, genetics	Diet, exercise, hypoglycemic agents, transporter-stimulating drugs
Gestational	First diagnosed during pregnancy	Increased metabolic demands, family history of diabetes, decreased insulin sensitivity	Diet, hypoglycemic agents, insulin
Other types	Other specific cause	Dependent on specific cause	Dependent on cause
Prediabetes	Above normal FPG or OGTT, but not abnormal enough to meet criteria for diabetes	Insulin resistance	Regular monitoring

Latent autoimmune diabetes of adulthood (LADA) is a type of diabetes that is frequently misdiagnosed because it has characteristics of both type 1 and type 2. The body mistakenly responds to insulin-producing beta cells of the pancreas as it does to foreign cells. This mistaken identity causes the body to attack and destroy the beta cells. They typically present with an insidious onset of hyperglycemia and no evidence of insulin resistance. Because beta cell destruction is fairly slow, the need for insulin occurs much later than with type 1 diabetes, but sooner than with type 2 diabetes.

Type 1 Diabetes Mellitus

Hyperglycemia caused by an absolute lack of insulin is known as type 1 diabetes mellitus. Previously, this type of diabetes has been referred to as insulin-dependent diabetes mellitus (IDDM) because individuals who have this disease must receive insulin replacement. Type 1 diabetes is most commonly seen in nonobese individuals less than 30 years old and occurs in a slightly higher proportion of males than females. Because the incidence of type 1 diabetes peaks in the early teens, in the past it was referred to as juvenile diabetes. However, type 1 diabetes mellitus can occur at any age. See page C13 for illustrations and further explanation.

Causes of Type 1 Diabetes.

Type 1 diabetes results from autoimmune destruction of the beta cells of the islets of Langerhans. It appears that individuals who have a genetic tendency to develop this disease experience an environmental trigger that initiates the autoimmune process. Examples of possible triggers include viral infections such as mumps, rubella, or chronic cytomegalovirus (CMV). It also has been suggested that exposure to certain drugs or toxins may trigger an attack. Because type 1 diabetes develops over several years, there is often no clear stimulating event. Antibodies to islets of Langerhans cells are present in most individuals at the time of diagnosis of type 1 diabetes.

Why an individual develops antibodies against the islet of Langerhans cells in response to a triggering event is unknown. One mechanism may be that the environmental agent antigenically changes the cells such that they stimulate the production of autoantibodies. It is also possible that individuals who develop type 1 diabetes mellitus share antigenic similarities between their pancreatic beta cells and certain triggering microorganisms or drugs. In the course of responding to a virus or drug, the immune system may fail to distinguish the pancreatic cells as self.

Genetic Tendency for Type 1 Diabetes Mellitus.

There appears to be a genetic tendency for individuals to develop type 1 diabetes mellitus. Certain individuals appear to have diabetogenic genes, meaning a genetic profile that predisposes them to type 1 diabetes (or possibly any autoimmune disease). Genetic loci that pass an inherited tendency for type

1 diabetes are part of the histocompatibility complex genes (see Chapter 4). The histocompatibility complex controls the recognition of self-antigens by the immune system; loss of self-tolerance is core to developing autoantibodies. The histocompatibility genes are primarily coded on chromosome 6. Another specific insulin-related gene on chromosome 11 has been implicated in the development of type 1 diabetes through its effects on beta cell development and replication. Siblings of individuals who have type 1 diabetes and children of a parent who has type 1 diabetes have an increased risk of developing the disease compared with those without an affected first-degree relative. In clinical studies, nonsymptomatic siblings show a higher incidence (2% to 4%) of antibodies against pancreatic beta cells compared to those who do not have a first-degree relative with diabetes; the earlier the onset of antibodies and the higher the level, the greater the likelihood of those siblings developing the disease later in life.

Characteristics of Type 1 Diabetes.

Individuals who have type 1 diabetes show normal glucose handling before disease onset. In the past, it was thought that type 1 disease developed suddenly and with little warning. Currently, however, it is thought that type 1 diabetes usually develops slowly over the course of many years, with the presence of autoantibodies against the beta cells and their steady destruction occurring well in advance of diagnosis.

By the time type 1 diabetes is diagnosed, there is usually little or no insulin being secreted from the pancreas, and more than 80% of the pancreatic beta cells have been destroyed. Blood glucose levels increase because glucose cannot enter most cells of the body without insulin. At the same time, the liver begins to undertake gluconeogenesis (new glucose synthesis) using the available substrates of amino acids, fatty acids, and glycogen. These substrates are present in high concentrations in the circulation because the catabolic action of glucagon is unopposed by insulin. This results in functional cell starvation in the face of high glucose levels. Only the brain and red blood cells are spared glucose deprivation because they do not require insulin for glucose entry.

All other cells switch to the use of free fatty acids for energy. Metabolism of free fatty acids in the Krebs cycle (see Chapter 1) supplies cells with the adenosine triphosphate (ATP) necessary to run cell functions. Extensive reliance on fatty acids for energy production increases production of various ketones by the liver. Ketones are acids, which cause plasma pH to decrease.

Type 2 Diabetes Mellitus

Hyperglycemia caused by cellular insensitivity to insulin is called type 2 diabetes mellitus. In addition, there is a corresponding insulin secretory defect that results in the pancreas being incapable of secreting enough insulin to maintain normal level of plasma glucose. Although insulin levels may be only slightly reduced or even be within the normal range, they are inappropriately low, considering the elevated level of plasma glucose. Because insulin is still produced by the pancreatic beta cells, type 2 diabetes mellitus was previously called non–insulin-dependent diabetes mellitus (NIDDM), a misnomer because many individuals who have type 2 diabetes are treated with insulin. In type 2 diabetes mellitus, women are overrepresented compared to men. A strong genetic predisposition and obvious environmental factors contribute to the development of type 2 diabetes. See page C14 for illustrations and further explanation.

Causes of Type 2 Diabetes.

For most individuals, the number one risk factor for type 2 diabetes mellitus is obesity. In addition, the genetic tendency to develop the disease is strong. It is possible that an unidentified genetic trait causes the pancreas to secrete altered insulin or causes the insulin receptors or second messengers to fail to respond to insulin adequately. It is also possible that a genetic link is associated with obesity and prolonged stimulation of the insulin receptors. Prolonged stimulation of receptors may lead to a decrease in the number of receptors for insulin present on body cells. This decrease is called **downregulation**. It is also possible that individuals who develop type 2 diabetes produce insulin autoantibodies that bind to the insulin receptor, blocking insulin's access to the receptor, but do not stimulate carrier activity. Other studies suggest that a deficit in the hormone leptin, due to a lack of the leptin-producing gene or its dysfunction, may be responsible for type 2 diabetes in some individuals. Without the leptin gene, sometimes called the obesity gene, animals, perhaps including humans, fail to respond to satiety cues, and thus are more likely to become obese and develop insulin insensitivity.

Although obesity is the main risk factor for type 2 diabetes, there are certain individuals who develop type 2 diabetes at a young age and who are thin or of normal weight. One example of this type of disease is maturity-onset diabetes of the young (MODY), an autosomal dominant condition related to a genetic defect in the pancreatic beta cell such that it is unable to produce insulin. In this circumstance and a few others, there appears to be an even stronger genetic link than in most types of type 2 diabetes.

Characteristics of Type 2 Diabetes.

An individual with type 2 diabetes still secretes insulin. However, there is often a delay in the initial secretion and a reduction in the total amount released. This trend worsens as a person ages. In addition, the cells of the body, especially muscle and adipose cells, show a resistance to the insulin that does circulate. As a result, the glucose carrier (the glut-4 glucose transporter) is inadequately present on cells, and glucose is not available for cells to use. As cells are starved for glucose, the liver initiates gluconeogenesis, further increasing blood glucose levels as well as stimulating the breakdown of triglyceride, protein, and glycogen stores to provide alternative sources of fuel, raising the levels of these substances in the blood. Only the brain and red blood cells continue to use glucose as an effective energy source. Because there is usually some insulin, however, individuals who have type 2 diabetes seldom rely totally on fatty acids for energy production and so are not prone to ketosis.

Gestational Diabetes

Gestational diabetes is defined as diabetes that occurs in a previously nondiabetic pregnant woman. Risk factors include marked obesity, personal history of gestational diabetes, glycosuria and a family history of diabetes. Although this type of diabetes often resolves after delivery, approximately 50% of affected women will not revert to the nondiabetic state after the pregnancy is over. Even in those who do, the risk of developing type 2 diabetes after about 5 years is higher than normal.

Causes of Gestational Diabetes.
The increased energy demands during pregnancy and the continually high levels of estrogen and growth hormone are believed to be the causes of gestational diabetes. Growth hormone and estrogen stimulate insulin release and may result in an oversecretion of insulin, leading to decreased cellular responsiveness. Growth hormone also has some anti-insulin effects, for example, the stimulation of glycogenolysis, the breakdown of glycogen, and the breakdown of adipose tissue. Adinonectin, a plasma protein derived from adipose tissue, plays a role in regulating insulin concentration and resistance; reduced levels of this substance may also contribute to the impaired glucose metabolism and hyperglycemia seen in gestational diabetes. Women who develop gestational diabetes may have subclinical problems with glucose control even before diabetes develops.

Consequences of Gestational Diabetes.
Gestational diabetes can negatively affect the pregnancy by increasing the risk of congenital malformations, stillbirths, and large-for-date babies, which can result in problems during delivery. Gestational diabetes is routinely tested for during prenatal medical examinations. Good obstetrical outcomes are dependent on good maternal glycemic control as well as prepregnancy weight. Women who have gestational diabetes usually are treated with diet, insulin, or both, as necessary. The use of oral antihyperglycemic agents such as sulfonylurea (glyburide) instead of insulin for pregnant women unable to achieve glycemic control with diet alone has been investigated. Findings suggest glyburide may be as effective as insulin in reducing obstetric complications, without increasing the risk of congenital malformations, although further studies are required to ensure the safety of this or other agents.

The Role of Glucagon in Diabetes Mellitus

Glucagon appears to have a role in the development of diabetes mellitus. Although glucagon is not considered a cause of diabetes mellitus, slightly elevated or normal glucagon levels in the face of high blood glucose and fatty acids suggest that the regulation of glucagon release is amiss. The presence and catabolic effects of glucagon, and its stimulation of gluconeogenesis when blood glucose is already high, offer an interesting focus for research on the cause of diabetes mellitus.

Clinical Manifestations

- Polyuria (increased urine output) as water follows glucose loss in the urine.
- Polydipsia (increased thirst) caused by the high urine volume and loss of water, leading to extracellular dehydration. Intracellular dehydration follows extracellular dehydration because intracellular water diffuses out of cells, down its concentration gradient, and into the hypertonic (highly concentrated) plasma. Intracellular dehydration stimulates antidiuretic hormone (ADH; vasopressin) release and causes thirst.
- Fatigue and muscle weakness caused by catabolism of muscle protein and the inability of most cells to use glucose for energy. Poor blood flow seen in long-term diabetics also contributes to fatigue.
- Polyphagia (increased hunger) caused by the chronic catabolism of fat and protein, and relative cellular starvation. Weight loss frequently occurs without treatment.
- Type 1 diabetics may present with nausea and severe vomiting.

Although both type 1 and 2 diabetics may show the clinical manifestations outlined above, and both types may develop the symptoms and complications listed below, individuals who have type 2 diabetes frequently present with one or more nonspecific symptoms, including:

- Increased rate of infections because of increased glucose concentration in mucus secretions, poor immune function, and reduced blood flow.
- Visual changes related to changes in water balance or, in more severe cases, retinal damage.
- Paresthesias, or abnormalities in sensation.
- Vaginal candidiasis (yeast infection), resulting from increased glucose levels in vaginal secretions and urine, and poor immune function. Candidiasis may lead to vaginal itching and discharge. Vaginal infections are a common condition presenting in women previously unsuspected of having diabetes.
- Muscle wasting may develop as muscle protein is broken down to meet the body's energy needs.

Diagnostic Tools

- In most cases, the suspicion of type 1 diabetes arises clearly with a history of polyuria, polydipsia, polyphagia, and weight loss. The individual may experience repeated vomiting and appear very sick. Type 1 disease is confirmed by plasma glucose testing.
- Suspicion and testing for type 2 diabetes may be delayed, because symptomology is often nonspecific. Type 2 diabetes is also confirmed by plasma glucose testing.

- Throughout pregnancy, women are tested for gestational diabetes by being screened for urine glucose, and at 28 weeks' gestation, their FPG or plasma glucose level after a glucose load (glucose tolerance test) is measured. Women who do not receive prenatal care will not be tested for gestational diabetes.

- Having an FPG level greater than 126 mg/100 mL on two separate occasions is diagnostic of diabetes mellitus. Fasting is defined as at least 8 hours without caloric intake. Fasting glucose is elevated because most cells cannot move glucose intracellularly without insulin, and gluconeogenesis is stimulated. Postprandial (after eating) glucose levels are elevated as well.

- Glucose present in the urine is suggestive of diabetes. Glucose handling in the kidney depends on carrier-mediated transport. As described in Chapter 18, glucose is freely filterable across the renal glomerular capillaries. In nondiabetics, all glucose that is filtered into the urine is actively transported back into the blood via stimulation of glucose carriers, resulting in a normal urine glucose of zero. When glucose levels are greater than approximately 180 mg/100 mL of blood, however, as can occur with moderate or severe diabetes mellitus, the renal carriers that move glucose out of the urine and back into the blood become saturated. This saturation means that they can carry no additional glucose and any excess is then lost in the urine (Fig. 16-3). Interestingly, long-term diabetics may have a slightly higher renal threshold for glucose excretion, as much as 200 mg/100 mL of blood, because the

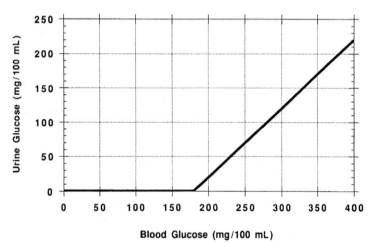

FIGURE 16-3 Urine glucose concentration as affected by blood glucose concentration. Note that no urine glucose is found until the blood glucose concentration exceeds a threshold value of 180 mg/10 mL.

tubules tend to adapt and reabsorb glucose more efficiently. Reabsorbing extra glucose, however, puts a strain on the kidneys. In addition, because glucose is osmotically active in the urine filtrate, water stays in the filtrate and is excreted in the urine with glucose, resulting in polyuria, a frequent symptom of diabetes. Although glucose in the urine is very common among diabetics, absence of urine glucose does not rule out diabetes.

- Ketones may be present in the urine. This is especially true for individuals who have poorly controlled type 1 diabetes.

- Elevated levels of glycosylated hemoglobin indicate poorly controlled diabetes. HbA1c levels maintained below 8% appear to be sufficient for the avoidance of most complications of diabetes. Levels less than 6% are considered in the normal range.

Acute Complications

- **Diabetic Ketoacidosis:** Almost always restricted to type 1 diabetics, diabetic ketoacidosis is an acute complication characterized by a worsening of all symptoms of diabetes. Diabetic ketoacidosis may occur after physical stress such as pregnancy or an acute illness or trauma. Sometimes it is the presenting symptom of type 1 diabetes.

   With diabetic ketoacidosis, blood glucose levels rise rapidly as a result of gluconeogenesis and a progressive increase in fat breakdown. Polyuria and dehydration follow. Ketone levels also rise (ketosis) as a result of the nearly total use of fatty acids to produce ATP. The ketones spill into the urine (ketonuria) and cause a recognizable fruity smell to the breath. With ketosis, pH decreases below 7.3. The low pH results in metabolic acidosis and stimulates hyperventilation, called Kussmaul respiration, as the individual attempts to compensate for the acidosis by blowing off carbon dioxide (a volatile acid).

   A person with diabetic ketoacidosis frequently experiences nausea and abdominal pain. Vomiting may occur and may contribute to the extracellular and intracellular dehydration. Total body levels of potassium fall as a result of prolonged polyuria and vomiting.

   Diabetic ketoacidosis is life threatening and is treated by hospitalization and the correction of fluid and electrolyte balances. Administration of insulin is required for reversal of the hyperglycemia. Because insulin sensitivity increases with decreasing pH, the dose and rate of administration of insulin must be carefully monitored. Studies have shown that the fast-acting insulin analog called lispro (Humalog) is an effective and less costly treatment for diabetic ketoacidosis compared to other types of insulin.

- **Hyperosmolar Hyperglycemic Nonketotic Coma:** Also called hyperosmolar nonacidotic diabetes, hyperosmolar hyperglycemic nonketotic coma is an acute complication seen in individuals with type 2 diabetes. This condition indicates a worsening of disease. Although not ketosis prone, type 2 diabetics may develop severe hyperglycemia, with blood glucose levels well in excess of over 300 mg/100 mL. This level of hyperglycemia causes plasma osmolality, normally tightly controlled at 275 to 295 mOsm/L, to increase to more than 310 mOsm/L. As a result, liters of urine are lost, resulting in massive thirst, severe potassium deficit, and, in approximately 15% to 20% of patients, coma and death. Treatment is geared toward fluid and electrolyte replacement. Hyperosmolar hyperglycemic nonketotic coma is usually seen in elderly diabetics after consumption of a high-carbohydrate meal.

- **Somogyi Effect:** The Somogyi effect is an acute complication characterized by a fall in blood glucose levels during the night, followed by a rebound increase in the morning. The cause of the nighttime hypoglycemia is most likely related to the evening insulin injection. The resulting hypoglycemia in turn causes a reflex increase in glucagon, catecholamines, cortisol, and growth hormone. These hormones stimulate gluconeogenesis, leading to the morning hyperglycemia. Treatment of the Somogyi effect is aimed at manipulation of the evening insulin injection so as not to initiate hypoglycemia. Dietary interventions can also reduce the Somogyi effect. The Somogyi effect is most common in children.

- **Dawn Phenomenon:** Dawn phenomenon is an early-morning (between 5 and 9 AM) hyperglycemia that results from a circadian increase in glucose levels in the morning. It can be seen in type 1 or 2 diabetics. Hormones that show circadian variation in the morning include cortisol and growth hormone, both of which stimulate gluconeogenesis. In type 2 diabetics, a decrease in insulin sensitivity might also occur in the morning, either as a normal circadian variation of its own or in response to the circadian increases in growth hormone and cortisol.

- **Hypoglycemia:** Type 1 diabetics may experience the complication of hypoglycemia after an insulin injection. Symptoms may be light-headedness or loss of consciousness. Coma may develop if hypoglycemia is severe. Tightly controlled type 1 patients, that is, patients who perform multiple insulin injections throughout the day and maintain HbA1c levels equal to or less than 7%, are at increased risk of experiencing hypoglycemic events. For some, the benefits of excellent HbA1c levels must be balanced by the risks of hypoglycemia.

Long-Term Complications

Diabetes mellitus has many long-term complications. Most seem directly caused by high blood glucose concentration. All contribute to the morbidity and mortality of the disease. These complications affect almost all body organs.

- **Cardiovascular System:** Long-term diabetes mellitus has a severe effect on the cardiovascular system. Microvascular damage occurs to the small arterioles, the capillaries, and the venules. Macrovascular damage occurs to the large and medium arteries. All organs and tissues of the body suffer as a result of these microvascular and macrovascular injuries.

Microvascular complications arise from a thickening of the basement membrane of the small vessels. The cause of the thickening is unknown, but seems directly related to high blood glucose levels. Microvascular thickening leads to ischemia and a decreased passage of oxygen and nutrients to the tissues. In addition, glycosylated hemoglobin has an increased affinity for oxygen, resulting in the hemoglobin molecule binding more tightly to oxygen, making it less available to meet tissue needs. Acidosis causes a decrease in red blood cell 2, 3-diphosphoglycerate (2, 3-DPG), which also increases hemoglobin's affinity for oxygen, making it less likely that tissues will be adequately oxygenated.

The resulting chronic hypoxia can directly damage or destroy cells. Chronic hypoxia also can lead to the development of hypertension by causing the heart to increase its cardiac output in an attempt to deliver more oxygen to ischemic tissues. The kidneys, retina, and peripheral nervous system, including both somatic motor and sensory neurons and the peripheral autonomic nerves, are severely affected by diabetic microvascular disease. Poor microvascular circulation impairs the immune and the inflammatory reactions because these depend on good tissue perfusion for delivery of immune cells and inflammatory mediators.

Macrovascular complications primarily arise from the development of atherosclerosis (hardening of the arteries) and contribute to poor blood flow, long-term complications, and high mortality. Macrovascular damage can occur even without the presence of overt diabetes mellitus (plasma glucose levels less than 126 mg/100 mL).

Damage to the endothelial layer of the arteries occurs in diabetes and may result directly from the high circulating levels of blood glucose, a glucose metabolite, or high levels of circulating fatty acids commonly seen in individuals who have diabetes. With injury, endothelial cell permeability increases, and lipid-laden molecules enter the artery. Damage to the endothelial cells initiates an immune and inflammatory reaction, leading to the deposition of platelets, macrophages, and fibrous tissue. Smooth muscle cells proliferate. The thickened arterial wall leads to hypertension, which further damages the endothelial lining of the arteries by exerting increased shear forces on the cells. (Refer to Chapter 13 for a full discussion of atherosclerosis.) Vascular effects of long-term diabetes include coronary artery disease, stroke, and peripheral vascular disease. Diabetic patients who suffer a myocardial infarct have a poorer prognosis than nondiabetics who suffer an infarct. Coronary artery disease is a main cause of morbidity and mortality in the diabetic population.

Stroke, or a cerebral vascular accident, also is a common outcome of diabetes. This outcome is especially true for type 2 diabetes as a result of the combined risks of atherosclerosis of the cerebral vessels and hypertension, which weaken and may ultimately burst the vessels.

Peripheral vascular disease also occurs from severe atherosclerosis. It contributes to the amputations and erectile dysfunction often experienced by long-term diabetics.

- **Vision Loss:** A common long-term complication of diabetes is vision loss. The most serious threat to vision is retinopathy, or damage to the retina, resulting from the lack of oxygen. The retina is highly active metabolically, and with chronic hypoxia, it progressively demonstrates breakdown in capillary structure, microaneurysm formation, and spots of hemorrhage. Areas of infarcts (dead tissue) develop; neovascularization (new vessel formation) and sprouting of old vessels occur. Unfortunately, the new vessels and sproutings are thin walled and frequently hemorrhagic, leading to activation of the inflammatory system and scarring of the retina. Interstitial edema occurs and intraocular pressure rises, leading to the collapse of the capillaries and the remaining nerves, and blindness may ensue. Diabetes is the number one cause of blindness in the United States. It is also associated with frequent development of cataracts and glaucoma.

- **Renal Damage:** Long-term diabetes resulting in renal damage is extremely common, and diabetic nephropathy is the number one cause of kidney failure in the United States and in other Western nations. In the kidney, damage to the glomerular capillaries from hypertension and high plasma glucose causes thickening of the basement membrane and glomerular enlargement. Nodular, sclerotic lesions, called Kimmelstiel–Wilson nodules, develop among the glomeruli, blocking blood flow and further damaging the nephrons.

  With glomerular enlargement, patients who have diabetes, especially type 1, begin to spill protein into the urine. Although the initial amount of protein lost in the urine may be small (microproteinuria), the damage continues, and progresses in a positive-feedback cycle: protein leakage across the glomeruli further damages the nephron, leading to more protein leakage. Eventually, marked proteinuria develops. This occurrence is associated with a predictable decrease in kidney function and life expectancy.

  The loss of plasma proteins in the urine also causes a decrease in capillary osmotic pressure, leading to a decrease in the reabsorption of fluid from the interstitial space. With net filtration of plasma into the interstitial space, generalized edema, called **anasarca**, occurs. This leads to compression of small capillaries and nerves and to further tissue hypoxia and nerve damage throughout the body, including in the kidney. The kidneys begin to deteriorate rapidly, and fluid overload and severe hypertension develop. With kidney deterioration, the ability to secrete hydrogen ions into the urine decreases, causing metabolic acidosis. Decreased renal production of vitamin D leads to bone breakdown, and decreased renal production of erythropoietin leads to red blood cell deficiency and anemia. Glomerular filtration decreases progressively, and renal failure may develop. Diabetics account for over 30% of renal dialysis transplant patients in the United States. For a full description of renal failure, see Chapter 18.

- **Peripheral Nervous System:** Diabetes mellitus damages the peripheral nervous system, including sensory and motor components of both the somatic and autonomic divisions. Neural disease related to diabetes mellitus is called **diabetic neuropathy**. Diabetic neuropathy is caused by chronic hypoxia of the nerve cells as well as by the effects of hyperglycemia, including hyperglycosylation of proteins involved in neural function. It also appears that nerve support cells, in particular the Schwann cells, begin to use alternative methods to handle the chronically high glucose load, which eventually results in segmental demyelination of the peripheral nerves. Some components of diabetic neuropathy are reversible or preventable with good glucose control; others are not. This suggests that unknown mechanisms of injury in diabetes besides those related to high blood glucose also occur. A 7-year European Diabetes Prospective Complications Study reported neuropathy in 23.5% of patients with type 1 diabetes. The risk of neuropathy was positively correlated with the duration of diabetes and inversely with glycemic control. Increased body mass index and smoking were associated with increased rates of neuropathy as well.

  Demyelination causes slowing of nerve conduction and loss of feeling. Loss of temperature and pain sensation predisposes an individual to severe and often unnoticed injury. Such injuries, coupled with poor blood flow and an impaired immune system, are responsible for the fact that the number one cause of foot amputations in the United States, other than trauma, is diabetes mellitus.

  Damage to the peripheral autonomic nerves can lead to postural hypotension; changes in gastrointestinal function; impaired bladder emptying, with resultant urinary tract infection; and, in men, erectile dysfunction.

- **Autonomic Neuropathy** can cause gastrointestinal, genitourinary, and cardiovascular symptoms as well as sexual dysfunction.

- **Metabolic Syndrome:** Metabolic syndrome describes a combination of cardiovascular and metabolic characteristics often associated with type 2 diabetes and macro- and microvascular pathology. According to the World Health Organization (WHO), a diagnosis of the disorder is based on a combination of insulin resistance and two other factors that may include hypertension, high plasma triglycerides, low levels of HDL cholesterol, central (or apple-shaped) obesity, microalbuminuria, or high urinary albumin-to-creatinine ratio. From the year 2000 census, it is estimated that 47 million U.S. residents meet the criteria for metabolic syndrome. The consequences of the syndrome are severe and include atherosclerosis, cerebrovascular disease, myocardial infarction, renal failure, and other disorders related to vascular impairment.

- Gestational diabetes is associated with increased risks of congenital malformation and obstetrical complications.

Treatment

Figure 16-4 presents an overview of treatment for type 2 diabetes on the basis of recommendations of the American Diabetic Association.

- The most important goal of those who study or treat diabetes mellitus is prevention. Although there is no known mechanism to prevent type 1 diabetes, attempts are under way to identify individuals at high risk of developing type 1 diabetes (e.g., siblings of affected individuals) by monitoring for anti–beta-cell antibodies and to devise interventions. Different experimental protocols (e.g., providing insulin injections before the demonstration of any symptoms of type 1 with the expectation that antibody development against the beta cells may be prevented) are being tried with this population. For type 2 diabetes, prevention of obesity, especially childhood obesity, is imperative for reducing the incidence of the disease. For those who have gestational diabetes, early identification of risk factors and prompt dietary intervention or other treatments can minimize infant and maternal morbidity and mortality.

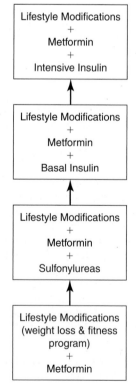

FIGURE 16-4 Treatment for type 2 diabetes.

- If diabetes mellitus does occur, the goal of treatment becomes consistent normalization of blood glucose levels with minimum day-to-day, hour-to-hour variability. Recent studies demonstrate that keeping blood glucose levels as normal as possible and as often as possible can successfully reduce the morbidity and mortality of diabetes mellitus. This goal is accomplished by different means, each suited precisely to the individual and the type of diabetes he or she has.

- **Insulin:** Type 1 diabetics require insulin therapy. Different types of insulin with different origins and purity are available. Today, human insulin is most commonly used and is associated with the fewest side effects and complications. Insulin preparations vary in terms of time to onset of action, peak time of action, and duration of action. Insulin injections are typically given subcutaneously one to four times a day after baseline blood glucose levels are measured. With studies showing the definite advantage of more frequent insulin injections, it is recommended that individuals test their plasma glucose levels frequently and use at least three to four injections per day. More frequent testing is required if there is a change in activity, during periods of growth, in pregnancy, or if an individual becomes ill.

  Other means of administration include subcutaneous insulin pumps that can be programmed to release a given amount of insulin at given times of the day. More or less than a usual amount of insulin may be programmed to be released if changes in routine (activity or diet) are planned or during times of illness. Insulin pumps have the advantage that injections need not be administered, which is an important consideration for all diabetics and especially children. Disadvantages of using the pump involve mistakes in programming, which can cause hypoglycemia or hyperglycemia, and pump failures, which can result in death. In addition, infection is a danger with the implant, especially given the poor blood flow and compromised immune system of most diabetics. In addition, the pumps are expensive.

- The first stage of treatment for type 2 diabetics is usually the improvement of insulin sensitivity and secretion by diet, weight loss, and exercise. Studies have shown that with the modification of diet and the initiation of an exercise program, many type 2 diabetics can normalize their blood sugar. If glucose normalization cannot be achieved by diet and exercise alone, or if patients cannot follow the regimen required, many type 2 diabetics benefit from oral hypoglycemic drugs. Table 16-3 includes a summary of the six oral medication classes approved for the treatment of type 2 diabetes. These drugs (e.g., biguanide, sulfonylurea) work by stimulating the beta cells of the pancreas to increase insulin secretion and/or by inhibiting hepatic gluconeogenesis. They also appear to increase the sensitivity of cells to insulin. For this type of drug to work, there must be some residual insulin secretion by the pancreas. Other drugs effective for type 2 diabetes work by stimulating the production of the glut-4 glucose transporters directly. By increasing the glucose transporters, these agents increase the cellular response to insulin. Specific oral hypoglycemic drugs

TABLE 16-3 Oral Medication Classes for the Treatment of Type 2 Diabetes

Medication Class	Mechanism of Action
Sulfonylureas	Binds with sulfonylurea receptor site causing closure of potassium channels and depolarization of cell membrane which opens calcium channels and stimulates insulin release from pancreatic beta cells
Meglitinides	Causes rapid secretion of insulin from pancreatic beta cells
Alpha-glucosidase inhibitors	Inhibits alpha-glucosidase, the enzyme necessary to break down carbohydrates, thereby delaying absorption of carbohydrates in the intestine and reducing the rise in blood sugar following a meal
Biguanides	Inhibits glucose production in the liver, decreases glucose absorption in the gut, and increases tissue response to insulin
Thiazolidinediones	Decreases insulin resistance thus increasing glucose uptake by the muscle, decreases glucose production by the liver
Dipeptidyl peptidase-4 (DPP-4) inhibitors	By inhibiting DPP-4, incretin activity is prolonged and enhanced which inhibits glucagon release, increases insulin secretion, and decreases gastric emptying

differ in time to onset of action, time to peak onset, and duration of action. Some are contraindicated in individuals who have renal disease. Often combinations of different types of drugs are more effective than a single drug alone.

- Type 2 diabetics, although considered non–insulin-dependent, also may benefit from insulin therapy. In type 2 diabetes, release of insulin may be deficient or the insulin produced may be subtly altered to be less effective than normal. In the latter case, exogenous insulin may be more effective than that which patients naturally produce. Some studies suggest that with provision of insulin exogenously, the course of type 2 diabetes may be slowed because of the elimination of stress on the pancreatic beta cells.

- **Dietary Plans:** Dietary regimens are individually calculated, depending on growth needs, weight-loss goals (usually for type 2 diabetics), and activity levels. Distribution of calories is generally 50% to 60% from complex carbohydrates, 20% from protein, and 30% from fat. Fiber, vitamins, and minerals are included. It is especially important for children who have type 1 diabetes to ingest adequate calories and minerals to ensure optimum growth.

- **Exercise:** An exercise program coupled with weight loss has been shown to increase insulin sensitivity and to reduce the need for pharmacologic intervention. For both types of diabetes, exercise has been demonstrated to increase cellular glucose utilization, thereby reducing blood glucose levels.

  Type 1 diabetics must be careful while exercising because the exercise-induced decrease in blood glucose may precipitate hypoglycemia. This is especially true if insulin administration is not matched to the exercise regimen.

- For diabetic ketoacidosis, the most important aspect of care is prevention. Prevention consists of careful monitoring of blood glucose levels and diet, especially in times of added stress or during a viral illness. If diabetic ketoacidosis occurs, it is treated with carefully administered insulin and interventions to balance fluid and electrolytes. Hospitalization is required.

- For hyperosmolar hyperglycemic nonketotic coma, care is centered upon fluid replacement and slow correction of potassium deficits. It can be prevented with good dietary control.

- **Other Pharmacologic Interventions:** Antihypertensive medications are among the pharmacologic interventions considered for all diabetics. For patients with diabetes, blood pressure recommendations are lower than that for the nondiabetic population, with systolic blood pressures above 115 mm Hg considered elevated. Antihypertensives, especially the angiotensin II–converting enzyme inhibitors (ACE inhibitors) or the angiotensin receptor blockers (ARBs), have been shown to reduce blood pressure in patients with diabetes and to delay the onset of renal disease. Even patients who do not have clinical hypertension or clinically obvious renal disease appear to develop less renal pathology when placed on ACE inhibitors. The addition of an ACE inhibitor should be considered in the care plan of all patients with diabetes. Although traditional beta blockers have been shown to worsen glycemic control, third-generation beta blockers added on top of an ACE inhibitor may prove beneficial for patients with refractory hypertension.

- Pancreatic transplantation has the potential to normalize glucose homeostasis. It also appears to reverse some of the established complications of diabetes, including improving diabetic neuropathy (but not diabetic retinopathy). Although clearly of benefit in normalizing plasma glucose levels, pancreatic transplantation carries with it the risks of surgery, the risks of rejection, and the necessity for lifelong immunosuppressive therapy.

- Advances in pancreatic islet cell replacement techniques have resulted in several thousand individuals worldwide being treated with islet cell transplantations. This treatment offers a significant hope for a diabetes cure in the future. At present, however, only 20% or so of patients become completely insulin-free, and immunosuppression is required. This approach is less invasive than total pancreatic transplantation.

- Experiments designed to allow for the insertion of the gene coding for insulin in individuals who have type 1 diabetes are under way. This procedure would offer a cure for diabetes rather than drug therapy.
- Eighty percent of obese patients who undergo bariatric (gastric bypass) surgery demonstrate a dramatic recovery from diabetes within days to weeks. The mechanism by which diabetes so rapidly remits is unclear, although it appears there is a significant improvement in insulin sensitivity that may be mediated by gut hormones. For example, glucagon-like peptide-1 (GLP-1), a hormone released from the small intestine in response to the rapid passage of food from the stomach, appears to increase insulin release and sensitivity; GLP-1 may be excessively stimulated after gastric bypass. Besides diabetes, 2-year rates of recovery from hypertriglyceridemia, low levels of high-density lipoprotein cholesterol, hypercholesterolemia, and hypertension were more favorable in patients who underwent gastric bypass surgery versus a comparable group who did not, although 10-year benefits were less clear. Gastric bypass surgery itself, however, carries significant risks, including bleeding, embolism, thrombosis, infection, and other complications. In addition, hypertrophy of pancreatic beta cells, a condition known as nesidioblastosis, may develop and result in serious postprandial hypoglycemia.

ACUTE PANCREATITIS

Acute pancreatitis is an inflammation of the pancreas characterized by autodigestion of the pancreas by pancreatic enzymes. Pancreatic cells are injured or killed, leading to areas of cell necrosis and hemorrhage. Stimulation of the immune and inflammatory systems contributes to the swelling and edema of the organ.

Causes of Pancreatitis

Gallstones and alcohol abuse are the leading causes of acute pancreatitis. Gallstones account for approximately 45% of cases, alcohol abuse accounts for 35%, 10% is idiopathic, and the remaining 10% is attributed to conditions such as hypercalcemia, infections, medications, toxins, trauma, or inflammatory disease. Chronic alcoholism is associated with pancreatitis, perhaps because of stimulation of pancreatic enzyme release or because of damage caused to the sphincter of Oddi at the opening of the small intestine from the common bile duct.

Pancreatitis may occur as a result of blockage of the pancreatic duct, usually caused by a gallstone in the common bile duct. Hyperlipidemia is a risk factor for the development of pancreatitis. Hyperlipidemia may overstimulate the release of pancreatic enzymes, or it may contribute to the development of gallstones.

Clinical Manifestations

- Pain, often in the epigastric area and radiating to the back, after a large meal or excess alcohol consumption is the usual presenting symptom. Pain is caused by the swelling and stretching of the pancreatic duct. Pain may be severe with sudden onset.
- Vomiting and nausea may accompany an attack of pancreatitis. The patient appears ill.
- Firm, distended, diffusely tender abdomen and possible rebound tenderness.
- If hemorrhage occurs, Cullen sign (bruising around umbilicus due to intraperitoneal bleeding) or Grey–Turner sign (flank bruising due to retroperitoneal bleeding).
- Tachycardia, tachypnea, hypertension secondary to pain or hypotension secondary to hypovolemic shock.
- Hyperglycemia.
- Decreased or absent bowel sounds.

Diagnostic Tools

- Blood analysis typically demonstrates elevated levels of serum amylase and lipase.
- Hyperglycemia and hyperlipidemia are common during an acute attack.
- Increased white blood cell count occurs with the inflammation and rises further with infection.
- Elevated C-reactive protein.
- Other diagnostic tests include abdominal CT, electrolytes, blood urea nitrogen, liver enzymes, serum albumin, bilirubin, coagulation panel, and arterial blood gases.

Complications

- Decreased blood pressure and cardiovascular shock may develop with a severe attack as a result of the systemic release of inflammatory mediators.
- A pancreatic abscess may occur if the pancreas becomes infected. Necrosis of the tissue may be widespread. Hemorrhage, circulatory collapse, and sepsis may follow.
- Fluid collection within or around the pancreas.
- Organ failure and metabolic abnormalities.

Treatment

- Withholding of food and fluids reduces pancreatic secretions.
- Fluids are given intravenously to maintain blood volume and pressure.

- Blood and/or albumin replacement may be necessary in some cases.
- Insulin to manage hyperglycemia.
- Narcotics, usually meperidine (Demerol), are administered to relieve pain. The use of Morphine is controversial because it may cause spasm of the sphincter of Oddi; however, it offers better pain control.
- Total parenteral nutrition may be used, but is not cost effective. Enteral feedings with a tube placed in the jejunum to avoid pancreatic enzyme stimulation may be necessary.

PANCREATIC CANCER

Pancreatic cancer is a relatively common cancer in the United States. The cause of pancreatic cancer is unknown, but it may develop from either exocrine or endocrine cells. Cancers of the exocrine cells of the small pancreatic ducts are most common and lead to blockage of the ducts. Possible causes include inhalation of carcinogens that are excreted by the kidneys such as food additive, industrial chemicals, or cigarette smoke. Predisposing factors may include chronic pancreatitis, diabetes, or chronic alcohol abuse. These tumors frequently penetrate the pancreas and invade surrounding tissue. Metastasis via the portal vein or lymphatic system is common and rapid. Metastases to the brain and lung are common. Mortality is nearly 100% within less than 5 years.

Clinical Manifestations

- Pancreatic cancer may be asymptomatic (until advanced) or may be associated with vague complaints of aversion to food. Pain may be an early complaint or may occur only with advanced disease.
- Clay-colored stools, abdominal or low back pain, pruritus, and skin lesions.
- Advanced disease is associated with jaundice, severe pain, and pronounced weight loss.

Diagnostic Tools

- Laparotomy (penetration of the abdomen with a fiberoptic tool for visualization and sampling) can confirm the diagnosis.
- Ultrasound and computed tomography (CT scan) may be used.

Treatment

- Surgery to relieve pain may include bypass of the blocked ducts.
- Possible chemotherapy and radiation for palliative purposes.

PEDIATRIC CONSIDERATIONS

- In the past, type 2 diabetes mellitus was referred to as adult-onset diabetes because it typically occurred in individuals older than 30 years of age. Unfortunately, this distinction is becoming less and less true as more teenagers and preteens are developing insulin resistance, most likely related to the increasing prevalence of obesity in childhood. Several studies suggest that over 20% of American children are obese; a finding having enormous implications for health and health care costs as these children reach adulthood and experience the complications of long-term hyperglycemia.

- Common childhood illnesses, especially viral infection, may precipitate ketoacidosis in a child with type 1 diabetes. A child is sometimes diagnosed for the first time as diabetic when he or she presents critically ill with ketoacidosis. Diabetic ketoacidosis, hypoglycemia, and the Somogyi effect are more common in children than adults because of especially labile glucose levels. Treatment of a toddler or young child who has diabetes is extremely demanding and difficult for parents. Encouragement, and often counseling for the entire family, is needed. Older children and teens may rebel against strict carbohydrate control and frequent insulin injections as expressions of normal developmental stages of independence and autonomy. Providers and parents who encourage and allow the older child and teen to make as many decisions as possible regarding his or her care may be able to defuse some of these demonstrations of independence. In addition, girls or boys trying to be as thin as possible may skip or reduce their insulin injections; this manifestation is in some ways similar to an eating disorder.

 GERIATRIC CONSIDERATION

- The risk for type 2 diabetes tends to increase with age. The risk is most likely related to increased adipose tissue, decreased lean body mass, decreased activity which causes increased insulin resistance, and decreased insulin secretion.

SELECTED BIBLIOGRAPHY

Abrahamson, M. J. (2009). Insulin intensification: A patient-centered approach. *Consultant*, 49(suppl. 7), S26–S31.

American Diabetes Association (2009). Diagnosis and classification of diabetes mellitus. *Diabetes Care*, 32(suppl. 1), S62–S67.

American Diabetes Association (2009). Summary of revisions for the 2009 clinical practice recommendations. *Diabetes Care*, 32(suppl. 1), S3–S5.

Appel, S. J., Wadas, T. M., & Ovalle, F. (2009). Latent autoimmune diabetes of adulthood (LADA): An often misdiagnosed type of diabetes mellitus. *Journal of the American Academy of Nurse Practitioners*, 21, 156–159.

Apte, M. V., Pirola, R. C., & Wilson, J. S. (2009). Pancreas: Alcoholic pancreatitis—it's the alcohol, stupid. *Nature Reviews Gastroenteology & Hepatology, 6*(6), 321–322.

Bahi-Buisson, N., Roze, E., Dionisi, C., Escande, F., Valayannopoulos, V., Feillet, F., et al. (2008). Neurological aspects of hyperinsulinism-hyperammonaemia syndrome. *Developmental Medicine and Child Neurology, 50*(12), 945–949.

Bartoszek, M. P. (2009). Recognizing polycystic ovary syndrome in the primary care setting. *The Nurse Practitioner, 34*(7), 22–23, 25–29.

Boyle, P. J., & Stolar, M. W. (2008). Demystifying type 2 diabetes management. *Clinician Reviews,* (suppl), 3–12.

Brunton, S. (2009). Safety and effectiveness of modern insulin therapy: The value of insulin analogs. *Consultant, 49*(suppl 7), S13–S19.

Bucher, D. (2008). Pressed for time: Treating type 2 diabetes in the real world. *Advance for Nurse Practitioners, 16*(11), 47–50, 52, 78.

Bugger, H., & Abel, E. D. (2008). The metabolic syndrome and cardiac function. *Advances in Pulmonary Hypertension, 7*(3), 332–336.

Colagiuri, S., Borch-Johnsen, K., Glumer, C., & Vistisen, D. (2005). There really is an epidemic of type 2 diabetes. *Diabetologia, 48,* 1459–1463.

Cox, D., & Polvado, K. J. (2008). Type 2 diabetes in children and adolescents. *Advance for Nurse Practitioners, 16*(11), 43–45.

Cummings, D. E. (2005). Gastric bypass and nesidioblastosis—Too much of a good thing for islets? *New England Journal of Medicine, 353,* 300–302.

Deatcher, J. V. (2008). Prediabetes: Are you or your patients at risk for type 2 diabetes? *American Journal of Nursing, 108*(7), 77–79.

Forsbach-Sanchez, G., Tamez-Perez, H. E., & Vazquez-Lara, J. (2005). Diabetes and pregnancy. *Archives of Medical Research, 36,* 291–299.

Fleury-Milfort, E. (2008). Practical strategies to improve treatment of type 2 diabetes. *Journal of the American Academy of Nurse Practitioners, 20,* 295–304.

Fleury-Milfort, E. (2008). Insulin replacement therapy: Minimizing complications and side effects. *Advance for Nurse Practitioners, 16*(11), 32, 34–40.

Greer, E. B., & Shen, W. (2009). Gender differences in insulin resistance, body composition, and energy balance. *Gender Medicine, 6,* 60–75.

Guyton, A. C., & Hall, J. (2006). *Textbook of medical physiology* (11th ed.). Philadelphia: W.B. Saunders.

Hill, A. N., & Appel, S. J. (2009). Signs of improvement: Diabetes update 2009. *The Nurse Practitioner, 34*(6), 12–22.

Hinnen, D., Kruger, D. F., & Pratley, R. E. (2008). Treating to success in type 2 diabetes: What to do when oral therapies fail. *Journal of the American Academy of Nurse Practitioners, 11*(suppl. 1), 6–21.

Jacobson, G. F., Ramos, G. A., Ching, J. Y., Kirby, R. S., Ferrara, A., & Field, D. R. (2005). Comparison of glyburide and insulin for the management of gestational diabetes in a large managed care organization. *American Journal of Obstetrics and Gynecology, 193,* 118–124.

Kerr, M. (2009). ADA 2009: New blood test bridges the gap between serum glucose and hemoglobin A1c. *Medscape Medical News.* Available at: http://medscape.com/viewarticle/704358. Accessed September 9, 2009.

Kruger, D. F., & Spollett, G. R. (2009). Addressing barriers to timely intensification of diabetes care: The relationship between clinical inertia and patient behavior. *Consultant*, 49(suppl. 7), S20–S25.

Lehne, R. A. (2010). *Pharmacology for nursing care* (7th ed.). St. Louis: Saunders Elsevier.

McCall, B. (2009). Treatment of gestational diabetes reduces risk for complications. *New England Journal of Medicine*, 361, 1339–1348.

Meigs, J. B., Shrader, P., Sullivan, L. M., & Mcateer, J. B. (2008). Genotype score in addition to common risk factors for prediction of type 2 diabetes. *The New England Journal of Medicine*, 359(21), 2208–2215.

Mitzner, L. (2009). Early recognition of diabetes complications. *The Clinical Advisor*, 12(1), 19–20, 23–24.

Neira, C. P., Hartig, M., Cowan, P. A., & Velasquez-Mieyer, P. A. (2009). The prevalence of impaired glucose metabolism in Hispanics with two or more risk factors for metabolic syndrome in the primary care setting. *Journal of the American Academy Nurse Practitioners*, 21, 173–178.

Philis-Tsimikas, A. (2009). Type 2 diabetes: Limitations of current therapies. *Consultant*, 49(suppl. 7), S5–S11.

Pool, D. (2008). Prevailing over acute pancreatitis. *American Nurse Today*, 3(3), 10–12.

Porth, C. M., & Matfin, G. (2009). *Pathophysiology: Concepts of altered health states* (8th ed.). Philadelphia: Lippincott Williams & Wilkins.

Sharma, T., Katz, C. M., Rutecki, G. W. (2008). Unexplained hypoglycemia: A focused approach to finding the cause. *Consultant*, 48(9), 665–667, 670–671.

Sherman, C. (2008). Advocating what works for diabetes. *The Clinical Advisor*, 11(12), 37–39.

Sjostrom, L., Lindroos, A.-K., Peltonen, M., Torgerson, J., Bouchard, C., Carlsson, B., et al. (2004). Lifestyle, diabetes, and cardiovascular risk factors 10 years after bariatric surgery. *New England Journal of Medicine*, 351, 2683–2693.

Tesfaye, S., Chaturvedi, N., Eaton, S. E. M., Ward, J. D., Manes, C., Ionescu-Tirgoviste, C., et al. (2005). Vascular risk factors and diabetic neuropathy. *New England Journal of Medicine*, 352, 341–350.

Umpierrez, G. E., Latif, K., Stoever, J., Cuervo, R., Park, L., Freire, A. X. E., et al. (2004). Efficacy of subcutaneous insulin lispro versus continuous intravenous regular insulin for the treatment of patients with diabetic ketoacidosis. *American Journal of Medicine*, 117, 291–296.

Vincent, D. (2009). Culturally tailored education to promote lifestyle change in Mexican Americans with type 2 diabetes. *Journal of the American Academy of Nurse Practitioners*, 21, 520–527.

Wade, M. (2008). Danger ahead: Identifying insulin resistance. *Advance for Nurse Practitioners*, 16(8), 61–65.

Weickhardt, A., & Michael, M. (2009). Pancreatic cancer: Advances in medical therapy. *Expert Review of Clinical Pharmacology*, 2(2), 173–180.

White, R. D. (2009). Lipids: Key to cardiovascular health in patients with diabetes. *Consultant*, 49(7), 410–412.

The Liver

The liver lies in the upper right quadrant of the abdominal cavity and is the largest organ in the body. The functions of the liver are diverse and essential and depend on the liver's unique blood flow system and its specialized cells (Table 17-1). When the liver is damaged, all body systems are affected.

● Physiologic Concepts

STRUCTURE

The liver has a smooth, firm surface and is encased in a fibroelastic capsule called **Glisson capsule**. It is grossly separated into **right** and **left lobes**. Glisson capsule contains blood vessels, lymph vessels, and nerves. The two liver lobes consist of many smaller units called **lobules**. The lobules contain the liver cells (**hepatocytes**) that line up together in plates. The hepatocytes are considered to be the functional units of the liver. Liver cells are capable of cell division and readily reproduce when needed to replace damaged tissue.

HEPATIC BLOOD FLOW AND PRESSURE

The liver receives its blood supply from two different sources. Approximately 2/3 or 1000 mL/min of the liver's blood supply, is venous blood draining from the stomach, the small and large intestines, the pancreas, and the spleen. This blood comes to the liver via the portal vein. Because it is venous blood, it is poorly oxygenated but has a rich supply of nutrients, including glucose, which

TABLE 17-1 Functions of the Liver	
Type	**Function**
Metabolic	
Absorptive period	Converts glucose to glycogen and triglycerides; stores glycogen. Converts amino acids to fatty acids or stores amino acids. Makes lipoprotein from triglycerides and cholesterol.
Postabsorptive period	Produces glucose from glycogen (glycogenolysis) and fatty acids and amino acids (glyconeogenesis). Converts fats to ketones (accelerated if fasting). Produces urea from protein catabolism.
Immunologic	Macrophages filter blood.
Metabolic transformation	Detoxifies or conjugates waste products, hormones, drugs.
Clotting functions	Produces several essential clotting factors.
Plasma proteins	Synthesizes albumin and other plasma proteins.
Exocrine functions	Synthesizes bile salts.
Endocrine functions	Involved in activation of vitamin D. Produces angiotensinogen. Secretes insulin-like growth factors (somatomedin).

the liver can convert into glycogen and immediately store. The blood may also contain intestinal bacteria, toxins, and ingested drugs. The other 1/3 of blood for the liver enters via the hepatic artery at a flow rate of approximately 500 mL/min. This is arterial blood and well saturated with oxygen. After perfusing the liver, both blood sources drain into the liver capillaries, called **sinusoids**. From the sinusoids, blood drains into a central vein in each lobule and from there into the hepatic vein. The hepatic vein empties into the inferior vena cava.

In healthy individuals, there is virtually no resistance to the flow of blood in the portal vein. As a result, blood pressure in the portal venous system is low, approximately 3 mm Hg. Blood flows easily out of the liver into the vena cava as well, where pressure is nearly 0 mm Hg.

METABOLIC FUNCTIONS OF THE LIVER

Metabolism refers to the cellular processes that occur when basic food molecules (sugars, amino acids, and fatty acids) are built into cell structures or energy stores and are broken down later to run cell functions. The buildup of cell structures and energy stores is called **anabolism**; the breakdown is called **catabolism**. The cells of the liver are key components in the interplay between anabolism and catabolism.

Glucose Handling by the Liver

After glucose is digested and absorbed into the bloodstream, it is delivered to all cells of the body to be used as an energy source. As discussed in Chapter 16, insulin is required for glucose to gain entry to most cells. If glucose is unnecessary for immediate energy, it can be stored in cells as glycogen. The liver is especially capable of storing large amounts of glucose as glycogen. Because the liver can store glycogen, it acts as a glucose buffer for the blood. When glucose levels rise in the blood, the liver's conversion of glucose to glycogen and the storage of glycogen increase. Glycogen formation, called **glycogenesis**, occurs in the **absorptive phase of digestion**, which is the period soon after a meal when glucose levels are high. Glycogenesis is insulin dependent. By increasing the conversion and storage of glucose in times of excess, the liver returns plasma glucose levels toward normal.

In times of fasting or between meals, the breakdown of glycogen to glucose occurs in the liver, again serving to normalize circulating levels of glucose. The breakdown of glycogen is called **glycogenolysis**. In addition, when glucose levels decrease between meals, the liver initiates **gluconeogenesis** (the new formation of glucose) to keep blood glucose levels constant. Gluconeogenesis is accomplished in the liver by conversion of amino acids to glucose after deamination (removal of the amino group) and by conversion of glycerol, a product of fatty acid breakdown, to glucose. The breakdown of glycogen and the formation of glucose occur in the **postabsorptive phase of digestion**, the time between meals when external food sources are not readily available. The postabsorptive stage of digestion is under the control of the pancreatic hormone glycogen and other gastrointestinal hormones, as discussed in Chapter 15.

Amino Acid Handling by the Liver

After digestion, amino acids enter all cells and are converted to proteins to be used by the cells to make either enzymes or structural components such as ribosomes, collagen, or muscle contractile proteins. Although a variety of organs (including the kidney and intestinal mucosa) participate in the storage of extra amino acids as proteins, the liver is the major storage tissue for protein. When amino acids are needed, the breakdown of stored protein occurs, and free amino acids are liberated. A decrease in plasma amino acids below a certain level triggers the breakdown of stored proteins.

All cells, including liver cells, have limits on how much protein they can store. When no further amino acids can be stored as protein, the liver deaminates the extra amino acids and either uses the products as energy or changes them into glucose, glycogen, or fatty acids. These substances can be stored in the liver—glucose as glycogen and fatty acids as triglycerides (fat). Fatty acids can also be stored in other cells of the body, especially adipose tissue.

During deamination of amino acids, ammonia is released. It is almost entirely converted in the liver to urea, which is then excreted by the kidneys.

Fatty Acid Handling by the Liver

Nearly all digested fats are absorbed into the lymphatic circulation as **chylomicrons**—conglomerates of triglycerides, phospholipids, cholesterol, and lipoprotein. The chylomicrons are delivered by the lymph to the thoracic duct, where they join the systemic circulation. Triglycerides are subsequently changed back into fatty acids and glycerol by enzymes in the walls of all capillaries, especially the capillaries that serve the liver and the adipose tissue. From the capillaries, fatty acids and glycerol can diffuse into most cells.

Once inside the liver and other cells, fatty acids and glycerol again combine to form triglycerides. Triglycerides are stored until needed during the postabsorptive stage. At this time they may be metabolized back to glycerol and free fatty acids. Glycerol and fatty acids can enter the Krebs cycle to produce ATP, so that cells are provided with energy. Elevations in the hormones glucagon, cortisol, growth hormone, and the catecholamines signal cells to break down stored triglycerides into free fatty acids and glycerol.

Instead of directly entering the Krebs cycle, some glycerol and free fatty acids may be used by the liver to produce new glucose. This can result in the production of ketones when triglyceride breakdown is excessive. The brain itself cannot use free fatty acids directly for energy production. Therefore, the liver's conversion of fats to glucose (gluconeogenesis) is essential for supporting the energy needs of the brain when glucose levels are low.

Cholesterol Handling by the Liver

Cholesterol is a lipid substance produced by the liver and used in the digestion of fat. During digestion, cholesterol is packaged with bile salts, phospholipids, and the triglycerides into small suspensions called micelles. Once the triglycerides are suspended as micelles, they can be digested by pancreatic enzymes and absorbed into the bloodstream. The cholesterol from the micelles is recirculated to the liver. The liver metabolizes some of the cholesterol and recycles it to be used again in digestion. The remainder is complexed with phospholipids and released into the bloodstream as **lipoproteins**. As lipoproteins, cholesterol is carried to body cells to be used for the production of cell membranes, intracellular structures, and steroid hormones. High levels of two types of lipoproteins, low-density lipoprotein (LDL) and very low-density lipoprotein (VLDL), suggest that the liver is handling high amounts of cholesterol. These types of lipoproteins may injure cells, including the endothelial cells lining the arteries, by releasing oxygen free radicals and high-energy electrons during their metabolism. High-density lipoprotein (HDL), on the other hand, carries

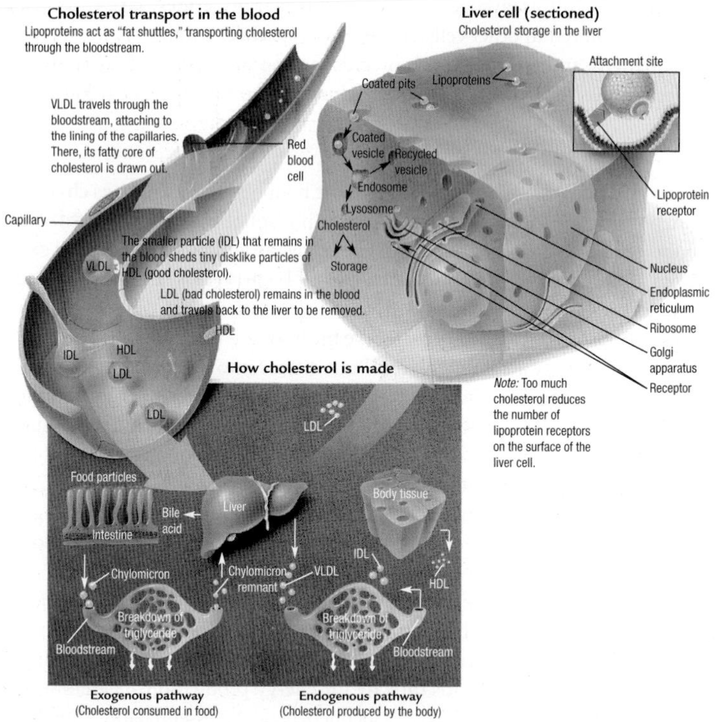

FIGURE 17-1 Cholesterol formation and storage. (From Anatomical Chart Company [2010]. *Atlas of pathophysiology.* [3rd ed.]. Philadelphia: Lippincott Williams & Wilkins.)

cholesterol away from cells to the liver and protects against arterial disease. Figure 17-1 illustrates the process of cholesterol transport and storage.

BILE SECRETION

Bile is made by all hepatocytes and consists of water, bile salts, bilirubin, cholesterol, fatty acids, lecithin, and electrolytes. Except for water, the most abundant substance in bile is bile salt. Bile salts are synthesized in the liver from cholesterol that has either been delivered to the liver from the small intestine or synthesized directly by the liver in the process of fat metabolism. All hepatic cells participate in making bile and each secretes bile into the small bile **canaliculi** that surround all liver cells. The canaliculi empty into progressively larger ducts that ultimately join into the **hepatic duct** and **common bile duct**. These ducts deliver bile either to the gallbladder for storage or directly into the intestine. Bile salts function in the digestion of fat (see Chapter 15) and are normally recycled after use in the small intestine. Without bile, as much as 40% of fats in the diet would not be absorbed across the intestine and so would be lost in the stool. The absorption of fat-soluble vitamins across the small intestine would be similarly affected. For example, without bile, a vitamin-K deficit would occur and be apparent in less than a week. Without adequate vitamin K, blood coagulation would be impaired.

The liver also functions in the handling of another component of bile, bilirubin. Bilirubin is formed as an end product of hemoglobin breakdown and must be metabolized by the liver for it to be excreted.

METABOLIC BIOTRANSFORMATION

The liver has an important role in transforming biologic substances that may be toxic at high levels or that cannot be excreted from the body without transformation. Substances acted upon in this manner by the liver may include both those ingested by an individual and those produced by the body itself. Examples of substances that are transformed by the liver include bilirubin, various hormones, drugs, and toxins. Metabolic biotransformation is also referred to as metabolic detoxification.

Bilirubin Biotransformation

Bilirubin is a product of red blood cell breakdown. When a red blood cell has lived out its 120-day life span, the cell membrane becomes fragile and ruptures. Hemoglobin is released and is acted upon by circulating phagocytic cells to form free bilirubin. Free bilirubin binds to plasma albumin and circulates in the bloodstream to the liver.

Free bilirubin is considered unconjugated in that, although it is bound to albumin, the binding is reversible. Once in the liver, bilirubin releases from albumin and, because free bilirubin is lipid soluble, moves easily into the hepatocytes. Once inside the hepatocytes, bilirubin is rapidly bound to another substance, usually glucuronic acid, and is now considered conjugated. Conjugated bilirubin is water soluble, not lipid soluble.

Most conjugated bilirubin is actively transported into the bile canaliculi. From there it is delivered along with the other components of bile to the gallbladder or small intestine. A small amount of conjugated bilirubin does not go to the intestine as a bile component, however, but rather is absorbed back into the bloodstream. Therefore, in the bloodstream, there is always a small amount of conjugated bilirubin present, along with unconjugated bilirubin on its way to the liver.

Once in the intestine, conjugated bilirubin is acted upon by bacteria and changed into urobilinogen. Most urobilinogen enters the bloodstream and is excreted by the kidneys in the urine, some is excreted in the stool,

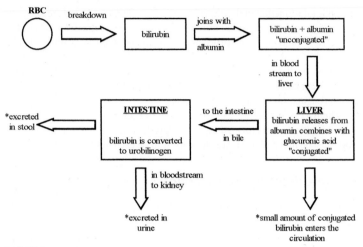

FIGURE 17-2 Conjugation of bilirubin.

and some is recycled back to the liver in the enterohepatic (intestinal to liver) circulation. Figure 17-2 shows the steps involved in the conjugation and excretion of bilirubin.

The conjugation of bilirubin is essential for its excretion. Without conjugation, bilirubin cannot be excreted by either the kidneys or the intestines. The handling of bilirubin by the liver is a form of metabolic detoxification. Without conjugation, unconjugated bilirubin would build up in the bloodstream to toxic levels.

Hormone Biotransformation

The liver inactivates or modifies many hormones of the body. It acts on steroid hormones, including cortisol, estrogen, testosterone, progesterone, and aldosterone, to make them water soluble rather than lipid soluble, allowing them to be excreted. If this biotransformation does not occur, these hormones tend to concentrate in the body and build up in tissues, especially adipose tissue.

Liver proteases inactivate or deaminate other hormones such as insulin, glucagon, and antidiuretic hormone (ADH, also called vasopressin). Thyroxine is deiodinated and inactivated. These actions allow the hormones to be excreted from the body.

Ammonia Biotransformation

Ammonia is a by-product of protein breakdown. It is transformed into urea in the liver and excreted in the urine. Without this liver function, ammonia levels build up in the blood and cause neurological dysfunction and possibly coma and death.

Drug and Toxin Metabolism

Drugs and toxins are often modified by the liver to be either inactivated or made water soluble by conjugation with another chemical compound. By these processes, the liver permits the body to excrete these substances. Without good liver function, many drugs and toxins accumulate in the body. Moreover, many of the chemical compounds used by the liver to conjugate lipid-soluble drugs and toxins, such as plasma proteins, are themselves synthesized by the liver. Therefore, they are in inadequate supply in the case of a poorly functioning liver.

Alcohol Handling by the Liver

Alcohol is an example of a drug that is primarily metabolized by the liver. Alcohol metabolism follows two pathways in the liver. The first pathway uses the enzyme alcohol dehydrogenase and results in the end product of acetaldehyde. Acetaldehyde is then changed to acetate and hydrogen ions. These reactions occur in the cytoplasm and the mitochondria of the hepatocyte.

The second metabolic pathway, called the **microsomal ethanol oxidizing system** (MEOS) pathway, named after the specific enzymes involved, occurs in the endoplasmic reticulum of the hepatocyte and is primarily used in the liver of individuals who have a long history of alcohol abuse. This pathway results in the production of acetaldehyde and free radicals. The free radicals and the acetaldehyde produced by either metabolic pathway are highly damaging to liver cells.

The MEOS pathway is also damaging to an individual because one of the enzymes required for running this pathway, cytochrome P450, is essential in the liver's transformation of many other toxins and drugs and excess fat-soluble vitamins. If this enzyme is preferentially used to detoxify alcohol, it is unavailable for its other roles. Thus, long-term alcohol abusers are susceptible to damage from many different toxins and drugs, and to the toxic effects of some vitamins.

Another coenzyme in alcohol metabolism is **nicotinamide adenine dinucleotide** (NAD). This coenzyme is also required for many other metabolic processes, including running the Krebs cycle to metabolize nutrients, making ATP, and allowing the liver to perform gluconeogenesis. Without NAD, hypoglycemia and lactic acid accumulation may develop. Hypoglycemia is a significant problem for many long-term alcohol abusers who typically have poor diets. Lactic acid accumulation can contribute to gout because increased lactic acid decreases the renal excretion of uric acid.

BLOOD STORAGE IN THE LIVER

The liver is a storage organ for blood. If blood volume decreases, for example, during a hemorrhage, the liver can release blood to the circulation. Likewise, the liver can increase its blood storage if volume is significantly increased or if blood backs up in the peripheral circulation in response to a failing right heart.

The amount of blood stored at any one time varies depending on an array of cardiovascular indices, but it may be as much as 400 to 500 mL.

PLASMA PROTEIN SYNTHESIS

The liver is responsible for synthesizing plasma proteins, including albumin. The albumin concentration in the plasma is the main source of plasma osmotic pressure, the primary force causing reabsorption of fluid from the interstitial space into the capillary (see Chapter 13). If the liver is incapable of making adequate amounts of plasma proteins, osmotic pressure in the capillary will be low, and plasma filtered out at the start of the capillary will not flow back in by the time the capillary reforms to a venule. Therefore, swelling and edema of the interstitial space will occur.

CLOTTING FACTOR SYNTHESIS

The liver functions in the production of several clotting factors, including factors I (fibrinogen), II (prothrombin), and VII (proconvertin). Without adequate production of these substances, blood clotting is impaired and bleeding may be extensive. In addition, vitamin K is a fat-soluble vitamin required for the formation of these and other clotting factors. Because bile salts are required for across-the-gut absorption of all fat-soluble vitamins, liver dysfunction resulting in decreased synthesis or supply of bile to the intestine can also lead to bleeding problems.

IMMUNOLOGIC FUNCTION

The many capillaries of the liver are called sinusoids. Blood flow in the sinusoids is a mixture of venous blood from the portal vein and arterial blood from the hepatic artery. The sinusoids are lined with phagocytic macrophage cells called **Kupffer cells**. These cells remove bacteria, dead cells, and other foreign substances from the blood, especially the portal blood, flowing into the liver from the intestines.

STORAGE OF VITAMINS AND MINERALS

The liver has the capability to store vitamins B_{12}, D, and A. Iron is stored in the liver as ferritin. The vitamins and iron can be released to the body from the liver when circulating levels decrease.

TESTS OF LIVER FUNCTION

Tests of liver function are frequently performed. Some of the most common ones are summarized in Table 17-2.

TABLE 17-2　Tests of Liver Function	
Test	**Significance**
Liver enzymes such as alkaline aminotransferase (ALT), aspartate aminotransferase (AST), alkaline phosphatase (ALP), serum glutamic pyruvic transaminase (SGPT), serum glutamic oxaloacetic transaminase (SGOT), lactate hydrogenase (LDH_5)	Enzyme released from injured liver cells
	Elevated with liver disease
Bilirubin (total, conjugated, and unconjugated)	Increase in various combinations with liver disease
Plasma protein concentration	Decreased with liver disease
Prothrombin time	Prolonged with liver disease
Ultrasound, magnetic resonance imaging (MRI), computed tomography (CT)	Indicates structural or defects or blockages such as stones
Serological tests for viral antigens, antibodies, or virus	Present with different types of hepatitis
Liver biopsy	Detection and confirmation of infection, fatty infiltration, fibrosis, or cancer

● Pathophysiologic Concepts

PORTAL HYPERTENSION

Portal hypertension is excessively high pressure in the portal vein. Normal portal venous pressure is approximately 3 mm Hg. Pressure greater than 9 to 10 mm Hg in the portal vein is considered portal hypertension. Portal hypertension develops when the resistance to blood flow through or out of the liver is high. Excessive blood flow going into the liver can also lead to portal hypertension.

Effects of Portal Hypertension

With the development of portal hypertension, blood normally going into the liver via the portal vein begins to bypass the liver in search of alternative routes that offer less resistance to flow. This bypass can result in collateral vessels opening from the portal vein to other lower-resistance vessels. When blood bypasses the liver, the hepatocytes cannot maintain their essential functions of biologic transformation, detoxification, and metabolism of foodstuffs. In addition, the opened collateral circulations frequently cannot handle the increased blood flow, and third spacing results (described below).

Causes of Portal Hypertension

Portal hypertension may develop if there is obstruction to flow through or out of the liver. Obstruction to flow *through* the liver can occur as a result of fibrosis and scarring of the liver, conditions that occur with repeated infections, or long-term liver disease such as cirrhosis. Obstruction to flow through the liver can also result from acute or chronic inflammation because swelling and edema in the interstitial space—which occurs as part of the processes of inflammation—provide resistance to blood flow. Hepatitis is an infection of the liver that is associated with acute or chronic inflammation. Likewise, a thrombus in the portal vein itself can block blood flow through the liver. If blood flow through the liver is impeded by any cause, portal pressure increases and portal hypertension can develop.

Obstruction to flow *out of* the liver can occur if there is a thrombus (arterial buildup) or an embolus (blood clot) in the hepatic vein draining the liver. Likewise, anything that blocks flow through the vena cava or into or out of the right side of the heart, including right-heart failure, cardiac myopathy, and pericarditis, can cause blood to back up into the liver, increasing the pressure in the portal venous system.

THIRD SPACING

Third spacing refers to fluid, primarily water, filtered from the plasma. This fluid accumulates in areas of the body other than inside cells or in the vascular system.

Types of Third Spacing

There are two types of third spacing that occur with liver pathology: ascites and interstitial edema. **Ascites** is the accumulation of serous (serum-like) fluid in the peritoneal cavity. The peritoneal cavity includes the abdominal cavity and the pelvic region up to the underside of the diaphragm, excluding the kidneys. The peritoneal cavity is lined by a thin membrane called the peritoneum.

Ascites usually occurs as a result of portal hypertension. With high resistance to blood flow through the liver, blood flow is diverted to mesenteric (abdominal–peritoneal) vessels. The increased flow causes increased capillary pressure in these vessels of the abdominal cavity, resulting in net filtration of fluid out of the vessels and into the peritoneal cavity. In addition, high pressure in the liver itself causes fluid to ooze across the liver into the peritoneal cavity. This fluid contains a high concentration of albumin. The loss of albumin from the vascular compartment (the blood) in ascites contributes to the depletion of blood proteins seen with advanced liver disease. It also contributes to the decrease in plasma osmotic pressure, leading to the development of interstitial edema.

Interstitial edema occurs throughout the body with advanced liver disease. It occurs as a direct result of the loss of serum albumin in ascites and from impaired protein synthesis. If plasma protein concentration is reduced, the force favoring reabsorption of fluid into all capillaries from the interstitial space is reduced, and edema of the interstitial compartment occurs (see Chapter 13).

Effect of Third Spacing on Blood Pressure

As a result of the accumulation of fluid in the peritoneal cavity and in the interstitial compartment throughout the body, circulating blood volume decreases. A significant decrease in blood volume can result in decreased blood pressure. When blood pressure decreases, the carotid and the aortic baroreceptors are activated (see Chapter 13), leading to various reflex responses aimed at returning pressure toward normal. One of these reflex responses (see Chapters 13 and 18) is an increase in the release of the hormone renin from the juxtaglomerular cells of the kidney.

Reflex Responses to Third Spacing

As described in previous chapters, increased renin ultimately results in an increase in the production of the hormone angiotensin II (AII). AII causes constriction of arterioles throughout the body, increasing total peripheral resistance and blood pressure. Increased AII also causes increased release of the hormone aldosterone from the adrenal cortex. Aldosterone increases the reabsorption of sodium ions across the kidney tubules and back into the blood. Because ADH (vasopressin) from the posterior pituitary is also released with a decrease in blood pressure, water follows the sodium ions back into the blood, expanding blood volume and increasing blood pressure. In fact, levels of ADH and aldosterone can become increasingly elevated with liver disease because a poorly functioning liver is less able to inactivate these and other hormones.

With increased plasma volume, even more fluid moves into the peritoneal cavity and the interstitial space, causing the ascites, swelling, and edema to increase. Eventually, hydrostatic (water) pressure in the peritoneal cavity and the interstitial space increases enough so that further filtration is opposed, and a new equilibrium of fluid pressures inside and outside of the capillaries is reached.

PORTAL-SYSTEMIC VENOUS SHUNTS

When portal hypertension reduces blood flow through the liver, collateral vessels, or **shunts**, also **varicies**, open between the portal vein and the systemic veins that drain the abdominal wall, esophagus, and rectum. The shunts divert blood flow, bypassing the liver. Unfortunately, these thin-walled vessels are poorly equipped to handle such high blood flow and begin to develop into varices (distorted, swollen veins). The varices are subject to rupture and, especially in the esophagus, significant bleeding may occur. Variceal rupture can lead to a fatal hemorrhage if shunt flow is high. Rectal varices can cause painful hemorrhoids. Complicating and worsening any hemorrhage is the fact that production of many coagulation factors is decreased with liver pathology, prolonging bleeding time.

SPLENOMEGALY

Splenomegaly is enlargement of the spleen. With portal hypertension, blood flow is diverted to the spleen via the splenic vein. Some extra blood (as much as a few hundred milliliters in an adult) can be stored in the spleen, leading to its enlargement. Because the blood stored in the spleen is unavailable to the general circulation, anemia (decreased red blood cells), thrombocytopenia (decreased platelets), and leukopenia (decreased white blood cells) can occur.

JAUNDICE

Jaundice is the yellowish discoloration of the skin and sclera of the eyes seen as a result of excess bilirubin in the blood (greater than 1.2 mg/dL). Bilirubin is a product of red blood cell breakdown. Jaundice is also referred to as **icterus**. There are three main types of jaundice: hemolytic jaundice, intrahepatic jaundice, and extrahepatic obstructive jaundice.

Hemolytic Jaundice

Caused by excessive red blood cell lysis (breakdown), hemolytic jaundice is a prehepatic cause of jaundice because it occurs as a result of factors not necessarily related to the liver. Hemolytic jaundice can occur anytime red blood cell destruction is excessive and the liver cannot conjugate (and so the body cannot excrete) all the released bilirubin. It is seen with transfusion reactions and with red cell lysis associated with faulty hemoglobin (e.g., sickle cell anemia and thalassemia). Autoimmune destruction of red cells can also lead to hemolytic jaundice.

In hemolytic jaundice, much of the bilirubin is still conjugated. Therefore, urine and stool color are normal. Unconjugated bilirubin levels (called free bilirubin or indirect hyperbilirubinemia) are elevated, because the liver's ability to conjugate bilirubin cannot keep up with the magnitude of the red cell destruction.

Intrahepatic Jaundice

Decreased hepatic uptake, conjugation, or excretion of bilirubin due to dysfunction of the hepatocytes or obstruction of the bile canaliculi are triggers of intrahepatic jaundice. Liver dysfunction can occur if the hepatocytes are infected by a virus, for instance, in hepatitis, or if the cells of the liver are damaged by cancer or cirrhosis. Some congenital disorders also affect the liver's ability to handle bilirubin. Certain drugs, including steroid hormones, some antibiotics, and the anesthetic halothane, can impair liver cell function. When the liver cannot conjugate bilirubin, unconjugated levels increase, leading to jaundice.

Intrahepatic jaundice caused by obstruction of the small bile canaliculi can occur with an intrahepatic tumor or stone, or it may result from widespread inflammation. Although the hepatocytes do conjugate bilirubin, obstruction in the canaliculi reduces the passage of the conjugated bilirubin into the bile duct. This obstruction results in an increase in the amount of conjugated bilirubin that enters the bloodstream. Depending on the degree of obstruction, stools may be pale or nearly normal in color. The urine is dark and frothy because large amounts of bilirubin are excreted by way of this route.

Extrahepatic Obstructive Jaundice

Blockage of bile flow through the bile duct also leads to obstructive jaundice. Extrahepatic obstruction can occur if the bile duct is blocked by gallstones or by a tumor. Again, as described above for intrahepatic jaundice due to obstruction, the liver continues to conjugate bilirubin, but the bilirubin cannot reach the small intestine. The result is reduced or absent stool excretion of urobilinogen, causing clay-colored stools. The conjugated bilirubin enters the bloodstream and much is excreted by the kidneys, giving the urine a dark, frothy appearance. If the obstruction is unrelieved, the bile canaliculi in the liver eventually become congested and rupture, spilling the bile into the lymph and the bloodstream.

CIRRHOSIS

Diffuse liver scarring and fibrosis characterize cirrhosis. Hard fibrous nodules replace normal liver tissue, and constrictive, fibrous bands encircle the hepatocytes. Normal liver architecture and function are disrupted.

Cirrhosis occurs in the liver in response to repeated incidents of cellular injury and the resultant inflammatory reactions. Causes of cirrhosis include infections such as hepatitis; bile duct obstruction, leading to bile buildup in the canaliculi and the subsequent rupture of the canaliculi; and toxin-induced injury to the hepatocytes. Alcohol is the toxin most often implicated in causing injury and inflammation in the liver (Fig. 17-3).

AII appears to play a role in the development of cirrhosis. Although normally involved in hepatic tissue repair, under some circumstances, AII stimulates hepatic inflammation and collagen synthesis. Individuals suffering from ascites frequently demonstrate elevated levels of AII, which may contribute to worsening of liver function.

HEPATITIS

Hepatitis is the inflammation of the liver. It can be caused by an infection or by toxins, including alcohol, and is seen with hepatic cancer. Signs and symptoms

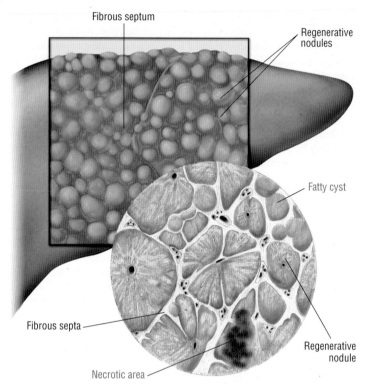

Fibrous septum

Regenerative nodules

Fatty cyst

Fibrous septa

Regenerative nodule

Necrotic area

FIGURE 17-3 Cirrhosis. The liver develops fatty pockets, or cysts, as well as hard fibrous nodules that intersperse among the cells and fibrous bands that encircle the hepatocytes. Resistance to blood flow increases and liver function is disrupted. Cells may die and be replaced by scar tissue. Inflammation is widespread.

for each type of hepatitis are similar. Modes of transmission and eventual outcomes may be different.

● Conditions of Disease or Injury

PHYSIOLOGIC JAUNDICE

A significant example of hemolytic jaundice is jaundice seen in the newborn, called physiologic jaundice. This condition is especially prevalent in premature infants and may be as high as 80%. It occurs as a result of increased breakdown of fetal hemoglobin in the first few days after birth combined with the immaturity of the liver at birth (especially in premature infants). Levels of unconjugated bilirubin build up in the blood, and because unconjugated bilirubin cannot be excreted in the urine, jaundice develops. Other pathologic events that may be involved according to Maisels (2005) include:

- Increased bilirubin delivery to the liver due to birth trauma along with faster RBC destruction.
- Impaired bilirubin uptake from the plasma if caloric intake is insufficient to form adequate amounts of protein.
- Defective bilirubin conjugation if intracellular binding protein does not remain adequately saturated.
- Delayed bilirubin excretion due to lack of bacterial flora and decreased intestinal motility.
- Altered hepatic circulation due to hypoxia or cardiac anomalies.
- Excessive bilirubin reabsorption from the intestine secondary to decreased bowel motility, intestinal obstruction or meconium.

Physiological jaundice is more common in breast-fed infants because the fatty acids in breast milk compete with bilirubin for albumin-binding sites. This is thought to alter bilirubin processing. Jaundice caused by breast-feeding may be a normal occurrence in the healthy infant. Levels of bilirubin and degree of jaundice are usually more pronounced and more prolonged in premature infants.

Clinical Manifestations

- Unconjugated bilirubin levels will be elevated in the newborn, usually peaking 2 to 4 days after birth, and subsiding on their own within 1 to 2 weeks after birth. Levels may remain elevated longer in premature infants.
- Jaundice accompanies the elevated bilirubin.

Diagnostic Tools

- Peak total bilirubin levels (conjugated and unconjugated) may reach 12 to 15 mg/dL, compared with normal levels of less than 6 mg/dL in a full-term infant. Levels of unconjugated bilirubin greater than 15 mg/dL are of concern.

Complications

- Because unconjugated bilirubin may precipitate out in the brain, brain damage from very high levels of unconjugated bilirubin, called **kernicterus**, may rarely occur (described below).

Treatment

- For most infants with mildly elevated bilirubin, treatment will include phototherapy. Phototherapy involves exposing an infant to fluorescent light in the visible spectrum (between 420- and 470-nm wavelengths) for extended periods (usually 1 to 3 days). This wavelength of light causes unconjugated bilirubin to be converted to a more water-soluble form, which, like conjugated bilirubin, can be excreted in the urine and feces.

- Maintain body temperature at or above 97.8°F *(36.5°C)*. Cold stress causes acidosis, which decreases the number and strength of albumin-binding sites resulting in higher unconjugated bilirubin levels.
- Early feedings to stimulate intestinal motility.
- Breast-feeding jaundice need not be treated.

HEMOLYTIC DISEASE OF THE NEWBORN

Hemolytic disease of the newborn is a more serious type of jaundice that appears at birth. This disease may result from either ABO or Rh incompatibility between the infant and the mother. ABO incompatibility is more common; Rh factor incompatibility is more serious. In Rh incompatibility, a mother who does not possess the Rh antigen on her red blood cells (i.e., she is Rh negative) makes antibodies against that antigen after being exposed to it on the red blood cells of her fetus. An Rh-negative woman could be exposed to the Rh antigen if the father of her child was Rh positive and her fetus carried that trait. With significant maternal antibody produced against fetal red blood cells, excessive lysis of the fetal cells can occur. Lysis of red blood cells leads to the release of bilirubin as well as agglutination (clumping) of the cells. This can occur before or during birth, overloading the already reduced capacity of the infant's liver to conjugate bilirubin. Typically, a woman develops antibodies against fetal Rh antigens only after several pregnancies or miscarriages in which she was repeatedly exposed to the antigen.

Clinical Manifestations

- Hemolytic disease of the newborn may be mild or severe, depending on the degree of maternal antibodies and the extent of infant red blood cell lysis. If the disease is mild, the skin is moderately pale and the infant's liver may be slightly enlarged.
- With severe disease, obvious jaundice, hepatomegaly, and splenomegaly are present. In addition, the classic symptoms of anemia, including increased heart rate and respiratory rates, are present.

Diagnostic Tools

- With pronounced disease, blood analysis demonstrates severe anemia and high levels of unconjugated bilirubin.
- An indirect Coombs' test that measures circulating maternal antibodies to the Rh antigen will be positive, demonstrating the mother has been exposed to the antigen.

- A direct Coombs' test measuring maternal antibodies actually bound to fetal or newborn red blood cells confirms hemolytic disease.

Complications

- If unconjugated bilirubin levels reach 25 to 30 mg/dL, infants may develop **kernicterus**. Kernicterus is a complex of neurologic symptoms related to high levels of unconjugated bilirubin crossing the neonatal blood–brain barrier and gaining access to the infant's central nervous system. Neurologic symptoms include behavioral changes and lethargy. If the condition persists or worsens, tremors, hearing loss, seizures, and death can occur. Survivors, if severely affected, may be mentally retarded, deaf, or prone to seizures.
- **Erythroblastosis fetalis** is an alloimmune hemolytic disease in which maternal antibodies attack fetal RBCs. In response, the fetus produces immature RBCs. Hydrops fetalis is the most severe form.
- With high levels of maternal antibodies, the fetus may die in utero of a condition called **hydrops fetalis**, which is characterized by gross edema of the entire fetus. Multiple organ system failure may occur.

Treatment

- For mild cases, phototherapy may successfully treat the disease.
- In cases of moderate or severe hyperbilirubinemia, infants are treated with exchange blood transfusions. Exchange blood transfusions involve transfusing the infant with Rh-positive blood containing no Rh antibody. Transfusions are continued until twice the baby's blood volume has been replaced and the bilirubin levels are decreased. This treatment also resolves anemia. Some Rh-positive fetuses at risk of dying in utero may be treated before birth with transfusions of red blood cells.
- The most important aspect of treatment of hemolytic disease of the newborn is prevention of the disease by identification of mothers at risk of developing Rh antibodies. At-risk mothers are Rh-negative women who are carrying a child by an Rh-positive father. It is now possible to administer a concentrated form of Rh-positive antibody, called Rh immune globulin, or RhoGAM, to women at risk. RhoGAM binds any Rh-positive antigen that gains entrance to the mother's bloodstream, thereby taking the antigen out of circulation before the mother develops her own permanent antibodies against it. Administration of RhoGAM produces a temporary, passive immunity to the Rh antigen in the mother. RhoGAM is typically given to women at 7 months' gestation if Rh incompatibility is suspected. Within 72 hours of delivery of an Rh-positive infant to an Rh-negative mother, RhoGAM is again administered to the mother to protect future pregnancies. RhoGAM cannot remove antibodies to the Rh antigens if the mother has already produced them in previously untreated

pregnancies (including miscarriages and abortions), but it might reduce the extent of new antibody production.

ALCOHOLIC CIRRHOSIS

Also called Laënnec cirrhosis, alcoholic cirrhosis occurs after years of alcohol abuse. Metabolic liver changes due to alcohol ingestion include:

- Decreased fat secretion from the liver.
- Decreased fatty acid utilization by the liver.
- Increased fatty acid esterification of fatty acids into triglycerides.
- Increased fatty acid synthesis.

The end products of alcohol digestion, especially the end products produced in the liver of a chronic alcohol abuser, include oxygen free radicals, which are toxic to hepatocytes. Poor nutrition, commonly seen in patients with an alcohol abuse problem, also contributes to liver damage, perhaps by overstimulating the liver to undergo gluconeogenesis and protein metabolism. Alcoholic cirrhosis has three stages: fatty liver disease, alcoholic hepatitis, and cirrhosis.

Fatty liver disease is the first, relatively benign stage of alcoholic cirrhosis. It is a reversible condition characterized by triglyceride accumulation in the hepatocytes and is believed to occur in up to 90% of individuals who abuse alcohol chronically. Alcohol may cause triglycerides to accumulate in the liver by acting as fuel for energy production such that cells use alcohol, and fatty acids are no longer needed. Alcohol end products, especially acetaldehyde, also interfere with the oxidative phosphorylation of fatty acids by the hepatocyte mitochondria, causing trapping of fatty acids inside the hepatocytes. In this first stage of cirrhosis, fatty infiltration of the liver is reversible if alcohol ingestion stops.

Alcoholic hepatitis is the second stage of alcoholic cirrhosis and is estimated to develop in approximately 20% to 40% of individuals abusing alcohol for an extended period of time. Hepatitis is the inflammation of liver cells. Inflammation and subsequent necrosis of some cells usually occurs after a serious increase in alcohol intake in long-term alcohol abusers. Damage to the hepatocytes probably occurs as a result of the cellular toxicity of the end products of alcohol metabolism, especially acetaldehyde and hydrogen ion. With alcoholic hepatitis, neutrophil infiltration of the liver and the secretion of the cytokine tumor necrosis factor alpha (TNF-α) drive the inflammation. Liver cells are stimulated to undergo apoptosis (programmed cell death) that can lead to scarring and fibrosis. This stage may also be reversible if alcohol intake stops.

Cirrhosis itself is the final, irreversible stage of alcoholic cirrhosis. In this stage, dead liver cells are replaced by scar tissue. Fibrous bands develop from the chronic activation of inflammatory responses and encircle and entwine between the remaining hepatocytes. The chronic inflammation results in substantial interstitial swelling and edema, which can collapse small blood vessels and cause increased resistance to blood flow through the liver, resulting in portal hypertension and ascites. Esophageal, rectal, and abdominal varices are common, and hepatocellular jaundice is apparent. Resistance to flow through the liver progressively increases and liver function further deteriorates.

Clinical Manifestations

- Early stages of cirrhosis may cause no specific symptoms, but hepatomegaly may be present.
- With continued progression, vague abdominal discomfort, anorexia, and nausea may occur. Fatigue is common. Edema, ascites, and jaundice begin.
- With advanced cirrhosis, manifestations of liver failure may appear.

Diagnostic Tools

- Liver function tests are altered with all stages of alcoholic cirrhosis except fatty liver.
- Elevated bilirubin levels are present.
- Prolonged prothrombin time resulting from decreased coagulation factors.
- Abdominal radiograph shows enlarged liver, calcification, and fluid accumulation.
- Decreased serum albumin and protein, decreased hemoglobin, hematocrit, and electrolytes.
- Liver biopsy indicates tissue destruction and fibrosis and can confirm cirrhosis.

Complications

- Inadequate nutrition. Vitamins A, C, and K deficiencies.
- Portal hypertension and esophageal varicies.
- Ascites.
- Hepatic encephalopathy.
- Liver failure, leading to transplantation or death, may develop.

Treatment

- A diet with adequate nutrition is recommended to reduce the metabolic load on the liver.
- Cessation of alcohol ingestion is essential.
- Rest is recommended.
- Beta-adrenergic blockers for portal hypertension.

- Endoscopic variceal ligation.
- Surgical shunt placement.
- Sclerosing agents.
- Esophageal balloon tamponade.
- Management of complications of liver failure if required.
- Corticosteroid administration appears to be beneficial in reducing inflammation for some patients.
- Inhibition of TNF-α as a means to slow apoptosis is receiving widespread attention as a therapy.

VIRAL HEPATITIS

Hepatitis, or inflammation of the liver parenchyma, can be acute or chronic and may range from mild to life-threatening. The viruses that cause hepatitis lead to hepatocyte injury primarily by stimulating host inflammatory and immune reactions that secondarily damage the hepatocytes; however, in some circumstances the viruses may directly injure the cells as well. The inflammatory reactions involve mast-cell degranulation and histamine release, cytokine production, complement activation, lysis of infected and neighboring cells, and edema and swelling of the interstitium. A later-occurring immune response supports the inflammatory responses. Further stimulation of complement and cell lysis and direct antibody attack against the viral antigens cause destruction of infected cells. The liver becomes edematous, collapsing capillaries and decreasing blood flow, leading to tissue hypoxia. Scarring and fibrosis of the liver can result.

Several viruses have been identified that are known to infect hepatocytes, the most common of which are hepatitis A, B, C, D, and E (Table 17-3). Other hepatitis viruses also have been identified, with new strains likely to become recognized in the future.

Hepatitis A

Hepatitis A (HAV) was formerly called infectious hepatitis. It is primarily passed by oral–fecal contamination resulting from poor hygiene or contaminated food. Sources of transmission may include ingestion of water contaminated with sewage, eating raw foods washed in contaminated water, consumption of shellfish from contaminated water, eating food prepared by an infected individual who did not perform proper hand hygiene after toileting, and oral sex. Individuals living in close quarters where hygiene may be inadequate, such as day care centers, mental institutions, prisons, and homeless shelters, are at risk of developing the disease. The virus may occasionally be passed in the blood. In some countries, HAV infection is endemic.

TABLE 17-3 Currently Identified Hepatitis Viruses

Type	Transmission	Prognosis	Diagnosis
Hepatitis A	Oral or fecal	Usually self-limiting	Hepatitis A antibody; IgM (early), IgG (later)
Hepatitis B	Bloodborne, especially maternal to child. Also sexual transmission	Usually self-limiting.10% may become chronic or fulminating	Hepatitis B surface antigen (HbsAg) and core antigen (HBeAg) followed by antibody against hepatitis B surface (HbsAb) and core (HbeAb) antigens
Hepatitis C	Bloodborne (low rate sexual transmission)	50% may become chronic infections	Hepatitis C antibody
Hepatitis D	Bloodborne. Coinfects with hepatitis B only	Increases the likelihood of hepatitis B progression	Hepatitis D antigen, hepatitis D antibody
Hepatitis E	Contaminated water, oral or fecal	Usually self-limiting, but high mortality in pregnant women	Measurement of hepatitis E virus

The time between exposure and onset of symptoms (incubation period) for HAV is between 2 and 6 weeks. Individuals who have the disease may be contagious for as long as 2 weeks before symptoms appear and up to one week following onset of symptoms. Antibodies against the hepatitis A virus are present with the onset of symptoms. The disease usually runs its course within approximately 4 months after exposure. No carrier (chronic) state exists, in which an individual remains contagious for an extended period after the acute illness, nor does a fulminating condition occur after the acute illness. Acute HAV infection in patients who have chronic hepatitis C (HCV) may worsen the progression of that disease.

Hepatitis B

Hepatitis B (HBV) is sometimes called serum hepatitis. It is a serious disease throughout the world, with over 300 million people suffering from chronic infection. In some countries, notably Southeast Asia, China, and Africa, HBV is endemic, with more than one-half of the population infected at some point in their lives and more than 8% of the population being chronic carriers of the virus. In countries with high rates of HBV, transmission usually occurs either by way of mother to infant before or during birth or from one child to another in early childhood. Worldwide public health campaigns to immunize infants and children are having dramatic effects on childhood infection rates in endemic countries. In countries with low levels of infection, including the United States, transmission is usually through sexual exposure or blood exposure in young adults. HBV may also be present in saliva and wound drainage. During the last few decades, public health campaigns to immunize teens and school-aged children have reduced the incidence in this population as well. Others still at high risk of developing HBV are unvaccinated injection drug users, health care workers, laboratory and dialysis workers who are in frequent contact with blood and blood products and nonmonogamous sexually active heterosexuals and homosexuals. The virus can survive up to a week in the open environment. Transmission during tattooing and body piercing in unvaccinated individuals may also occur if hygienic practices are not followed.

HBV has a long incubation period, between 1 and 7 months with an average onset of 1 to 2 months. The acute stage of an active infection may last up to 2 months. Approximately 5% to 10% of adults with HBV develop chronic hepatitis and continue to experience hepatic inflammation for longer than 6 months. Chronic hepatitis may be slowly progressive or may be fulminant, leading to hepatic necrosis, cirrhosis, liver failure, and death. An individual infected with HBV might also develop a persistent carrier state, causing him or her to be contagious without demonstrating symptoms. Especially likely to become chronic carriers are those infected during infancy and those who are immunosuppressed.

The HBV virus is a double-stranded DNA virus called a Dane particle. It has a number of well-described surfaces and viral core antigens that can be identified in the laboratory from a blood sample. In a primary infection, the viral antigen that is usually measurable first in a blood sample is a surface antigen on the viral coat labeled HBsAg. The presence of antibodies against the HBV core antigen (anti-HBc antibodies) follows; early in an infection, these antibodies are mainly of the IgM type. The presence of virus in the blood (viremia) is well established by the time antibodies are produced, making this acute phase of infection a time of high transmissibility. Identification of the core antigen (HBcAg) or the hepatitis DNA itself in the serum is diagnostic of active infection with HBV. Blood donations are routinely screened for the presence of HBV antigens.

In response to the different viral antigens, different antibodies develop in individuals in a predictable sequence, beginning from the acute stage of illness until the beginning of recovery. Some forms of antibody to HBV last the lifetime of an individual who has experienced infection. If one continues to harbor HBV, however, there will be continual expression of viral antigens, including a second core antigen, HBeAg; the continued presence of viral antigens suggests the person is suffering from chronic hepatitis. With new, highly sensitive assay techniques, individuals with persistent infection still may have measurable antiviral antibodies; therefore anyone demonstrating viral surface or core antigens, regardless of antibody status, should be presumed to have ongoing viremia. Although in adults most primary infections resolve, approximately 5% of infections will develop into persistent infections; this percentage is much higher in infants and children.

Hepatitis C

HCV was identified in 1989 and up to now 3.2 million Americans may be chronically infected. The virus has a high rate of replication and easily mutates. This RNA virus is passed in the same manner as HBV and primarily entered the U.S. population through blood transfusions before screening was available. In addition, soldiers and other personnel who have served in Southeast Asia have an increased incidence of infection compared with those who have not. Many individuals infected earlier in life are only now finding out they have the disease. Others who have confirmed infection have no knowledge of infection and no outstanding medical or social history indicative of high risk. Although the virus is present in semen and vaginal secretions, it is uncommon for long-term sexual partners of HCV carriers to become infected with the virus, although individuals who have multiple sexual partners or who engage in high-risk behaviors such as unprotected anal sex are more likely to become infected. Currently, the most common source of transmission in the United States is intravenous drug use. Percutaneous exposure via tattooing, body piercing, folk practices, and barbering also poses a slight risk of transmission.

The incubation period for HCV ranges from 15 to 150 days, with an average of about 50 days. Because symptoms tend to be milder than for HBV, individuals may not recognize they have a serious infection and thus may not seek health care or be diagnosed. Unlike HBV, HCV seldom leads to fulminating hepatitis. Unfortunately, there is a high rate of chronic infection that may go undiagnosed for years. In addition, coinfection of individuals with both HCV and the human immunodeficiency virus (HIV) is common and is a major cause of morbidity and mortality in the 21st century. Globally, at least 30% of HIV-positive individuals are coinfected with HCV. Both antibody to HCV and the virus itself are measurable in blood, allowing for effective screening of donated blood. Although offering a quicker turn-around than viral tests, antibody tests may falsely read negative when run early in the course of disease, since the individual may not feel or appear ill, and because there is a relatively long time lapse between when an individual who has the disease is contagious and when he or she begins to express antibodies. The presence of antibodies to HCV does not imply the lack of a chronic state. There is no vaccine available at this time against HCV.

Hepatitis D

Hepatitis D (HDV) is called the delta hepatitis agent and is actually a defective virus that cannot infect the hepatocyte on its own to cause hepatitis. Instead, it coinfects with HBV, leading to a worsening of the HBV infection. Infection with HDV might also develop later in an individual who has mild chronic HBV. Intravenous drug users have a higher rate of occurrence and a mortality rate of approximately 3%. The delta agent increases the risk of developing fulminating hepatitis, liver failure, and death. The HDV virus is passed similarly to HBV virus with an incubation period of 1 to 6 months. HDV antigen and antibodies can be tested in blood donations. Prevention is based on avoidance of HBV.

Hepatitis E

Hepatitis E (HEV) was identified in 1990. It is an RNA virus primarily transmitted by ingestion of contaminated water and has symptoms similar to HAV infection. Most reported cases are in developing countries. It neither results in a carrier state nor causes chronic hepatitis. However, fulminating disease leading to liver failure and death have occurred, with women who become infected during pregnancy at highest risk.

Hepatitis G

Hepatitis G (HGV) is an RNA virus that can be transmitted sexually or percutaneously. Little is known about the virus although it has been detected in intravenous drug users, hemodialysis patients, and individuals with chronic HBV or HCV.

Clinical Manifestations

Clinical manifestations of viral hepatitis can range from asymptomatic to profound illness, hepatic failure, and death. There are three stages of illness for all types of hepatitis: the prodromal stage, the icterus (jaundice) stage, and the convalescent (recovery) period.

The prodromal stage, called the preicterus period, begins after the viral incubation period ends and the person begins to have signs of illness. This stage is preicterus because jaundice (icterus) has not yet developed. An individual is highly infectious at this time. Antibodies to the virus are usually not present. This stage lasts 1 to 2 weeks. It is characterized by

- General malaise
- Fatigue
- Symptoms of upper respiratory tract infection
- Myalgia (muscle pain) and arthralgia
- An aversion to most foods, weight loss

- Nausea and vomiting
- Altered sense of taste and smell
- Right upper quadrant tenderness
- Dark urine and clay-colored stools.

The icterus or jaundice stage is the second stage of viral hepatitis, and it may last 2 to 3 weeks or much longer. It is characterized in most people, as its name suggests, by the development of jaundice. Other manifestations include:

- Worsening of all symptoms present during the prodromal stage
- Hepatic tenderness and enlargement
- Splenomegaly
- Possible itchiness (pruritus) of the skin

The recovery stage is the third stage of viral hepatitis and usually happens within 4 months for HBV and HCV and within 2 to 3 months for HAV. During this period:

- Symptoms subside, including jaundice.
- Appetite returns.

Diagnostic Tools

- Liver enzymes are abnormal, beginning in the prodromal stage.
- Antibodies to the virus are elevated, starting in the icterus stage. Some antibody levels subside during the recovery stage; others remain elevated for years.
- Viral antigen is detectable in blood of newly infected individuals and those chronically infected.
- Liver biopsy.

Complications

- A complication of hepatitis is the development of chronic hepatitis that occurs when individuals continue to report symptoms and viral antigens persist for more than 6 months. Symptoms of chronic active or fulminating hepatitis may include those of liver failure, with death occurring anywhere from 1 week to several years later. Chronic hepatitis is most common following infection with HCV and HBV.
- Individuals who are immunocompromised have poorer outcomes.
- Individuals infected with both HBV and HCV are at increased risk of developing cirrhosis, hepatocellular carcinoma, and death. Frequent screening of chronically infected patients for signs of advancing liver disease is warranted.
- Liver failure.

Treatment

- Treatment for viral hepatitis includes supportive measures such as rest as needed, small high-calorie meals, and antiemetics.

- Patients who have hepatitis should avoid consumption of alcohol. Alcohol worsens the degree and accelerates the progression of HBV and especially HCV. Alcohol use in patients who have HCV increases the risk of hepatocellular carcinoma and decreases the response to treatment. Hepatotoxic drugs should also be avoided.

- Individuals with hepatitis should be educated concerning modes of transmission to sexual partners and family members.

- Drug therapy for individuals with infection usually is reserved for those with chronic infection. Injections of interferon alpha (IFN-α), a potent cytokine, have been used to treat both HBV and HBC. Injections are typically given three times a week for at least 3 months. The efficacy of IFN-α for either disease is variable. Even in individuals who do show improvement in liver enzymes with treatment, relief may be temporary, with sustained disappearance of HBV occurring in approximately 30% of patients, while long-term disappearance of HCV occurs less often. Interferon is generally contraindicated for individuals with very advanced liver disease. It is also associated with significant side effects, including myalgia, fever, thrombocytopenia, and depression, all of which lead many to be disqualified for this treatment and others to discontinue treatment early.

- Nucleotide analogues that selectively target the viral enzyme reverse transcriptase have become important medications for the treatment of chronic hepatitis. These drugs were originally developed for use in patients with HIV, and are especially appealing for the large number of patients suffering both HIV and viral hepatitis. The response rate to drugs of this category is high although the cost is a disadvantage. Nucleotide analogues, for example, lamivudine and ribavirin, are usually well tolerated, often making them the first-choice therapy for patients. Other drugs of this type have been developed as well. One limitation is the potential development of resistance to the medication.

- Combination therapies of modified interferons plus nucleotide analogues are the most successful treatments at this time. The modified interferons, called pegylated interferons or peginterferons, have a longer half-life than IFN-α and require less-frequent dosing. Combination therapy is expensive and side effects are distressing and common as with the traditional interferons.

- Relatives of individuals diagnosed with hepatitis are offered a purified gamma globulin specific against HAV or HBV, which may offer passive immunity against infection. This is a temporary immunity. A vaccine against HAV is available. This vaccine is made from inactivated hepatitis virus. Studies have shown that it is 96% effective after one dose.

- A vaccine against HBV is also available. Given the highly contagious nature of the virus and its potentially deadly effects, it is strongly recommended that all individuals, but especially those in high-risk categories, including all health care workers or others exposed to blood products, be vaccinated. It is also recommended that other individuals at high risk for becoming infected by the virus, including homosexuals and heterosexuals sexually active with more than one partner and injection drug users, be vaccinated as well. There do not appear to be any significant side effects following immunization against HBV.

- Since infants infected with HBV are at very high risk of developing chronic infection, it is essential that infants be vaccinated against HBV. While this is imperative for those born in countries with endemic rates of infection, infants worldwide benefit from vaccination soon after birth. There do not appear to be any serious adverse effects of infant vaccination, and in many countries a series of three HBV vaccinations is begun soon after birth. This practice has resulted in a large decrease in the transmission of virus from mother to child and a corresponding decrease in chronic HBV infection and worldwide liver cancer in children.

- Vaccines against HBV are produced by way of recombinant DNA administered intramuscularly three times at predetermined intervals. The first and second doses are given 1 month apart, and the third dose is given 2 to 6 months after the second. Vaccination is 85% effective in producing immunity. Individuals who do not show immunity after three doses, as evidenced by negative HBV antibody titers, are revaccinated. After a third or fourth vaccination, most individuals respond.

LIVER FAILURE

Liver failure is the ultimate outcome of any severe, unrelenting liver disease including liver cancer and cirrhosis. Liver failure may follow years of low-grade HCV infection or may occur suddenly with the onset of fulminating HBV. Acute liver failure may also follow from an overdose of certain medications, including acetaminophen, taken either during a suicide attempt or inadvertently at high doses by individuals using the drug for pain relief. Liver failure is a complex syndrome characterized by the impairment of many different organs and body functions. Two conditions associated with liver failure are hepatic encephalopathy and hepatorenal syndrome.

Hepatic Encephalopathy

Hepatic encephalopathy is a complex of central nervous system disorders seen in individuals suffering from liver failure. It is characterized by memory lapses and personality changes. A flapping tremor can develop. Other jerking movements and poor balance may also be present. An individual suffering from hepatic encephalopathy may ultimately lapse into a coma and die.

Hepatic encephalopathy likely results from the accumulation of toxins in the blood, which occurs when the liver fails to transform or detoxify them adequately. A failing liver is not only unable to detoxify the blood because of poor hepatocyte function, but it receives less blood to detoxify than usual because much of the portal flow is diverted by high resistance and portal hypertension. As toxins and metabolic by-products accumulate, osmotic pressure increases, leading to brain swelling and cerebral edema.

One of the main toxins that accumulates and is implicated in causing many of the symptoms of hepatic encephalopathy is ammonia. Ammonia is a by-product of protein metabolism and intestinal bacterial action. An important function of the liver is to transform ammonia to urea. Unlike ammonia, urea is easily excreted by the kidneys. When the ammonia is not transformed into urea, blood levels increase and ammonia is delivered to the brain. Other substances such as hormones, drugs, and gastrointestinal toxins also accumulate in the blood with advanced liver disease and undoubtedly contribute to hepatic encephalopathy.

Hepatorenal Syndrome

Hepatorenal syndrome refers to the occurrence of renal failure seen in association with advanced liver disease. The kidneys of individuals who have advanced liver disease frequently cease producing urine and fail to function, although the kidneys appear to be physically capable of functioning. Oliguria (decreased production of urine) usually occurs suddenly and is most commonly seen in individuals suffering from alcoholic cirrhosis or fulminating hepatitis. With hepatorenal syndrome, blood volume expands, hydrogen ion accumulates, and electrolyte balance is disturbed.

Suspected causes of functional renal failure associated with liver disease include significant variceal hemorrhage, leading to vascular collapse and shock. All types of shock can lead to a decrease in renal blood flow, which can irreversibly damage the kidney (see Chapter 18). Decreased blood flow to the kidneys might also occur as a result of the peripheral vasoconstriction that occurs in response to ascites and the interstitial accumulation of fluid. Finally, the accumulation of toxins specifically damaging to the kidneys increases because the failing liver is unlikely to be performing biotransformation or detoxification adequately.

Clinical Manifestations

Clinical manifestations of liver failure may be initially subtle but may become extreme as liver failure progresses. Manifestations include:

- Jaundice from impaired ability to conjugate bilirubin.
- Abdominal pain or tenderness from inflamed liver.

- Nausea and anorexia with a profound distaste for certain foods.
- Fatigue and weight loss from deficiencies in the performance of many of the liver functions of metabolism.
- Splenomegaly.
- Ascites.
- Mild confusion to stupor as ammonia accumulates.
- Asterixis or liver flap is a classical finding associated with hepatic encephalopathy.
- Peripheral edema caused by a decrease in the forces favoring reabsorption of fluid into the capillary from the interstitial space, which results from a decrease in plasma protein production and a loss of albumin in ascites.
- Varices of the esophagus, rectum, and abdominal wall resulting from portal hypertension.
- Bleeding tendencies caused by thrombocytopenia (decreased levels of platelets) resulting from blood accumulation in the spleen and prolonged prothrombin time caused by impaired production of several coagulation factors.
- Petechiae (small hemorrhagic spots on the skin) caused by thrombocytopenia.
- Amenorrhea in women, caused by alterations in steroid hormone production and metabolism.
- Gynecomastia (breast enlargement) in males caused by estrogen buildup as the liver fails to perform its biotransformation functions. Testosterone levels usually decrease in men, accompanied by impotence and loss of libido (sex drive).

Diagnostic Tools

- Altered liver function tests.
- Blood analysis demonstrates anemia owing to various small and large bleeds, sequestration of red blood cells in the spleen, and impaired production of red blood cells.
- Bleeding and clotting studies are abnormal.
- Hypoglycemia may occur because gluconeogenesis is impaired.

Complications

- Hepatic encephalopathy.
- Hepatorenal syndrome.
- Variceal bleeding.
- Coma and death may result.

Treatment

Although there is no cure for liver failure short of liver transplant, individual symptoms and clinical manifestations can be treated. Treatments are specific for various manifestations. Ascites is treated as follows:

- Dietary restriction of salt and a potassium-sparing diuretic increase water excretion.
- Potassium supplementation may be necessary to reverse the effects of high aldosterone.
- Measures to remove ascitic fluid to relieve discomfort may be performed and include placing a shunt between the peritoneal cavity and the vena cava or paracentesis (aspiration drainage of fluid out of the peritoneal cavity with a large-bore needle). Both measures increase the risk of infection, and paracentesis can cause hypotension. Neither treatment is a cure for the ascites, which returns as long as liver disease continues.

Portal hypertension is treated as follows:

- A connection or shunt between the portal vein and another systemic vein can be made to relieve the diversion of blood to the esophagus and other collateral vessels. This maneuver does not restore liver function, but it may reduce collateral flow and the complication of variceal bleeding. It may also reduce ascites. One example of such a connection is a transjugular intrahepatic portosystemic shunt. Careful selection and monitoring of patients for this procedure is essential.

Variceal bleeding is treated as follows:

- A vasoconstrictor drug may be given to decrease flow. Balloon tamponade—the insertion of a balloon catheter into the esophagus to exert pressure on the bleeding varicele—may be performed. Surgical treatment to tie off the collateral vessels sprouting from the portal vein may be attempted. Vitamin K supplementation can help control bleeding.

Hepatic encephalopathy treatments are as follows:

- Ventilation and sedation to protect the airway and to reduce psychomotor agitation, and bolus injections of mannitol to reduce cerebral edema are administered. Blood glucose is closely monitored because hypoglycemia may occur with liver failure.
- Most dietary advice is concerned with restriction of dietary protein and inclusion of high-carbohydrate sources.
- Prevention of infections and rapid treatment is important.
- Liver dialysis (artificial extracorporeal liver support) is increasingly being used.
- Liver transplants are becoming more common for the treatment of advanced liver disease. There is variable success for this procedure, depending on the

cause of liver failure and the individual patient. The increase in transplants over the past 20 years has reduced chronic liver disease mortality in the United States.

LIVER CANCER

Primary liver cancer is uncommon in the United States but much more common worldwide. When it does occur, it is usually seen in individuals who have a history of HBV or HCV infection or who have chronic liver disease, for example, cirrhosis. Others known to be at high risk for developing liver cancer include those exposed to high levels of known carcinogens, including aflatoxins found on moldy corn or peanuts. Primary liver cancers may be of the hepatocytes themselves (hepatocellular carcinoma) or of the bile ducts (cholangiocarcinoma). The prognosis is poor and death usually occurs within 6 months of diagnosis due to gastrointestinal hemorrhage, cachexia, liver failure, or metastasis.

Secondary liver cancer is the result of a metastasis of cancer from areas of the body (e.g., the intestine or the pancreas) that drain into the liver through the portal vein or from other cancers. In the Unitied States it is significantly more prevalent than primary liver cancer. Both primary and secondary liver cancers themselves frequently metastasize outside the liver, especially to the heart and lungs, because hepatic drainage encounters these organs first. All types of liver cancer have poor prognoses, often related to intrahepatic recurrence of the cancer. Less than 5% of individuals with liver cancer survive longer than 5 years.

Clinical Manifestations

- Initially symptoms may be vague such as weakness, fatigue, and malaise.
- Dull abdominal pain.
- A feeling of abdominal fullness.
- Nausea and vomiting.
- Jaundice.
- Anorexia (decreased appetite) and aversion to certain foods.
- Palpable mass in the right upper quadrant.
- If the tumor obstructs the bile duct, portal hypertension and ascites may develop. Jaundice worsens, and colicky pain may develop.
- Hepatomegaly.

Diagnostic Tools

- Elevated liver enzymes.
- Elevated levels of a protein normally not present in adult serum, alpha-fetoprotein.
- Magnetic resonance imaging reveals a tumor.
- Liver biopsy.

Treatment

- Surgery for some tumors is possible, although outcomes tend to be poor related to intrahepatic metastases that lead to recurrence. Recent evidence suggests that downregulation of the immune response–related genes (HLA genes) that encode MHC class II antigens may occur in patients and contribute to cancer recurrence, suggesting a possible target for future therapy.
- Chemotherapy.
- Liver transplant if the tumor is small and there is no evidence of spread.

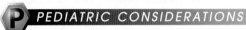

PEDIATRIC CONSIDERATIONS

- Infants and children are particularly dependent on fatty acid oxidation during periods of fasting as a result of reduced glycogen storage, immature activity of enzymes involved in glycolysis and gluconeogenesis, and increased basal metabolic needs. Ketone bodies are produced and can serve as alternative fuel for cardiac and skeletal muscles. Excess ketones, however, can lower blood pH.
- Especially at risk of developing HAV are toddlers and children who have poor toilet hygiene and children who are cared for by individuals (in day care centers or at home) who do not follow rigorous hand-washing practices after diaper changing.
- Especially at risk of developing HBV are infants born to mothers who have HBV. The virus responsible for HBV may pass from mother to fetus through the placenta if the mother becomes infected in the third trimester of pregnancy or suffers from chronic HBV infection. Exposure of an infant to infected blood before or during birth may also result in the infant developing the disease. There is a 90% risk of chronic hepatitis developing in infants infected with HBV before or during birth, making it a serious neonatal infection. Therefore, all infants, regardless of the known HBV status of the mother, are recommended to receive vaccination against HBV within 7 days of birth. Those born to mothers known to be infected are also recommended to receive the HBV immunoglobulin (gamma globulin).
- Liver failure in children is an uncommon occurrence but is devastating when it does happen. Most cases result from acute autoimmune hepatitis, drug toxicity, or an unknown etiology. Wilson disease, a genetic disorder resulting in the retention of copper in various organs of the body including the liver, is also a known cause of pediatric liver failure.

GERIATRIC CONSIDERATIONS

- Decreased liver size, weight and blood flow is associated with aging.
- The older adult is more susceptible to effects of toxins and drugs. Medication dosage adjustments may be necessary to accommodate for decreased liver function and to prevent toxicity.

SELECTED BIBLIOGRAPHY

Agency for Healthcare Research and Quality (AHRQ). (2008). *Management of chronic hepatitis B*. Retrieved August 21, 2009, from http://www.ahrq.gov/clinic/tp/hepbtp.htm.

Alonso, E. M. (2005). Acute liver failure in children: The role of defects in fatty acid oxidation. *Hepatology*, 41, 696–699.

Atlas of Pathophysiology (3rd ed.). (2010). Philadelphia, PA: Lippincott Williams & Wilkins.

Bataller, R., Sancho-Bru, P., Gines, P., & Brenner, D. A. (2005). Liver fibrogenesis: A new role for the renin–angiotensin system. *Antioxidants and Redox Signalling*, 7, 1346–1355.

Blei, A. T. (2005). The pathophysiology of brain edema in acute liver failure. *Neurochemistry International*, 47, 71–77.

Boyer, T. D., & Haskal, Z. J. (2005). American Association for the Study of Liver Diseases practice guidelines: The role of transjugular intrahepatic portosystemic shunt creation in the management of portal hypertension. *Journal of Vascular and Interventional Radiology*, 16, 615–629.

Burke, B. L., Robbins, J. M., Bird, T. M., Hobbs, C. A., Nesmith, C., & Tilford, J. M. (2009). Trends in hospitalizations for neonatal jaundice and kernicterus in the United States, 1988–2005. *Pediatrics*, 123(2), 524–532.

Centers for Disease Control and Prevention (CDC). (2008). *Viral hepatitis*. Retrieved October 17, 2009, from http://www.cdc.gov/hepatitis/.

Copstead, L. C., & Banasik, J. L. (2010). *Pathophysiology*. St. Louis, MO: Saunders Elsevier.

Guyton, A. C., & Hall, J. (2006). *Textbook of medical physiology* (11th ed.). Philadelphia, PA: W.B. Saunders.

Jonas, M. M. (2009). Hepatitis B and pregnancy: An underestimated issue. *Liver International*, 29(s1), 133–139.

Jones, R., Dunning, J., & Nelson, M. (2005). HIV and hepatitis C co-infection. *International Journal of Clinical Practice*, 59, 1082–1087.

Kennedy, P. T., Phillips, N., Chandrasekhar, J., Jacobs, R., Jacobs, M., & Dusheiko, G. (2008). Potential and limitations of lamivudine monotherapy in chronic hepatitis B: Evidence from genotyping. *Liver International*, 28(5), 699–704.

LaVecchia, C. (2005). Coffee, liver enzymes, cirrhosis and liver cancer. *Journal of Hepatology*, 42, 444–446.

Maisels, M. J. (2005). Jaundice. In M. G. MacDonald, M. D. Mullett, & M. Seshia (Eds.). *Avery's neonatology: Pathophysiology and management of the newborn* (6th ed., pp. 768–846). Philadelphia, PA: Lippincott Williams & Wilkins.

Osborn, K. S., Wraa, C. E., & Watson, A. B. (2010). *Medical-surgical nursing: Preparation for practice*. Upper Saddle River, NJ: Pearson.

Porth, C. M., & Matfin, G. (2009). *Pathophysiology: Concepts of altered health states* (8th ed.). Philadelphia, PA: Lippincott Williams & Wilkins.

Profit, J., Cambric-Hargrove, A. J., Tittle, K. O., Pietz, K., & Stark, A. R. (2009). Delayed pediatric office follow-up of newborns after birth hospitalization. *Pediatrics*, 124(2), 548–554.

Radovich, P. (2008). Buting time for patients with acute liver failure. *American Nurse Today*, 3(11), 10–12.

Reau, N. S. (2009). The hepatitis C virus: Prospecting for specifically targeted therapies. *Medscape CME Gastroenterology*. Retrieved October 17, 2009, from http://cme.medscape.com/viewarticle/709545.

Tabloski, P. A. (2010). *Gerontological nursing*. Upper Saddle River, NJ: Pearson.

Teutsch, H. F. (2005). The modular microarchitecture of human liver. *Hepatology*, 42, 317–325.

Thomas, D. J. (2007). Abdominal problems. In L. M. Dunphy, J. E. Winland-Brown, B. O. Porter, & D. J. Thomas (Eds.). *Primary care: The art and science of advanced practice nursing* (2nd ed., pp. 473–561). Philadelphia, PA: F. A. Davis.

The Genitourinary System

Although the kidney is sometimes thought of as simply being an organ for waste elimination, it is much more than that. Major functions of the kidney include:

- Regulation of fluid and electrolyte balance.
- Maintenance of pH balance.
- Regulation of calcium/phosphate balance.
- Activation of intestinally absorbed vitamin D.
- Excretion of waste products.
- Regulation of blood pressure.
- Production of erythropoietin.

● Physiologic Concepts

STRUCTURE

The kidneys lie outside the peritoneal cavity in the upper posterior portion of the abdominal wall, one on each side of the body. Each kidney is made up of approximately one million functional units, each of which is called a **nephron**. As shown in Figure 18-1, the nephron begins as a capillary tuft, called the glomerulus. Plasma is **filtered** across the glomerulus by the process of bulk flow and enters the twisting, looping tubule of the nephron. Of the plasma that enters the tubule, only a small fraction is excreted as urine. The remaining

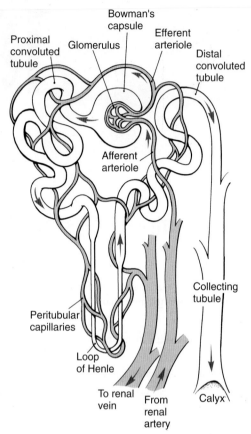

FIGURE 18-1 Structure of the nephron. (From Bullock, B.A., & Henze, R.L. (2000). *Focus on pathophysiology.* Philadelphia, PA: Lippincott Williams & Wilkins.)

plasma, compared with what entered the tubule across the glomerular capillary, has its final composition and volume drastically altered by the processes of renal **reabsorption** and **secretion**.

Each kidney is divided anatomically into an outer cortex containing all the glomerular capillaries and some short tubular segments, and an inner medulla where most of the tubular segments are located. The progression of tubular segments from the glomerulus to the proximal tubule, to the distal tubule, and finally to the collecting tubule is shown in Figure 18-1. Each nephron's collecting tubule joins other collecting tubules to become several hundred large collecting ducts. The large collecting ducts are located in the renal papillae, which are located in the innermost portion of the kidney, the renal medulla.

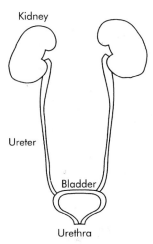

FIGURE 18-2 Urinary tract.

The large collecting ducts feed into a central draining area, called the renal pelvis, and from there empty into the ureter. The ureter from each kidney is connected to the bladder (Fig. 18-2). The bladder stores urine until it is released outside the body by the process of micturition (urination). Micturition occurs through a single tube called the urethra.

RENAL BLOOD FLOW

The kidneys receive approximately 1000 to 1200 mL of blood per minute which is 20% to 25% of the cardiac output. Of that amount, only 1% to 2% goes to the medulla while the remainder circulates through the cortex. This high rate of blood flow is not required for meeting extraordinary energy demands, but for allowing the kidney to adjust the blood composition continually. By adjusting the blood composition, the kidney is able to maintain blood volume; ensure sodium, chloride, potassium, calcium, phosphate, and pH balance; and eliminate products of metabolism such as urea and creatinine.

Blood flows to the kidneys via the renal arteries, one renal artery to each kidney. In the kidney, the renal artery branches many times, ending as several afferent arterioles. Each afferent arteriole becomes the glomerular capillary that supplies a nephron with blood.

The glomerular capillary reforms not to become a venule as most capillaries do, but to form the efferent arteriole. This is shown in Figure 18-1. The efferent arteriole soon branches into a second capillary network, the peritubular capillaries, which surround and support the nephron tubules themselves. At the end of each nephron, the peritubular capillaries finally reform to venules. The venules join to become veins. Blood leaves the kidney and heads back to the vena cava to be recirculated. The peritubular capillaries surrounding the long loop of the nephron (the loop of Henle) are called the **vasa recta**.

FILTRATION, REABSORPTION, AND SECRETION

Filtration refers to the bulk flow of plasma across the glomerular capillary into the interstitial fluid space surrounding the start of the nephron, an area called the *Bowman space*. At the glomerulus, approximately 20% of the plasma is continually filtered into the Bowman space. This filtrate is of the same composition as the plasma, except that protein molecules are not usually filtered. The initial filtrate diffuses across the Bowman space and into the beginning section of the tubule, *Bowman capsule*, to begin its journey through the rest of the tubule.

Most of the substances that enter the tubule at the Bowman capsule do not remain in the tubule. Instead, they move (or are moved) back into the blood across the peritubular capillaries by the process of **reabsorption**. Other substances are added to the urine filtrate, also across the peritubular capillaries, by the process of **secretion**. It is by reabsorption and secretion that the nephrons manipulate the composition and volume of the initial urine filtrate to produce the final urine.

GLOMERULAR FILTRATION

Glomerular filtration is the process by which approximately 20% of the plasma entering the glomerular capillary moves across the capillary into the interstitial space and from there into the Bowman capsule. Neither red blood cells nor plasma proteins are more than minimally filtered in healthy kidneys.

The process of filtration across the glomerulus is similar to that which occurs across all capillaries, as described in Chapter 13. What is different in the kidney is that the glomerular capillaries have increased permeability to small solutes and water. Also, unlike other capillaries, the forces favoring filtration of plasma across the glomerular capillary into the Bowman space are greater than the forces favoring reabsorption of fluid back into the capillary. Therefore, net filtration of fluid into the Bowman space occurs. This fluid then diffuses into the Bowman capsule and begins its journey through the rest of the nephron.

In the glomerulus, the primary force favoring filtration is capillary pressure. In most other capillaries, this pressure averages 18 mm Hg; in the glomerulus the average pressure is almost 60 mm Hg. This higher capillary pressure occurs as a result of decreased resistance to flow offered by the afferent arteriole feeding the glomerulus, compared with arterioles elsewhere. Therefore, the hydrostatic pressure reaching the glomerulus is greater, as shown in Figure 18-3.

Interstitial fluid pressure in the Bowman space is also much greater than in normal interstitial spaces (approximately 15 mm Hg vs. approximately −3 mm Hg). This greater pressure is a result of the high fluid volume entering

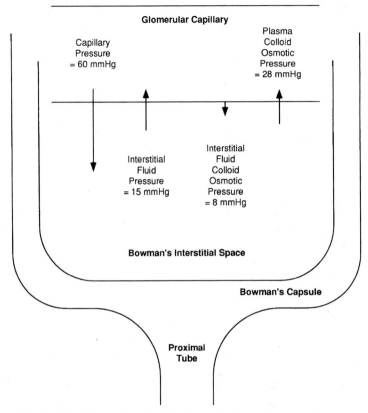

FIGURE 18-3 Forces favoring filtration and reabsorption across the glomerular capillary.

the Bowman space from the glomerulus, thus opposing further glomerular filtration. Capillary concentration of protein (plasma colloid osmotic pressure) is the same in the glomerulus as in other capillaries. The plasma colloid osmotic pressure increases throughout the length of the glomerulus as the protein-free filtrate is pushed into the Bowman space, averaging approximately 28 mm Hg overall; this force opposes glomerular filtration. The interstitial fluid colloid osmotic pressure (the pressure exerted by interstitial proteins) is normally approximately 8 mm Hg; this pressure favors glomerular filtration.

Adding up the forces favoring filtration across the glomerulus (60 + 8 mm Hg) and the forces favoring reabsorption (28 + 15 mm Hg), a net force of approximately 25 mm Hg results favoring the filtration of plasma into the Bowman space. This filtrate enters the Bowman capsule, moves through the tubule, and a portion of it becomes urine.

Glomerular Filtration Rate

The glomerular filtration rate (GFR) is defined as the volume of filtrate entering the Bowman capsule per unit of time. GFR is nearly constant and gives a good indication of the health of the kidneys. GFR depends on the four forces determining filtration and reabsorption (capillary pressure, interstitial fluid pressure, plasma colloid osmotic pressure, and interstitial fluid colloid osmotic pressure). Therefore, any change in these forces can alter GFR. Likewise, GFR depends on the available surface area of the glomerulus for filtration. Therefore, a loss of glomerular surface area decreases GFR.

An average value for GFR in an adult is 180 L/day (125 mL/min). A normal plasma volume is approximately 3 L (out of a total blood volume of approximately 5 L). This means that the kidney filters the plasma approximately 60 times each day! Equally remarkable is the fact that of the 180 L/day filtered into the Bowman capsule, only approximately 1.5 L/day are excreted from the body as urine. The rest is reabsorbed back into the blood across the peritubular capillaries.

Measurement of Glomerular Filtration Rate

GFR measurement is possible if one has a substance (call it x) that is freely filterable at the glomerulus and then is not reabsorbed, secreted, or changed in any way before it appears in the urine. To calculate the GFR from this substance, one would measure its concentration in a plasma sample (P_x), its concentration in a urine sample (U_x), and the urine volume over a certain period of time (V). Given these values, the equation for GFR, in milliliters per minute, can be solved as shown in the following equation:

$$\text{GFR(mL/min)} = \frac{U_x(\text{mg/mL})V(\text{mL/min})}{P_x(\text{mg/mL})} \qquad (18\text{-}1)$$

The classic substance that fits the criteria described above for substance x is the polysaccharide inulin. However, inulin is not normally present in the body, which means using inulin to measure GFR involves infusing it into an individual for an extended period. This offers a highly accurate but impractical method for measuring GFR. Instead, what is usually measured in plasma and urine is the concentration of creatinine, which is a naturally produced protein.

Creatinine is produced as a result of normal daily protein metabolism, a process that is assumed to occur at a nearly constant rate. This assumption may not hold true, for example, it may increase after muscle trauma or intense exercise. To measure GFR using creatinine, a blood sample is drawn along with a timed urine sample, and creatinine concentrations in the blood and urine are measured.

GFR measured from creatinine concentration and urine volume is only an estimate of the true GFR, because a small amount of creatinine is actually secreted into the lumen of the tubule from the peritubular capillaries. Therefore, GFR estimated by creatinine will be slightly high, because more creatinine will be excreted in the urine than was filtered at the glomerulus. Measurement of GFR is important because it offers a clue to nephron function. In conditions of disease leading to renal failure, GFR falls.

RENAL CLEARANCE

The concentration of a substance totally cleared from the blood into the urine over time is known as the renal clearance. The GFR described above for inulin is actually the clearance of inulin, because all filtered inulin is cleared by the kidneys (it is neither reabsorbed nor secreted). For creatinine, clearance is actually slightly greater than the GFR, because some creatinine is secreted into the urine as well as filtered.

Other substances not normally excreted in the urine, such as glucose, have zero clearance. Although glucose is freely filtered across the glomerulus, it is normally totally reabsorbed by the tubules and none appears in the urine (i.e., none is cleared). Substances that are partially reabsorbed back into the plasma, for example, sodium and chloride ion, are cleared at a rate less than the GFR but greater than zero. Substances that are secreted from the blood into the tubule are cleared at a rate greater than the GFR.

Measuring the clearance of any substance is done by the same technique as measuring GFR. The concentration of the substance in the plasma and urine is determined, as is the urine volume over a given period. The equation expressing the clearance of any substance is UV/P, where U is the concentration of the substance in the urine (milligrams [mg] per milliliter [mL]), V is the volume per time of urine (mg/mL), and P is the concentration of the substance in the plasma (mg/mL).

Only for a substance like inulin (freely filtered, neither reabsorbed nor secreted) is the GFR equal to the clearance. For all other substances, clearance is either more or less than the GFR. Measuring the clearance of a plasma substance that is 100% excreted by the kidneys allows one to estimate renal plasma flow, and from there, renal blood flow.

MEASUREMENT OF RENAL PLASMA FLOW AND RENAL BLOOD FLOW

Measuring renal plasma flow usually involves measuring the clearance of a substance called *para*-aminohippurate (PAH). PAH is freely filtered at the glomerulus. It is not reabsorbed, but is actively secreted into the urine filtrate. Therefore, all PAH in the plasma (100%) is cleared by the kidneys. The clearance of PAH gives an estimate of renal plasma flow. Because the plasma is approximately 40% to 50% of the total blood volume, this allows one to estimate renal blood flow.

It is only possible to estimate renal blood flow from clearance of PAH because not all plasma entering the kidney goes through a glomerular capillary. Approximately 10% to 15% of renal blood flow feeds nonfiltering tissue such as renal fat and connective tissue. Therefore, clearance of PAH is said to give the **effective renal plasma flow** (ERPF), which is 10% to 15% less than the total renal plasma flow, as shown in the following equation:

$$C_{pah} = \frac{U_{pah}V}{P_{pah}} = ERPF \qquad (18\text{-}2)$$

From the ERPF, the effective renal blood flow (ERBF) can be found with the following equation:

$$ERBF = \frac{ERPF}{1 - Vc} \qquad (18\text{-}3)$$

where Vc is the measured hematocrit of the blood sample (the amount of blood occupied by red blood cells, not plasma).

REGULATION OF RENAL BLOOD FLOW

Maintenance of adequate renal blood flow is essential for kidney survival and for control of plasma volume and electrolytes. Changes in renal blood flow may increase or decrease the glomerular hydrostatic pressure, affecting GFR. The kidney has several mechanisms for controlling renal blood flow. These mechanisms serve to maintain both kidney function and GFR constant in spite of systemic blood pressure changes.

Renal blood flow is controlled by intrarenal and extrarenal mechanisms. Intrarenal mechanisms include the inherent ability of the afferent and the efferent arterioles to dilate or constrict, thereby controlling blood flow through the kidney. This inherent ability is called **autoregulation**. Extrarenal mechanisms regulating renal blood flow include the direct effects of increased or decreased mean arterial pressure and the effects of the sympathetic nervous system. A third mechanism regulating renal blood flow that has both intrarenal and extrarenal components involves a hormone produced by the kidney that affects the entire systemic circulation. This hormone, called renin, exerts its effects through the production of a potent vasoconstrictor, angiotensin II (AII).

Autoregulation

Autoregulation is the intrinsic response of vascular smooth muscle to changes in blood pressure. Like many arterioles, smooth muscle cells of the afferent and the efferent arterioles respond to their own stretch with reflex constriction. When systemic blood pressure is increased, stretch on afferent arterioles is increased. Stretching the afferent arterioles causes them to constrict, reducing the blood flow and returning renal blood pressure back toward normal. In contrast, when systemic blood pressure is decreased, stretch on the afferent and the efferent arterioles is reduced, and the arterioles respond by relaxing and dilating to increase flow. As a result of autoregulation, renal blood flow remains nearly constant over a range of blood pressures between 80 and 180 mm Hg.

Autoregulation is especially effective during blood pressure increases. The bottom limit of autoregulation, 80 mm Hg, however, is reached more frequently than the upper limit. Therefore, GFR may decrease with severe hypotension.

Sympathetic Nervous System

Sympathetic nerves innervate both the afferent and the efferent arterioles of the kidney and can override autoregulation when stimulated. As is true in most arterioles, stimulation of the sympathetic nerves causes constriction of the afferent arterioles, leading to increased resistance to flow. As a result, blood flow through the glomerulus decreases, causing a decrease both in capillary hydrostatic pressure and in GFR. Simultaneous sympathetic stimulation of the efferent arterioles, however, and their subsequent constriction, causes blood flow to back up in the glomerulus. This backup can actually increase capillary hydrostatic pressure and glomerular filtration. The net result of sympathetic stimulation to the kidneys is a significant decrease in renal blood flow (because blood going both in and out is reduced) but a lesser decrease in GFR. The sympathetic nervous system is stimulated when there is a decrease in systemic blood pressure.

Decreased renal blood flow in response to decreased systemic blood pressure is adaptive and helps the organism survive a hypotensive crisis. With hypotension, less water and salt are filtered at the glomerulus, causing less to be lost in the urine. This helps to increase blood volume and restore blood pressure.

In conditions of increased blood pressure, sympathetic stimulation to all arterioles is reduced. The afferent and the efferent arterioles dilate, and renal blood flow and GFR both increase. This change results in increased loss of water and salt in the urine, which helps to reduce blood volume and return blood pressure toward normal.

Note that sympathetic input dominates over autoregulatory mechanisms of the kidney. If sympathetic stimulation increases, renal blood flow decreases despite attempts by the kidney to autoregulate its flow.

Renin

Renin is a hormone released from the kidney in response to either a decrease in blood pressure or a decrease in plasma sodium concentration. Cells that synthesize and secrete renin and control its release are a particular group of cells of the nephron called the **juxtaglomerular (JG) apparatus**. This group of cells includes smooth muscle cells of the afferent arteriole and cells of the macula densa. The smooth muscle cells synthesize renin and act as baroreceptors monitoring blood pressure. Macula densa cells are part of the thick ascending limb of the nephron. These cells sense plasma sodium concentration. The macula densa cells and the afferent arteriolar cells are in close approximation to each other where the ascending limb of the distal tubule nearly touches the glomerulus. When the macula densa cells sense a change in plasma sodium, they pass that message on to the renin-secreting cells.

When blood pressure falls, the smooth muscle cells increase renin release. When blood pressure increases, the smooth muscle cells decrease their release of renin. If plasma sodium levels decrease, macula densa cells signal the renin-producing cells to increase their activity. If plasma sodium levels increase, macula densa cells signal the smooth muscle cells to decrease renin release.

Sympathetic nerves also stimulate the JG apparatus to secrete renin. Thus, decreased blood pressure causes increased renin both directly, via the JG baroreceptors, and indirectly, via the sympathetic nerves.

Once released, renin circulates in the blood and acts to catalyze the breakdown of a small protein, angiotensinogen, to a 10–amino-acid protein, angiotensin I (AI). Angiotensinogen is produced by the liver and is highly concentrated in the blood. Renin release is thus the rate-limiting step in the reaction. The conversion of angiotensinogen to AI occurs throughout the plasma, but primarily in the pulmonary capillaries. AI has few effects of its own, but it is quickly acted upon by another enzyme readily available in the bloodstream—angiotensin-converting enzyme (ACE). ACE splits AI into an 8–amino-acid peptide, angiotensin II (AII).

Angiotensin II

AII is a potent vasoconstrictor that acts throughout the vascular system to increase smooth muscle contraction, thereby decreasing vessel diameter and increasing total peripheral resistance (TPR). An increase in TPR directly increases systemic blood pressure (see Chapter 13). AII is also a potent hormone that circulates in the blood to the adrenal glands, causing the synthesis of the mineralocorticoid hormone aldosterone.

Aldosterone

Aldosterone circulates in the blood and binds to cells of the cortical collecting duct. The binding of aldosterone increases sodium reabsorption from the urine filtrate, causing sodium to return into the peritubular capillaries. Since water often follows sodium movement, increased sodium reabsorption allows for increased water reabsorption, causing increased plasma volume. An increase in plasma volume increases venous return to the heart, thereby increasing the stroke volume and cardiac output. Increased cardiac output, like increased TPR, directly increases systemic blood pressure.

Other stimuli for aldosterone release, besides AII, are high plasma potassium level and a hormone from the anterior pituitary, adrenocorticotropic hormone (ACTH). In addition to affecting sodium reabsorption, aldosterone stimulates the secretion (and therefore the excretion) of potassium from the cortical collecting duct into the urine filtrate. Aldosterone affects sodium and potassium transport across the gut, in the same manner as it does across the collecting duct.

Renin–Angiotensin Reflex Response to Changes in Blood Pressure

With a decrease in blood pressure, the JG cells release renin, which in turn causes an increase in AII. AII constricts arterioles throughout the body, including the afferent and the efferent arterioles. AII-induced constriction increases TPR and a return of blood pressure back toward normal (Fig. 18-4). Renal blood flow is reduced, which causes less urine to be produced. Decreased urine output contributes to increased plasma volume and blood pressure.

The opposite occurs with increased blood pressure. With an increase in blood pressure, renin release decreases, as do AII levels. This leads to dilation of systemic arterioles, a reduction of TPR, and a return of blood pressure back toward normal. Decreased AII causes afferent and efferent arterioles to relax, leading to an increase in renal blood flow and urine output, which also serves to decrease blood pressure.

Renin–Angiotensin–Aldosterone Response to Decreased Sodium

The second stimulus for renin release is plasma sodium concentration. Decreased sodium in the tubular fluid passing the cells of the macula densa causes increased

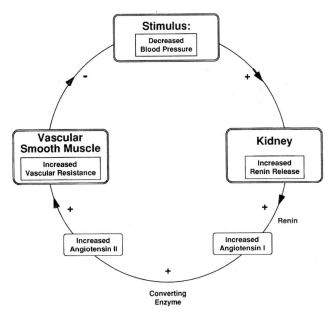

FIGURE 18-4 Response of renin, AI, and AII to a decrease in blood pressure.

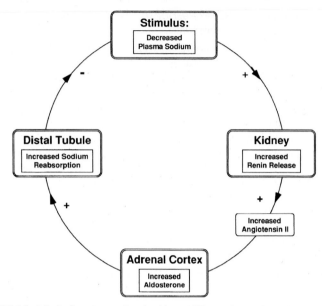

FIGURE 18-5 Response of renin, AI, and AII to a decrease in plasma sodium.

renin release. As shown in Figure 18-5, increased renin leads to increased AII, which stimulates aldosterone synthesis and therefore increases sodium reabsorption. Increased sodium reabsorption reduces the stimulus for further renin release. The opposite is true if there is increased plasma sodium passing the macula densa cells.

RENAL REABSORPTION

Reabsorption is the second process by which the kidney determines the concentration of a substance filtered from the plasma. Reabsorption refers to the active (requiring energy and always being mediated by a carrier) or the passive (no energy required) movement of a substance filtered at the glomerulus back into the peritubular capillaries. Reabsorption may be total (e.g., glucose) or partial (e.g., sodium, urea, chloride, and water).

Reabsorption of Glucose

Glucose is freely filtered at the glomerulus. All of the filtered glucose is normally reabsorbed by active transport, primarily in the proximal tubule.

Because carriers are involved, a transport maximum (Tm) for glucose can be reached. The Tm is the amount of a substance that can be transported per unit of time. For glucose, at a certain filtered load (GFR × plasma concentration), all carriers become occupied. Any glucose filtered beyond that load is not reabsorbed, but is instead excreted in the urine. The Tm for glucose is approximately 375 mg/min of filtered glucose. The concentration of glucose which results in this filtered load, given a GFR of 125 mL/min, is 3.0 mg/mL of plasma because glucose concentration clinically is frequently expressed as per 100 mL of blood, or, 300 mg/dL. However, glucose begins to appear in the urine even before this plasma level is reached, because each nephron has a slightly different Tm and the carrier transport rate may accelerate at the highest glucose concentrations. Plasma glucose seldom gets high enough that glucose Tm is reached unless an individual has diabetes mellitus (see Chapter 16). Note that the kidney does not control blood glucose levels; it simply filters and reabsorbs all it can. The pancreas, via insulin release, controls blood glucose.

In the kidney, glucose reabsorption is coupled with the reabsorption of sodium ions from the urine filtrate into the tubular cells. At some point this movement is driven by the splitting of adenosine triphosphate (ATP) by the sodium–potassium ATPase. It is a process that requires energy. It is this secondary use of energy that makes glucose transport an active (energy-requiring) process.

Reabsorption of Sodium

Sodium reabsorption occurs throughout the tubule by a combination of simple diffusion and active transport. Approximately 65% of sodium reabsorption occurs across the proximal tubule and 25% across the loop of Henle. Therefore, only approximately 10% of the filtered sodium remains in the tubule by the time the filtrate reaches the distal convoluted tubule. The final concentration of sodium in the urine is usually less than 1% of the total amount filtered at the glomerulus.

Unlike glucose, plasma sodium concentration is regulated by the kidney. Although sodium is freely filtered and 98% to 99% is normally reabsorbed, the final 1% to 2% of its reabsorption can vary. Plasma sodium concentration is 145 mmol/L, and the amount of filtered sodium is approximately 18 mmol/min (supposing a GFR of approximately 180 L/day). This amounts to approximately 1500 g of sodium filtered each day. Even if only 2% of this amount—30 g/day—is excreted, it is a considerable amount. This final 1% to 2% is controlled by the presence or absence of the hormone aldosterone.

Transport of sodium out of the nephron and back into the capillaries may either be coupled in the same direction to the reabsorption of another substance (cotransport), or it may be coupled in the opposite direction with another substance (counter-transport). Substances cotransported with sodium include glucose, amino acids, and chloride. Hydrogen ion (H^+) is counter-transported and thus secreted into the urine when a sodium ion is reabsorbed.

Reabsorption of Chloride

Chloride reabsorption can be active or passive and is nearly always coupled to sodium transport. It is affected by the electrical gradient across the tubule. Like sodium, most chloride reabsorption (65%) occurs across the proximal tubule, less across the loop of Henle (25%), and the rest (10%) between the distal convoluted tubule and the collecting-duct system.

Reabsorption of Potassium

Most potassium in the body is present intracellularly. Therefore, although plasma potassium is freely filtered across the glomerulus, its concentration in the Bowman capsule is low. Most potassium that is filtered is reabsorbed: 50% across the proximal tubule, 40% in the thick ascending limb, and the remaining 10% in the final part of the nephron, the medullary collecting duct. Most potassium reabsorption occurs by passive diffusion.

Potassium is also *secreted* into the tubule by active transport across the cells of the proximal tubule, the descending limb of the loop of Henle, and the collecting ducts. The amount of secreted potassium is variable and depends on the amount of potassium ingested in the diet. An individual on a high-potassium diet filters, reabsorbs, *and* secretes potassium. An individual on a low-potassium diet only filters and reabsorbs, but does not secrete, potassium. Potassium secretion by the collecting ducts is stimulated by the hormone aldosterone released from the adrenal cortex.

Reabsorption of the Amino Acids

Amino acids filtered at the glomerulus are actively reabsorbed in the proximal tubule. All reabsorption of amino acids is carrier-mediated. The Tm for the carriers is well above the amounts of amino acids normally filtered, so none are normally present in the urine.

Reabsorption of Plasma Proteins

Very few plasma proteins are filtered across the glomerulus. Those that are filtered are actively reabsorbed across the proximal tubule. Because the GFR is so high, the filtration of even a few molecules of plasma protein, such as albumin, would result in a significant daily loss of protein if reabsorption did not occur.

The few proteins filtered at the glomerulus are not reabsorbed. They are degraded by tubular cells and excreted in the urine. Examples of these proteins include the protein hormones, such as growth hormone and luteinizing hormone, both of which are secreted from the anterior pituitary.

Reabsorption of Urea

Urea is produced in the liver as an end-product of protein metabolism. It is freely filtered at the glomerulus. Because urea is highly permeable across most (but not all) of the nephron, it diffuses back into the peritubular capillaries. It follows water as water is reabsorbed from the urine filtrate moving through the nephron. By the end of the proximal tubule, approximately 50% of the filtered urea has been reabsorbed. From the end of the proximal tubule to the medullary collecting ducts, the proximal tubule is impermeable to urea. Along this route, some portions of the tubule begin to secrete urea into the filtrate. Thus, at the point the filtrate reaches the medullary collecting ducts, urea concentration has again reached what it was in the original glomerular filtrate. At the medullary collecting ducts, urea once more becomes permeable and again follows water reabsorption out of the tubule. As the filtrate leaves the kidney, approximately 40% of the original filtered urea remains and is excreted.

Note that urea reabsorption depends on water reabsorption. If water reabsorption is low, more urea will be excreted, and vice versa.

ACID–BASE HANDLING

The kidney plays a pivotal role in maintaining acid–base balance. Most metabolic processes in the body produce acid (see Chapter 19). These processes include oxidative phosphorylation, which produces the volatile acid carbon dioxide, and the metabolism of proteins, which produce nonvolatile acids such as sulfuric and phosphoric acids. Although the lungs normally excrete all carbon dioxide produced by oxidation, the kidney is the only organ capable of eliminating nonvolatile acids. More importantly, the kidneys have the essential job of reabsorbing large quantities of the base bicarbonate, which is freely filtered at the glomerulus. Without this function, fatally low blood pH would occur. The kidneys assist in eliminating acid produced by cell metabolism in individuals who have lung disease by increasing the secretion and excretion of acid and by reabsorbing increased amount of base.

Reabsorption of Bicarbonate

Reabsorption of bicarbonate is an active process that occurs primarily in the proximal tubule (and to a lesser extent in the collecting ducts). As shown in Figure 18-6, reabsorption occurs when a molecule of water breaks down in the proximal tubular cell into an H^+ and a hydroxyl molecule (OH^-). The H^+ is actively secreted into the lumen of the tubule and joins with a bicarbonate molecule that has been filtered at the glomerulus. Hydrogen plus bicarbonate results in carbonic acid (H_2CO_3), which, in the presence of the enzyme carbonic anhydrase, breaks down to carbon dioxide and water. These diffuse back into the proximal tubular cell to be used again as this cycle repeats.

By this process, the filtered bicarbonate is saved from being excreted in the urine. The reaction of hydrogen with bicarbonate is reversible, as shown in the following equation:

$$CO_2 + H_2O \rightleftharpoons H_2CO_3 \rightleftharpoons H^+ + HCO_3^- \qquad (18\text{-}4)$$

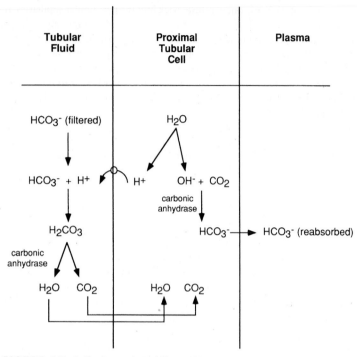

FIGURE 18-6 Reabsorption of filtered bicarbonate by the proximal tubular cells.

The OH^- produced in the proximal tubule cell joins with an intracellular carbon dioxide molecule. In the presence of the enzyme carbonic anhydrase, it too proceeds to a bicarbonate ion. This bicarbonate also returns into the peritubular capillary as shown in Figure 18-6. The enzyme carbonic anhydrase is readily available.

Secretion and Excretion of Acid

The above reactions only serve to reabsorb filtered bicarbonate. They do not eliminate acid. The kidney does actively secrete and excrete H^+ in the urine as well, which allows it to rid the blood of metabolically produced nonvolatile acids. As shown in Figure 18-7, H^+ excretion occurs after most of the filtered bicarbonate has been reabsorbed. In this case, the H^+ produced in the proximal tubule cell from the breakdown of water moves into the lumen of the tubule and combines with filtered phosphate ions (or to a lesser extent, sulfate ions) and is then excreted in the urine.

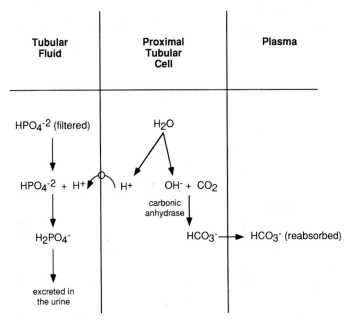

FIGURE 18-7 Excretion of H^+ bound to filtered phosphate.

The effect of excreting hydrogen bound to phosphate is not only the loss of acid in the urine but *a net gain of bicarbonate*. This net gain occurs because a bicarbonate ion is still produced in the proximal tubule when carbon dioxide joins with OH^-. This bicarbonate is returned to the plasma.

A second mechanism by which the kidney excretes acid is by active secretion of ammonium ion (NH_4^+) into the tubular fluid (Fig. 18-8). Ammonium ion is produced in the proximal tubular cell as a result of the metabolism of glutamine. Glutamine enters the cell from the peritubular capillary and from the tubular lumen, after being filtered across the glomerulus. Once in the tubule, ammonium ion cannot return into the proximal tubular cells; therefore, it is excreted in the urine. The bicarbonate produced from glutamine metabolism diffuses back into the peritubular capillary, thereby returning base to the blood. Finally, a small amount of H^+ is excreted free in the urine, causing the urine to normally have an acidic pH.

Secretion of Bicarbonate

Under conditions of alkalosis (excess base), the kidney can secrete bicarbonate, thus ridding the plasma of base and returning the pH toward normal. Secretion

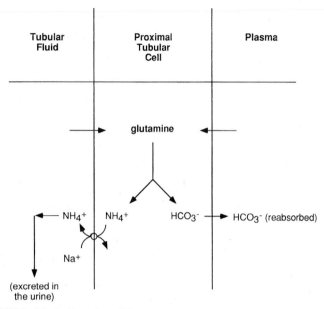

FIGURE 18-8 Excretion of H+ as ammonium ion. Glutamine diffuses into the proximal tubular cell from the plasma and from the tubular fluid. The active transport of ammonium into the tubular fluid occurs as a result of a sodium–ammonium counter-transport system.

of bicarbonate is an active process occurring in the cortical collecting duct. However, even under conditions of alkalosis, bicarbonate reabsorption in the proximal tubule is ongoing and essential. Loss of all filtered bicarbonate would be fatal.

RENAL CONCENTRATING MECHANISM: THE COUNTERCURRENT SYSTEM

To survive periods without water, animals, including humans, must excrete a concentrated (hypertonic) urine. They must eliminate waste products, including urea, without losing much water in the process. In contrast, under conditions of water excess, animals must excrete large amounts of water in a dilute (hypotonic) urine. The kidney has adapted to handle day-to-day variations in water consumption by developing the **countercurrent multiplier system**. For this system to work, the hormone antidiuretic hormone (ADH), also called vasopressin, is required.

The countercurrent multiplier system exists in the loop of Henle, a long, curving portion of the nephron located between the proximal and distal tubules. The multiplier system has five basic steps and depends on active transport of

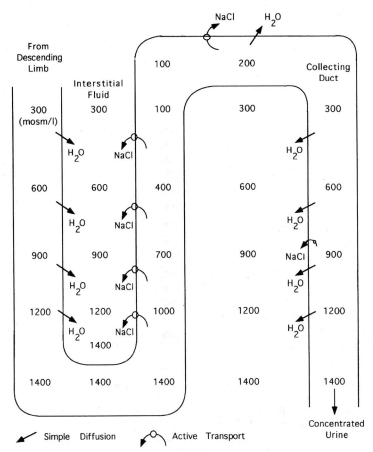

FIGURE 18-9 Formation of a concentrated urine in the presence of ADH. With ADH, water diffuses out of the collecting duct into the concentrated interstitium.

sodium (and chloride) out of the ascending part of the loop. It also depends on impermeability of this part of the loop to water, which keeps water from following sodium out. Finally, this system relies on the permeability of collecting ducts to water. The five steps are outlined in the following section and are shown graphically in Figure 18-9.

Steps of the Countercurrent Multiplier System

1. When sodium is transported out of the ascending limb, the interstitial fluid surrounding the loop of Henle becomes concentrated.

2. Because water is impermeable across the ascending limb, water cannot follow sodium out of the ascending limb. Thus, the remaining filtrate becomes progressively diluted.

3. Water *is* permeable across the descending limb of the loop. Water leaves this section and flows down its concentration gradient into the surrounding interstitial space. This concentrates the descending limb fluid. As the fluid loops into the ascending limb, it is progressively diluted as sodium is pumped out.

4. The net and key result is the concentration of the interstitial fluid surrounding the loop of Henle. Concentration is highest surrounding the bottom of the loop, becoming more dilute as the ascending limb is followed up.

5. At the top of the ascending limb, tubular fluid is isotonic (equal in concentration to the plasma) or even hypotonic (more dilute compared with plasma).

Result of the Countercurrent Multiplier System

The goal of the countercurrrent system is to concentrate the interstitial fluid surrounding the loop of Henle (as described in step 4). This is vital because the final filtrate passes down the collecting ducts through this fluid. Permeability of the collecting ducts to water is variable. If permeability to water is high (as shown in Fig. 18-9), as the water moves down through the concentrated interstitium, it will diffuse out of the collecting duct and back into the peritubular capillary. The result is little water excretion and concentrated urine. In contrast, if permeability to water is low at this portion of the nephron, water will not diffuse out of the collecting duct and instead will be excreted in the urine. The urine will be dilute, as shown in Figure 18-10.

Role of Antidiuretic Hormone in Concentrating the Urine

Whether the collecting ducts are permeable to water or not is determined by the circulating level of the posterior pituitary hormone, ADH (also called vasopressin). Release of ADH from the posterior pituitary is increased in response to a decrease in blood pressure or an increase in extracellular osmolarity (decreased water concentration). ADH acts on the collecting tubules to increase water permeability. If blood pressure is low or plasma osmolarity is high, ADH release will be stimulated and water will diffuse into the peritubular capillaries, increasing blood volume and pressure, and decreasing extracellular osmolarity. In contrast, if blood pressure is too high or extracellular fluid is too dilute (decreased osmolarity), ADH release will be inhibited, causing the collecting ducts to be impermeable to water, and thus more water will be excreted in the urine, decreasing blood volume and pressure, and increasing extracellular osmolarity.

Sensors that measure blood pressure and control ADH release include the carotid and the aortic baroreceptors and a group of receptors in the left atrium. Sensors that measure extracellular osmolarity lie in the hypothalamus, adjacent to the cells that actually synthesize ADH. After synthesis in the hypothalamus, ADH is stored in the posterior pituitary.

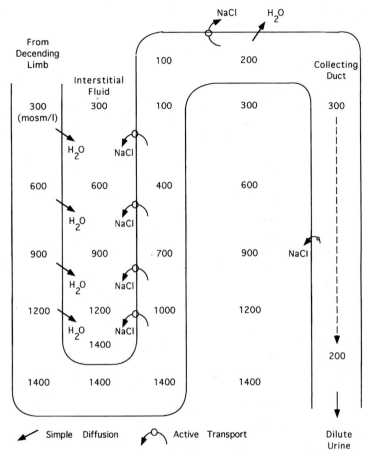

FIGURE 18-10 Formation of a dilute urine if ADH is absent. Note that because there is actually some NaCl transported out of the collecting duct, urine osmolality can be less than 300 mOsm/L.

Approximately 1400 mOsmol/L is the most concentrated human urine can become. The most dilute concentration is less than 200 mOsmol/L.

RENAL ENDOCRINE FUNCTION

The kidney functions as an endocrine organ, not only with the production and release of renin but also with the production and release of two other hormones: 1,25-dihydroxyvitamin D_3, important for bone mineralization; and erythropoietin, required for red blood cell production.

1,25-Dihydroxyvitamin D$_3$

The kidney acts in conjunction with the liver to produce an active form of vitamin D, called 1,25-dihydroxyvitamin D$_3$, from an inactive precursor consumed in the diet. The inactive form of vitamin D can also be produced in a reaction catalyzed by sunlight on a precursor present in the skin. Vitamin D is essential for maintenance of plasma calcium levels required for bone formation. The active form of vitamin D acts as a hormone by circulating in the blood and stimulating absorption of calcium and, to a lesser extent, phosphate across the small intestine and across the kidney tubules. Vitamin D also stimulates bone resorption (breakdown). Bone resorption releases calcium, and thus plasma calcium is increased by this mechanism as well.

Parathyroid hormone is the stimulus for the kidney to play its role in activating vitamin D$_3$. Parathyroid hormone is released from the parathyroid gland in response to decreased plasma calcium. This is an example of a negative feedback cycle: decreased plasma calcium leads to increased parathyroid hormone, which leads to increased renal activation of vitamin D$_3$. Activation of vitamin D$_3$ increases gut and kidney absorption of calcium, increasing plasma calcium and removing the stimulus for parathyroid release. Parathyroid hormone also directly stimulates bone resorption to release calcium into the plasma when necessary. Individuals who have renal disease frequently develop brittle, easily broken bones as a result of too little active vitamin D$_3$.

Erythropoietin

The hormone that stimulates the bone marrow to increase the production of erythrocytes (red blood cells) is called erythropoietin. The cells of the kidney responsible for synthesizing and releasing erythropoietin respond to renal hypoxia. Individuals who have renal disease frequently demonstrate chronic and debilitating anemia.

MICTURITION

Micturition is the process of urination, which is the elimination of urine from the body. Micturition occurs when the internal and the external urethral sphincters at the base of the bladder are relaxed.

The bladder is composed of smooth muscle (the detrusor muscle), innervated by sensory neurons that respond to stretch, and parasympathetic fibers that travel from the sacral area to the bladder. An area of smooth muscle at the base of the bladder (the internal sphincter) is also innervated by parasympathetic nerves. An external sphincter composed of skeletal muscle is just below the internal sphincter and at the top of the urethra. The external sphincter is innervated by motor neurons from the pudendal nerve. When urine accumulates, stretch of the bladder is sensed by afferent fibers that send the information to the spinal cord. Parasympathetic nerves to the bladder are activated, causing contraction of the smooth muscle and opening of the internal sphincter. At the same time, the motor neurons going to the external sphincter are inhibited and the external sphincter is relaxed, causing micturition to occur.

Micturition, however, can be voluntarily inhibited. This is possible because at the same time that the afferent nerves are conveying information on bladder stretch to the spinal cord, they are also sending information up the cord to the brainstem and cortex, allowing one to be conscious of the need to void. Descending neurons from the brain can inhibit or stimulate the spinal reflex to void. These descending pathways inhibit urination by causing contraction of the skeletal muscles of the pelvis as well as the external sphincter. Descending pathways also block the firing of parasympathetic nerves to the internal sphincter. For urination to be facilitated, skeletal muscles can be voluntarily relaxed. Voluntary control over micturition becomes functional in children by or before the time they become 3 or 4 years of age. However, it may become interrupted at any time by central nervous system disease or injury or from spinal cord trauma.

TESTS OF RENAL FUNCTION
Blood Urea Nitrogen

Urea is a nitrogenous waste product of protein and amino acid metabolism. One important job of the kidney is to eliminate this potentially toxic substance from the body. With declining renal function, blood urea nitrogen (BUN) levels increase. Measuring BUN therefore provides an indication of kidney health. The normal BUN for infants and children is 5 to 18 mg/dL. The normal range for adults is 10 to 20 mg/dL although it may be slightly higher in older adults.

BUN, however, is not only determined by renal function. It can also be affected by circumstances not associated with the kidney, such as increased or decreased dietary protein intake, or any unusual cause of an increased protein breakdown, such as a muscle injury. Likewise, liver disease may *decrease* BUN, because the liver is required to convert ammonia to urea. Because BUN levels are affected by these other factors, BUN level alone may be an indiscriminate indicator of renal disease. Therefore, often the ratio of BUN to serum creatinine is reported as well. Normally BUN and creatinine covary, keeping this ratio at approximately 10:1. If BUN is affected by factors other than renal factors, however, this ratio may change. Ratios greater than 15:1 suggest a nonrenal cause of urea elevation. Ratios less than 10:1 occur with liver disease.

Serum Creatinine

Creatinine is a product of muscle breakdown. Creatinine is excreted by the kidney through a combination of filtration and secretion. The concentration of creatinine in the plasma remains nearly constant from day to day. It varies slightly from approximately 0.7 mg/100 mL of blood in a small woman to 1.5 mg/100 mL in a muscular man. Levels greater than these suggest that the kidney is not clearing creatinine and indicate renal disease. Serum creatinine is very indicative of renal function. As a rough guide, a doubling of serum creatinine levels indicates a 50% reduction in renal function. Likewise, a tripling of normal creatinine levels indicates a 75% reduction in renal function. The clearance of creatinine may be used to estimate GFR.

Urinalysis

A urine sample may be easily obtained and evaluated for the presence of red blood cells, protein, glucose, and leukocytes, all of which are normally minimal to absent in the urine. Urine casts, which occur in the presence of high amounts of urine protein, may also be observed under some conditions of renal disease or injury. Urine osmolality (specific gravity) is measurable and should range between 1.015 and 1.025. Dehydration causes increased urine osmolality as more water is reabsorbed back into the peritubular capillaries. Overhydration results in decreased urine osmolality. Microorganisms can be identified using urine microscopy and culture and sensitivity tests. A 24-hour urine collection is useful for measuring hormones, creatinine, protein, urea, glucose, and other substances that are excreted in varying concentrations throughout the day.

Cystoscopy

Cystoscopy is the process in which a lighted scope (cystoscope) is inserted up the urethra into the bladder. Bladder lesions, stones, and biopsy samples may be taken.

Voiding Cystourethrography

Voiding cystourethrography involves bladder catheterization and infusion of a radioactive dye to study the shape and size of the bladder. It can be used to detect and grade the degree of vesicoureteral reflux. If used inappropriately, cystourethrography may spread an unresolved bladder infection into the ureters or kidney.

Intravenous Urography

Intravenous urography, also referred to as intravenous pyelography (IVP), is a technique in which a radiologic dye is injected intravenously, and x-ray films are taken sequentially as the dye filters through the kidney. Obstructions to flow in the glomeruli or tubules, vesicoureteral reflux, and stones may be visualized. A drawback to the use of this technique is the finding that some individuals are allergic to the dye and may suffer an anaphylactic reaction. High doses of radiation are involved.

Renal Ultrasound

Renal ultrasound uses the reflection of sound waves to identify renal abnormalities, including structural abnormalities, kidney stones, tumors, and other masses. Because it is noninvasive and does not involve radiation exposure, this technique is frequently used to evaluate renal function in children who have had a urinary tract infection. It does not, however, offer sufficient detail to evaluate vesicoureteral reflux, renal scarring, or inflammation.

Other Diagnostic Tools

A radiograph of the kidney, ureter, and bladder (KUB) is useful for baseline screening to determine if additional diagnostic testing is indicated. The structure, location, size, and shape of the KUB can be visualized along with the presence of foreign bodies, stones, and neoplasms. Magnetic resonance imaging and computed tomography offer information about masses, vascular problems, and filling defects. Renal biopsy is helpful for diagnostic and evaluative purposes.

● Pathophysiologic Concepts

ALTERATIONS IN GLOMERULAR FILTRATION

Glomerular filtration depends upon the summation of forces favoring filtration of plasma out of the glomerulus and forces favoring reabsorption of filtrate into the glomerulus. Anything that affects the forces of filtration or the forces of reabsorption affects net glomerular filtration. Forces favoring filtration are capillary pressure and interstitial fluid colloid osmotic pressure. Forces favoring reabsorption are interstitial fluid pressure and plasma colloid osmotic pressure.

Alterations in Capillary Pressure

Capillary pressure depends on mean arterial pressure. Increased mean arterial pressure increases capillary pressure, tending to increase glomerular filtration. A decrease in mean arterial pressure decreases capillary pressure and tends to decrease glomerular filtration. Autoregulation of afferent and efferent arterioles minimizes these changes unless the mean arterial blood pressure becomes too high (180 mm Hg) or too low (80 mm Hg).

Increased sympathetic activity and increased AII constrict afferent and efferent arterioles. These stimuli decrease the capillary pressure somewhat. However, because afferent and efferent arterioles are both affected, the responses tend to cancel each other out and GFR is nearly unaffected. Because the efferent arteriole response to sympathetic stimulation is especially sensitive, with heavy sympathetic stimulation, GFR may actually increase, as blood in the glomerulus backs up due to greater constriction of the efferent compared to afferent arteriole.

Alterations in Interstitial Fluid Colloid Osmotic Pressure

Interstitial fluid colloid osmotic pressure is low because very few plasma proteins or red blood cells filter out of the glomerulus into the interstitial space.

With injury to the glomerulus or the peritubular capillaries, interstitial fluid colloid osmotic pressure may increase. If the interstitial fluid osmotic pressure increases, fluid is drawn out of the glomerulus and peritubular capillaries, and swelling and edema occur in the Bowman space and the interstitial space surrounding the tubule. Swelling in the Bowman space or around the tubule can interfere with further glomerular filtration and tubular reabsorption because of increasing interstitial fluid pressure. Swelling and edema may also collapse the delicate glomeruli or peritubular capillaries, leading to hypoxia and death of the nephrons in extreme situations.

Alterations in Plasma Colloid Osmotic Pressure

Plasma colloid osmotic pressure depends on the protein concentration of plasma. Plasma protein levels can decrease as a result of liver disease, protein loss in the urine, or protein malnutrition. Plasma colloid osmotic pressure is the major force favoring reabsorption of fluids back into the capillaries. If it decreases, less fluid reenters the capillaries. Fluid accumulates in the tubular and the peritubular (surrounding) areas. Again, swelling around the tubule can collapse the tubule and the surrounding peritubular capillaries, leading to hypoxia and death of the nephron.

Alterations in Interstitial Fluid Pressure

Interstitial fluid pressure in the Bowman space and surrounding the tubule can increase dramatically if the glomerular or peritubular capillaries are damaged. Increased interstitial fluid pressure opposes further glomerular filtration. Increased interstitial fluid pressure can cause collapse of the surrounding nephrons and the peritubular capillaries, leading to hypoxia and renal cell injury or death. When cells die, they release intracellular enzymes that stimulate immune and inflammatory reactions (see Chapter 4), which further contribute to swelling and edema. Edema worsens interstitial fluid pressure. With loss of glomerular filtration, blood volume and electrolyte composition cannot be regulated.

Tubular Obstruction

One cause of increased interstitial fluid pressure is tubular obstruction. Obstruction present in the nephron causes fluid to back up into the Bowman capsule and the interstitial space. Unrelieved tubular obstruction can collapse the nephrons and capillaries and can lead to irreversible damage, especially to the renal papillae, which are the final site for urine concentration. Causes of obstruction include renal calculi (stones) and scarring from repeated kidney infections.

AZOTEMIA

Azotemia refers to the abnormal elevation of nitrogenous waste products in the blood such as urea, uric acid, and creatinine. Azotemia indicates a decrease in GFR, occurring either acutely or with chronic renal failure. Azotemia is an early sign of renal damage.

UREMIA

Uremia is not a single event, but rather a syndrome (a constellation of symptoms) that develops in an individual who has end-stage renal disease. Because the kidney is pivotal in maintaining water, acid–base, and electrolyte balance and in removing toxic waste products, the symptoms of uremia are widespread and affect all the organs and tissues of the body. Common symptoms include fatigue, anorexia, nausea, vomiting, and lethargy. Intractable itching (pruritus) may occur. Hypertension, osteodystrophy, and uremic encephalopathy develop as well, with central nervous system changes, including confusion and psychosis, characterizing end stages. The range of symptoms appears to be caused by acidosis, anemia from decreased erythropoietin, and the buildup of all waste products.

NEPHROTIC SYNDROME

Nephrotic syndrome is the loss of 3.5 g or more of protein in the urine per day. Under normal circumstances, virtually no protein is lost in the urine. Nephrotic syndrome usually indicates severe glomerular damage. Diabetic nephropathy is the most common cause of nephrotic syndrome. In individuals who do not have diabetes, different glomerular diseases may account for the disorder.

Increased glomerular capillary permeability allows protein to leave the vascular space and be eliminated in the urine. The resulting hypoalbuminemia stimulates hepatic synthesis of cholesterol and clotting factors thus causing hyperlipidemia and increased risk for thrombus formation. Hypoalbuminemia also causes decreased plasma osmotic pressure that results in generalized edema and decreased circulating volume, which stimulates the renin–angiotensin–aldosterone system to retain sodium and water causing further edema formation.

Clinical manifestations may include increased susceptibility to infections (caused by hypoimmunoglobulins) and generalized edema, called **anasarca**. Hyperlipidemia (elevated plasma lipids) is associated with hypoalbuminemia, perhaps as a hepatic response to low levels of albumin. Possible complications include renal vein thrombosis, pulmonary embolism, deep vein thrombosis, and transient ischemic attacks.

Treatment consists of mechanisms to reduce proteinuria. These mechanisms include a soy-based protein, low-fat diet, with salt restrictions. ACE inhibitors reduce proteinuria and have become a mainstay of treatment. Hypertension is treated with AII receptor blockers. Diuretics may be prescribed to increase fluid loss. Protein supplements may be provided to prevent malnutrition unless renal failure is suspected, in which case they are contraindicated as protein worsens renal failure. Lipid-lowering agents may be prescribed although hyperlipidemia typically resolves with remission.

ANASARCA

Defined as a generalized edema in individuals suffering from hypoalbumine-mia as a result of nephrotic syndrome or other conditions, anasarca is caused by a systemic decrease in capillary osmotic pressure. With a decrease in this major force favoring reabsorption of interstitial fluid back into the capillaries, edema of the interstitial space throughout the body occurs. The edema is usually soft and pitting and occurs early in the periorbital (surrounding the eye) regions, the ankles, and the feet.

RENAL OSTEODYSTROPHY

Demineralization of bone occurring with renal disease is known as renal osteodystrophy. Renal osteodystrophy has many causes, including decreased renal activation of vitamin D_3, leading to decreased calcium absorption across the gut, and subsequent reduced serum calcium levels. In addition, decreased renal function leads to an accumulation of phosphate ions, and hyperphosphatemia causes the secretion of parathyroid hormone, which leads to bone breakdown (resorption). Decreased serum calcium levels also stimulate parathyroid hormone release. An elevated bone breakdown contributes to easy bone fracturing.

Renal osteodystrophy also occurs as a result of the role bone plays in acting as a buffer for plasma H^+. Bone buffering means bone takes up H^+ and removes it from the general circulation to help maintain plasma pH. In taking up H^+, calcium (which is also positively charged) is leached from the bone to maintain electrical balance in the bone. With chronic acidosis of advanced renal disease, bone buffering of H^+ increases and the leaching of bone calcium becomes significant.

Treatment of renal osteodystrophy is aimed toward calcium and vitamin D supplementation. A phosphate-restricted diet is necessary.

METABOLIC ACIDOSIS/RENAL ACIDOSIS

Metabolic acidosis is a decrease in plasma pH not caused by a respiratory disorder. Chronic renal disease results in metabolic acidosis as a result of reduced H^+ excretion and altered bicarbonate reabsorption. The result is increased plasma H^+ and lowered pH.

Increased H^+ concentration contributes to bone resorption and causes neural and muscular function changes. The respiratory system is stimulated by the increase in hydrogen. Tachypnea (increased respiratory rate) occurs in an attempt to blow off the excess hydrogen as carbon dioxide. The respiratory response to renal acidosis is called respiratory compensation.

UREMIC ENCEPHALOPATHY

Uremic encephalopathy refers to neurologic changes seen in severe renal disease. Symptoms include fatigue, drowsiness, lethargy, seizures, muscle twitching, peripheral neuropathy (pain in the legs and feet), decreases in memory, and coma. Uremic encephalopathy appears to be caused by accumulation of toxins, alterations in potassium balance, and decreased pH. Treatment involves renal replacement with dialysis or transplantation if the condition is irreversible.

RENAL DIALYSIS

The process of adjusting blood levels of water and electrolytes in a person who has poor or nonfunctioning kidneys is called renal dialysis. In this procedure, blood is directed past an artificial medium containing water and electrolytes in predetermined concentrations. The artificial medium is the dialyzing fluid. In the United States, more than 300,000 people require dialysis to survive.

By simple diffusion across a selectively permeable membrane, water and electrolytes in the blood move down their individual concentration gradients into or out of the dialyzing solution. As a result of simple diffusion, the final blood levels of these substances can be manipulated to be near normal. For example, sodium concentration in the dialyzing fluid can be adjusted to cause net loss or gain of sodium from the blood. Glucose is added to dialyzing fluid, at the same concentration present in blood, to ensure that glucose is not lost during dialysis. Urea is kept very low in the dialyzing fluid so that urea diffuses down its concentration gradient, out of the blood and into the artificial medium. There are two types of dialysis: hemodialysis and peritoneal dialysis.

Hemodialysis

In hemodialysis, dialysis is performed outside the body. Blood is passed from the body, through an arterial catheter, into a large machine. Two chambers separated by a semipermeable membrane are inside the machine. Blood is delivered to one chamber, dialyzing fluid is placed in the other, and diffusion is allowed to occur. Blood is returned to the body via a venous shunt.

Hemodialysis takes about 3 to 5 hours and is required approximately three times per week. By the end of the 2- to 3-day interval between treatments, salt, water, and pH balance are again abnormal, and the individual usually does not feel well. Hemodialysis contributes to problems of anemia because some red blood cells are destroyed in the process. Infection is also a risk.

Peritoneal Dialysis

In peritoneal dialysis, the individual's own peritoneal membrane is used as a natural, semipermeable barrier. Prepared dialysate solution (approximately 2 L) is delivered into the peritoneal cavity through an indwelling catheter placed under the skin of the abdomen. The solution is allowed to remain in the peritoneal cavity for a predetermined amount of time (usually between 4 and 6 hours). During this time, water and electrolytes diffuse back and forth between the circulating blood. The person can usually continue activity while the exchange takes place.

Peritoneal dialysis must be performed approximately four times per day. Because the procedure is performed daily (at home or at work), the fluctuations in plasma composition seen between hemodialysis treatments are minimized and convenience is increased. Unlike with hemodialysis, individuals usually feel well on a daily basis. However, peritoneal dialysis may lead to infections from the indwelling catheter or catheter malfunction.

Heart disease is common among patients who have renal failure for several reasons, including increasing age and the high incidence of diabetes mellitus or hypertension in patients on dialysis. Recent studies have shown that patients on dialysis who suffer a myocardial infarct have high mortality and poor long-term survival.

KIDNEY TRANSPLANTATION

Defined as a form of kidney replacement available to patients who have renal failure, kidney transplantation involves placement of a donor kidney into the abdominal cavity of an individual suffering from end-stage renal disease. Transplanted kidneys can come from living or dead donors. The more similar the antigenic properties of the donated kidney are to the patient, the more likely the transplantation will be successful. With appropriate follow-up, approximately 94% of kidneys transplanted from cadavers and 98% from living donors function well after surgery. Long-term graft survival (10 years) is similar for both (approximately 78% for grafts from living donors vs. 76% for grafts from cadavers). Each year, about 4000 kidney patients die while waiting for an organ transplant.

Individuals receiving kidney donation must remain on a variety of immunosuppressant medications for life to prevent organ rejection. Ideally, immunosuppressive therapy should be individualized to match the characteristics of the donor kidney (donor source, age, status of the donor kidney) and the characteristics of the recipient (age, race, reactive antibodies present, transplant number, and tolerance toward immunosuppressive therapy). In addition, the degree of histocompatibility between donor and recipient must be considered. If rejection does occur, it may happen during the very early postoperative period, through the first 3 months, or it may be delayed months or years after the transplantation. All individuals on immunosuppressive therapy are subject to increased risk of infection. Infections may be kidney related or independent of the renal system.

● Conditions of Disease or Injury

RENAL AGENESIS

Failure of the kidneys to develop during gestation is called renal agenesis. A familial tendency may exist with inheritance as a dominant trait. Drugs affecting AII, poorly controlled diabetes, and chemical exposure have been implicated as possible teratogens. Renal agenesis may be unilateral, which is more common, or bilateral. Bilateral agenesis is incompatible with life.

Unilateral agenesis results in hypertrophy of the remaining kidney as it adapts to compensate functionally for the absent kidney. If the remaining kidney is malformed, successful compensation may not be possible. Lifelong monitoring of renal function is highly recommended.

Clinical Manifestations

- Bilateral renal agenesis, called Potter syndrome, is associated with facial anomalies and pulmonary disease. Infants with Potter syndrome die in utero or soon after birth.
- With unilateral renal agenesis, no symptoms are apparent if the remaining kidney is healthy. The remaining kidney may compensate and grow almost twice as big as otherwise expected. If the remaining kidney functions poorly, however, various disease manifestations may be present.

Diagnostic Tools

- Prenatal ultrasound can often detect renal agenesis.
- After birth, computerized axial tomography (CAT) scan or renal ultrasound is used to diagnose the condition.

Treatment

- No treatment is required for unilateral agenesis if the remaining kidney is healthy.
- If structural or functional defects are present in the remaining kidney, surgery may be required.

VESICOURETERAL AND URETHROVESICAL REFLUX

Vesicoureteral reflux is the retrograde (backward) flow of urine from the bladder into the ureters and the kidney. Urethrovesical reflux is the backward flow of urine from the urethra into the bladder. Vesicoureteral reflux usually occurs as a result of congenital misplacement of the ureters or urethra, which increases the likelihood of retrograde flow. The valvular mechanism at the ureter–bladder junction may also be incompetent and thus contribute to the problem. Secondary causes include neurogenic bladder and repeated infections that cause structural scarring and impediment to the normal flow of urine. Although seen more commonly in children with urinary tract infections, it may also occur in adults as a result of increased volume or pressure in the bladder. Urethrovesical reflux can occur during coughing or other activities that increase intra-abdominal pressure, especially in women because of the short length of the urethra.

Clinical Manifestations

- Repeated urinary tract infections. These are especially suggestive of reflux in children younger than 5 years old.
- Irritability and poor feeding in infants.

Diagnostic Tools

- Intravenous urography and cystourethrography can help diagnose reflux. Grading of reflux determines treatment.

Complications

- Renal obstruction and failure from repeated urinary tract infections may occur.

Treatment

- Spontaneous remission may occur, in which case no treatment is required.
- Surgery may be necessary to correct the defect if it is severe anatomically or functionally.
- Prophylactic antibiotic therapy starting at birth (if the condition is known) may prevent repeated kidney infections.

RENAL CALCULI

Nephrolithiasis, or renal calculi, refer to stones that occur anywhere in the urinary tract although the renal pelvis or the calyces of the kidney are the most common sites. Males are affected more often than females. Calculi are most commonly made up of calcium crystals, but may be composed of struvite or magnesium, ammonium, uric acid, or combinations of these different substances. When these substances are not dissolved in the urine, they form precipitates and grow in size.

Renal calculi can be caused by increased urine pH (e.g., calcium carbonate stones), decreased urine pH (e.g., uric acid stones), high concentration of stone-forming substances in the blood and urine, certain dietary habits or drugs, anything that obstructs urine flow, leading to urine stasis in the urinary tract, conditions that cause bone resorption, such as immobilization and renal disease (calcium stones), gout, a disease of increased uric acid production or decreased excretion (uric acid stones), obesity and weight gain due to increased excretion of overabundant calcium, oxalates, and uric acid, and dehydration.

Clinical Manifestations

- Pain is often colicky (rhythmic), especially if the stone is in the ureter or below. The pain may be intense. The location of pain depends on the site of the stone.

- Severe pain associated with obstruction accompanied by nausea and vomiting.
- A stone in the kidney itself may be asymptomatic unless it causes obstruction or an infection develops.
- Hematuria, caused by irritation and injury of the renal structures, is common with calculi.
- Decreased urine output results if obstruction to flow occurs.
- Dilute urine also results if obstruction to flow occurs, because the ability to concentrate urine may be interrupted by swelling around the peritubular capillaries.

Diagnostic Tools

- Blood and urine tests may identify stone-forming substances.
- Radiograph (KUB), ultrasound, or intravenous urography may locate a stone.

Complications

- Urinary obstruction can occur upstream from a stone anywhere in the urinary tract. Obstruction above the bladder can lead to **hydroureter**, that is, abnormal distension of ureter with urine. Unrelieved hydroureter, or obstruction at or above the site where the ureter exits from the kidney, can lead to **hydronephritis**, swelling of the renal pelvis and collecting-duct system. Hydronephritis can cause the kidneys to be unable to concentrate the urine, leading to electrolyte and fluid imbalance.
- Obstruction causes increased interstitial hydrostatic pressure and can lead to a decrease in GFR. Unrelieved obstruction can cause collapse of the nephrons and the capillaries, leading to ischemia of the nephrons as the blood supply is interrupted. Renal failure may develop if both kidneys are involved.
- Anytime there is obstruction to the flow of urine (stasis), the chance of a bacterial infection increases.
- Renal cancer may develop from repeated inflammation and injury.

Treatment

- Increased fluid intake increases urine flow and helps wash out the stone. High fluid intake in individuals prone to calculi may prevent their formation.
- Pain management with narcotic analgesics for severe pain.
- If the stone content is identified, dietary modification may reduce the levels of the stone-forming substance. Urine needs to be strained to collect stones for composition analysis.
- Appropriate alteration of urine pH may encourage stone breakdown.

- Extracorporeal (outside the body) lithotripsy (shock wave therapy) or laser therapy may be used to break apart the stone.
- Surgery may be necessary to remove a large stone or to place a diversion tube around the stone to relieve obstruction.

NEUROGENIC BLADDER

A neurogenic bladder is one that has experienced disruption of its neural connections. Neurologic disruption can be of the sensory or motor neurons; motor neurons affected may be located at the upper or lower level of the nervous system.

Interruption of sensory neurons leaves an individual unable to sense the need to void. Interruption of efferent nerves at the cortical or upper motor neuron level causes voluntary control of micturition to be lost. Because higher centers also facilitate micturition, voiding will be incomplete (spastic bladder dysfunction). If the interruption is of the lower motor neurons at the sacral area or below, the spinal reflex controlling micturition will be blocked and the bladder will not empty spontaneously (flaccid bladder dysfunction).

Causes of neurogenic bladder include multiple sclerosis, which affects the cortical level; spinal cord transection; trauma; or tumors anywhere in the spinal cord. Poliomyelitis especially injures lower motor neurons, whereas diabetes mellitus is a common cause of sensory neuron damage. Other causes may include stroke, advanced age, metabolic disorders, chronic alcoholism, collagen diseases, vascular diseases, herpes zoster, and Parkinson disease.

Clinical Manifestations

- Sensory neuron interruption leads to dribbling and overflow incontinence because bladder fullness cannot be felt.
- Upper motor neuron and cortical interruption with an intact reflex arc leads to incontinence, small urine volume, and incomplete emptying. Infections may develop owing to urinary retention.
- Lower motor neuron interruption, below the level of the reflex arc, leads to overflow incontinence.

Diagnostic Tools

- History and physical examination will assist diagnosis.
- Neuromuscular studies may help locate a lesion.
- Cystometry to assess bladder's nerve supply, detrusor muscle tone, and bladder filling pressures.
- Uroflow studies.

Complications

- Repeated urinary tract infections may occur.
- Incontinence.
- Chronic renal failure may develop from repeated infections and scarring.

Treatment

- Sensory neuron interruption is treated with bladder training. The bladder is emptied at predetermined (2- to 4-hour) intervals either naturally or with a catheter.
- Upper motor neuron and cortical interruption are treated by catheter drainage or manual initiation of the reflex arc by stroking the abdominal or the perineal area.
- Lower motor neuron interruption is treated by catheter drainage or manual compression of the bladder.
- Various pharmacologic options include antimuscarinics to decrease detrusor muscle tone and increase bladder capacity; cholinergics to stimulate parasympathetic receptors to increase bladder tone; muscle relaxants to decrease external sphincter tone.
- Surgical options to resect reflex nerves or create urinary diversions.
- Research is currently being conducted related to implanted electrodes for restoration of voluntary control.

URINARY TRACT INFECTION

A urinary tract infection is an infection anywhere in the urinary tract, including the kidney itself, caused by proliferation of a microorganism. Most urinary tract infections are bacterial in origin, but fungi and viruses also may be implicated. The most common bacterial infection is by *Escherichia coli*, a fecal contaminant commonly found in the anal area.

Urinary tract infections are especially common in girls and women. One cause is the shorter urethra in the female, which allows the contaminating bacteria to gain access more easily to the bladder. The short urethra increases the likelihood that microorganisms deposited in the urethral opening during intercourse gain access to the bladder. Other factors that contribute to the frequency of urinary tract infections in girls and women include the cultural tendency for girls to delay urination and the irritation to the skin of the urethral opening that occurs during sexual intercourse. Pregnant women have a progesterone-dependent relaxation of all smooth muscle, including the bladder and the ureters, so they tend to retain urine in these parts of the tract, increasing the risk of bacterial growth. The pregnant uterus might also obstruct urine flow in some situations.

A protective factor against urinary tract infections in women is the estrogen-dependent production of a mucous coating of the bladder, which has antimicrobial functions. With menopause, estrogen levels fall and this protection is lost. Protection against urinary tract infections in both sexes is offered by the usually acidic nature of urine, which acts as an antibacterial agent.

Although urinary tract infections are less common in males, they can occur. A frequent cause in older men is benign prostatic hyperplasia (BPH) or prostatitis. The prostate is a walnut-sized gland that sits immediately below the opening of the bladder. Hyperplasia of the prostate may cause obstruction to flow, which predisposes an individual to an infection. Normally, prostatic secretions have an antimicrobial, protective effect.

Individuals who have diabetes also are at risk of frequent urinary tract infections because of the high glucose content of the urine, poor immune function, and increased frequency of neurogenic bladder. Persons who have a spinal cord injury or anyone using a urinary catheter to void are at increased risk of infection.

Types of Urinary Tract Infections

Urinary tract infections may be divided into cystitis and pyelonephritis. Cystitis is an infection of the bladder, the most common site for an infection. Pyelonephritis is an infection of the kidney itself and can be either acute or chronic.

Acute pyelonephritis usually occurs as a result of an ascending bladder infection. It may also occur as a result of a blood-borne infection. Infections may be in both or in one kidney.

Chronic pyelonephritis may result from repeated infections and is usually found in individuals who have frequent calculi, other obstructions, or vesicoureteral reflux. With all kidney infections, inflammatory and immune responses cause interstitial edema and possible development of scar tissue. The tubules are most often affected and may atrophy. With chronic pyelonephritis, extensive scarring and obstruction of the tubules result. The ability of the kidneys to concentrate urine decreases as tubules are lost. The glomeruli are usually unaffected. Chronic renal failure may develop.

Clinical Manifestations

- Cystitis typically presents with dysuria (pain on urination), increased frequency of urination, and a sense of urgency to urinate.
- Lower back or suprapubic pain may occur, especially with pyleonephritis.
- Fever accompanied by blood in the urine in severe cases.
- Symptoms of infection in infants or young children may be nonspecific and include irritability, fever, lack of appetite, vomiting, and very strong-smelling diapers.

- Symptoms of infections in the elderly may be subtle; any elderly person who has abdominal symptoms such as nausea or vomiting should be assessed for urinary infection. Fever may or may not be present. Sometimes only increased agitation or confusion may develop, which means that those caring for the elderly need to be especially cognizant of the frequency and subtleness of geriatric urinary tract infection. Asymptomatic infections in the elderly are also very common; there does not appear to be a benefit in treating elderly patients who have asymptomatic infection.
- Acute pyelonephritis typically presents with
  - Fever.
  - Chills.
  - Flank pain.
  - Dysuria.

Chronic pyelonephritis may have manifestations similar to acute pyelonephritis. However, it can also include hypertension and may eventually lead to signs of renal failure.

Diagnostic Tools

- Urine culture and sensitivity of the microorganism allow for identification and treatment.
- White blood cells will be present in the urine with infection anywhere. White cell casts present in the urine suggest pyelonephritis rather than cystitis, since they indicate that white cells have been lysed in the tubules.
- Voiding cystoureterography or excretory urography detects congenital abnormalities.

Complications

- Renal or perirenal abscess formation may occur.
- Renal failure may develop after repeated infections if both kidneys are involved.

Treatment

- Women and girls in particular should be encouraged to drink fluids frequently (cranberry juice has been shown to reduce the incidence of cystitis) and go to the bathroom as needed to wash out microorganisms that may ascend the urethra.
- Girls should be taught at a young age to wipe from front to back after urination to avoid contamination of the urethral opening with fecal bacteria.
- Women should be encouraged to urinate after sexual intercourse to wash out ascending microorganisms.

- Bubble baths are discouraged in young girls because of the irritation of the urethral opening that may occur, leading to access of bacteria to the urethra. Likewise, young girls should be discouraged from playing in the bathtub after shampooing.
- Antimicrobial therapy with a repeat urinalysis during or after drug therapy is required.
- Urinary analgesic such as phenazopyridine for painful urination.
- If chronic pyelonephritis is caused by an obstruction or reflux, surgical treatment specific to relieve these problems is necessary.

INCONTINENCE

Urinary incontinence is the involuntary loss of urine. It may be chronic or transient and can be related to inability of the bladder to store urine, inability of the bladder to adequately empty, a combination of the two, or sensory problems that interrupt stimuli transmission to and from the bladder. Women tend to be affected more than men and the occurrence tends to increase with age. Risk factors may include, but are not limited to: immobility, smoking, fecal impaction, delirium, estrogen depletion, diabetes mellitus, urinary tract infection, spinal cord injury, and certain medications.

An acute onset of incontinence is typically due to a reversible cause. Chronic incontinence can be classified as urge, stress, mixed, overflow, or functional. A sudden sensation of urgency with involuntary leakage is classified as urge incontinence. Stress incontinence is characterized by involuntary leakage associated with increased abdominal pressure which may be caused by sneezing, coughing, or lifting heavy objects. The combination of stress and urge incontinence is referred to as mixed incontinence. It commonly occurs in older females and involves larger amounts of urine leakage. Overflow incontinence can be the result of a urethral obstruction that prevents normal bladder emptying or with a neurogenic bladder. Functional incontinence occurs when physical, cognitive, or mental impairments interfere with toileting.

Clinical Manifestations

- Involuntary loss of urine.

Diagnostic Tools

- Thorough history and physical examination to identify patterns and causes (bladder diary).
- Thorough assessment of risk factors.

Complications

- Embarrassment and feelings of poor self-esteem.
- Depression.

Treatment

- Manage any underlying cause.
- Bladder training.
- Pelvic muscle strengthening exercises.
- Anticholinergics and or musculotropic relaxants.
- Surgical interventions such as urethropexy or pubovaginal sling.

INTERSTITIAL CYSTITIS

Interstitial cystitis (IC), often referred to as interstitial cystitis/painful bladder syndrome (IC/PBS), is a chronic condition of pain, urgency, and frequency. Activation of the inflammatory process injures the protective lining of the bladder causing pain in several locations. Symptoms tend to be more severe with certain foods and bladder filling. Offensive food substances may include chocolate, alcohol, citrus fruit, coffee, and carbonated beverages. Vulvodynia is often a comorbidity making it difficult to determine that IC/PBS is the only problem. The comorbidity is most likely due to the fact that innervation from the sacral and pudendal nerves innervate the bladder and the vulva.

Clinical Manifestations

- Chronic pelvic pain.
- Urinary frequency and urgency.
- Nocturia.

Diagnostic Tools

- Symptom-based diagnosis after other pathologies are eliminated.
- Positive potassium sensitivity test. Intravesical potassium instillation will cause an increase in urgency and pain in the presence of defective bladder epithelial function.
- Biopsy and urodynamics to rule out other problems.

Complications

- Interference with daily activities, work, sleep, sexual activities.

Treatment

- Avoid aggravating factors.
- Pentosan polysulfate sodium for bladder urothelial function.
- Supportive treatment may include antihistamines and tricyclic antidepressants.
- Intravesical instillation of anesthetic (dimethyl sulfoxide is the only FDA-approved therapy) or heparin for acute, severe pain.

GLOMERULONEPHRITIS

Glomerulonephritis is an inflammation of the glomerulus. Types of glomerulonephritis include acute, rapidly progressive, and chronic.

Acute Glomerulonephritis

A sudden inflammation of the glomerulus is called acute glomerulonephritis. Acute inflammation of the glomerulus occurs as a result of deposition of antibody–antigen complexes in the glomerular capillaries. Complexes usually develop 7 to 10 days after a pharyngeal or skin streptococcal infection (post-streptococcal glomerulonephritis) but may follow any infection. See page C15 for illustrations.

An inflammatory reaction is initiated in the glomerulus after the deposition of antibody–antigen complexes. Inflammatory reactions in the glomeruli (or anywhere else in the body; see Chapter 4) cause complement activation and mast-cell degranulation, leading to increased blood flow, increased glomerular capillary permeability, and increased glomerular filtration. Plasma proteins and red blood cells leak through the damaged glomeruli. The eventual breakdown of the glomerular membrane causes swelling and edema of the Bowman space. This swelling and edema increase interstitial fluid pressure, which can collapse any functioning glomeruli in the area. Eventually, increased interstitial fluid pressure opposes further glomerular filtration.

Activation of the inflammatory reaction also draws white blood cells and platelets into the area of the glomerulus. Activation of coagulation factors occurs with inflammation, which can lead to fibrin deposits, scarring, and the loss of functional glomeruli. Glomerular membranes thicken and GFR decreases further.

Acute glomerulonephritis usually resolves with specific antibiotic therapy, especially in children. Some adults may not recover and may develop rapidly progressive glomerulonephritis or chronic glomerulonephritis.

Rapidly Progressive Glomerulonephritis

Rapidly progressive glomerulonephritis is an inflammation of the glomeruli that occurs so rapidly that there is a 50% decrease in GFR within 3 months of disease onset. Rapidly progressive glomerulonephritis can occur from a worsening of acute glomerulonephritis, from an autoimmune disease, or may be idiopathic (unknown) in origin.

Rapidly progressing glomerulonephritis is associated with diffuse proliferation of glomerular cells within the Bowman space. Such proliferation gives rise to the appearance of a crescent-shaped structure obliterating the Bowman space. GFR decreases, leading to renal failure.

Goodpasture syndrome is a type of rapidly progressing glomerulonephritis caused by autoantibodies produced against the glomerular cells themselves.

Pulmonary capillaries are also attacked. Extensive scarring of the glomeruli results. Renal failure frequently occurs within weeks or months. The cause of Goodpasture syndrome is unknown.

Chronic Glomerulonephritis

Chronic glomerulonephritis is the long-term inflammation of the glomerular cells. It may occur as a result of unresolved acute glomerulonephritis, or it might develop spontaneously. Chronic glomerulonephritis commonly occurs after years of subclinical glomerular injury and inflammation, associated with only slight hematuria (blood in the urine) and proteinuria (protein in the urine).

Common causes include diabetes mellitus and long-standing hypertension. Both of these diseases are associated with significant and repeated glomerular injury. The outcome of this slowly progressive disorder is sclerosis, diffuse scarring, and glomerular deterioration. Tubular atrophy frequently accompanies glomerular breakdown. Individuals with chronic glomerulonephritis who have diabetes or who are even mildly hypertensive have a poor prognosis for long-term renal function. Chronic glomerulonephritis may also accompany long-standing systemic lupus erythematosus.

Clinical Manifestations

All types of glomerulonephritis are associated with

- Decreased urine volume.
- Blood in the urine (brownish-colored urine), either gross or subtle.
- Protein in the urine.
- Fluid retention due to decreased GFR.
- Periorbital and peripheral edema.
- Mild to severe hypertension.

Diagnostic Tools

- Hematuria as measured by urinalysis.
- Red blood cell casts in the urine.
- Proteinuria greater than 3 to 5 g/day.
- Decreased GFR as measured by creatinine clearance.
- If the condition is caused by acute poststreptococcal glomerulonephritis, antistreptococcal enzymes, such as antistreptolysin-O and antistreptokinase, will be present.
- KUB reveals bilateral kidney enlargement.
- Renal biopsy confirms the diagnosis.

Complications

- Renal failure may develop.
- Cardiac hypertrophy.
- Heart failure.

Treatment

- If the condition develops following acute poststreptococcal glomeru-lonephritis, antibiotic therapy is required.
- Autoimmune destruction of the glomeruli may be treated with corticos-teroids for immunosuppression.
- Anticoagulants to decrease fibrin deposits and scarring can be used in rap-idly progressive glomerulonephritis.
- Plasmapheresis to suppress rebound antibody production in those with rap-idly progressive glomerulonephritis.
- Loop diuretics, fluid and sodium restriction for fluid overload.
- Strict glucose control in diabetics has been shown to slow or reverse the progression of glomerulonephritis. Research has shown that the ACE inhibitors can reduce glomerular damage in diabetics even if frank hyper-tension is not evident.
- ACE inhibitors can reduce glomerular damage in individuals with chronic hypertension.
- Dialysis or kidney transplant may be necessary for chronic glomeru-lonephritis.

MYOGLOBINURIA

Myoglobinuria or rhabdomyolysis is the presence of high levels of myoglobin in the urine. Myoglobin is an intracellular protein found in muscle. With muscle-cell damage, especially a crush injury or major body trauma, myoglo-bin levels in the blood can rise precipitously. A severe electrical burn may cause significant muscle damage and myoglobinuria as well. Normally, myoglobin is filtered in the urine and is then totally reabsorbed into the peritubular cap-illaries by active transport. However, when large amounts of myoglobin are present in the blood, its threshold for reabsorption is exceeded and it spills in the urine. Large amounts of myoglobin in the urine filtrate clog the tubules, leading to obstruction, inflammation, and tubular and glomerular injury. Renal failure can result.

Individuals have reported myoglobinuria after intense episodes of athletics or long-distance running. It appears that besides muscle breakdown, the pounding or jarring effect on the kidney may contribute to the filtration of proteins in these circumstances. Sepsis, malignant hyperthermia, extreme exertion, prolonged seizures, potassium or phosphate depletion, hyperthermia, statin drugs, alcoholism, and drug abuse may also lead to myoglobinuria.

Clinical Manifestations

- Dark reddish brown pigmentation of the urine.
- Hematuria.

Diagnostic Tools

- Red blood cells, protein, and protein casts are present in the urine.
- Elevated levels of plasma creatine phosphokinase, a product of muscle metabolism, can be measured.

Complications

- Electrolyte imbalance, as a result of potassium and phosphate release from injured muscle cells, may occur.
- Renal failure may develop.

Treatment

- Administration of sodium bicarbonate to facilitate renal elimination of myoglobin.
- Flushing the kidney with an osmotic diuretic (mannitol).
- Correction of electrolyte and volume imbalances.
- Short-term dialysis, allowing time for the kidneys to recover, may be necessary.

HEMOLYTIC UREMIC SYNDROME

Hemolytic uremic syndrome is a condition of injury to the endothelial cells of the glomeruli as a result of a viral, rickettsial, or bacterial infection, frequently infection by the bacteria *E. coli* O157 from inadequately cooked meat, especially hamburger. Damage to the glomerular endothelial cells results in swelling and edema and in a narrowing of the capillary to blood flow. Narrowing of the capillary causes injury to passing red blood cells, which are then broken down in the spleen, resulting in hemolytic anemia. Damage to the glomerular cells stimulates inflammatory reactions, including complement activation, fibrin deposition, accumulation of white blood cells, and the release of a variety of vasoactive peptides. Platelets accumulate, leading to clotting and to a decrease in their circulating levels. Blood flow to the kidney may decrease, and scarring may occur. Hemolytic anemia, thrombocytopenia, and acute renal failure characterize this disorder.

Clinical Manifestations

- Fever, anorexia, vomiting, and abdominal pain.
- Bloody diarrhea.
- Bruising, from thrombocytopenia (decreased platelets).
- Pallor.
- Irritability.
- Seizures and lethargy with central nervous system involvement.
- Oliguria (decreased urine output).

Diagnostic Tools

- Urine culture may identify the causative organism.
- Obstruction and inflammation may be visible using ultrasound or radiographs.

Complications

- Renal failure may occur. It may be either temporary or permanent.

Treatment

- Dialysis is required if renal failure develops.
- Blood transfusions may be used.
- Correction of fluid and electrolyte imbalance is required.
- Kidney transplant in severe cases.

RENAL FAILURE

Renal failure is the loss of function in both kidneys to the point that they can no longer clear waste products of protein metabolism from the blood. Because the kidneys have such a vital role in maintaining homeostasis, renal failure is associated with multiple systemic effects. All attempts at preventing renal failure are essential. If renal failure does occur, it must be treated aggressively.

The U.S. National Kidney Foundation's Kidney Disease Outcomes Quality Initiative has revised and defined the stages of chronic kidney disease. Stages are based on the presence or absence of symptoms and on progressively decreasing GFR, corrected for body size (per 1.73 m^2). Normal GFR for a healthy adult is approximately 120 to 130 mL/min. The stages of kidney disease are as follows:

- **Stage 1**: Kidney damage (pathological abnormalities or markers of damage including abnormalities in blood or urine tests or in imaging studies) with normal or near-normal GFR, at or above 90 mL/min (≥75% of normal).

- **Stage 2**: GFR between 60 and 89 mL/min (approximately 50% of normal), with evidence of kidney damage. This stage is considered one of diminished renal reserve. Remaining nephrons are highly susceptible to failing themselves as their load becomes overwhelming. Additional renal insults hasten the decline.
- **Stage 3**: GFR between 30 and 59 mL/min (25% to 50% of normal). This stage is considered one of renal insufficiency. Nephrons continue to die.
- **Stage 4**: GFR between 15 and 29 mL/min (12% to 24% of normal), with fewer nephrons remaining.
- **Stage 5:** End-stage renal failure; GFR of less than 15 mL/min (<12% of normal). Few functioning nephrons remain. Scar tissue and tubular atrophy are present throughout the kidneys.

Renal failure is also categorized as **acute renal failure**, which occurs suddenly and is usually reversible, or **chronic renal failure**, which is associated with progressive, irreversible loss of renal function. Acute renal failure is often complicated by multiorgan failure making management more complex. Chronic renal failure usually develops after years of renal disease or damage, but may occur rapidly in some situations. Chronic renal failure inevitably leads to renal dialysis, transplantation, or death.

Acute Renal Failure

Causes of acute renal failure have been separated into three general categories: prerenal, intrarenal, and postrenal. Identifying the cause of acute renal failure is accomplished by a study of the patient's history and the quantity and quality of his or her urine.

Prerenal failure, the most common cause of acute renal failure, develops as a result of decreased kidney perfusion. It occurs as a result of conditions unrelated to the kidney but that damage the kidney by affecting renal blood flow. Diminished renal blood flow may be the result of an absolute decrease in circulating volume (i.e., dehydration, hemorrhage); a relative decrease in circulating volume (i.e., third-spacing, myocardial infarction, etc.); or primary renal hemodynamic dysfunction (i.e., renal artery stenosis, drug-induced renal autoregulation impairment). Possible causes include anything that severely reduces systemic blood pressure, leading to shock, such as an anaphylactic reaction, severe blood loss or volume depletion, a burn, or sepsis (a blood-borne infection). Surgical procedures resulting in a prolonged decrease in renal blood flow can also cause prerenal failure. Renal autoregulation is unsuccessful with a mean systemic blood pressure below 80 mm Hg.

Interruption of renal blood flow, and therefore oxygen delivery, can irreversibly damage the kidneys within 30 minutes. The tubules are most susceptible to the effects of hypoxia, and ischemic tubular necrosis (tubular cell death caused by decreased oxygenation) frequently develops.

Intrarenal failure, also referred to as intrinsic or parenchymal renal failure, is a type of acute renal failure that occurs as a result of primary damage to kidney tissue itself. It may be vascular, interstitial, glomerular, or tubular in nature. Specific causes include glomerulonephritis, acute pyelonephritis, myoglobinuria, and most commonly, acute tubular necrosis. Damage to the basement membrane damages the filtering capabilities of the kidney.

With intrarenal failure, kidney cell damage usually occurs as a result of ischemic tubular necrosis. This tends to blur the distinction between prerenal failure and intrarenal failure because a main cause of ischemic tubular necrosis is decreased renal blood flow.

Tubular necrosis can also result from the direct action of nephrotoxic (damaging to the nephron) drugs, such as heavy metals and organic solvents. Aminoglycoside antibiotics, such as gentamicin, are also nephrotoxic. Radiopaque contrast media used for viewing the cardiac chambers or the gastrointestinal (GI) tract can be nephrotoxic in susceptible individuals. Ingestion of toxic amounts of analgesic mixtures, especially codeine and caffeine, may lead to acute tubular necrosis. Sporadic reports of elderly individuals who use nonsteroidal anti-inflammatory drugs (NSAIDs) having acute renal failure after an intense athletic event (e.g., a marathon run in heat) are cause for concern.

Postrenal failure is a type of acute renal failure that occurs as a result of conditions that affect the flow of urine out of the kidneys and includes injury to or disease of the ureters, bladder, or urethra. The usual cause of postrenal failure is obstruction. Obstruction can occur in response to many factors, including untreated calculi, a tumor, repeated infections, prostatic hyperplasia, blocked catheter, or a neurogenic bladder.

Most cases of renal failure are associated with low urine output. Occasionally, high-output failure may occur. In this case, urine production continues and is usually associated with a better outcome.

Recovery from acute renal failure typically occurs after a few weeks, but occasionally takes as long as 6 weeks after the onset of oliguria (decreased urine output). Recovery begins with diuresis (increased urine output). Although urine is being produced, alterations in electrolyte balance continue. After the diuretic phase, the recovery phase of acute renal failure follows, during which renal function and electrolyte balance return. Full recovery usually occurs within 1 to 2 years. Some individuals may never recover total renal functioning.

Clinical Manifestations

- Oliguria may occur, especially if the failure is caused by ischemia or by obstruction. Oliguria results from decreased GFR.
- Toxic tubular necrosis may be nonoliguric (high output) and is associated with the production of an adequate volume of dilute urine.
- Tachycardia and hypotension.
- Dry mucus membranes, cool and clammy skin, lethargy.
- Edema, confusion, seizures, and coma may occur as the disease progresses.

Diagnostic Tools

- A good history identifies precipitating causes of renal failure.
- Laboratory finding of azotemia (increased nitrogenous compounds in the blood), and elevated BUN and creatinine confirm diagnosis.
- Laboratory findings of hyperkalemia (increased potassium in the blood) and acidosis are common.
- Other laboratory findings may include decreased hematocrit and hemoglobin, decreased bicarbonate, and low pH.
- Ultrasound, computed tomography, and KUB radiographs are helpful in identifying the cause.

Complications

- Fluid retention from nonfunctioning kidneys may lead to edema, congestive heart failure, or water intoxication.
- Alterations in electrolytes and pH may cause uremic encephalopathy.
- If the hyperkalemia is severe (≥6.5 mEq/L), dysrhythmia and muscle weakness may occur.
- Hypertensive crisis.
- Infection.

Treatment

- Prevention of acute renal failure is essential. Individuals experiencing shock should be quickly treated with fluid replacement to support blood pressure. Individuals at risk of developing acute renal failure, for instance, those about to undergo heart surgery, may be given an osmotic diuretic before surgery to increase renal function. Likewise, adequate hydration before nephrotoxic drugs are administered may prevent acute renal failure. For patients at high risk of suffering renal failure, the use of nephrotoxic drugs and intravenous radioactive dyes must be shown to be essential before they are employed, and their use may be contraindicated in some cases.
- If renal failure does occur, data suggest that prevention of the oliguric phase results in a better prognosis. Prevention of oliguria involves:
  - Aggressive plasma volume expansion.
  - Diuretics to increase urine production.
  - Vasodilators, especially dopamine, given to increase renal blood flow.
- Dietary restrictions on potassium and protein are often implemented in acute renal failure. High-carbohydrate intake prevents the metabolism of proteins and reduces nitrogenous waste production.
- Antibiotic therapy to prevent or treat infections may be necessary because of the high rate of sepsis seen with acute renal failure.

- Continuous peritoneal dialysis is often employed during the oliguric stage of acute renal failure to give the kidneys time to recover. Dialysis also prevents the buildup of nitrogenous wastes, stabilizes electrolytes, and reduces fluid overload.
- Continuous renal replacement therapy (CRRT) is a modified form of dialysis that occurs over a longer period of time with less fluid removal. It minimizes fluctuations of hemodynamic stability in critically ill patients.

Chronic Renal Failure

Chronic renal failure is the progressive, relentless destruction of renal structure. Chronic renal failure can result from virtually any of the diseases described in this chapter. In addition, analgesic nephropathy, the destruction of the renal papillae related to the daily use of analgesic medications for many years, may lead to chronic renal failure in susceptible individuals. Another major cause is diabetic nephropathy which causes functional and structural kidney changes that result in metabolic and hemodynamic problems. Thickening of the glomerular basement membrane, increased glomerular permeability, and decreased GFR are more likely with poor glycemic control and hypertension. Regardless of the cause, unremitting deterioration of the kidneys occurs as indicated by a progressive fall in GFR.

Early in its course, fluid balance, salt handling, and waste accumulation are variable and depend on the part of the kidney in failure. Until renal function has decreased to less than 25% of normal, clinical manifestations of chronic renal failure may be minimal as surviving nephrons take over the functions of those lost. Surviving nephrons increase their rates of filtration, reabsorption, and secretion, and undergo hypertrophy in the process. As more nephrons progressively die, the remaining ones have an increasingly difficult job, which leads to their own damage and eventual death. Part of this cycle of death appears to be related to the demands on remaining nephrons for increased protein reabsorption. With progressive loss of nephrons, scar tissue accumulates and renal blood flow may be reduced. Renin release may increase, which, coupled with fluid overload, can lead to hypertension. Hypertension accelerates renal failure, perhaps by increasing the filtration (and therefore the demands for reabsorption) of plasma proteins and by causing oxidative stress.

Failure of adequate production of erythropoietin by the kidneys frequently leads to anemia and a resultant fatigue that negatively impacts the quality of life. In addition, chronic anemia leads to decreased tissue oxygenation throughout the body and activates reflexes aimed at increasing cardiac output to improve oxygenation. These reflexes involve activation of the sympathetic nervous system and an increase in cardiac output. Ultimately, these changes predispose an individual with renal failure to develop congestive heart failure, making chronic kidney disease an independent risk factor for cardiovascular disease.

Clinical Manifestations

- In stage 1 renal failure, no symptoms may be apparent.
- As disease progresses, reduced production of erythropoietin causes chronic fatigue, and early signs of tissue hypoxia and cardiovascular compromise may develop.
- As disease progresses, polyuria (increased urine output) occurs as the kidneys are unable to concentrate the urine.
- During the final stages of renal failure, urine output decreases because of low GFR.

Diagnostic Tools

- Radiographs or ultrasound will show small, atrophied kidneys.
- Serum BUN, creatinine, and GFR will be abnormal.
- Hematocrit and hemoglobin are reduced.
- Plasma pH is low.
- An elevated respiratory rate indicates respiratory compensation for metabolic acidosis.

Complications

- With progression of renal failure, volume overload, electrolyte imbalance, metabolic acidosis, azotemia, and uremia occur.
- In stage 5 renal failure (end-stage disease), severe azotemia and uremia are present. Metabolic acidosis worsens, which significantly stimulates respiratory rate.
- Hypertension, anemia, osteodystrophy, hyperkalemia, uremic encephalopathy, and pruritus (itching) are common complications.
- Decreased production of erythropoietin may lead to cardiorenal anemia syndrome, a self-perpetuating triad of anemia, cardiovascular disease, and renal disease that ultimately leads to increased morbidity and mortality.
- Congestive heart failure may develop.
- Without treatment, coma and death result.

Treatment

- Prevention of renal failure is the most important goal. Prevention includes lifestyle changes and drugs when necessary to control hypertension, good glycemic control in diabetics, and the avoidance of nephrotoxic drugs whenever possible. Long-term use of codeine-containing analgesics and possibly NSAIDs should be avoided, especially in persons who have renal compromise. Early diagnosis and treatment of systemic lupus erythematosus and other diseases known to damage the kidneys is essential.

- Treatments are modified as progression worsens.
- For stages 1, 2, and 3 renal failure, the goals are to slow further nephron loss, primarily by the use of protein restriction and antihypertensive medications. ACE inhibitors are especially helpful in slowing progression.
- Because of the relationship between congestive heart failure and anemia associated with chronic kidney disease, the Renal Anemia Management Period (RAMP) has been proposed. RAMP is defined as the time following the onset of chronic kidney disease when early diagnosis and treatment of anemia will slow kidney disease progression, delay cardiovascular complications, and improve quality of life. Treatment of anemia is by administration of recombinant human erythropoietin (rHuEPO). This drug has been shown to dramatically improve quality of life and reduce the need for transfusions. It also significantly improves cardiac function.
- For later stages, treatment is geared toward correcting fluid and electrolyte imbalances.
- For end-stage disease, treatment includes dialysis or renal transplantation.
- At all stages, prevention of infection is important.

CHILDHOOD KIDNEY CANCER: WILMS TUMOR

Wilms tumor is a cancer of any part of the kidney that typically develops in children younger than 4 years of age. Because of its early onset, Wilms tumor likely develops after one or more mutations in important tumor suppressor genes.

Wilms tumor is a solid tumor that can grow to a large size. Mutations of the gene that code for the protein necessary for transcription in the embryonic kidney have been associated with the tumor. It may be encapsulated (contained within the capsule of the kidney). Staging and prognosis of the disease depend on encapsulation and spread. Encapsulation is associated with a favorable prognosis, whereas spread of the tumor outside of the abdominal area to the lungs is associated with a poorer outcome. Overall, prognosis is good, with an approximately 90% survival rate.

Clinical Manifestations

- A large abdominal mass may be noted by parents or a health care provider.
- Vomiting, abdominal pain, hypertension, and hematuria may be present.

Diagnostic Tools

- A careful history can raise the suspicion of Wilms tumor.
- Physical examination may identify the mass.
- CT scan or ultrasound may confirm the diagnosis.

Treatment

There is currently a cure rate of approximately 85%.

- Removal of the involved kidney.
- Chemotherapy and radiation.

ADULT KIDNEY CANCER

Most adult kidney cancer is a result of renal cell carcinoma. This cancer is especially common in the sixth or seventh decade of life, and is more common in males than in females. Risk factors for kidney cancer include repeated kidney stone irritation, smoking, obesity, and occupational chemical exposure. The risk is also increased in those with a first-degree relative who has the disease. The incident seems to be higher in African Americans and Hispanics.

Renal cancers develop from the tubular epithelium and can occur anywhere in the kidney. At diagnosis, tumors are staged. Treatment and outcomes depend on staging, with outcomes ranging from 85% survival for stage I tumors to less than 10% survival for stage IV tumors.

Clinical Manifestations

- Often symptomless in its early stages.
- Hematuria is the most common manifestation. It may be frankly visible or may be microscopic and sporadic.
- A flank mass may be palpable. Flank pain may be present as well.
- Polycythemia may be present, reflecting alteration in the renal control of hematopoiesis.
- Fever may accompany the cancer.

Diagnostic Tools

- The use of CT scanning has improved the diagnosis of suspected renal cancer.
- Ultrasound, renal angiography, and MRI may confirm the diagnosis.

Complications

- Metastasis to the lungs or elsewhere may precede diagnosis.
- Hemorrhage.

Treatment

- Surgery to remove the affected kidney is usually performed. In patients who already have only one functioning kidney, surgical techniques to preserve renal function in the affected kidney may be attempted.

- Chemotherapy and immunotherapy may be used as well.
- Biotherapy with interferon or interleukin in advanced disease to induce remission.
- Hormone therapy.
- Use of antiangiogenic agents such as inhibitors of vascular endothelial growth factor is being evaluated in clinical trials.
- Analgesics for pain management.

 PEDIATRIC CONSIDERATIONS

- Children who receive kidney transplantation frequently experience growth retardation. Whether this is a result of immunosuppressive therapy or a loss of a vital renal function such as erythropoietin production or vitamin D_3 activation is unclear. Studies suggest that erythropoietin replacement can reduce growth complications of kidney transplantation. For all patients, medical therapy with rHuEPO can also drastically reduce the symptoms of anemia, especially fatigue, and can improve the quality of life.

- In children, urinary tract infections are usually due to fecal–renal migration of *E. coli*. Although common, even one urinary tract infection in a child of either sex who is younger than 5 years of age is suggestive of vesicoureteral reflux and thus the child should be evaluated with renal ultrasound, cystourethrography, or intravenous urography to prevent subsequent renal damage.

- Enuresis, or bed wetting, is a form of incontinence in children. Most cases are caused by maturational delay and resolve by adolescence.

- Children are especially susceptible to renal damage after infection with *E. coli* O157. Many children infected with this bacterium require dialysis or even die.

 GERIATRIC CONSIDERATIONS

- GFR declines with age due to a 30% to 50% loss of functional nephrons and reduced renal blood flow. Such a decline means that when drugs normally cleared by the kidneys are given to an elderly individual, their dosage should be adjusted to reflect declining renal function. However, because muscle mass, and therefore serum creatinine, also declines with age, the increase in serum creatinine level that normally indicates a fall in GFR may not be apparent. Since serum creatinine levels are frequently used to determine drug dosing, elderly individuals may receive inappropriately high doses of drugs despite reduced kidney function. This problem can have severe toxic consequences. In order to adjust for age on GFR, the following equation has been developed by Cockcoft and Gault:

$$\text{Creatinine clearance} = \frac{(140 - \text{age}) \times (\text{body weight in kg})}{72 \times \text{serum creatinine in mg/dL}} \qquad (18\text{-}5)$$

- Age is a primary risk factor for urinary tract infections in both men and women, and urinary tract infections are the most common cause of infection in nursing home residents. The elderly are especially susceptible because of prostatic hypertrophy; neurogenic bladder associated with long-term diabetes mellitus; poor muscle functioning, leading to incomplete voiding; and delayed voiding because of reduced mobility getting to a bathroom.

SELECTED BIBLIOGRAPHY

Bradway, C., Coyne, K. S., Irwin, D., & Kopp, Z. (2008). Lower urinary tract symptoms in women—A common but neglected problem. *Journal of the American Academy of Nurse Practitioners, 20*, 311–318.

Bradway, C., & Rodgers, J. (2009). Evaluation and management of genitourinary emergencies. *The Nurse Practitioner, 34*(5), 37–44.

Carrico, D. J., Sherer, K. L., & Peters, K. M. (2009). The relationship of interstitial cystitis/painful bladder syndrome to vulvodynia. *Urologic Nursing, 29*(4), 233–238.

DiMuzio, C. (2008). CRRT spells success against acute renal failure in critically ill patients. *American Nurse Today, 3*(5), 9–11.

Dowling-Castronovo, A., & Specht, J. K. (2009). Assessment of transient urinary incontinence in older adults. *American Journal of Neurology, 109*(2), 62–71.

Guyton, A. C., & Hall, J. (2006). *Textbook of medical physiology* (11th ed.). Philadelphia, PA: W.B. Saunders.

Helming, M. B. (2009). Genitourinary disorders in children: A review of less common presentations. *Advance for Nurse Practitioners, 17*(3), 24–29.

Johnson, V. Y. (2008). Urinary incontinence: No one should suffer in silence. *American Nurse Today, 3*(11), 21–25.

Kramer, B. J. (2009). Arterial blood gases. *Registered Nurses Journal, 72*(4), 22–24.

Lerma, E. V. (2008, September). A comprehensive look at kidney stones. *The Clinical Advisor, 22*, 26, 29–32.

McCrary, E. B. (2008). The road to renal failure: An overview of diabetic nephropathy. *Advance for Nurse Practitioners, 16*(7), 61–63.

National Kidney Foundation. (2005). *25 facts about organ donation and transplantation.* Retrieved October 15, 2005 in http://www.kidney.org/news/newsroom/fsitem.cfm?id=30.

Oh, H., & Seo, W. (2007). Alterations in fluid, electrolytes and other serum chemistry values and their relations with enteral tube feeding in acute brain infarction patients. *Journal of Clinical Nursing, 16*(2), 298–307.

Osborn, K. S., Wraa, C. E., & Watson, A. B. (2010). *Medical-surgical nursing: Preparation for practice.* Upper Saddle River, NJ: Pearson.

Pasero, C., Eksterowicz, N., Primeau, M., & Crowley, C. (2008). Using catheter techniques to deliver analgesia. *American Nurse Today, 3*(11), 14–15.

Porth, C. M., & Matfin, G. (2009). *Pathophysiology: Concepts of altered health states* (8th ed.). Philadelphia, PA: Lippincott Williams & Wilkins.

Russell, C. L. (2009). Defining high risk in adult kidney transplantation. *Progress in Transplantation*, 19(3), 252–258.

Scales, K., & Pilsworth, J. (2008). The importance of fluid balance in clinical practice. *Nursing Standard*, 22(47), 50–57.

Schreuder, M. F., Langemeijer, M. E., Bokenkamp, A., Delemarre-Van de Waal, H. A., & Van Wijk, J. A. (2008). Hypertension and microalbuminuria in children with congenital solitary kidneys. *Journal of Pediatrics and Child Health*, 44, 363–368.

Siegel, J. F., Sand, P. K., & Sasso, K. (2008). Vulvodynia and pelvic pain? Think interstitial cystitis. *The Nurse Practitioner*, 33(10), 41–45.

Watring, N., & Mason, J. D. (2008). Deciphering dysuria. *Clinician Reviews*, 18(12), 16–22.

Wilcox, C. S. (2005). Oxidative stress and nitric oxide deficiency in the kidney: A critical link to hypertension? *American Journal of Physiology* (*Regulatory, Integrative and Comparative Physiology*), 289, R913–R935.

Fluid and Electrolyte and Acid–Base Balance

The maintenance of water, electrolyte, and acid–base balance is a daily requirement of all living organisms. In humans, water and electrolyte intake and output are regulated through hormonal and neural interactions that overlie behavioral and dietary practices. As for acid–base balance, most metabolic processes occurring in the body result in the production of acid. It is essential that these acids be removed from the body. The removal of carbon dioxide is performed by the lungs. The removal of other, nonvolatile (nongaseous) acids is performed by the kidneys. The lungs and the kidneys, together with various buffer systems in the body, maintain plasma acid concentration within narrow, physiologic limits.

● Physiologic Concepts

WATER BALANCE

Water makes up approximately 60% of total body weight. Of this amount, two thirds (66%) is intracellular and one third (33%) is extracellular (i.e., in the plasma or interstitial space) (Fig. 19-1). Water is essential to life because of the role it plays in energy production, the maintenance of osmotic pressure, and the transport of substances in the body and across cell membranes. Maintaining the correct balance between water intake and output is critically important; if an individual becomes overhydrated, dilution of plasma electrolytes and solutes, cell swelling, and

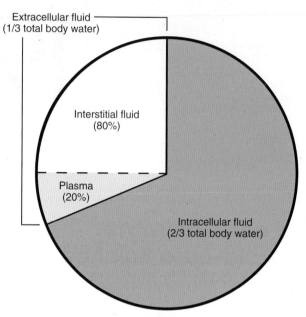

FIGURE 19-1 Body water percentages.

possibly death can result. Likewise, if one becomes severely dehydrated, plasma solute and electrolyte overconcentration and cell shrinkage occur and can lead to nervous system dysfunction and death. Stimuli to take in fluid may be physiologic or social. Outputs vary, related to ambient temperature, exercise, and clothing. Ultimately, the thirst drive centered in the hypothalamus and the output of urine by the kidneys maintain the harmony between intake and output.

Normal Water Intake and Output

Adults ingest between 1.5 and 2.5 L of fluid a day. Another 300 to 400 mL are produced daily via metabolic reactions. Daily outputs exactly balance these inputs in healthy individuals: 1.0 to 2.0 L excreted in urine, 100 mL excreted in the feces, 50 mL excreted in sweat, and approximately 1000 mL excreted through exhalation of air and surface evaporation. **Insensible fluid loss** refers to the loss of fluid from respiration, evaporation, sweat, and other drainage. As highlighted in Figure 19-2, fluid ingestion and urine excretion are the only variables under the precise control of neural and hormonal stimuli.

Control of Fluid Ingestion

Although the amount of fluid we drink each day is influenced by dietary and social influences, the ultimate control over whether we ingest an adequate

INPUT

H₂O ingestion

produced in metabolism of food

OUTPUT

insensible loss with ventilation

loss in sweat and evaporation

lost in feces
lost in urine

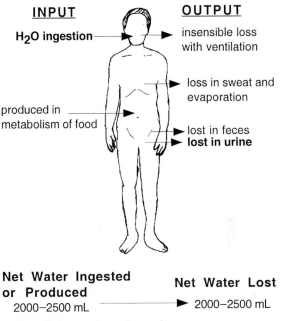

Net Water Ingested or Produced
2000–2500 mL

Net Water Lost
2000–2500 mL

FIGURE 19-2 Fluid ingestion and excretion.

amount of fluid is exerted by the thirst center located in the hypothalamus at the level of the third ventricle. Thirst is sensed by hypothalamic osmoreceptors that increase their rate of firing with increased plasma osmolarity (i.e., decreased water concentration). When activated, these osmoreceptors, along with neighboring cells that sense blood pressure, signal the hypothalamus to increase the release of antidiuretic hormone (ADH, also called vasopressin) from the posterior pituitary gland (see Chapters 9, 13, and 18). ADH has two major effects. The first and most important is to increase the permeability of the renal collecting ducts of the kidney to water (see Chapter 18). Increased permeability of the collecting ducts allows water to be reabsorbed out of the urine back into the blood, thereby diluting the plasma back toward normal (and so reducing the stimulus for ADH release). The second effect of ADH is to act as a pressor, an agent causing a rise in blood pressure; its other name is vasopressin. In this role, ADH causes a constriction of vascular smooth muscle and an increase in blood pressure (see Chapter 13). The increase in blood pressure also reduces the stimulus for continued release of ADH.

A second hormone, angiotensin II, also has a direct effect on the cells of the hypothalamus to increase the sensation of thirst. It, too, is an important dipsogenic (thirst-stimulating) hormone.

ELECTROLYTE BALANCE

Sodium

As the major extracellular ion in the body, sodium is responsible in large part for determining plasma osmolality and is also important in maintaining membrane potential and neural conductance. The regulation of plasma sodium is mainly achieved by the kidney, which freely filters and then reabsorbs at least 98% of filtered sodium. The remaining 2% is reabsorbed or excreted into the urine, depending on the presence or absence of the hormone **aldosterone**; increased aldosterone increases sodium reabsorption back into the blood by acting at the level of the distal tubule of the kidney (see Chapter 18). Low levels of aldosterone lead to the excretion of all or some of the final 2% of sodium in the urine.

Aldosterone is secreted from the adrenal cortex following stimulation by the hormone angiotensin II. A brief summary of this hormonal system, presented in detail in Chapter 18, is as follows: **Angiotensin II** is produced after a cascade of reactions initiated by the hormone renin released from the juxtaglomerular cells of the kidney. Renin is released in response to low plasma sodium and low blood pressure. As a result of an increase in angiotensin II levels, aldosterone release is stimulated, and sodium balance and blood pressure return toward normal; this process is an excellent example of a negative feedback cycle.

Sodium output also occurs through small amounts lost in the sweat and in the feces. In times of excessive sweating or diarrhea, depletion of sodium from these routes can be life threatening.

Sodium ingestion is influenced by taste as well as by a homeostatic drive (salt appetite) to maintain sodium balance. Humans and other animals have a drive to ingest salt that is triggered by low plasma sodium. Humans and other animals also show a distinct preference for salt ingestion, a circumstance that for a minority of humans may contribute to salt-sensitive hypertension.

Potassium

Potassium, the major intracellular ion in the body, plays a vital role in determining cell membrane potential. Although extracellular potassium concentration is low, potassium level in the extracellular fluid is carefully regulated, because changes in extracellular concentration can result in life-threatening disturbances in neural and cardiovascular function. Potassium can shift between the intracellular and extracellular compartments, depending on various neural and hormonal influences and the pH of the extracellular fluid. For example, beta-adrenergic nervous stimulation and insulin secretion both increase the movement of potassium intracellularly by stimulation of the Na^+/K^+ pump. In contrast, decreasing the pH of the plasma may increase the movement of potassium out of the cell.

The source of potassium in the body is that ingested in the diet. Excretion of potassium is primarily through the urine, with a small amount lost in the sweat and the feces. The major controlling factor over total body stores of potassium is the hormone aldosterone.

As described in Chapter 18, the maintenance of potassium balance is achieved by the kidney. Potassium is freely filtered across the glomerulus and then at least 80% is reabsorbed. If excess potassium has been ingested in the diet, the kidney can also *secrete* potassium into the urine to return to balance. If potassium is deficient in the diet, none is secreted into the urine and all is reabsorbed. Increased secretion (and so excretion) occurs in response to stimulation of the distal tubules of the kidney by the hormone aldosterone. Aldosterone is released from the adrenal cortex in response to angiotensin II, as described previously. Aldosterone release is also, to a lesser extent, stimulated directly by low plasma potassium and by an increase in the pituitary hormone adrenocorticotropin (ACTH).

Calcium

Calcium is primarily an intracellular ion, with nearly 99% of its total body stores in bone and most of the remaining 1% stored intracellularly in other tissues. A very small amount of extracellular calcium either circulates bound to albumin; is complexed to nonorganic substances such as citrate, phosphate, or sulfate; or exists in an ionized form. Calcium in the ionized form is important for muscle contraction and a variety of enzymatic reactions. It is also required for most steps of the coagulation pathway. Calcium is ingested in the diet, filtered, reabsorbed, and excreted by the kidney. It is not secreted.

The control of serum calcium results primarily from changes in the secretion of parathyroid hormone from the parathyroid gland (see Chapter 9); decreased serum calcium stimulates increased parathyroid hormone secretion. Increased parathyroid hormone then acts in one of three ways to return serum calcium back toward normal: it (1) increases renal reabsorption of calcium; (2) stimulates bone breakdown to release bone calcium; or (3) stimulates the activation of vitamin D, thereby increasing calcium reabsorption across the gut. A second hormone, calcitonin, secreted from specialized cells of the thyroid gland, also exerts control over serum calcium levels. Calcitonin is released in response to increased serum calcium, and it acts to reduce serum calcium by causing a decrease in bone breakdown. Calcitonin also decreases calcium reabsorption by the kidney, further lowering serum levels. Serum calcium is inversely related to serum phosphate.

Phosphate

Phosphate is an intracellular ion that is vital for most metabolic reactions and is an essential component of ATP, DNA, and RNA. Phosphate also serves as a hydrogen ion buffer in plasma and urine. Approximately 85% of phosphate is stored in bone, with 14% in all other cells; less than 1% is extracellular. Phosphate is ingested in the diet and, in proportion to its ingestion, is filtered and excreted in the urine. In the serum, it varies inversely with calcium. With renal failure, phosphate levels rise precipitously and result in low serum calcium levels.

Magnesium

Magnesium is primarily an intracellular ion that is stored in bone (50%), in body cells (49%), and in blood (1%). Magnesium is required for a variety of enzymatic reactions and is an important ion for DNA synthesis and RNA transcription, for translation, and for protein synthesis. Magnesium can bind to calcium receptors, either turning on the calcium response (mimicking) or blocking the effects of calcium. Magnesium is ingested in the diet and is filtered and excreted in the urine.

ACID–BASE BALANCE

pH

pH is a reflection of the ratio of acid to base in extracellular fluid. The pH in serum can be measured with a pH meter, or one can calculate it by measuring serum bicarbonate and carbon dioxide concentrations and placing these values into the Henderson–Hasselbalch equation, as shown in the following equation:

$$pH = (pK + \log HCO_3^-)/CO_2 \qquad (19\text{-}1)$$

In this equation, HCO_3^- is the concentration of bicarbonate in the serum, and CO_2 is the concentration of dissolved carbon dioxide in the serum. The pK refers to the negative logarithm of the dissociation constant, K. The dissociation constant is a fixed value for the bicarbonate/carbon dioxide system at normal body temperature. It reflects the degree to which bicarbonate and carbon dioxide dissociate to accept or donate a hydrogen ion. For the bicarbonate/carbon dioxide system, pK is 6.1.

The pH reflects the hydrogen ion concentration of the solution. The greater the hydrogen ion concentration, the greater the acidity of the solution and the lower the pH. In contrast, the higher the pH, the lower the hydrogen ion concentration, and the more basic the solution.

Acids

An acid is any substance capable of liberating a hydrogen ion. Examples of acids include the substances in bold in the following formulas, all of which are shown giving up a hydrogen ion:

$$\mathbf{HCl} \rightleftharpoons H^+ + Cl^-$$
$$\mathbf{H_2CO_3} \rightleftharpoons H^+ + HCO_3^-$$
$$\textbf{Lactic acid} \rightleftharpoons H^+ + \text{lactate}$$
$$\mathbf{NH_4^+} \rightleftharpoons H^+ + NH_3$$

An acid can be strong or weak, depending on the degree to which it breaks down to liberate hydrogen ions. For example, hydrogen chloride (HCl) rapidly and totally breaks down into hydrogen and chloride ion; therefore, it is considered a strong acid. In contrast, few lactic acid molecules break down to hydrogen ion and lactate; therefore, lactic acid is considered a weak acid. The double arrow in each equation indicates that the reactions are reversible.

Bases

In each reaction above showing the dissociation (breakdown) of an acid, the substance produced in addition to the hydrogen ion is considered a base. A base is any substance that can accept a hydrogen ion, thereby taking it out of solution. Because each of these reactions is reversible, each substance produced with the hydrogen ion can rejoin with it and move the reaction in the opposite direction. Thus, these substances can be considered bases. These reactions are rewritten in the following formulas with the base in bold:

$$\mathbf{Cl^-} + H^+ \rightleftharpoons + HCl$$
$$\mathbf{HCO_3^-} + H^+ \rightleftharpoons + H_2CO_3$$
$$\mathbf{Lactate} + H^+ \rightleftharpoons Lactic\ acid$$
$$\mathbf{NH_3} + H^+ \rightleftharpoons NH_4^+$$

A base can be strong or weak, depending on the degree to which it accepts a hydrogen ion. Most acids and bases found in the body are weak.

Buffers

Weak acids and weak bases make good buffers. A buffer is a substance that can either take free hydrogen ions from a solution or release hydrogen ions to a solution, thereby preventing large fluctuations in pH. There are three important buffer systems in the body: the bicarbonate–carbonic acid buffer system, the phosphate buffer system, and the hemoglobin buffer system.

Bicarbonate-Carbonic Acid Buffer System

The main buffer system in the body is the bicarbonate–carbonic acid buffer system. This system acts in the blood to buffer plasma pH. When free hydrogen ions are added to blood containing bicarbonate, the bicarbonate ions bind with the hydrogen ions, becoming carbonic acid (H_2CO_3). This binding ensures that there will be few free hydrogen ions remaining in solution, thereby preventing a significant decrease in blood pH. Carbonic acid is considered a weak acid; bicarbonate ion is considered its weak, conjugate (complementary) base. As shown in Equation 19-2, carbonic acid can also dissociate to form carbon dioxide and water; therefore, the bicarbonate buffer system is primarily used to eliminate hydrogen ion from the body through the elimination of the volatile gas carbon dioxide. The breakdown of carbonic acid to carbon dioxide and water requires the enzyme carbonic anhydrase, which is present in red blood cells. The reaction of carbonic acid to carbon dioxide and water is reversible, and carbon dioxide and water can rejoin to form carbonic acid. This process also requires the action of carbonic anhydrase. This reversible reaction is shown in the following equation.

$$CO_2 + H_2O \rightleftharpoons H_2CO_3 \rightleftharpoons H^+ + HCO_3^- \qquad (19\text{-}2)$$

Phosphate Buffer System

The second buffer system used by the body is the phosphate buffer system. Phosphoric acid ($H_2PO_4^-$) is a weak acid; it dissociates in plasma to phosphate (HPO_4^{2-}) and hydrogen ion (H^+). Phosphate is a weak base. The kidney uses this system to buffer the urine as it excretes hydrogen ion. A sulfuric acid–sulfate buffer system is used to a lesser degree.

Hemoglobin Buffer System

The third main buffer system in the body, the hemoglobin buffer system, is provided by proteins in the blood, especially hemoglobin present in red blood cells. Hemoglobin binds to free hydrogen ions as the red blood cells circulate past metabolically active cells. As a result of the binding of free hydrogen ions by hemoglobin, increases in free hydrogen ion concentration in the blood are minimized, and venous blood pH decreases only slightly compared with arterial blood. As the blood flows through the lungs, hydrogen ions dissociate from the hemoglobin and join with bicarbonate to become carbonic acid (Equation 19-2), which breaks down to carbon dioxide and water. Carbon dioxide is exhaled, resulting in the elimination of the metabolically produced hydrogen ions. Most of the water is reabsorbed, and some is exhaled in the breath.

Respiratory Control of Acid–Base Balance

The lungs rid the body of carbon dioxide. Although carbon dioxide itself is not an acid, it becomes one when it joins with water to form carbonic acid (Equation 19-2). The minute-by-minute regulation of plasma pH is controlled by an increase or decrease in the rate of respiration, thereby increasing or decreasing the exhalation of carbon dioxide. This system is possible because of the sensitivity of the respiratory center in the brain to free hydrogen ions (see Chapter 14), which usually vary in accordance with carbon dioxide.

Carbon Dioxide Production and Carriage in the Blood

Carbon dioxide is produced in all cells as a result of oxidative metabolism. From the cells, it diffuses into the bloodstream. Carbon dioxide is carried in the blood in three different ways: dissolved, bound in the red cell, and as bicarbonate. Approximately 7% is carried dissolved in the blood. The amount of carbon dioxide dissolved in the blood depends on the product of its partial pressure in the blood and its solubility constant (how well it dissolves). The solubility constant of carbon dioxide in blood is 0.57. Although the partial pressure of carbon dioxide in the atmosphere at sea level is almost zero and thus is nearly zero in inspired air, venous blood carries carbon dioxide away from metabolizing cells and has a carbon dioxide partial pressure of 45 mm Hg. Partial pressure of carbon dioxide in arterial blood is nearly 40 mm Hg. Therefore, the amount of carbon dioxide dissolved in the blood differs between the arterial and venous circulations.

As shown in Equation 19-3, 23% of carbon dioxide diffuses into red blood cells and is carried bound to hemoglobin.

$$Hemoglobin + CO_2 = Carboxyhemoglobin \qquad (19\text{-}3)$$

After reacting with water, as shown in Equation 19-2, 70% of carbon dioxide is carried in the blood. This reaction primarily occurs in red blood cells, where carbonic anhydrase is plentiful. As a result of this reaction, a very large amount of carbon dioxide first forms carbonic acid and then bicarbonate. The reaction is driven to bicarbonate, because as each hydrogen ion is produced, it is rapidly buffered in the cell by hemoglobin. Therefore, free hydrogen concentration remains low, and the reaction continues to move to the right, until nearly all of the carbon dioxide has reacted to bicarbonate. Hemoglobin buffering of hydrogen ion ensures that there is no significant fall in pH. Carbonic anhydrase is present in the gut and kidney as well as in the red cells.

Elimination of Carbon Dioxide by the Lungs

As dissolved carbon dioxide diffuses into the lungs and is exhaled, the reactions shown in Equation 19-2 reverse and flow to the left. When dissolved carbon dioxide diffuses out of the blood and into the lungs to be exhaled, carbon dioxide bound to hemoglobin becomes dissociated, dissolves in the blood, and is exhaled. Likewise, as carbon dioxide is blown off, bicarbonate ions react with hydrogen ions to form carbonic acid, which dissolves to carbon dioxide and water, and again, the carbon dioxide is exhaled.

Mass Action of Carbon Dioxide and Hydrogen

Mass action is the process in which a decrease in the product on one side of a reversible reaction causes all reactions to flow in that direction. Mass action also occurs in the opposite circumstance. For instance, if there is an increase in the amount of a substance on one side of a reversible reaction, the reaction is driven to flow away from that substance.

Mass Action (Equation 19-2):

$$CO_2 + H_2O \rightleftharpoons H_2CO_3 \rightleftharpoons H^+ + HCO_3^-$$

When carbon dioxide is produced by the cells and diffuses into the blood to join with water, mass action serves to drive all reactions to the right. As long as carbon dioxide is still diffusing into the blood and hydrogen ion produced from its breakdown continues to bind to hemoglobin, preventing free hydrogen ions from accumulating, mass action pushes the reaction to the right. When free hydrogen ions begin to accumulate, mass action begins to drive the reaction in the opposite direction. Equilibrium for this reaction is reached when there is no longer a concentration gradient for carbon dioxide between cells and plasma or when all hemoglobin binding sites for hydrogen are filled and free hydrogen ions begin to accumulate.

Renal Control of Acid–Base Balance

Urine Buffers

Nonvolatile acids produced during metabolism are excreted in the urine as described in Chapter 18. Their excretion occurs as a result of active *secretion* of hydrogen ions by cells of the kidney into the urine filtrate. In the filtrate, hydrogen ions join with phosphate, sulfate, or ammonia (NH_3) buffers and are then excreted in the urine as salts of phosphoric acid, sulfuric acid, or ammonium ion (NH_4^+).

Bicarbonate Handling by the Kidneys

The kidney actively reabsorbs bicarbonate ion, which is easily filtered across the kidney capillaries back into the bloodstream so that it is not lost in the urine. Extensive loss of bicarbonate—which is both a base and a primary buffer for the body—would cause severe acidosis (decrease in plasma pH). Under conditions of base excess, the kidney has the opposite capability: it actively secretes bicarbonate ion into the urine, thereby reducing plasma pH as necessary.

ELECTROLYTE INTERACTIONS AND EXCHANGES

Cells of the body carefully balance the number of cations (positively charged ions) and anions (negatively charged ions) they contain. Therefore, if one cation increases intracellularly, another cation leaves the cell to keep the charge balance constant. Cations most often juggled include potassium, hydrogen, and, to a lesser extent, calcium ion. Anions juggled include chloride and bicarbonate.

Cation Balance

If plasma potassium concentration increases as a result of increased dietary intake or extensive cell death or trauma, more potassium diffuses into all cells of the body, including the kidney tubule cells. In response, hydrogen ion leaches out of all the cells into the plasma, leading to increased plasma hydrogen ion concentration and a decrease in plasma pH. The high plasma potassium in the kidney cells causes those cells to increase potassium secretion into the urine filtrate. In response, less hydrogen ion is secreted into the urine by the kidney cells, further increasing hydrogen ion levels in the plasma. Therefore, high plasma potassium can actually lead to a decrease in plasma pH, which can result in a metabolic acidosis.

The opposite situation may occur if plasma hydrogen ion concentration increases for any reason. In this case, increased hydrogen ion diffuses into all cells, causing potassium to leach out into the plasma. Increased hydrogen ion concentration in the kidney cells leads to an increased secretion of hydrogen into the urine, whereas potassium secretion and excretion in the urine decrease. Thus, chronic acidosis can lead to hyperkalemia (increased potassium in the blood). It should be noted, however, that other inputs to potassium balance, for example insulin, can counteract the effect of hydrogen concentration on potassium efflux from cells, leading to a stable potassium concentration.

Increased plasma hydrogen also causes hydrogen ion to move into bone cells. Because of the presence of phosphate and other minerals, bone serves as an important buffer for free hydrogen ions. With accumulation of hydrogen ions in bone, bone cells leach calcium out into the plasma. Loss of bone calcium can weaken bones, increasing the risk of osteoporosis and fractures. This is common in renal failure when acid increases.

Anion Balance

The anions most frequently juggled between intracellular and extracellular compartments are chloride and bicarbonate ions. When chloride levels in the plasma fall, bicarbonate concentration in the plasma rises, causing alkalosis. This balancing act happens daily as chloride is extracted from blood passing through the stomach after a meal and is used by cells of the stomach to produce hydrochloric acid (HCl). Thus, plasma leaving the stomach is alkalotic (basic). The HCl secreted into the stomach is used to begin the digestive process. Just the opposite happens in the small intestine, where chloride ions move back into the plasma as blood passes through the small intestine. This process serves to lower the bicarbonate level in blood leaving the small intestine, thus returning plasma pH to normal before the blood leaves the gut.

TESTS OF BLOOD ELECTROLYTES AND GASES

Normal lab values of blood electrolytes and gases in an adult are listed in Table 19-1.

● Pathophysiologic Concepts

FLUID VOLUME DEFICIT

A fluid volume deficit is a reduction in extracellular fluid volume. Such a deficit may occur after acute hemorrhage, diarrhea, prolonged vomiting, or excessive sweating, or it may occur because of a shift of fluid from the extracellular to

TABLE 19-1 Normal Blood Electrolytes and Gases in an Adult	
Plasma Osmolality	**275–295 mOsm/kg**
Plasma Electrolyte Values	
• Plasma sodium	135–148 mEq/L (also written 135–148 mmol/L)
• Plasma potassium	3.5–5.0 mEq/L (3.5–5.0 mmol/L)
• Serum calcium	8.5–10.5 mg/dL
• Serum phosphate	2.5–4.5 mg/dL
• Serum magnesium	1.8–2.7 mg/dL
Blood Gas Values	
• Partial pressure of carbon dioxide in arterial blood	Between 35 and 45 mm Hg
• Partial pressure of carbon dioxide in venous blood	45 mm Hg
• Bicarbonate concentration in venous blood	Between 22 and 28 mEq/L (22–28 mmol/L)
• pH of arterial blood	Between 7.35 and 7.45
• Partial pressure of oxygen in arterial blood	100 mm Hg
• Partial pressure of oxygen in venous blood	40 mm Hg

the intracellular compartment. A fluid volume deficit may result from the loss of both salt and water, making it an isotonic deficit, or it may result from water deficiency only. A water-only deficiency would be characterized by hypernatremia (excessive sodium) in the blood. One measures fluid volume deficit by determining acute weight loss. Weight loss is calibrated, with 2% signifying a mild deficit, between 2% and 5% signifying a moderate deficit, and greater than 8% signifying a severe deficit.

FLUID VOLUME EXCESS

A fluid volume excess is typically isotonic, that is, it is characterized by increased salt and water accumulation. The most common cause of fluid volume excess is renal dysfunction. Heart failure, liver disease or failure, and corticosteroid excess may also lead to volume excess. Fluid excess is characterized by an acute weight gain of over 5% of body weight. Lung congestion with respiratory rales, cough, and dyspnea may occur, as may dependent edema. Diuretic therapy may be required.

HYPONATREMIA

Plasma sodium concentration of less than 135 mEq/L with plasma osmolality less than 280 mOsm/kg is called hyponatremia. Sodium loss can occur after vomiting, diarrhea, or excessive sweating. Hyponatremia may also occur if fluid loss is replaced with pure water instead of an electrolyte-containing fluid. Kidney disease characterized by excess reabsorption of water, as seen with syndrome of inappropriate ADH (SIADH; see Chapter 9), may also lead to hyponatremia, as may excessive use of sodium-losing diuretics.

Hyponatremia is characterized by alterations in central nervous system functioning, including confusion, depression, headache, stupor, and coma. Gastrointestinal complaints of cramping, diarrhea, and vomiting occur. Peripheral edema may result. Treatment is based on the cause and may include limiting water intake, discontinuing or changing a diuretic, and prescribing medications that block the function of ADH. Administration of a saline solution may be required.

HYPERNATREMIA

Plasma sodium concentration greater than 148 mEq/L, with plasma osmolality greater than 295 mOsm/kg, is called hypernatremia. Hypernatremia usually occurs from a disproportionate loss of water relative to sodium (e.g., during watery diarrhea or sweating). Renal inability to reabsorb water (diabetes insipidus; see Chapter 18) would also lead to hypernatremia, as would near drowning in seawater.

Clinical manifestations of hypernatremia include increased thirst and concentrated urine of low volume. Alterations in central nervous system functioning include decreased reflexes, seizures, and coma in extreme cases. Cardiovascular effects may include a decrease in blood pressure accompanied by an increase in heart rate. Treatment is oral rehydration. Serum osmolality must be carefully monitored so as not to disrupt central nervous system functioning.

HYPOKALEMIA

Plasma potassium concentration less than 3.5 mEq/L is called hypokalemia. Hypokalemia may result from decreased dietary intake; from increased loss either from the kidneys, gut, or through sweating; or from a shift of potassium from the extracellular to the intracellular compartment.

The clinical manifestations of hypokalemia depend on the degree of the disorder and the previous health status of the individual. Mild hypokalemia (serum potassium 3.0 to 3.5mEq/L) may not produce any symptoms in otherwise healthy persons. With more severe hypokalemia, symptoms of weakness, fatigue, nausea and vomiting, and constipation can occur. Muscle necrosis can occur with potassium less than 2.5 mEq/L, and with severe hypokalemia (potassium levels less than 2.0 mEq/L), paralysis can develop, leading to respiratory failure. Central nervous system dysfunction characterized by confusion or stupor may result. Hypokalemia can also lead to cardiac dysrhythmia, especially in patients who have pre-existing cardiac disease or in those who take a wide range of drugs, including digoxin. Because hypokalemia inhibits aldosterone release, the kidneys are unable to concentrate the urine, resulting in polyuria. Treatment is aimed at increasing dietary intake or at the use of supplements or infusion.

HYPERKALEMIA

Plasma potassium concentration greater than 5.0 mEq/L is called hyperkalemia. Hyperkalemia usually occurs with renal failure when the kidneys are unable to secrete potassium. It may also happen with major trauma or burns, during which damaged cells release their intracellular potassium stores. Instances of hyperkalemia have been reported after accidental intravenous administration of highly concentrated potassium solutions or intravenous administration of potassium in patients who have low urine output.

Clinical manifestations of hyperkalemia include changes in muscle function, including cramping and weakness. Cardiac dysfunction may result in changes in the electrocardiogram (ECG), leading to cardiac arrest and death. Treatment depends on the cause and the extent. For excess ingestion, dietary changes are advised. Individuals who have kidney failure may require dialysis. Rapid movement of potassium out of the extracellular fluid may be accomplished by the administration of insulin, which increases intracellular transport of potassium.

HYPOCALCEMIA

Hypocalcemia is a serum calcium concentration of less than 8.5 mg/dL. Hypocalcemia may result from an inability to access bone calcium stores as a result of the dysfunction, suppression, or removal of the parathyroid gland. Hypocalcemia may also result from vitamin D deficiency, leading to decreased absorption of dietary calcium. Increased protein binding of serum calcium as a result of decreased H^+ may lead to hypocalcemia, as may elevation of phosphate levels resulting from renal failure.

The consequences of hypocalcemia include changes in neuromuscular function, including muscle spasms and cramping, and numbness and tingling of the extremities. The cardiovascular system may be affected, resulting in hypotension and decreased cardiac output. Bone pain, deformities, and fractures may result. Osteomalacia and childhood rickets can develop. Treatment of acute hypocalcemia involves intravenous infusion of a calcium compound. For long-term conditions, increased calcium and vitamin D in the diet are recommended.

HYPERCALCEMIA

A serum calcium concentration greater than 10.5 mg/dL is known as hypercalcemia. Hypercalcemia usually results from excess release of bone calcium that typically happens with hyperparathyroidism or bone neoplasm. Other cancers may affect bone remodeling and result in hypercalcemia as well. Hypercalcemia may also occur after prolonged immobilization. Excess intake of vitamin D unaccompanied by increased dietary intake of calcium may lead to hypercalcemia. Lithium, used to treat manic-depressive disorder, increases serum calcium levels.

The clinical consequences of hypercalcemia include alterations in kidney function, with an increased risk of kidney stones and polyuria related to an inability of the kidney to concentrate the urine. A variety of neuromuscular manifestations develop, including muscle weakness, loss of tone, and muscle atrophy. The cardiovascular system is affected, leading to increased blood pressure and alterations in the ECG. Central nervous system dysfunction, including lethargy, stupor, and coma, may occur. Treatment is aimed at reducing the further release of calcium from bone and at rehydration.

HYPOPHOSPHATEMIA

A concentration of serum phosphate less than 2.5 mg/dL is called hypophosphatemia. Hypophosphatemia may occur as a result of malnutrition and is common in those who abuse alcohol; it is at least partially related to poor nutrition in this population. Shifts of phosphate from the extracellular to the intracellular compartment may also lead to hypophosphatemia. Because intracellular phosphate transport is stimulated by insulin, prolonged glucose administration or hyperalimentation may lead to depletion of extracellular phosphate. Similarly, insulin administration, either at too high a dose or in an attempt to treat an episode of diabetic ketoacidosis, may lead to hypophosphatemia. Decreased intestinal absorption of phosphate may accompany either prolonged diarrhea or the use of aluminum- or calcium-containing antacids, because these substances bind phosphate and increase its excretion in the stool.

Manifestations of hypophosphatemia include neuromuscular dysfunction characterized by tremors, muscle weakness, seizures, and sometimes coma and death. Because phosphate is a vital component of ATP, all energy stores are affected. Red blood cell, white blood cell, and platelet function are diminished as well. Treatment is replacement therapy.

HYPERPHOSPHATEMIA

A serum phosphate concentration greater than 4.5 mg/dL is called hyperphosphatemia. Most commonly, hyperphosphatemia is a result of diminished renal function, but it may also occur from a redistribution of intracellular phosphate, most commonly after a major trauma. Chemotherapy that destroys cancer cells may lead to hyperphosphatemia as the cancer cells are destroyed. Increased phosphate may occur from phosphate-containing laxatives or enemas.

Serious consequences of hyperphosphatemia include neuromuscular (tetany, weakness) and cardiovascular (dysrhythmia, hypotension) changes resulting from reciprocal hypocalcemia. Treatment is aimed at correcting the cause of the disorder. Dialysis may be required.

HYPOMAGNESEMIA

A magnesium concentration less than 1.8 mg/dL is called hypomagnesemia. Hypomagnesemia may result from reduced intake related to malnutrition or alcohol abuse, or from gut malabsorption of magnesium related to laxatives or diarrhea. Overingestion of calcium may impair magnesium absorption across the gut because calcium and magnesium compete for the same transport site. Renal loss of magnesium may be excessive with the use of certain diuretics or with different magnesium-wasting kidney diseases such as diabetes mellitus, hyperaldosteronism, and hypoparathyroidism.

Clinical consequences of hypomagnesemia include personality changes, neuromuscular tetany or spasms, hypertension, and cardiac dysrhythmia. Treatment is replacement therapy.

HYPERMAGNESEMIA

Serum magnesium concentration greater than 2.7 mg/dL is called hypermagnesemia. This condition is relatively uncommon because the kidney can greatly increase magnesium excretion when required. Therefore, if hypermagnesemia does occur, it usually does so in individuals who have renal dysfunction. Overingestion of magnesium as a laxative, especially in those who have poor renal function, may lead to the condition. Magnesium sulfate is provided to women who have toxemia of pregnancy, and hypermagnesemia may be a serious complication in this population.

Hypermagnesemia is associated with a variety of severe neurologic effects, including muscle weakness or paralysis, confusion, coma, and death. Because magnesium can compete for calcium-binding sites in the smooth muscle and heart, hypermagnesemia may result in symptoms of hypocalcemia, including hypotension and cardiac dysrhythmia, leading to cardiac arrest in severe cases. Treatment is cessation of magnesium administration. The administration of calcium is also used to counter the effects of hypermagnesemia. Dialysis may be needed to clear the blood.

ACIDOSIS/ACIDEMIA

A systemic increase in hydrogen ion concentration is called acidosis. Hydrogen ion concentration can increase as a result of a failure of the lungs to eliminate carbon dioxide or if there is excess production of volatile or nonvolatile acids. Acidosis can also occur if there is a loss of bicarbonate base caused by persistent diarrhea or by a failure of the kidney either to reabsorb bicarbonate or to secrete hydrogen ions.

The decrease in arterial pH to less than 7.35 is called acidemia. Acidemia may result from respiratory, renal, or metabolic causes.

ALKALOSIS/ALKALEMIA

Alkalosis is a systemic decrease in hydrogen ion concentration. Hydrogen ion concentration can decrease as a result of excess loss of carbon dioxide during hyperventilation, excess loss of nonvolatile acids during vomiting, or excess ingestion of a base.

Alkalemia is the increase in arterial blood pH above 7.45. Alkalemia may result from respiratory, renal, or metabolic causes.

COMPENSATION

The lungs and kidneys work together to maintain plasma pH within the range of 7.35 to 7.45. If acidosis or alkalosis results from a respiratory disorder, the kidneys respond by altering their handling of hydrogen ion and bicarbonate base to return the pH back toward normal. Renal actions aimed at reversing acidosis or alkalosis caused by a respiratory disorder are called renal compensation. Renal compensation begins to have an effect approximately 24 hours after a respiratory alteration in pH. Despite this delay, renal compensation is powerful and long-lasting.

If acidosis or alkalosis results from a metabolic or a renal disorder, the respiratory system responds by increasing or decreasing respiratory rate, to return the pH to normal. Respiratory actions aimed at reversing acidosis or alkalosis caused by a metabolic or renal disorder are called respiratory compensation. Respiratory compensation occurs immediately upon changes in hydrogen ion concentration, because hydrogen ion is the determining influence controlling the respiratory center in the brain. However, respiratory compensation is not long term.

● Conditions of Disease or Injury

Many of the conditions and diseases that result in fluid and electrolyte disturbance are described elsewhere in this book, including diabetes insipidus and SIADH. Likewise, the effects of diarrhea and vomiting and renal, cardiac, and hepatic failure on fluid, electrolyte, and acid–base balance are presented in detail elsewhere. Therefore, only a few of the causes of fluid and electrolyte disturbance are reviewed in the following sections.

PSYCHOGENIC POLYDIPSIA

Excessive water intake caused by a psychiatric abnormality already present in a patient, usually schizophrenia, is called psychogenic polydipsia. This disorder occurs for no known reason, but seems to worsen during times of exacerbation of psychotic symptoms. It may be worsened by medication-induced stimulation of ADH in this population.

Clinical Manifestations

- Compulsive water ingestion coupled with high urine outflow.

Diagnostic Tools

- Hyponatremia and hypo-osmolarity apparent on laboratory analysis.
- Urine osmolarity very low.

Complications

- Neurologic dysfunction leading to seizure or coma may result.

Treatment

- Behavioral intervention to decrease water intake may be effective.
- Drugs to reduce ADH may be prescribed.
- For severe water intoxication, hypertonic saline may be infused carefully.
- Treatment of the underlying psychotic disorder may improve the condition.

PRIMARY HYPERALDOSTERONISM

Excessive synthesis and release of aldosterone from the adrenal gland is called primary hyperaldosteronism. Its causes may include an aldosterone-secreting tumor or the condition may occur for no known reason (idiopathic). Other hormonal abnormalities, such as Cushing disease related to elevated ACTH or adrenal hypoplasia, may also lead to aldosteronism.

Because aldosterone increases renal reabsorption of sodium while at the same time increasing potassium excretion by the kidneys, hypokalemia may result.

Clinical Manifestations

- Symptoms of hypernatremia and hypokalemia.
- Blood volume expansion.

Diagnostic Tools

- Laboratory analysis reveals the electrolyte abnormalities.
- Serum aldosterone levels measure high. Plasma renin activity is low.

Complications

- Neurologic dysfunction, cardiac irregularity, and hypertension may develop.

Treatment

- A salt-restricted diet or a potassium-sparing diuretic.
- Treatment of any underlying cause may cure the disorder.
- Spironolactone promotes sodium excretion and potassium retention.

RESPIRATORY ACIDOSIS

Respiratory acidosis is the decrease in arterial pH resulting from a primary respiratory disorder. The lungs are responsible for eliminating volatile acid in the form of metabolically produced carbon dioxide. If respiration is impaired and carbon dioxide levels increase, Equation 19-2 is driven to the right by mass action, causing an increase in hydrogen ion concentration. Initially, the increase in hydrogen ion is buffered. However, if exhalation of volatile acid is significantly impaired, free hydrogen ion levels increase, causing pH to decrease.

Causes of Respiratory Acidosis

All obstructive pulmonary disorders (chronic obstructive lung disease, asthma), as well as hypoventilation of any origin, including drug overdose or airway obstruction, can cause respiratory acidosis. Severe pulmonary congestion may lead to decreased diffusion of carbon dioxide into the lungs from the blood, reducing its elimination in expired air. Likewise, infant or adult respiratory distress syndrome from any cause is associated with reduced pulmonary blood flow and poor exchange of carbon dioxide and oxygen between the lungs and the blood, resulting in the accumulation of carbon dioxide.

Compensation for Respiratory Acidosis

When acidosis is caused by a respiratory problem, renal compensation occurs. Renal compensation results in the kidney increasing its secretion and excretion of acid and increasing its reabsorption of base. Little or no bicarbonate is secreted into the urine. Renal compensation takes at least 24 hours to begin. Therefore, although a powerful remedy, renal compensation occurs only in cases of respiratory acidosis lasting that long. If successful, plasma pH will remain in the normal range.

Clinical Manifestations

- Neurologic symptoms such as headache, behavioral changes, and tremors.
- Respiratory depression from increased carbon dioxide may occur.

Diagnostic Tools

- The partial pressure of carbon dioxide is greater than 45 mm Hg (because increased carbon dioxide is the cause of the problem).
- For respiratory acidosis lasting longer than 24 hours, plasma bicarbonate levels are increased (greater than 28 mEq/L), reflecting the fact that the kidney is excreting more hydrogen ion and reabsorbing more base.
- If renal compensation is successful, plasma pH will be low, but in the normal range. If compensation is unsuccessful or if the respiratory acidosis is more acute than 24 hours, plasma pH will reflect high hydrogen ion concentration (pH > 7.35). Urine pH is acidic as the kidneys excrete more hydrogen ion and return pH toward normal.

Complications

- Paralysis and coma may result from cerebral vasodilatation in response to increased carbon dioxide concentration if levels become toxic.

Treatment

- Improvement of ventilation is essential. Mechanical ventilation may be required.

RESPIRATORY ALKALOSIS

The increase in arterial pH resulting from any primary respiratory disorder is called respiratory alkalosis. Respiratory alkalosis results when carbon dioxide levels decrease to less than 38 mm Hg. With decreased carbon dioxide, Equation 19-2 is driven to the left, resulting in a decrease in free hydrogen ion concentration and an increase in pH.

Causes of Respiratory Alkalosis

Hyperventilation is the main cause of respiratory alkalosis. Causes of hyperventilation include fever and anxiety. Hypoxemia can stimulate hyperventilation if the partial pressure of oxygen in arterial blood decreases to less than 50 mm Hg (normal is approximately 100 mm Hg). Salicylate toxicity and brain infections can directly stimulate the respiratory center in the brain to increase the respiratory rate, which can lead to respiratory alkalosis.

Compensation for Respiratory Alkalosis

Alkalosis caused by a respiratory problem stimulates renal compensation. Renal compensation involves the kidney returning pH toward normal by decreasing its secretion and excretion of hydrogen ion and actively secreting bicarbonate ion into the urine. Again, renal compensation requires 24 hours to become effective.

Clinical Manifestations

- The rapid respirations responsible for alkalosis are the major clinical man-ifestation.
- Central nervous system disturbances include dizziness, muscle contractions, and changes in consciousness.

Diagnostic Tools

- Blood gases reveal decreased partial pressure of carbon dioxide of less than 35 mm Hg (because decreased carbon dioxide is the cause of the alkalosis). For respiratory alkalosis lasting longer than 24 hours, bicarbonate levels are decreased (less than 22 mEq/L), reflecting the fact that the kidney is reab-sorbing less base or secreting base into the urine.
- If renal compensation is successful, plasma pH will be high, but within the normal range. If compensation is unsuccessful or if the respiratory alkalosis is more acute than 24 hours, plasma pH will reflect the low plasma hydrogen ion concentration (pH > 7.35). Urine pH is basic as the kidneys attempt to excrete more bicarbonate base and return pH toward normal.

Complications

- Convulsions and coma if the condition persists or becomes very severe.

Treatment

- Determining and treating the cause of hyperventilation is the most success-ful therapy.
- Increasing partial pressure of carbon dioxide by breathing into a bag and rebreathing the expired air may reverse the alkalosis in an acute situation.

METABOLIC ACIDOSIS

The decrease in arterial pH resulting from a nonrespiratory problem is called metabolic acidosis. Metabolic acidosis is characterized by the accumulation of nonvolatile acids.

Causes of Metabolic Acidosis

Metabolic acidosis may occur if there is an increase in the production of a non-volatile acid, a decrease in the renal clearance of any nonvolatile acid, or a loss of bicarbonate.

Increase in Nonvolatile Acids

Lactic acid produced during prolonged hypoxia, ketones produced as a by-product of fat metabolism in diabetics, and acids resulting from overdose of drugs such as salicylates (a product of aspirin metabolism) are examples of nonvolatile acids; an increase in the production of any of these may lead to metabolic acidosis. Excess protein metabolism during starvation or protein malnutrition also results in increased nonvolatile acid production.

Decrease in the Renal Clearance of Hydrogen Ion

During renal failure or if there is any interruption in renal blood flow, a decrease in the renal clearance of hydrogen ions occurs. As a result of these conditions, the kidney, which normally reabsorbs all filtered bicarbonate and actively secretes hydrogen ion into the urine, cannot function properly, causing hydrogen ion to accumulate. Nitrogenous waste accumulation, such as urea during renal failure or renal hypoxia, acidifies the blood.

Loss of Bicarbonate

With decreased renal function, the kidneys fail to reabsorb bicarbonate and loss of bicarbonate occurs. Loss of bicarbonate, a base, leads to acidosis. Bicarbonate levels also decrease with chronic diarrhea because bicarbonate is concentrated in intestinal secretions. High levels of extracellular chloride (hyperchloremia) cause metabolic acidosis because bicarbonate ions shift intracellularly. This type of metabolic acidosis is called hyperchloremic acidosis.

Compensation for Metabolic Acidosis

When acidosis is caused by a metabolic problem, respiratory compensation occurs. Respiratory compensation for metabolic acidosis involves the lungs expiring more carbon dioxide through increases in the rate and depth of respirations. Plasma pH returns toward normal. Respirations present during metabolic acidosis caused by diabetic ketoacidosis are called Kussmaul respirations. Respiratory compensation begins almost immediately with the onset of acidosis. Whether respiratory compensation can be fully successful depends on the severity of the acidosis. For metabolic acidosis not caused by kidney disease, the kidneys will also compensate and excrete more acid.

Clinical Manifestations

- Weakness and fatigue occurring from poor muscle function.
- Anorexia, nausea, and vomiting.
- Warm flushed skin resulting from a pH-sensitive decrease in vascular response to sympathetic stimuli.
- If metabolic acidosis is caused by diabetic ketoacidosis, additional manifestations will include:
  - Ketone smell (fruity) on breath
  - Anorexia, nausea and vomiting, abdominal pain
  - Kussmaul respirations
  - Decreasing level of consciousness, leading to coma

- If metabolic acidosis is caused by chronic renal failure, additional manifestations will include:
  - Pruritus (itching)
- If metabolic acidosis is caused by diarrhea, additional manifestations will include:
  - Signs of dehydration, including decreased blood pressure and loss of skin turgor
  - Abdominal pain and cramping
  - Frequent, loose stools

DIAGNOSTIC TOOLS

- Table 19-2 and Box 19-1 include a summary of simple blood gas analysis.
- Blood gases reveal decreased bicarbonate levels of less than 22 mEq/L (because decreased bicarbonate either is the direct cause of the acidosis or reflects an increase in hydrogen ion concentration).
- Because respiratory compensation occurs immediately, carbon dioxide levels quickly decrease, reflecting that the lungs are increasing the rate of respiration to exhale more acid. Partial pressure of carbon dioxide is less than 35 mm Hg. Respirations are rapid and deep.
- If respiratory compensation is successful, plasma pH is low but in the normal range. If compensation is unsuccessful, plasma pH will reflect high plasma acidity and be less than 7.35, even in the face of reduced carbon dioxide. Urine pH will be acidic if renal function is normal, because the kidneys will attempt to excrete more acid to return pH toward normal.
- If metabolic acidosis is caused by diabetic ketoacidosis, additional diagnostic tools will include:
  - Increase in blood and urine glucose
  - Ketonuria and decreased urine pH
- If metabolic acidosis is caused by chronic renal failure, additional diagnostic tools will include:
  - Urine pH only slightly acidic or non-acidic
  - Increased blood urea nitrogen (BUN), reflecting excess protein catabolism (breakdown) and decreased GFR

TABLE 19-2 Simple Arterial Blood Gas Analysis		
pH	**Carbon Dioxide**	**Bicarbonate**
<7.35 = acidosis	>45 = Respiratory	<22 = Metabolic
>7.45 = alkalosis	<35 = Respiratory	>28 = Metabolic

B O X   1 9 - 1   Steps to Interpret Simple ABGs

1. Look at the pH and determine if it is acidosis or alkalosis.
2. If it is acidosis, the CO_2 will be high or the bicarbonate will be low. If it is alkalosis, the bicarbonate will be high or the CO_2 will be low.
3. Look at the table to determine which finding is consistent with metabolic or respiratory acidosis or alkalosis.

Complications

- If metabolic acidosis is caused by chronic renal failure, complications may include renal osteodystrophy (bone dissolution due to renal disease) and renal encephalopathy.
- If pH falls below 7.0, cardiac dysrhythmia can occur. This happens as a result of changes in cardiac conduction, which occur in direct response to a decrease in pH and because of the effects of increased hydrogen ion concentration on plasma and intracellular potassium.

Treatment

- Treatment for metabolic acidosis is specifically based on treating the cause of the disorder.
- For patients with renal disease, treatment should include providing excess base in the diet.
- Administration of sodium bicarbonate may be used to raise pH rapidly if the person is at risk of dying. This procedure must be undertaken carefully because sodium bicarbonate infusion may cause brain swelling.

METABOLIC ALKALOSIS

The increase in arterial pH resulting from a nonrespiratory problem is called metabolic alkalosis. There are several causes of metabolic alkalosis.

Causes of Metabolic Alkalosis

If there is excessive loss of acid or if base ingestion increases, metabolic alkalosis may occur. Dehydration and alterations in extracellular electrolyte levels, causing shifts in plasma electrolytes, can lead to metabolic alkalosis as well.

Loss of Acid

Because stomach contents are usually acidic, excessive vomiting can result in acid loss. Vomiting also causes alkalosis indirectly because of the loss of chloride in the vomit.

Increased Bicarbonate Levels

Ingestion of bicarbonate in the form of bicarbonate-containing antacids used to treat indigestion or heartburn can cause increased bicarbonate levels. Bicarbonate solutions may be used during cardiopulmonary resuscitation and can lead to metabolic alkalosis.

Decreased Extracellular Fluid Volume

Volume contraction or decreased extracellular fluid volume can lead to increased plasma bicarbonate levels and to metabolic alkalosis by causing less bicarbonate to be filtered across the glomerulus. A greater percentage of the filtered bicarbonate is reabsorbed back into the peritubular capillaries if the rate of blood flow is also reduced.

Alterations in Extracellular Electrolyte Levels

Alkalosis as a result of hydrogen ions shifting intracellularly is caused by alterations in extracellular electrolyte levels. For example, a decrease in extracellular chloride may cause metabolic alkalosis as chloride diffuses out of the cell and hydrogen ion shifts into the intracellular compartment. This is called hypochloremic alkalosis. Likewise, hypokalemia (decreased plasma potassium) may cause metabolic alkalosis because of increased hydrogen excretion by the kidneys.

Compensation for Metabolic Alkalosis

When alkalosis is caused by a metabolic problem, respiratory compensation occurs. Respiratory compensation for metabolic alkalosis involves a decrease in the rate and depth of respirations. Respiratory compensation serves to return plasma pH toward normal and can occur almost immediately upon onset of alkalosis. The kidneys will also participate in compensation when possible.

Clinical Manifestations

- Neurologic manifestations are slow to develop, but may include confusion, hyperactive reflexes, spasms, and tetany (sustained muscle contraction).

Diagnostic Tools

- Blood gases reveal increased bicarbonate levels greater than 28 mEq/L (because increased bicarbonate either is the direct cause of the alkalosis or reflects a decrease in hydrogen ion concentration).
- Because of respiratory compensation, carbon dioxide levels are increased, reflecting the fact that the lungs are slowing the rate of respiration to retain more acid in order to return pH toward normal. The partial pressure of carbon dioxide is greater than 45 mm Hg. The rate and depth of respirations are reduced, possibly causing hypoxemia.

- If respiratory compensation is successful, plasma pH will be high but in the normal range. If compensation is unsuccessful, plasma pH will reflect the high plasma base concentration and will be greater than 7.45 in the face of elevated carbon dioxide.
- Urine pH will be basic if renal function is normal, because the kidneys will attempt to excrete less acid and more base to return pH toward normal.

Complications

- With pH greater than 7.55, dysrhythmia and coma may result from alterations in neuronal and cardiac muscle cell depolarization.

Treatment

- If the cause is due to chloride or potassium deficiency, these ions must be replaced.
- If decreased extracellular volume is the cause, saline solution replacement is required.

PEDIATRIC CONSIDERATIONS

- Infants and children are at high risk of serious fluid volume deficit with prolonged diarrhea or vomiting. Worldwide, a main cause of infant mortality is infectious diarrhea leading to circulatory collapse. The use of replacement fluids for children at risk can significantly improve morbidity and mortality. Vaccination against rotavirus, a major cause of infant and early childhood diarrhea, is available.
- Children with renal failure who are on dialysis show improved growth if bicarbonate levels can be normalized. Peritoneal dialysis appears better able to normalize bicarbonate than hemodialysis and thus improve growth outcomes for children.

GERIATRIC CONSIDERATION

- The older adult is at a greater risk for dehydration due to decreased thirst mechanism, decreased total body water, and decreased kidney function.

SELECTED BIBLIOGRAPHY

Bailey, J. L. (2006). Metabolic acidosis: An unrecognized cause of morbidity in the patient with chronic kidney disease. *Kidney International*, 96, S15–S23.

Broccard, A. F. (2006). Respiratory acidosis and acute respiratory distress syndrome: Time to trade in a bull market? *Critical Care Medicine*, 34, 229–231.

Copstead, L. C., & Banasik, J. L. (2010). *Pathophysiology*. St. Louis, MO: Elsevier Mosby.

Guyton, A. C., & Hall, J. (2006). *Textbook of medical physiology* (11th ed.). Philadelphia, PA: W.B. Saunders.

Herd, A. M. (2005). An approach to complex acid–base problems. Keeping it simple. *Canadian Family Physician*, 51, 226–232.

Irland, N. B. (2009). Late decelerations and acid–base balance. *Nursing for Women's Health*, 13(4), 335–340.

Kramer, B. (2009). Arterial blood gases. *Registered Nurses Journal*, 72(4), 22–24.

Oh, H., & Seo, W. (2007). Alterations in fluid, electrolytes and other serum chemistry values and their relations with enteral tube feedings in acute brain infarction patients. *Journal of Clinical Nursing*, 16(2), 298–307.

Porth, C. M., & Matfin, G. (2009). *Pathophysiology: Concepts of altered health states* (8th ed.). Philadelphia, PA: Lippincott Williams & Wilkins.

Reynolds, I. G. (2007). Discovering and stopping hyperkalemia. *American Nurse Today*, 2(11), 52.

Scales, K., & Pilsworth, J. (2008). The importance of fluid balance in clinical practice. *Nursing Standard*, 22(47), 50–57.

Touhy, T. A., & Jett, K. F. (2010). *Ebersole and Hess' gerontological nursing & healthy aging*. St. Louis, MO: Mosby Elsevier.

The Reproductive System

Perhaps one of the most important functions of humans is the ability to re-produce. While there is a plethora of literature related to the topic, many still find it a difficult and even embarrassing topic of conversation. Pathology of the reproductive system can interfere with an individual's ability to contribute to the genetic pool.

● Physiologic Concepts (Male)

MALE REPRODUCTIVE ANATOMY

The reproductive role of the human male is to produce and deliver sperm to impregnate a female. To carry out these functions, a male has internal and external sexual organs. These structures include the testes, several tubules that carry sperm out of the testes, various glands, and the penis (Fig. 20-1).

The Testes

The **testes** are the male gonads. Testes develop during gestation in response to the production of androgenic hormones by the male embryo. The primary androgen is testosterone, the synthesis of which begins at approximately 8 weeks' gestation.

During early gestation, the fetal testes are located in the abdominal cavity. At approximately 6 months' gestation, the testes descend from the abdominal cavity through the inguinal canal into an external sac, called the **scrotum**. Associated blood vessels, nerves, and a supporting cord descend from the

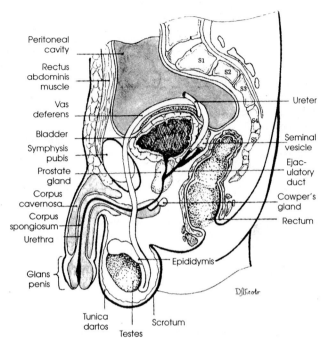

FIGURE 20-1 Side view of male genitourinary anatomy. (From Bullock, B. L. & Rosendahl, P. P. (1992). *Pathophysiology: Adaptations and alterations in function* (3rd ed.). Philadelphia, PA: Lippincott Williams & Wilkins.)

abdominal cavity simultaneously. After descent, the abdominal opening of the canal closes. The scrotum sits dorsal to the **penis**, the male sexual organ and the male structure for urination. Because of their location outside the body, the testes remain at a lower-than-body temperature. This provides optimal conditions for **spermatogenesis**, or sperm formation.

Seminiferous Tubules

Each testis is filled with hundreds of long, coiled tubules, called **seminiferous tubules.** Immature sperm arise from stem cells present in the tubular walls and then migrate into the tubule lumen. The seminiferous tubules include two types of cells: **Sertoli cells**, which line the inside of the tubules, and **Leydig interstitial cells**, which surround the outside of the tubules. The developing sperm receive essential support and nourishment from the Sertoli cells during their long maturation. The Leydig interstitial cells synthesize and secrete testosterone during gestation and after puberty. Testosterone is essential both for sperm maturation and Sertoli cell function.

The Epididymis, Vas Deferens, and Urethra

From the seminiferous tubules, sperm journey into another long tubule, the **epididymis**. The epididymis curves around the posterior side of the testes and ascends toward the peritoneal cavity. The epididymis leads into the **vas deferens**. The vas deferens enters the peritoneal cavity and widens to form a space called the **ampulla**, which has a glandular, convoluted structure on each side called the **seminal vesicle**.

At the ampulla, the vas deferens forms the **ejaculatory duct**. The ejaculatory duct passes through the **prostate gland** and joins with the **internal urethra** below the **bladder**. The internal urethra enters the penis and forms the **urethra**. Mucus-secreting glands line the urethra.

Sperm Maturation

Sperm at the entrance to the epididymis are immature and unable to fertilize an egg. By the time the sperm have traveled through the vas deferens (approximately 2 weeks), the sperm will have become fully mature. Mature sperm can be stored in the vas deferens and ampulla, where they remain viable for more than a month.

The Seminal Vesicles

With sexual excitement, the seminal vesicles secrete a mucuslike substance containing sugar, prostaglandins, and fibrinogen into the ejaculatory duct. The sperm use the sugar for energy, and the prostaglandins assist sperm in penetrating the female cervix. Prostaglandins may also cause contractions of the female genital tract, which propel the sperm in their journey to reach the egg.

The Prostate

The prostate is a walnut-shaped gland that sits beneath the bladder. During sexual excitement, the prostate secretes a thin, milky fluid containing various enzymes and ions into the ejaculatory duct. This mixture joins the sperm and seminal vesicle fluid. Prostate fluid is alkaline (basic). When it, along with the rest of the ejaculate, is deposited in the vagina of the female, it neutralizes the acidic vaginal secretions; this is important because sperm have poor motility in a low pH environment.

Neural Innervation of the Male Reproductive System

Afferent sensory neurons and efferent parasympathetic and sympathetic fibers are found throughout the male genitalia. Afferent sensory fibers are activated in response to tactile stimulation and send their information to the spinal cord. Parasympathetic nerves exit the spine at the level of the sacral area and innervate the arteries and arterioles of the penis. Parasympathetic fibers release the neurotransmitter acetylcholine, causing dilation of the blood vessels. Sympathetic nerves exit the spine from the upper lumbar areas and innervate the smooth muscle of the vas deferens and ampulla. Sympathetic fibers release the neurotransmitter norepinephrine, which causes smooth muscle contraction. Sympathetic fibers also innervate and cause contraction of the prostate and the seminal vesicles. Descending neurons from higher centers of the brain, including the cerebral cortex, influence the firing of the parasympathetic and sympathetic fibers.

THE MALE SEXUAL ACT

Physical manipulation of the penis or sexual thoughts activate the parasympathetic and sympathetic nerves, causing sexual excitement. There are four stages of the male sexual act: erection, emission, ejaculation, and resolution. All stages can occur as simple spinal reflexes initiated by sensory stimulation. They do not require central nervous system involvement. Normally, however, both mental and physical stimuli contribute to sexual excitement. Inhibitory cerebral stimulation may interrupt the spinal reflexes at any point.

Erection

The penis hardens and becomes elongated during sexual excitement. An erection occurs following activation of the parasympathetic fibers to the penis that cause vasodilation and increased blood flow. As the arteries and arterioles of the penis fill up with blood, the veins draining the penis become compressed and occluded. Venous occlusion causes the spongy tissue in the shaft of the penis, the **corpus cavernosum** and **corpus spongiosum**, to become engorged. Engorgement of these tissues results in an erection. Parasympathetic stimulation also causes the glands lining the urethra to secrete mucus. Mucus lubricates the glans (head) of the penis, which facilitates and increases the pleasure associated with penetration of the female. During this stage, heart rate and respiratory rate increase.

Emission

When sexual excitement reaches a critical level, activation of the sympathetic nerves to the penis causes contraction of the vas deferens and ampulla. This contraction results in **emission**—the propulsion of the sperm out of the vas deferens and ampulla through the ejaculatory duct and into the internal urethra. During emission, sympathetic stimulation to the prostate and seminal vesicles causes release of prostate and seminal vesicle secretions into the ejaculatory duct. The combination of sperm, prostate secretions, and seminal vesicle secretions is called **semen**.

Ejaculation

With the addition of semen in the internal urethra, a feeling of fullness occurs. Sensory fibers traveling to the spinal cord transmit this feeling, resulting in further activation of the sympathetic fibers and smooth muscle contraction of the ducts. Motor neurons to skeletal muscles at the base of the penis are also activated, leading to contraction of these muscles. The culminating responses are wavelike, rhythmic contractions associated with intense pleasure. During these contractions, semen is forcefully propelled through the urethra and out of the urethral opening. Emission and ejaculation comprise the male **orgasm**. Heart rate and respiratory rate reach a maximum at this time.

Resolution

After experiencing an orgasm, a male shows a reversal of sexual excitement, including disappearance of the erection and a return of heart rate and breathing patterns to normal.

SPERMATOGENESIS

Spermatogenesis (the formation of sperm) begins during puberty and continues throughout the lifetime of a male. Undifferentiated germ cells lining the seminiferous tubules undergo a programmed number of mitotic cell divisions, resulting in the production of the **primary spermatocytes** (immature sperm), which ultimately develop into the **spermatozoa** (mature sperm). Spermatogenesis requires approximately 2 months. From each primary spermatocyte, four viable sperm (each with 23 chromosomes) are produced. Spermatogenesis occurs in the seminiferous tubule under the control of two pituitary hormones—follicle-stimulating hormone (FSH) and luteinizing hormone (LH)—and the sex hormones, primarily testosterone.

Follicle-Stimulating Hormone

FSH is a protein hormone released from the anterior pituitary in response to a stimulating hormone from the hypothalamus: gonadotropin-releasing hormone (GnRH) (see Chapter 9). FSH binds to receptors present on the membranes of the Sertoli cells that line the seminiferous tubules, and activates a cyclic adenosine monophosphate (cAMP) second messenger system. The final effect of FSH is to cause Sertoli cells to proliferate and secrete various nutrients, ions, and proteins into the tubule that stimulate the continued proliferation and differentiation of the immature sperm.

Sertoli cells exert feedback on the hypothalamus and pituitary to control the further release of FSH by secreting the hormone **inhibin**. Inhibin levels rise with increased cell activity and inhibit the further release of FSH.

Luteinizing Hormone

LH is the second protein hormone released from the anterior pituitary in response to stimulation by GnRH. LH binds to the Leydig cells that surround the tubule, and again through the activation of a cAMP second messenger system, stimulates the synthesis of the steroid hormone testosterone. Testosterone diffuses into the seminiferous tubules and binds to the Sertoli cells, stimulating them to continue to secrete the proteins, ions, and nutrients required to maintain proliferation and differentiation of the sperm. One protein that is manufactured by the Sertoli cells, androgen-binding protein, ensures that levels of testosterone remain high in the lumen of the seminiferous tubule. Mature Leydig cells usually develop at approximately 10 years of age in a boy.

Testosterone feeds back on the hypothalamus, and to a lesser extent on the anterior pituitary, to inhibit the further release of GnRH and LH. This feedback keeps the levels of circulating testosterone relatively constant. Besides being required for the successful formation of sperm, testosterone is also essential for the production of the male secondary sexual characteristics and the maintenance of the male libido (sex drive).

Stimuli Controlling GnRH Release

GnRH is released in small pulses throughout the day, resulting in relatively constant daily levels. Increases or decreases in GnRH release may occur seasonally and with different physical and psychological conditions such as anxiety or depression. Changes in the secretion of GnRH may affect sperm formation by affecting LH and FSH and may alter libido.

MALE SECONDARY SEXUAL CHARACTERISTICS

Male secondary sexual characteristics are under the control of the male androgens, especially testosterone. The effects of testosterone are described fully in Chapter 9. The male secondary sexual characteristics include the following:

- Increased protein anabolism and muscle mass.
- Increased bone growth and strength.
- Male pattern of hair on the face, axillary, and pubic regions. Hair growth is thick on most areas of the body.
- Increased metabolic rate, probably as a result of increased protein anabolism (buildup) and muscle mass formation. Increased metabolic rate raises the caloric needs of males, beginning at puberty, compared to females.
- Proliferation and activation of sebaceous glands in the skin, which produce an oily substance called sebum. Increased amounts of sebum can cause acne, especially during teenage years.
- A deepening voice, as a result of hypertrophy of the larynx.
- Male pattern baldness, typically beginning with a bald spot on the top of the head. A genetic tendency influences male pattern baldness.

● Pathophysiologic Concepts (Male)

ERECTILE DYSFUNCTION

Erectile dysfunction (ED), previously called impotence, is the inability of a male to achieve or maintain an erection. ED can occur infrequently, frequently, or every time a man attempts sexual intercourse. When asked, approximately 35% of men 40 years of age and older, and more than 80% of men 70 years of age and older, report at least sporadic ED. Although in the past it was believed that ED was due mostly to psychological factors, it is now recognized that for most men physical causes are paramount (discussed later). With a greater awareness of the medical causes of ED, more open discussion of its prevalence, its effects on a man's quality of life, and its treatment is becoming mainstream. Still, however, men frequently avoid seeking help for ED, thus making further education and services to promote men's health and wellness necessary. Use of a tool such as *The Sexual Health Inventory For Men*, developed by Capparelli and Rosen, will encourage more dialogue. When ED is identified, extensive screening for coronary heart disease (CHD) should be initiated because of the high correlation between ED and CHD.

Physical Causes of Erectile Dysfunction

One of the main physical causes of ED is atherosclerosis of the penile arteries. With atherosclerosis, blood flow to the penis is reduced and there is an inability of the penile arteries to dilate during sexual excitement, thus limiting tumescence. Other physical causes of ED include systemic diseases such as hypertension, hyperlipidemia, renal failure, multiple sclerosis, Parkinson disease, stroke, hypothyroidism, acromegaly, and, most commonly, diabetes mellitus. Diabetes in particular is associated with atherosclerosis as well as neuropathy (nerve damage). At the cellular level, pathophysiologic changes contributing to ED include autonomic hypersensitivity, reduced production of nitric oxide by the prostate and the vascular smooth muscle of the penis, and endothelial cell dysfunction.

Besides physical factors, many drugs are known to interfere with a man's ability to achieve an erection and/or an orgasm, including some antihypertensive and psychotropic medications. ED also may occur following surgery in the genital region, for example, after treatment for prostate cancer. Chronic or acute fatigue may also cause ED.

Psychological Causes of Erectile Dysfunction

Psychologically based ED occurs with activation of descending inhibitory impulses originating in the cerebral cortex. Psychological conditions associated with ED include stress, anger, worry, bereavement, fear of sexual failure, and depression.

Lifestyle Causes of Erectile Dysfunction

Lifestyle factors that may contribute to ED include smoking, alcohol abuse, recreational drug use, stress, and obesity. Smoking cessation and weight reduction have been shown to be effective in reducing the risk for CHD as well as ED.

Treatment of Erectile Dysfunction

There are many treatments available for ED, including mechanical aids and pumps and penile injections that cause local vasodilation. In addition, pharmaceutical advances have resulted in the production and marketing of several highly effective oral ED medications, the first of which was sildenafil citrate (Viagra). This type of drug acts to inhibit the enzyme phosphodiesterase that normally inactivates a second messenger required for relaxation of the penile arteries. By blocking phosphodiesterase, relaxation of the penile arteries is prolonged, allowing the penis to fill more fully with blood. An erection is achieved and augmented. ED medications are taken before attempting intercourse and enhance the normal sexual response; they do not stimulate an erection on their own. Side effects of oral ED medication may include headache, facial flushing, and visual abnormalities. Oral ED medications are contraindicated for men with certain types of heart disease or those taking other vasodilators such as nitroglycerin. Other medications may include adrenergic antagonists to potentiate parasympathetic neurotransmission and testosterone supplements.

For ED related to the side effects of prescribed medications, reevaluation of drug dosage or drug choice may reduce symptoms. ED associated with systemic disease or depression must be addressed directly. ED related to other psychological factors may be relieved by relaxation techniques, counseling, or sexual therapy. Studies suggest that in some men with ED, a strict weight loss and exercise program may help restore sexual function.

GYNECOMASTIA

Gynecomastia is the enlargement of breast tissue in males. It can result from excess production of estrogen in the male or the liver's inability to break down normal male estrogen secretions. Gynecomastia is frequently seen during early puberty in some males and may be a normal development or may be related to excess body weight or a hormonal imbalance.

● Conditions of Disease or Injury (Male)

Table 20-1 includes a summary of male reproductive organ alterations. More detailed information about other alterations is included below.

TABLE 20-1 Summary of Male Reproductive Organ Alterations	
Alteration	**Overview**
Cryptorchidism	• Failure of one or both testicles to descent into the scrotum • Much greater risk for development of testicular cancer • May result in fertility issues • Causes: usually unknown; prematurity; testosterone deficiency; structural factors that impede gonadal descent; genetic predisposition • Clinical manifestations: testicle not palpable in scrotum • Treatment: hCG may stimulate descent; surgery; regular testicular self-exam
Hydrocele	• Collection of plasma filtrate in the scrotum, outside the testes • Scrotal swelling causes reduced blood flow to testes • Causes: congenital, genital trauma, testicular tumor, idiopathic • Clinical manifestations: asymptomatic or scrotal swelling and discomfort • Treatment: identify cause and drain fluid
Varicocele	• Abnormal dilation of vein in spermatic cord (usually left side) • Altered blood flow may cause infertility • Typically occurs between 15 and 25 years of age • Causes: valvular incompetence of spermatic vein or vena cava obstruction causing backflow and accumulation of blood; may be due to a renal tumor in older men • Clinical manifestations: asymptomatic or slight feeling of discomfort and testicular heaviness; torturous, dilated veins may be palpable • Treatment: testicular support garment; surgical ligation of the vein
Hypospadias/ Epispadias	• Hypospadias: Urethral opening located on ventral surface of the penis; in severe cases the opening may be in the scrotal or perineal area • Penis may be bowed downward (chordee), penile shaft may be rotated (torsion), foreskin may be altered • Complications may include infections, hematuria, calculi, painful intercourse

Alteration	Overview
	• Causes: Congenital; genetic factors; hormonal variations; maternal ingestion of progestin; advanced maternal age
	• Treatment: surgical repair depending on severity; circumcism is not advised so the foreskin can be used for repair
	• Epispadias: congenital misplacement of urethral opening to the dorsal side of the penis; less common than hypospadias
Phimosis	• Foreskin cannot be retracted back over the glans
	• Causes: poor hygiene; chronic infections
	• Clinical manifestations: edema, erythema, tenderness, purulent drainage
	• Treatment: circumcision
Paraphimosis	• Foreskin is retracted; cannot be moved to cover the glans
	• Clinical manifestations: edema due to constriction
	• Treatment: surgery
Peyronie Disease	• Lateral curvature of the penis during erection
	• Fibrous thickening of fascia in corpora cavernosa
	• May be associated with diabetes, keloids, beta-blockers
	• Clinical manifestations: painful erection, painful intercourse, erection problems distal to the fibrotic area
	• Treatment: surgery
Priapism	• Prolonged penile erection
	• Idiopathic or associated with spinal cord trauma, sickle cell, leukemia, pelvic tumors, injections for impotence
	• Clinical manifestations: sustained, painful erection not associated with sexual arousal
	• Treatment: iced saline enemas, ketamine, phosphodiasterase 5 inhibitors, spinal anesthesia, aspiration of blood from corpus
Testicular Torsion	• Rotation of the testicle on its vascular pedicle
	• Twisting of arteries and veins in the spermatic cord occludes circulation to the testicle
	• Most common in neonates and in adolescents
	• Clinical manifestations: pain and swelling
	• Treatment: surgical emergency if it cannot be reduced manually with scrotal elevation

BENIGN PROSTATIC HYPERPLASIA

Benign prostatic hyperplasia (BPH) is the noncancerous enlargement of the prostate gland. BPH is seen in more than 80% of men 80 years and older. BPH may cause compression of the urethra as it passes through the prostate, making urination difficult, reducing force of the flow of the urine stream, or causing dribbling of urine to occur. The cause of BPH is unclear but may be related to an imbalance between estrogen and testosterone in the prostate. The decrease in androgenic hormone production associated with aging produces an increase in dihydrotestosterone, the major prostatic intracellular androgen, and results in an androgen and estrogen imbalance. This imbalance causes changes in the periurethral glandular tissue of the prostate producing masses of fibrous glandular tissue that compresses the normal prostate tissue causing a nodular hyperplasia.

Clinical Manifestations

- Increased frequency of urination, with delay in initiating urination and a reduction in the force of the urine stream.
- Decreased diameter of the urinary stream.
- As the condition progresses, the bladder may not empty completely, causing dribbling or urine overflow. The time required to void increases.

Diagnostic Tools

- Diagnosis involves a good history and physical examination coupled with the use of imaging techniques. Biopsy of the prostate may be required to rule out neoplasia.

Complications

- With advanced BPH, urinary tract obstruction may occur as urine is unable to pass through the prostate. Urinary obstruction can lead to urinary tract infections and, if unrelieved, renal failure.

Treatment

- Mild prostate enlargement may not be treated, but followed in a "wait and see" manner.
- Active surveillance involves annual monitoring for disease progression including a history, physical examination, and symptom score.
- With more significant enlargement, medical therapy will be initiated. Alpha-blockers antagonize alpha-adrenergic receptors in the smooth muscle of the prostate causing relaxation of the muscle fibers thereby decreasing tension in

the prostate. 5-alpha reductase inhibitors block the conversion of testosterone to dihydrotestosterone causing the prostate to shrink in size. A combination of the two types of medications significantly increases symptom improvement as opposed to monotherapy.

- Surgical approaches that involve minimal invasiveness include transurethral incision of the prostate (TUIP). In this procedure, the gland is split in half surgically to reduce pressure on the urethra. Lasers may be used to split the prostate.

- Other minimally invasive procedures to reduce the size of the prostate include transurethral needle ablation, transurethral vaporization, and transurethral microwave therapy.

- If obstruction to urine flow is severe, transurethral prostatectomy (TURP) may be required to remove the enlarged prostate. Complications may include ED and incontinence.

- A permanent catheter might be placed in patients unwilling to undergo or unable to tolerate surgery.

- Annual digital rectal examinations and screening for prostate-specific antigen (PSA) are encouraged to identify a malignancy that may arise from hyperplastic cells.

INFLAMMATORY DISORDERS OF THE MALE REPRODUCTIVE TRACT

Inflammation of the male genital tract can occur anywhere between the testes and the urethral opening. Inflammation is usually due to a sexually transmitted disease or a urinary tract infection and is most commonly seen in sexually active men. Other causes of inflammation include systemic disease, such as mumps or trauma. Inflammation of the prostate may occur in older men with BPH. Common inflammatory conditions of the genitalia in men include the following.

Urethritis is an inflammation of the urethra. Urethritis is usually caused by a sexually transmitted microorganism, commonly *Neisseria gonorrhoeae* or *Chlamydia trachomatis*.

Epididymitis is an inflammation of the epididymis. Epididymitis is usually caused by a sexually transmitted microorganism, commonly *N. gonorrhoeae* or *C. trachomatis*. Epididymitis usually occurs from ascending urethral infection.

Orchitis is an acute inflammation of the testes. Orchitis usually develops following epididymitis or a systemic disease such as mumps.

Prostatitis is an inflammation of the prostate gland. Prostatitis is especially common in older men. It is often caused by an acute or chronic infection, usually ascending from the urethra. Prostatitis may be noninfectious and idiopathic in origin.

Clinical Manifestations

- Urethritis may present with pain and burning on urination. A discharge from the penis may be present.
- Epididymitis may present with acute scrotal or inguinal pain. Flank pain may be present. The scrotum may be inflamed and tender on the affected side.
- Orchitis usually presents acutely with a very high fever (104°F) and swelling and redness of the testicle and scrotum. The individual appears very ill, and malaise is obvious.
- Prostatitis from an ascending urinary tract infection usually presents with painful and frequent urination. Interrupted or slow urine stream and nocturia (urination at night) may be present. Fever and malaise are common. Low back or perineal pain is common, especially when standing. Digital examination reveals a very tender and enlarged prostate.

Diagnostic Tools

- Diagnosis involves a thorough history and physical examination. Blood and urine cultures for the identification of an infectious organism may be required.

Complications

- Epididymitis and orchitis may cause infertility, related to poor testicular blood flow, and infarct of the testicular cells.

Treatment

- Antibiotic therapy is required for all bacterial or chlamydial infections.
- Orchitis is treated with bed rest, analgesics for pain, and elevation of the testicles to increase venous drainage. Cold compresses may reduce initial inflammation. If a testicular abscess occurs, surgical removal of the testicle may be necessary.

CANCER OF THE MALE REPRODUCTIVE TRACT

Cancer of the male reproductive tract may develop in the penis, testes, or prostate.

Penile Cancer

Primary cancer of the penis is rare in the United States. It usually occurs in noncircumcised men, possibly related to accumulation of thick secretions (smegma) under the foreskin that increase the risk of sexually transmitted infections. It is slow growing and may occur anywhere on the penis. Primary penile cancer usually develops in men between 40 and 80 years of age and is more common in African Americans than in Caucasians. Secondary penile cancer may occur from metastasis of bladder, rectal, or prostate cancer.

Testicular Cancer

Testicular cancer is rare, mostly occurring in young men between the ages of 15 and 35. It is usually a germ-cell (gamete) cancer but may develop from Leydig or Sertoli cells. The cause of testicular cancer is unknown, but there appears to be a genetic factor. Testicular cancer is more common in Caucasians and occurs more frequently in men with a history of cryptorchidism. Trauma and prenatal exposure to the synthetic estrogen diethylstilbestrol (DES) may increase risk.

Prostate Cancer

Prostate cancer is the number one cancer among American males and the second leading cause of death due to cancer in that population (the first is lung cancer). Prostate cancer is usually diagnosed in men older than 65 years of age; however, it is being diagnosed increasingly in younger men, perhaps as a result of more aggressive screening. Autopsy studies show that approximately 50% of men older than 50 years of age have some cancerous prostate cells; this finding has led to significant debate over recommended treatment, especially for elderly men with slow-growing, early-stage tumors.

The cause of prostate cancer is unknown, although both genetic and environmental factors are believed to play a role. The risk of prostate cancer is increased in men who have a first-degree relative with the disease, in African American men, and in men exposed to certain environmental or occupational toxins, such as cadmium. Prostate cancer appears to be related to lifelong levels of testosterone. Prostate cancers are testosterone dependent until late in the course of the disease.

Using clinical and biopsy results, prostate tumors are staged from A to D. **Stage A** tumors are well differentiated (A1) or moderately/poorly differentiated (A2) but restricted to the prostate gland. These tumors are asymptomatic, and their presence is reported in more than 80% of men older than 80 years of age. Stage A tumors cannot be felt on digital examination. **Stage B** tumors include a single nodule (B1) or a group of discrete nodules (B2) palpable on digital examination and confined to the prostate. **Stage C** tumors are large masses that fill the entire prostate gland (C1) and may extend beyond the edges of the gland (C2). **Stage D** tumors are metastatic, with cancerous cells found in the lymph nodes draining the pelvis (D1) and in other sites (D2), often the bone.

Clinical Manifestations

- Penile cancer is characterized by a painless wartlike growth or an ulcerative lesion under the prepuce. It may also be a reddened lesion with plaque.

- Testicular cancer is characterized by the development of a mass in the testis, which may become painful as it grows. Testicular heaviness or aching may occur. Gynecomastia may develop.
- Prostate cancer may be asymptomatic or associated with increased frequency and urgency of urination, and a decrease in the force of the urine stream. Blood may be passed in the ejaculate, and in advanced disease, back pain may be present.

Diagnostic Tools

- Biopsy of cells of the penis can diagnose and stage penile cancer.
- Transillumination of the testes, ultrasound, and MRI may identify a testicular mass and support clinical findings of a testicular cancer.
- Tumor markers commonly associated with testicular cancer include alpha-fetoprotein (AFP), beta human chorionic gonadotropin (hCG), and lactate dehydrogenase (LDH).
- A digital rectal examination (DRE) may reveal a fixed, firm mass in the prostate, suggestive of a tumor. The mass is often painless with irregular borders and results in asymmetry of the prostate gland. Ultrasound may be used to pinpoint the location of a prostate tumor. A biopsy of prostate cells taken via a transurethral resection can confirm the diagnosis of prostate cancer. DRE should be conducted annually beginning at 50 years of age.
- Prostate-specific antigen (PSA), a blood test that measures the level of a glycoprotein released by the prostate gland, can be used to identify the presence of even early-stage prostate cancer. Current recommendations are to perform a biopsy if the PSA level is greater than 4 nanograms per milliliter (ng/mL) of blood; levels greater than 10 ng/mL suggest cancer. However, PSA elevation may occur with noncancerous conditions such as prostatitis or benign prostatic hyperplasia (BPH). Likewise, in approximately 25% of men, PSA measurements may be in the normal range even when cancer is present. The need to treat stage A cancers detected by PSA assay is controversial, especially in elderly men.

A recently suggested strategy to address the issue of false-negative and false-positive PSA readings is to evaluate PSA levels on a sliding scale, depending on if the male is young (younger than 50 years) or older. For young men, a PSA of even 2.6 ng/mL may be considered significant, especially if a previous lower baseline measurement is available. In older men, a moderately elevated level may not call for aggressive follow-up. In addition, measuring free versus protein-bound PSA may allow for better discrimination of cancer versus benign source, with a lower ratio of free-to-bound PSA expected in men with cancer.

- Measurement of PSA levels coupled with findings from a digital exam offer the most sensitive screening results. PSA levels should be drawn prior to the

digital exam to minimize the risk of a false-positive reading due to manipulation of the prostate.
- Transrectal ultrasound can be used to view the prostate using sound waves.
- Diagnosis is confirmed with a biopsy.

Complications

- Untreated, progressive penile cancer has an extremely high mortality rate (about 90%).
- Testicular cancer may metastasize to the lungs, lymph nodes, liver, bone, or central nervous system.
- Survival with prostate cancer depends on the stage at diagnosis. Most men diagnosed with stage D cancer die within 3 to 5 years.
- ED and incontinence may develop as a result of any of the male reproductive cancers or may develop following treatment of the cancers.

Treatment

- For penile cancer, treatment may range from excisional biopsy to a total penectomy. Radiation and chemotherapy may also be required.
- For testicular cancer, surgery to remove the affected testis is performed. Radiation and chemotherapy are provided.
- A chest radiograph and a lymph node biopsy are performed on men with testicular cancer to rule out metastasis.
- Watchful waiting may be adequate for some elderly men with stage A prostate cancer.
- Radical prostatectomy (surgical removal of the prostate) or radiation therapy is usually used to treat all stage B and C prostate tumors and all stage A tumors in young men. Treatment options can include proton-beam radiation, implanted radiation seeds, and cryotherapy. Stage D tumors are treated with hormonal therapy to slow the spread of the disease and palliative measures to reduce pain. Hormonal therapy includes antiandrogen drugs, estrogen therapy, and drugs that block the release of the hypothalamic GnRH (leuprolide). Orchiectomy (removal of the testes) may accompany hormonal therapy.

● Physiologic Concepts (Female)

FEMALE REPRODUCTIVE ANATOMY

The reproductive roles of the female include the monthly development and release of an ovum (egg), the provision of an appropriate internal environment if the ovum is fertilized by a sperm, and the carriage and nourishment of an embryo and fetus until survival outside the womb is possible. Internal reproductive structures that allow a female to meet these roles include the **ovaries, fallopian tubes, uterus,** and **vagina.** After the birth of her infant, the female's role continues as she nourishes the infant with milk produced in her **breasts.** The breasts are usually considered accessory reproductive organs. The **clitoris** is composed of erectile tissue and is located at the anterior portion of the female external genitalia. Although not essential for reproduction, the clitoris is important in providing a woman's pleasure during the sexual act. The external genitalia consist of fatty tissue called the **mons pubis** and **outer** and **inner** folds of tissue, called the **labia majora** and **labia minora,** respectively. The opening of the urethra is located between the vagina and the clitoris. Internal female reproductive anatomy is shown in Figure 20-2.

The Ovaries

A female is born with two ovaries located bilaterally in the lower abdominal cavity beside the uterus. The ovaries are the gonads of the female and contain the female sex cells—the ova (singular term is ovum). At birth, the female infant has approximately 2 million ova, down from a maximum of about 7 million present at 20 weeks' gestation. The ova have undergone numerous mitotic, but no meiotic, divisions. They remain latent in the ovary until a girl enters puberty

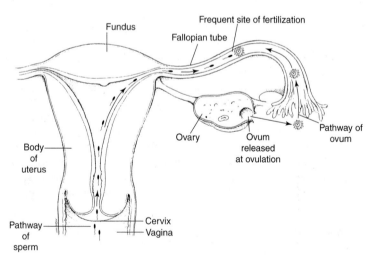

FIGURE 20-2 Female reproductive organs, showing the path of the oocyte as it moves from the ovary into the fallopian (uterine) tube; the path of sperm is also shown, as is the usual site of fertilization. (From Porth, C. M. (2005). *Pathophysiology: Concepts of altered health states* (7th ed.). Philadelphia, PA: Lippincott Williams & Willkins.)

between approximately 11 and 16 years of age, by which time the number of ova has fallen to 300,000.

The Follicle

Each individual ovum is surrounded in the ovary by a group of support cells, called **granulosa** cells. The ovum plus its surrounding granulosa cells is called a **follicle**. In childhood, the immature follicle, called a **primordial follicle**, consists of an ovum and a single layer of granulosa cells surrounding it. When a female enters puberty, the entire ovary and many of the primordial follicles enlarge. This enlargement includes increasing layers of granulosa cells and an increase in the size of each ovum. The enlarged follicle is called a **primary follicle**. Each month during a woman's reproductive life, one of the primary follicles responds to hormonal stimulation with **ovulation**—the release of a mature ovum.

The Fallopian Tubes

The fallopian tubes, also called the oviducts, are smooth muscle passageways that open at one end into the body of the uterus and at the other end into the peritoneal cavity. The opening into the peritoneal cavity has fingerlike projections, called **fimbriae**, that surround the ovary. These projections are covered with **cilia**. The cilia wave toward the fallopian tube, drawing an ovum released from the ovary into the fallopian tube. The movement of the fimbriae is so effective that an ovum released by one ovary can enter the fallopian tube on the opposite side if the same-side fallopian tube is blocked or absent.

Once in the fallopian tube, the ovum travels a short distance to enter a widened area called the **ampulla**. If fertilization of the ovum by a sperm does happen, it typically occurs in the fallopian tube at the ampulla. From the ampulla, the fertilized or unfertilized ovum travels over the next 3 to 4 days to the uterus. If the ovum has been fertilized by a sperm, the newly fertilized egg is called a **zygote**. Cell division of the zygote occurs during transit through the fallopian tube to the uterus. By the time the zygote reaches the uterus, it will consist of approximately 100 cells; at this point, a fertilized egg is called a **blastocyst**.

The Uterus

The uterus is a hollow organ composed of three layers: an inner endometrial layer, a middle smooth muscle layer, and an outer connective tissue layer. During the first half of the menstrual cycle, the endometrium hypertrophies and becomes highly vascular and secretory to prepare for the arrival of the fertilized ovum. If fertilization of the ovum has not occurred, the endometrial layer is sloughed off each month in the process of **menstruation**. If fertilization has occurred, the arriving blastocyst must implant in the wall of the uterus for the pregnancy to continue.

The nonpregnant uterus is pear shaped and approximately the size of a woman's fist. During pregnancy the uterus increases significantly in size. The uterus consists of two parts: the **body** and the **cervix**. The body of the uterus is the upper portion, sitting in the midpelvis. The upper part of the uterine body is called the **fundus**. The fallopian tubes are extensions from the fundus. The cervix is the lower part of the uterus and is the only part anchored by ligaments to the abdominal cavity. The cervix protrudes into the vagina. A canal down the center of the cervix, called the **cervical canal**, allows sperm deposited in the vagina to gain access to the uterus and fallopian tubes. The opening of the cervical canal into the uterus is called the **internal os**. The opening of the cervical canal into the vagina is called the **external os**. A newborn passes out of the uterus through the cervical canal.

The Vagina

The vagina is a muscular passageway lined with mucus-secreting cells. The muscular layer is highly vascularized. Muscles of the vagina are innervated by the **pudendal motor nerve**. The vagina is normally a collapsed chamber that expands during sexual intercourse to accommodate the penis and, while giving birth, to allow infant passage.

The Female Breast

The breast is the mammary gland. Under appropriate hormonal influence, the breast is capable of secreting milk after the birth of an infant. The breasts are located on the upper anterior portion of the chest and consist of 15 to 30 lobes of glandular tissue. Each lobe drains into a lactiferous (milk) duct, which opens at the tip of the nipple.

Before puberty, a girl's breasts are small and undeveloped. The nipple is flat against the chest. With onset of puberty, and under the influence of estrogen, the breasts increase in size, fatty deposits, and ductal structure. During pregnancy, under the influence of pregnancy hormones, the ductal system develops further, and the glandular cells become capable of producing milk.

THE MENSTRUAL CYCLE

The menstrual cycle is the cyclic maturation and release of an ovum. It involves the growth of a follicle, ovulation of the ovum, and characteristic changes in the endometrial lining of the uterus. For a point of reference, the first day of the menstrual cycle is considered the first day of menstruation (bleeding). Each menstrual cycle is approximately 28 days in length. There are two distinct phases of the menstrual cycle: the **follicular phase** and the **luteal phase**. These two phases are separated by **ovulation** (see Fig. 20-3, discussed in the following sections). During the follicular phase, the follicle develops and secretes estrogen. The uterine endometrial cells reproduce and grow. During the luteal phase, prog-

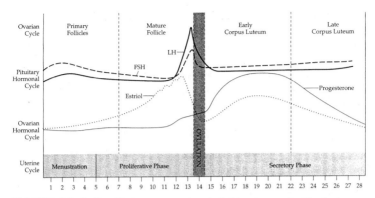

FIGURE 20-3 The 28-day menstrual cycle (without ovum fertilization).

esterone is secreted by the remaining cells of the follicle while the lining of the uterus becomes highly vascularized and secretory. Hormones from the hypothalamus, anterior pituitary, and ovary work together in an intricate balance to control the menstrual cycle.

The Follicular Phase of the Menstrual Cycle

The development of the follicle depends on the release of FSH and LH from the anterior pituitary. FSH begins to increase slightly in the first few days after the start of menstruation. LH levels show a moderate rise. Under the influence of FSH, and to a lesser extent LH, 6 to 12 primary follicles begin to develop during the first week of the menstrual cycle.

By the beginning of the second week, the growth of one of the primary follicles dominates and the others begin to deteriorate in a process called **atresia**. The granulosa cells of the dominant follicle respond to FSH and LH with secretion of **estrogen**. A second class of follicular cells, called **thecal cells**, grows to surround the granulosa layers. Estrogen secretions accumulate in the follicle, causing an **antrum** (cavity) to form. Increasing levels of estrogen act locally to increase the number of FSH receptors on the follicle, which when bound by FSH further stimulate the secretion of estrogen, thus initiating a positive feedback cycle. Toward the end of the second week of the menstrual cycle, the ovum inside the follicle completes its first meiotic division. As a result of the first meiotic division, one daughter cell becomes a mature ovum, containing 46 chromosomes (23 pairs). The other daughter cell, called a polar body, is discarded.

Ovulation

On approximately day 12 of the menstrual cycle, there is a dramatic rise (6- to 10-fold) in the release of LH from the anterior pituitary. This rise is called a preovulatory LH surge. FSH increases to a lesser degree. Rising LH levels initiate a profound, final growth of the follicle, which begins to swell with its accumulated secretions. At this time, LH begins to convert the thecal cells from estrogen-secreting cells to mostly progesterone-secreting cells. By day 13, estrogen levels have fallen and progesterone levels begin to rise. On day 14, the continued swelling of the follicle causes it to ooze secretions and then rupture, releasing the ovum into the abdominal cavity. Some granulosa cells are released as well, and they continue to surround the released ovum.

The Luteal Stage of the Menstrual Cycle

After ovulation, the granulosa and thecal cells remaining in the follicle enlarge and undergo the process of **luteinization**, a change to yellowish, lipid-laden cells. The complex of granulosa and thecal cells left behind in the ruptured follicle is known as the **corpus luteum**. The corpus luteum continues to secrete large amounts of progesterone and estrogen that act in a negative feedback manner on the hypothalamus to reduce the further secretion of LH and FSH. Progesterone and estrogen production by the corpus luteum, however, appears to be partially dependent on the remaining, but falling, levels of LH. Within approximately 10 days, LH and FSH levels are very low, and if fertilization of the ovum has not occurred, the corpus luteum degenerates. With degeneration of the corpus luteum, progesterone and estrogen levels rapidly fall and reach their lowest point on the last day (day 28) of the menstrual cycle. A lack of progesterone initiates menstruation.

If the ovum is successfully penetrated by a sperm, the second meiotic division occurs in the ovum. One final daughter cell, containing 23 chromosomes, is produced. Fusion of the 23 chromosomes present in both the egg and sperm results in the formation of a 46-chromosome cell, the zygote. This first cell divides rapidly, and early embryogenesis begins.

Uterine Changes During the Menstrual Cycle

During the follicular stage of the menstrual cycle, estrogen causes **proliferation** (reproduction and growth) of the endometrial and smooth muscle cells of the uterus, to prepare the uterus in case an egg is fertilized later in the cycle. Estrogen also causes the mucus-secreting cells of the cervix to secrete a large amount of clear, thin fluid that facilitates easy passage of sperm through the cervix.

After ovulation, progesterone effects on the uterus dominate. The endometrial cells that proliferated earlier in the cycle begin to **secrete** glycogen-rich fluid and various enzymes. The myometrial (smooth muscle) cells become highly vascularized and engorged with blood as the uterus further prepares for the arrival of a fertilized ovum. Cervical mucus secretions become thick and plug the cervical openings to prevent the ascent of anything that might disrupt fertilization or implantation of an embryo.

If fertilization of an egg does not occur, progesterone and estrogen levels fall toward the end of the cycle, causing the swollen blood vessels to constrict and deprive the uterine cells of oxygen and nutrients. As a result, the uterine lining disintegrates and menstrual flow begins. Within 2 to 3 days of the onset of menstruation, the cycle starts over as the levels of FSH and LH rise, initiating a new follicular phase. If fertilization does occur, the uterine lining remains well oxygenated and well nourished, and menstruation will not occur. The hormonal and uterine profiles seen during a menstrual cycle are shown in Figure 20-3.

Control of the LH Surge

The cause of the preovulatory LH surge is not completely understood. It has been hypothesized that positive feedback stimulation on the hypothalamus or pituitary hormones occurs when estrogen levels get very high. The very high levels of estrogen that develop by day 12 of the menstrual cycle are believed to be responsible for the burst of LH.

Hypothalamic Control of the Menstrual Cycle

The hypothalamus controls the release of FSH and LH by the secretion of GnRH. GnRH secretion is pulsatile and precise during a menstrual cycle. It is likely that GnRH levels undergo fluctuations during the month that immediately precedes the fluctuations in FSH and LH levels, including the LH surge. GnRH secretion increases at puberty. Inhibition of GnRH release can occur with physical or emotional stress.

IMPLANTATION OF THE BLASTOCYST

If the ovum is fertilized and conception occurs, the fertilized egg travels through the fallopian tubes and, as it reaches the blastocyst stage, implants in the uterine lining that has been prepared for its arrival. Implantation happens as a result of the development of special enzyme-secreting **trophoblast cells** on the surface of the blastocyst. The secreted enzymes break down the lining of the uterus, allowing the early embryo's entrance to the endometrial layer. Cells of the endometrium swell to nourish the embryo, becoming specialized cells, called **decidual cells** (the decidua). The decidua nourishes the growing embryo for the next 8 weeks. The decidual layer closest to the developing embryo appears to be antigenically neutral, thereby protecting the developing embryo from attack by the maternal immune system which otherwise might see the embryo as foreign.

THE PLACENTA

The trophoblast cells that attach to the uterus form the placenta, an organ consisting of fetal and maternal tissue. With implantation, invading trophoblasts begin to secrete the placental hormone, hCG. hCG prolongs the life of the corpus luteum, continuing the secretion of progesterone and estrogen required for maintenance of the uterine lining. Placental secretion of hCG is measurable in the serum within 24 hours of implantation and remains elevated for the duration of pregnancy. By approximately the third month of pregnancy, the placenta has taken over all hormonal roles of the corpus luteum, and the corpus luteum disintegrates.

In addition to functioning as an endocrine organ, the placenta functions in **gas and nutrient exchange** between the fetal and maternal circulations. In the placenta, blood flows through fetal arteries to a fetal capillary network, which lies in close approximation to a maternal capillary network. Across this capillary interface, oxygen and nutrients are delivered from the mother to the fetus, and fetal waste products are removed to the maternal circulation. The fetal capillaries regroup to form veins, and the oxygen-rich and nutrient-rich blood returns to the fetal heart. Maternal capillaries reform to veins that deliver fetal waste to the mother's lungs and kidneys. The fetus grows and develops in this nourishing and protective environment for approximately 38 to 42 weeks.

PARTURITION

Parturition is the delivery of the infant at the end of pregnancy. At this time, the placenta is also delivered. Parturition occurs when a combination of maternal and fetal factors increases the excitability of the uterus, initiating contractions of the smooth muscle. The contractions increase in frequency and intensity, resulting in softening and widening of the cervix to allow for delivery of the infant. The factors involved in exciting the uterus include an increasing ratio of estrogen to progesterone, starting at approximately the seventh month of pregnancy. Estrogen excites uterine smooth muscle, whereas progesterone relaxes uterine and other smooth muscle. An increase in the ratio of estrogen to progesterone will therefore increase uterine contractility. In addition, as the fetus grows, the uterus and cervix stretch. Stretching causes the smooth muscle of the uterus to contract in response, with the contractions becoming more forceful as the fetal size increases. Maternal release of the posterior pituitary hormone oxytocin near the end of pregnancy also stimulates uterine smooth muscle contraction. The release of fetal hormones, especially prostaglandins and oxytocin, as well as fetal cortisol, also appears to stimulate parturition. Some of the factors that stimulate parturition are outlined in Figure 20-4.

LACTATION

Lactation is the secretion of milk from the breast. Under the influence of estrogen, progesterone, and prolactin during pregnancy, the breasts increase in size and undergo growth and branching of the breast ductal system. Once the ducts are fully developed, secretory cells in the breasts prepare to produce milk.

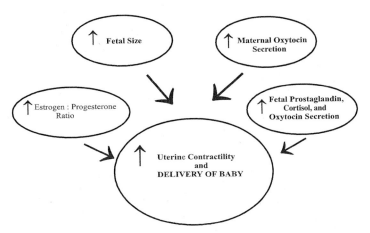

FIGURE 20-4 Factors that stimulate parturition.

Estrogen and progesterone, although essential in preparing the breasts to lactate, inhibit actual milk production. Prolactin, a hormone from the anterior pituitary, is stimulatory for both breast development and milk production. This hormonal interplay means that milk production does not occur to any significant degree until pregnancy is over and the source of estrogen and progesterone (the placenta) is removed. This removal leaves the lactogenic (milk-producing) effects of prolactin unopposed. Prolactin levels increase in the woman each time she nurses her baby, for as long as she continues to breastfeed. Release of prolactin is under the control of two opposing hypothalamic hormones: prolactin-inhibitory hormone (PIH) and prolactin-stimulatory hormone. PIH appears to be the neurotransmitter dopamine. Release of both PIH and prolactin-stimulatory hormone can be influenced by emotional and physical factors. Prolactin inhibits the release of LH and FSH from the pituitary, reducing the likelihood that a lactating woman will release another egg and become pregnant. This scenario does not always hold true, however, especially if the infant is bottle-fed as well as breastfed, and many nursing women do become pregnant.

Ejection of the milk from the nipples occurs as a result of the release of oxytocin from the posterior pituitary in response to sucking on the nipple of a prolactin-primed breast. Oxytocin stimulates contraction of the smooth muscle of the breast ducts and causes expulsion of milk. Oxytocin is under hypothalamic control and is influenced by emotional and physical factors.

FEMALE SEXUAL RESPONSE

The female sexual response includes excitement, orgasm, and resolution. It involves physical and psychological responses.

Excitement

Excitement occurs when physical manipulations of the genitalia or sexual thoughts activate the parasympathetic nerves supplying the female genital region. The clitoris is especially sensitive to physical manipulation. Activation of the parasympathetic nerves causes dilation of the blood vessels, leading to engorgement of erectile tissue in the vagina and clitoris. Mucus-secreting cells of the vagina are stimulated to secrete mucus, lubricating the vagina. For women, higher brain centers usually play a major role in facilitating parasympathetic activation. Heart rate and respiratory rate increase.

Orgasm

When sexual excitement reaches a very high level, muscles of the vagina and perineal area (posterior to the vagina) begin to contract rhythmically. Uterine and fallopian smooth muscles also appear to undergo waves of contraction. Intensely pleasurable sensations accompany the muscle contractions. Vaginal and uterine contractions may help propel sperm toward the fallopian tubes.

Resolution

After orgasm, the period of resolution occurs. This period is characterized by a reduction in genital blood flow and a return of heart rate and respirations to normal.

FEMALE SECONDARY SEXUAL CHARACTERISTICS

The female secondary and associated sexual characteristics are under the control of estrogen and to a lesser extent progesterone (see Chapter 9). The female secondary sexual characteristics include:

- Fully developed breasts.
- The female pattern distribution of pubic hair. The growth of pubic and axillary hair in women is not estrogen dependent, but occurs as a result of adrenal gland androgen release.
- Bone growth and closure of the epiphyseal plates.

PUBERTY

Puberty is the beginning of sexual maturation. Puberty typically occurs at a younger age in girls than boys. It begins in girls between 8 and 14 years of age, and in boys between 10 and 16 years of age. The menstrual cycle is the culmination of puberty in girls. In boys, puberty culminates in the ability to ejaculate mature sperm.

Puberty is initiated when the hypothalamus begins to secrete pulsatile bursts of GnRH. The hypothalamus apparently responds to cues concerning body mass index, diurnal signals, and the maturation of other brain areas, including the limbic system. Hormonal stimuli to the hypothalamus, from leptin and other hormones related to body size, may play a role as well. Even prior to puberty, the anterior pituitary and the gonads are capable of responding to hormonal stimulation, making hypothalamic activation the pivotal event.

MENOPAUSE

By the time a woman nears 50 years of age, she has only a few thousand ova remaining; when this number falls below a threshold of about 1000, she will enter menopause. Menopause is defined only in retrospect, as a lack of menstrual cycles for the previous 12 months. It occurs in a woman when her ovaries no longer respond to LH and FSH with estrogen and progesterone production, and no longer release an ovum. Menopause usually occurs between the ages of 40 and 50, and typically spans 8 to 10 years. During the long process of menopause, fluctuations in the timing and duration of a woman's menstrual cycle occur, ultimately resulting in cessation of the menses. Current data suggest that the onset of menopause, like fertility, follows a seasonal rhythm such that higher frequencies of menopause onset are observed in winter compared to the summer, spring, and fall. Surgically induced menopause or premature menopause may happen in women at younger ages.

The absence of estrogen causes symptoms of menopause. Symptoms may include poor sleep quality and fatigue, episodes of flushing of the skin (hot flushes), overwhelming, sudden rushes of body heat (hot flashes), sensations of dyspnea (difficulty in breathing), and occasional outbursts of irritability or emotionality. Vaginal atrophy and drying occur, which may make intercourse painful. Lack of estrogen causes the skin to lose its elasticity and become dry and loose. Without estrogen, decreases in bone mass occur and may lead to osteoporosis, with increased risk of bone fracture. Protective effects of estrogen on the cardiovascular system are lost, contributing to a dramatically increased risk of coronary artery disease and myocardial infarct. Estrogen also influences cognitive functioning, and a fall in estrogen may play a role in memory loss and perhaps even Alzheimer disease.

Because of the many changes that occur in a woman's body after the loss of estrogen, most notably hot flashes and the increased risk of osteoporosis, many women in the United States choose hormone replacement therapy (HRT) during and after menopause. While short-term HRT appears acceptable, especially during the perimenopausal years, studies suggest that extended use of HRT may increase the risks of cardiovascular disease and breast cancer. In addition, women who have experienced blood clot formation are discouraged from receiving hormone replacement.

● Pathophysiologic Concepts (Female)

DYSMENORRHEA

Dysmenorrhea is painful menstruation that occurs without evidence of pelvic infection or disease. Dysmenorrhea is usually caused by excessive release of a specific prostaglandin, prostaglandin F2 alpha, from the uterine endometrial cells. Prostaglandin F2 alpha is a potent stimulator of myometrial smooth muscle contraction and uterine blood vessel constriction. It worsens the uterine hypoxia normally associated with menstruation, causing significant pain. For most women, nonsteroidal anti-inflammatory drugs (NSAIDs) that inhibit prostaglandin production, such as ibuprofen, can effectively reduce cramping; acetaminophen is less helpful, since it works by a mechanism different from traditional anti-inflammatory drugs. Prostaglandin inhibitors should be used at the first sign of pain or at the first sign of menstrual flow. Because forceful menstrual cramping may contribute to the development of endometriosis (painful growth of uterine tissue outside of the uterus), complaints of dysmenorrhea should always be taken seriously, and attempts should be made to reduce its incidence.

AMENORRHEA

Amenorrhea is the absence of a menstrual cycle. It is considered primary if a woman has never had a menstrual cycle or secondary if she has had menstrual cycles in the past, but no longer. Amenorrhea exists naturally before puberty (primary amenorrhea) and after menopause (secondary amenorrhea). It also occurs during pregnancy, for a few to several weeks after delivery of an infant, and may occur during lactation. Emotional disturbances, physical stress, and low body mass index (such as experienced by female athletes) may also cause amenorrhea. Endocrine disorders, especially involving the ovaries, pituitary, thyroid, or adrenal glands, can cause amenorrhea, both primary and secondary.

● Conditions of Disease or Injury (Female)

PELVIC INFLAMMATORY DISEASE

Pelvic inflammatory disease (PID) is the infectious inflammation of any of the organs of the upper genital tract in women, including the uterus, fallopian tubes (salpingitis), or ovaries (oophoritis). The infectious agent is usually bacterial and is often acquired during sexual intercourse. A variety of microbial agents may be implicated, including *N. gonorrhoeae*, *C. trachomatis*, and *Escherichia coli*. In severe cases, the entire peritoneal cavity may be affected. Risk factors include multiple sexual partners, smoking, use of an intrauterine (IUD) device, and a history of sexually transmitted infections.

Clinical Manifestations

- Although occasionally a woman will be asymptomatic, she usually presents with a high fever and severe bilateral abdominal pain.
- Chills, malaise, nausea, vomiting, dysuria.
- Movement of the cervix or palpation of the adnexa elicits severe pain.
- Bleeding between periods may occur.
- Abdominal pain worsens with intercourse and physical activity.
- Profuse, purulent vaginal discharge.

Diagnostic Tools

- Palpating or moving the cervix during an internal pelvic examination is very painful.
- Purulent discharge at the external os may be apparent on inspection.
- Culture of the cervical discharge may indicate the infecting microorganism.
- White blood cell count and cell sedimentation rate are usually elevated.
- Visualization of the inflamed pelvis by laparoscopy, the insertion of a fiberoptic probe, can be used to confirm the diagnosis of PID.

Complications

- PID may lead to scarring and adhesions of the uterus or fallopian tubes, predisposing a woman to infertility.
- Pelvic adhesions and scarring increase the risk of a subsequent **ectopic pregnancy**. In an ectopic pregnancy, the embryo implants and grows at a site other than the uterus, usually the fallopian tube. Rupture of the fallopian tube may occur, leading to internal hemorrhage and maternal death.
- Pulmonary emboli.
- Approximately 5% to 10% of women with PID die, usually from septic shock.

Treatment

- Antibiotic therapy at home or in the hospital is required.
- Analgesics and intravenous fluids.
- Drainage of any abscess formation.
- Avoidance of sexual intercourse until the inflammation has subsided will allow healing to occur and will reduce the risk of repeated infection.

- Education on the use of barrier methods of contraception (condom, diaphragm with foam or jelly) to prevent future occurrences of sexually transmitted disease is important. Birth control pills may reduce PID by increasing the production of cervical mucus, but do not replace the need for a condom.
- The sexual partner(s) of an affected woman should be evaluated for infection and, if necessary, treated with antibiotics.
- Surgery may be indicated if an abscess ruptures.
- Appendicitis must be ruled out as the cause of abdominal pain.

ENDOMETRIOSIS

Endometriosis is the presence of uterine endometrial cells outside the uterus, anywhere in the pelvic or abdominal region. The endometrial cells respond to estrogen and progesterone with proliferation, secretion, and bleeding during the menstrual cycle. This can cause inflammation and severe pain. The inflammation may lead to scarring of pelvic or abdominal organs and infertility.

Retrograde menstruation is the main risk factor for endometriosis. Retrograde menstruation is the movement of some menstrual discharge *up* the fallopian tubes into the peritoneal cavity during menstruation, rather than down and out the vagina. However, retrograde menstruation occurs in most women without causing symptoms of endometriosis. A genetic predisposition and a depressed immune system that allows the debris to seed the peritoneal cavity may increase a woman's risk of endometriosis. Exposure to environmental toxins may contribute to the development of endometriosis in some women.

Clinical Manifestations

- Menstrual cramping and pain, ranging from mild to severe, before and/or during menstruation is the most common symptom of endometriosis. The intensity of the pain is not proportional to the absolute amount of endometrial tissue in extrauterine sites (e.g., women may have severe pain with little endometriosis visible during surgical inspection or may have only minor pain with significant spread).
- Abnormal uterine bleeding.
- Changes in bowel movements, either diarrhea or constipation, may occur around the time of menstruation. Nausea may also be present.
- Pain with intercourse (dyspareunia) or during defecation (if rectal tissue is involved). The pain is usually worse during menstruation, but in severe cases pain may be constant.

Diagnostic Tools

- Transvaginal ultrasound.
- Visualization of the peritoneal cavity using laparoscopic techniques can diagnose endometriosis and assign a stage to the disease.

Complications

- Infertility is a common (30% to 40%) complication of endometriosis. Endometriosis may cause infertility by causing scarring and obstruction of the fallopian tubes or by initiating a maintained state of inflammation. Hormonal disturbances may occur.
- Spontaneous abortion.
- Anemia.
- Emotional distress, family and marital problems, and low self-esteem may develop in some women, especially if infertility is a concern.

Treatment

Treatment is based on the stage and severity of the disorder and is focused on pain management, reducing disease progression, and preventing or reversing infertility. The following treatments contribute to these goals:

- Medications to interrupt the menstrual cycle and stop the proliferation and secretion of extrauterine cells are frequently used to treat endometriosis. Medications include birth control pills that reduce menstrual flow and cramping, NSAIDs such as aspirin or ibuprofen to reduce cramping, and GnRH agonists or androgen agonists to block the release of LH and FSH, thus preventing ovulation and menstruation. Treatments are aimed at providing time for extrauterine tissue to regress and inflammation to subside. After several months, a woman may discontinue therapy and, after a recommended period, attempt to become pregnant if desired.
- Conservative surgical treatments, including laser surgery, may be used to remove visible endometrial implants.
- Radical surgical interventions, including removal of the uterus (hysterectomy), fallopian tubes, and ovaries may be required if the pain is unbearable or significantly interfering with a woman's life. Such surgery would cause irreversible infertility.

POLYCYSTIC OVARIES

The presence of polycystic ovaries is one of the most common endocrinopathies of women. It is characterized by the presence of eight or more peripheral ovarian cysts, 10 mm or less in diameter. This ring of cysts is called the "black pearl necklace" sign. The cysts consist of preovulatory follicles that have undergone atresia (degeneration). In women with polycystic ovaries, the ovaries are intact and responsive to FSH and LH, but ovulation of an ovum does not occur. FSH levels are less than normal throughout the follicular stage of the cycle, while LH levels are higher than normal but do not show a surge. Research suggests that the imbalance in FSH relative to LH results from an abnormality of the GnRH "pulse generator" in the hypothalamus that controls the pulse rate of GnRH release. The GnRH pulse rate, in turn, determines the release of FSH relative to LH from the anterior pituitary. Ultimately, the consistently high LH increases androgen and estrogen production by the thecal cells of the follicle and by the adrenal gland. The anovulatory follicles degenerate and form cysts, giving the condition its name. This disorder is associated with unexplained hyperandrogenic characteristics and chronic anovulation. It is diagnosed by observation at surgery, bimanual exam, histopathology, and high-resolution transvaginal ultrasonography.

A somewhat different disorder, **polycystic ovarian syndrome** (PCOS), usually includes the presence of polycystic ovaries plus a constellation of other symptoms such as obesity, insulin resistance, and androgen excess characterized by hirsutism (development of male secondary sex characteristics). Insulin resistance is often accompanied by elevated levels of insulin, an occurrence that worsens the symptoms of PCOS, since insulin acts synergistically with LH to enhance thecal cell production of androgens. In addition, insulin decreases hepatic production of sex hormone–binding globulin, a key protein that binds testosterone in the blood. Having less of this protein leads to an increase in unbound, biologically active (i.e., free) testosterone, worsening the symptoms of PCOS. PCOS may coexist with or increase the risk for diabetes. It also tends to increase the risk for cardiovascular disease.

PCOS is estimated to occur in 5% to 10% of the female population; 30% to 40% of those individuals have impaired glucose tolerance, and 10% have type 2 diabetes by their 40s. Risk factors include a genetic tendency. Obesity often accompanies or precedes PCOS.

Clinical Manifestations

- Amenorrhea or dysfunctional uterine bleeding.
- The development of hirsutism, including a deepening of the voice, facial hair, and clitoral enlargement in response to high androgen levels, is common but not universal.
- Often women with PCOS are obese, but this is not absolute.

Diagnostic Tools

- Blood hormonal assay will show excess androgen and estrogen levels, with low FSH and no LH surge.

Complications

- Infertility may be present due to lack of ovulation.
- There is an increased risk of developing estrogen-dependent tumors of the breast and endometrium.
- Comorbidities include obesity, cardiovascular disease, and diabetes mellitus.

Treatment

- Antiestrogen drugs (e.g., clomiphene citrate) are provided to lower estrogen levels, causing FSH and LH to rise, and stimulating ovulation. Other drugs may be used to stimulate ovulation.
- Oral contraceptives, containing low-dose estrogen and progesterone, can limit cyst development.
- Surgical resection of the ovaries, or drug therapy to suppress ovarian function, may be required.
- Drugs such as metformin, an insulin-sensitizing drug, have been shown to be effective in improving insulin sensitivity.

UTERINE FIBROIDS

One of the most common health problems for women in the third and fourth decade of life is uterine fibroids, or leiomyomas. The estrogen-dependent benign tumors originate in the smooth muscle of the uterus. They are categorized by location that may include intramural, subserosal, or submucosal. Risk factors may include family history, African American heritage, obesity, hypertension, nulliparity, poor nutrition, and age over 30 to 40 years.

Clinical Manifestations

- May be asymptomatic.
- Dysfunctional uterine bleeding.
- Pelvic pain.
- Sense of fullness or pressure in the abdomen due to tumor bulk.
- Infertility or pregnancy loss.

Diagnostic Tools

- Bimanual exam reveals enlarged, firm, irregularly shaped, nontender uterus.
- Transabdominal or transvaginal ultrasound reveals solid areas.
- Hysterosonogram detects uterine cavity distortion. An infusion of saline into the uterine cavity enables visualization via transvaginal ultrasound.
- Magnetic resonance imaging is usually reserved for treatment planning.

Complications

- Anemia.
- Infertility.
- Increasing size can cause urinary symptoms, constipation, pelvic pain, or intestinal obstruction.
- Spontaneous abortion, premature labor, dystocia.

Treatment

- NSAIDs for pain management.
- Birth control pills or hormones to reduce the size of the fibroid.
- Myomectormy or surgical removal of the fibroids.
- Uterine artery embolization to obliterate arterial supply to the fibroid.
- MRI guided ablation of the fibroid.
- Hysterectomy.

FIBROCYSTIC DISEASE OF THE BREAST

Fibrocystic disease of the breast is also called benign breast disease. It is characterized by smooth, mobile, well-defined palpable lumps in the breasts that change in size and tenderness during different stages of the menstrual cycle. The swellings are very common among normal, healthy women. Intake of caffeine-containing food and drinks tends to increase the tenderness. The incidence of fibrocystic disease increases with advancing age until menopause occurs. Although the exact cause of the disease is unknown, it appears that estrogen is at least partially responsible. Although most lumps that vary through the menstrual cycle are benign, some of the lesions may proliferate and show atypical cellular growth. Women with repeated and large cyst development may be at a higher risk for breast cancer and should be screened regularly.

Clinical Manifestations

- Tenderness in the breasts, especially near menstruation, is the main symptom.
- Palpable lumps that increase in size during the menstrual cycle are common.

Diagnostic Tools

- Biopsies of the lumps may be performed to rule out carcinoma and to identify precancerous conditions.
- Mammography or ultrasound may be able to distinguish the fluid-filled cyst from a solid tumor. A biopsy may be necessary.

Complications

- Lesions that are proliferative and show atypical cells may progress to cancer. This progression is especially a risk for women with a personal or family history of breast cancer.

Treatment

- Pain may be relieved by changing dietary habits. For some women, eliminating caffeine from the diet reduces symptoms. Support bras, especially when the breasts are most sensitive, may reduce pain.
- Cysts may be drained in cases of severe pain.
- A synthetic androgen (e.g., danazol) may be prescribed in cases of severe pain.

CANCER OF THE FEMALE REPRODUCTIVE TRACT

Cancer of the female reproductive tract may develop in the vagina, vulvar, uterus, or ovaries.

Vaginal Cancer

Vaginal cancer is rare in the United States, usually occurring in women older than 60 years of age. The vaginal squamous cells are most often involved. Frequently, the cancer is a secondary metastasis. The risk of developing vaginal cancer increases in women who were exposed prenatally to DES or in those who have had previous cervical cancer.

Vulvar Cancer

The incidence of vulvar cancer has been on the rise, especially in women less than 50 years of age. The squamous epithelial cells are the most common origin of vulvar cancer. Although the exact cause is unknown, risk factors may include leukoplakia, obesity, hypertension, diabetes, lichen sclerosus, and infection with human papillomavirus.

Uterine Cancer

Uterine cancer includes cancer of the cervix and endometrium. **Cervical cancer** is often a result of a sexually transmitted disease of the cervix caused by certain strains of the human papillomavirus (HPV). Cervical cancer is most common in women who have had multiple sexual partners or whose sexual partners have had many partners. Women who are infected with HPV during their teenage years are especially at risk of developing cervical cancer, possibly related to the high rate of cell division occurring in the cervix during those years when exposed to the virus. Because of the ability of cervical mucus to concentrate carcinogens present in cigarette smoke, smoking is considered a cofactor in the development of cervical cancer. Premalignant changes in the cervix usually precede cervical cancer by many years. The premalignant changes, called dysplasia, can be identified and staged during cytologic studies of a cervical smear (the Papanicolaou smear, or Pap smear).

Uterine endometrial cancer is the most common female reproductive cancer and is usually an adenocarcinoma (from the epithelial cells). Endometrial cancer is related to lifetime exposure to estrogen and typically presents in post-menopausal women. Lifetime estrogen exposure increases in women who are obese (estrogen concentrates in adipose tissue), who have never been pregnant, or who experience early menarche and late menopause. Women with a high-fat diet are at increased risk, apparently related to associated obesity. Other risks include hormonal exposure in the diet and reduced intake of fruits and vegetables. Oral contraceptives reduce the risk of developing endometrial cancer by reducing lifetime estrogen exposure. Exposure to estrogen replacement therapy increases the risk of endometrial cancer in postmenopausal women; this risk is minimized by the coadministration of progesterone in combined HRT. Therefore, the use of estrogen alone is contraindicated in women with an intact uterus.

Ovarian Cancer

Although relatively rare, ovarian cancer is one of the leading causes of death from female reproductive cancer. Ovarian cancer is usually of the epithelial cells and is related to lifelong estrogen exposure. In children or adolescents, ovarian cancer may develop in the germ cells (ova). Ovarian cancer is highest among women with a strong family history of breast or ovarian cancer, although identifiable genetic risks are present in only 5% of women with ovarian cancer. Patients with mutations of BRCA1 or BRCA2 have a much higher lifetime risk. High-fat diet, obesity, and lack of childbearing increase the risk of ovarian cancer. Oral contraceptive use, pregnancy, breast feeding, and, in some studies, tubal ligation (severing of the fallopian tubes) seem to protect against ovarian cancer. Moderate exercise, which is related to lower estrogen levels, may decrease the risk of ovarian cancer.

Clinical Manifestations

- Vaginal cancer may be asymptomatic or associated with bleeding, discharge, or pain.
- Vulvar cancer may be asymptomatic initially. Vulvar pruritus and burning pain, bleeding. A small ulcer may progress to a vulvar mass with abnormal urination and defecation in severe cases.
- Cervical cancer may be asymptomatic or associated with bleeding after intercourse or spotting between menstrual periods. A vaginal discharge with odor may be present.

- Endometrial cancer may be asymptomatic or associated with abnormal bleeding.
- Ovarian cancer is usually asymptomatic until the disease is advanced. Late symptoms include abdominal swelling and pain. Gastrointestinal obstruction may cause vomiting, constipation, or small-volume diarrhea. Urinary frequency or urgency without an identifiable renal origin. Central obesity.

Diagnostic Tools

- The Pap smear can identify cervical and endometrial cancer.
- Direct cytologic sampling of the vagina, vulvar, and endometrium can diagnose vaginal, vulvar, and endometrial cancer.
- Ovarian cancer can be identified by use of MRI or vaginal ultrasound. The ovaries may be palpable. Surgery is required to stage the disease and identify metastases. Increased level of an ovarian tumor cell antigen, CA125, in a symptomatic woman or a woman with a family history of ovarian or breast cancer can be an early indication of disease.

Complications

- Death may occur with any of the reproductive cancers. Survival rates are highest (75% to 95%) with endometrial cancer and lowest (25% to 30%) with ovarian cancer. Early detection can improve survival rate significantly, especially for cervical cancer, which has a survival rate near 100% if identified while still in situ (before it has spread).

Treatment

- Surgery, with or without chemotherapy, is the treatment of choice for all the reproductive cancers. Laser surgery or cryosurgery (freezing) may be used for vaginal or cervical cancers. Improved chemotherapy has increased survival rate for all reproductive cancers, including ovarian cancer.
- Prophylactic bilateral **salpingo-oophorectomy**, the removal of both ovaries and fallopian tubes, may be performed on women at high risk of ovarian cancer who choose this option.

BREAST CANCER

Breast cancer is a relatively common cancer among women in the United States, and it is the leading cause of death in women between 45 and 64 years of age. Breast cancer may be discovered while in situ (localized), or it may be discovered as a malignant (spreading) neoplasm. Breast cancer is usually an adenocarcinoma found in the milk ducts.

The risk that a woman in the United States will develop breast cancer at some time in her lifetime is approximately one in eight. Breast cancer incidence increases with age and is influenced by genetic, hormonal, and environmental factors. Men may develop breast cancer, although the incidence is low.

Risk Factors for Breast Cancer

A strong risk factor for breast cancer is a history of the disease in one or more first-degree relatives (sisters or mother). Genetic studies have identified key genes, including BRCA1 found on chromosome 17 and BRCA2 found on chromosome 13, that contribute to familial breast cancer. BRCA1 and BRCA2 play important roles in DNA repair and act as tumor suppressors. Women who inherit a gene for breast cancer typically develop the disease at an earlier age than women who do not have a family history of the disease. The genes for breast cancer can be carried and passed by either parent, in an apparently autosomal-dominant manner. Women with inherited errors in BRAC1 have a 56% to 85% lifetime risk of acquiring breast cancer as well as an increased lifetime risk of ovarian cancer; women who inherit errors in the BRAC2 gene carry a similar risk for breast cancer. However, only about 10% of all women with breast cancer have a genetic risk for the disease. For most women, mutations in these or other common cancer genes, including mutated myc or p53 genes, are acquired after birth.

Lifetime estrogen exposure is also related to the development of breast cancer. Women who experience early menarche and late menopause are at increased risk. Ages of menarche and menopause are genetically influenced. Lack of or delayed childbearing also increases the risk of breast cancer, as may estrogen replacement therapy in some women. Fibrocystic disease of the breast characterized by epithelial hyperplasia is associated with increased risk. A high-fat diet and, in some studies but not others, alcohol consumption have also been linked to breast cancer. Lobular carcinoma in situ (LCIS) significantly increases the risk of breast cancer. HRT in postmenopausal women appears to increase the risk of breast cancer. Protection against breast cancer is possible by consumption of a diet rich in fruits and vegetables, regular exercise, and weight control.

Clinical Manifestations

- A painless lump or mass in the breast. Most cancers occur in the upper outer quadrant of the breast (50%) or in the center of the breast (20%). The lump is usually fixed (nonmobile), with irregular borders. It is unilateral and does not usually show variation in size with the menstrual cycle.
- Retraction of the nipple, nipple discharge, or puckering of the breast tissue may signal an underlying tumor.
- Lymph node swelling, either axillary or clavicular, may indicate metastasis.

Diagnostic Tools

- Breast self-examination (BSE) performed on a regular (monthly) basis is important for early detection of a tumor. BSE should be performed by all women older than 20 years.

- Mammography, a radiograph of the breast, is an important screening tool to identify breast cancer before a lump can be felt. The increased use of mammography has contributed to the fall in death rate due to breast cancer as a result of early detection. Currently annual or biannual mammography is recommended for all women older than 40 years of age and for younger women with a family history of the disease or other risk factors. New research is underway to determine if the current screening recommendation should be modified.

- Biopsy of a suspected lump will confirm the diagnosis. Determination of tumor size, tumor characteristics, and examination of surrounding lymph nodes allow for staging and histologic classification of the tumor. Staging is from I to IV and is important in determining treatment and estimating prognosis.

- Measurement of estrogen receptors on the tumor cells indicates the estrogen sensitivity of the tumor. A high level of estrogen receptors indicates the tumor may respond well to hormonal therapy that involves blocking the ability of estrogen to act on the tumor.

Complications

- Widespread metastases may occur. Sites of metastasis include the brain, lungs, bone, liver, and ovaries. Survival rates depend on staging: stage I (tumor < 2 cm, no metastases), 80%; stage II (tumor 2 to 5 cm, axillary node metastasis), 65%; stage III (tumor > 5 cm, axillary node metastasis and spread to skin or chest wall), 40%; stage IV (widespread metastases), 10%.

Treatment

- Surgery, including mastectomy or lumpectomy (the removal of the tumor plus a smaller amount of surrounding tissue) along with the dissection of the **sentinel** (primary drainage) node, is the first step for most women. If the sentinel node biopsy is positive, additional nodes are removed and tested. Nodal involvement indicates metastasis of the tumor and requires more aggressive postsurgical interventions.

- Adding radiotherapy or chemotherapy in conjunction with surgery improves survival and reduces the likelihood of recurrence. These therapies are based on the presence or absence of metastasis.

- Antiestrogens or estrogens specifically designed to interfere with the growth of breast tissue have been used for several years to treat breast tumors positive for estrogen receptors. These same drugs, including tamoxifen, are now being used to treat breast tumors that do not appear to be specifically estrogen sensitive. These drugs, often called designer estrogens or selective estrogen receptor modulators, improve survival and reduce the likelihood of recurrence.

- Drugs that specifically interfere with a tumor's ability to grow are available to treat breast cancer. For example, some tumors overexpress a surface receptor, called the HER2 receptor, that binds a circulating epidermal growth factor known to stimulate cancer cell growth. The drug trastuzumab (Herceptin) is designed to bind to and block the HER2 receptor, thereby slowing or stopping the growth of tumors that express this receptor. This drug has been shown to reduce the risk of breast cancer recurrence.

- Breast reconstruction may be performed following surgery to improve appearance.

- Counseling and support for the woman, her partner, and her family are essential.

Pathophysiologic Concepts (Male and Female)

INFERTILITY

Infertility is the inability or reduced ability to produce offspring. Infertility in a couple may result from female factors (40% to 50%), male factors (30% to 40%), or a combination (20%). Infertility in a couple may occur from the start of the relationship (primary infertility) or after the couple has already produced one or more offspring (secondary infertility).

Female Factors

Female factors leading to infertility include problems with follicular growth, anovulation (failure to ovulate), or ovulatory irregularities. Optimal fertility in women lasts upto about 30 years of age and then begins to fall sharply, primarily related to anovulation and/or ovulatory irregularities that occur with increasing frequency as a woman ages. The trend to delay childbirth in Western societies has increased the prevalence of infertility in those cultures. Structural abnormalities, vaginal or uterine infection, or inappropriately thick cervical mucus also may impact fertility. Blockage of the fallopian tubes following pelvic infection or the presence of uterine abnormalities that prevent implantation may be involved. Immune responses may destroy the implanted embryo if the woman is either hyperimmune to the embryo or fails to develop tolerance to it. Miscarriages later in gestation may occur if the placenta is poorly placed or poorly perfused with blood, or if the cervix cannot support the weight of a growing fetus.

Treatment of female infertility is specific to the cause. Drugs to induce ovulation or superovulation (more than one ovum) may be administered.

Harvesting of eggs from the woman for in vitro fertilization (outside of the body) may be attempted. Eggs fertilized outside the body may be implanted into the fallopian tube or uterus. For some women, eggs from a donor may be fertilized in vitro and then implanted into the infertile woman's uterus and carried there to term. Research findings have shown that for some previously infertile women, treatment with the normal pregnancy hormone hCG can enhance fertility and improve the success of therapeutic procedures.

Male Factors

Male factors causing infertility may include defects in spermatogenesis that result in deformed sperm or sperm too few in number to allow for successful penetration of the ovum. Sperm motility (movement) may be impaired as well. Male infertility may occur following infection and scarring of the testicles, epididymis, vas deferens, or urethra. Systemic infections, such as mumps, may cause swelling of the testicles and destruction of the seminiferous tubules. Obstruction of the blood vessels supplying the testes can cause hypoxia and a failure of the sperm to develop or survive. Autoantibodies produced against sperm may reduce sperm number and quality. Exposure of the testicles to high temperature may reduce spermatogenesis. Erection, emission, or ejaculation may be dysfunctional with nerve damage, atherosclerosis, or psychological disturbance. Congenital anomalies may affect the ability of the penis to deliver sperm inside the vagina.

Treatment of male factor infertility is specific to the cause. For example, for a man with a low sperm count, sperm may be obtained via masturbation and then introduced artificially into his female partner after techniques to increase the concentration of the highest-quality sperm have been performed. This process is called artificial insemination. Sperm from a known or unknown donor may also be collected and deposited inside a female. Other treatments include improving the overall health of a man, including eliminating the use of recreational drugs such as marijuana and alcohol that might impact fertility.

● Conditions of Disease or Injury (Male and Female)

PRECOCIOUS PUBERTY

Precocious puberty is the occurrence of puberty in girls before 6 to 8 years of age or in boys less than 9 years of age. Premature development of sexual characteristics appropriate to the sex of the child is called **isosexual precocious puberty**. Development of sexual characteristics appropriate to the opposite sex is called **heterosexual precocious puberty**. Heterosexual precocious puberty is rare and usually is caused by either a disorder in the fetal adrenal gland or decreased sensitivity of a genetically male fetus to androgens, which reverses during puberty (see Chapter 9). Although not considered precocious puberty, signs of early sexual development may be present at birth as a result of an oversensitivity of the fetus to sex hormones produced by the mother. In this case, after birth and the withdrawal of maternal hormones, these early signs of sexual development disappear.

Causes of Isosexual Precocious Puberty

True isosexual precocious puberty is more common and usually occurs when the hypothalamus prematurely begins to secrete GnRH. The anterior pituitary responds to GnRH with the secretion of FSH and LH. FSH and LH cause the gonads to secrete the sex hormones and signs of puberty appear. Hypothalamic prematurity may occur idiopathically (for no known cause), especially in girls, or may result from a central nervous system tumor or disease. Ectopic production of a gonadotropin and a hormone-secreting tumor of the gonads are other causes of precocious puberty.

Clinical Manifestations of Isosexual Precocious Puberty

- Premature development of breasts (thelarche), pubic or axillary hair (adrenarche), or menses (menarche) in girls.
- Premature growth of the penis, scrotum, beard, or pubic hair in boys. A deepening of the voice may occur.

Diagnostic Tools

- A physical examination and hormonal profile is used for diagnosis of precocious puberty.
- Imaging techniques, including computed tomography (CT) scans, ultrasound, and magnetic resonance imaging (MRI), are used to identify tumors.
- DNA testing may be used to determine gender in certain cases.

Complications

- Estrogen and testosterone can cause premature growth of the skeleton and early closure of the epiphyseal bone plates, leading to short height in adulthood.
- Psychosocial stress may occur for children and their families.

Treatment

- If a tumor is identified, surgical resection, radiation, or chemotherapy may be used.
- For precocious puberty of idiopathic origin, treatment may consist of administration of a long-lasting GnRH agonist. This agonist decreases pituitary

responsiveness to endogenous GnRH, causing LH and FSH levels to fall, shutting off the pubertal sequence.

- Some children will not be treated. Appropriate counseling for the family and child is important.

SEXUALLY TRANSMITTED INFECTION

Sexually transmitted infection (STI) may develop in anyone having sexual contact with multiple partners or with one partner who has had sexual contact with others. Microorganisms capable of causing an STI include the bacteria *N. gonorrhoeae*, responsible for causing gonorrhea, and *Treponema pallidum*, responsible for causing syphilis. *Chlamydia*, the most common STI in the United States, is caused by the intracellular bacterium *C. trachomatis*. The herpes simplex virus, human papillomavirus (HPV), hepatitis B virus, and human immunodeficiency virus (HIV) are also sexually transmitted. *Trichomonas vaginalis* is a protozoan responsible for causing trichomoniasis.

An STI may be passed via semen or vaginal secretions or by skin-to-skin contact. Clinical manifestations of an STI depend on the agent responsible, host characteristics, and the stage of infection. Treatments are specific to the causative agent. Herpes simplex, hepatitis B, HPV, and HIV infection are discussed elsewhere in this text. Effects of STIs can cause a wide range of systemic disorders that may include headache, brain damage, alopecia, conjunctivitis, blindness, neurologic disorders, meningitis, pharyngitis, thrush, canker sores, arthritic pain, bone ache, aortic stenosis, heart disease, *Pneumocystis carinii* pneumonia, hepatitis, Kaposi sarcoma, skin irritation, dysentery, urinary tract infection, pelvic scarring, genital damage, urethritis, urethral strictures, Reiter syndrome, pruritus, rash, warts, lymphadenitis, sterility, cervical cancer, PID, epididymitis, prostatitis, ED, and childbearing difficulties such as premature birth and birth defects.

Clinical Manifestations

Page C16 illustrates common clinical manifestations associated with STIs.

- Gonorrhea may be asymptomatic or may present with purulent discharge from the urethra or vagina and burning on urination. Some individuals, including infants born to infected mothers, may develop conjunctivitis or pharyngitis.
- Primary syphilis is characterized by the presence of a painless genital ulcer (chancre) that spontaneously regresses. Secondary syphilis develops weeks to months later and is characterized by a temporary skin rash, typically located on the palms of the hands and the soles of the feet. Tertiary syphilis may develop decades after the initial infection and is characterized by sensory loss, muscle weakness, and heart defects.

- *Chlamydia* may be asymptomatic or may present with urethritis or cervicitis characterized by discharge, itching, and burning on urination. In women, spotting between periods or after intercourse may occur.
- HPV infections are frequently asymptomatic. Itching, burning, and tenderness in genital area. Genital warts may be smooth, flat or raised and with a rough texture. Warts are located in vaginal and/or anal area.
- Trichomoniasis may be asymptomatic or may present with greenish discharge and itching. Pain with intercourse is common. Men are seldom symptomatic.

Diagnostic Tools

- Smears of vaginal or urethral discharge observed under the light microscope may indicate the presence of *N. gonorrhoeae* and *C. trachomatis*. Diagnosis may also be based on pH, odor, color, and the presence of white blood cells. The protozoan *T. vaginalis* may be visible with a light microscope.
- Vaginal or urethral cultures can identify the presence of *N. gonorrhoeae* and *C. trachomatis*. *T. pallidum* is identified in a blood test (VDRL or RPR).
- Colposcopy reveals cervical changes with HPV. Presence of genital warts, which are papular or pedunculated growths.

Complications

- **Untreated gonorrhea** may cause female sterility or PID and increases the risk of ectopic pregnancy. Both men and women may develop disseminated infection with arthritis, endocarditis, or conjunctivitis leading to blindness. If passed to a newborn during birth, blindness may result.
- **Untreated syphilis** may cause heart failure and neurologic deterioration. If passed to a fetus during pregnancy, fetal death or neonatal infection may occur.
- **Chlamydial** infection may cause infertility in men and women, and epididymitis in males. PID and ectopic pregnancy may occur in infected women. If passed to a newborn, conjunctivitis may occur.
- **HPV** increases the risk for anal, vaginal, penis, vulvar, mouth, and possibly sinus cancer.

Treatment

Extensive education about the importance of safe sex practices is imperative. All partners need to be notified, tested, and treated if indicated.

- Because of the prevalence of penicillin-resistant gonorrhea, gonorrhea is currently treated with a single intramuscular dose of ceftriaxone.
- Syphilis is treated with intramuscular penicillin. If the patient is pregnant, erythromycin or ceftriaxone is used. If the individual is allergic to penicillin but not pregnant, doxycycline or tetracycline is recommended.

- Chlamydial infection may be treated with a macrolide (clarithromycin, azithromycin, or erythromycin, the latter during pregnancy), doxycycline, or tetracycline. Since gonorrhea frequently occurs with *Chlamydia*, individuals suspected of having either disease are usually treated with both ceftriaxone and a second drug. A large dose (1 g) of azithromycin may be given in the office for a one-dose treatment.
- HPV vaccine protects against some types and is administered in a series of three injections to females between 9 and 26 years of age. It is most effective if administered prior to sexual intercourse.
- Genital warts can be treated with self-administered podofilox or imiquimod. Cryotherapy with liquid nitrogen or cryoprobe. Trichloroacetic or bichloroacetic acid, surgical removal.
- Trichomoniasis is treated with metronidazole (Flagyl), or topical clotrimazole during pregnancy.

 PEDIATRIC CONSIDERATIONS

- A congenital hydrocele typically resolves spontaneously during the first year of life.
- Cryptorchidism is present at birth and is especially common in premature infants. The testes will usually descend spontaneously within the first year of life.

 GERIATRIC CONSIDERATIONS

- As males age, the testes become less firm, the number of seminiferous tubules that contain sperm decreases, testosterone production decreases, but viable sperm may continue to be produced up to 90 years of age.
- In the older male and female, the only changes in sexual response should be timing. Libido may decrease, but total disappearance warrants further evaluation.

SELECTED BIBLIOGRAPHY

Albertsen, P.C., Hanley, J.A., & Fine, J. (2005). Twenty-year outcomes following conservative management of clinically localized prostate cancer. *Journal of the American Medical Association*, 293, 2095–2101.

Ahonen, K. A. Ovarian cancer. *Advance for Nurse Practitioners*, 17(1), 47–49.

American Cancer Society. *Cancer statistics 2009*. Available at http://www.cancer.org/docroot/PRO/_1_1_Cancer_Statistics_2009_Presentation.asp. Accessed 10/01/09.

Bartoszek, M. P. (2009). Recognizing polycystic ovary syndrome in the primary care setting. *The Nurse Practitioner*, 34(7), 22–23, 25–29.

Bertram, C. C. (2008). Informational needs and the experience of women with abnormal papanicolaou smears. *Journal of the American Academy of Nurse Practitioners*, 20(9), 455–462.

Bradway, C., & Rodgers, J. (2009). Evaluation and management of genitourinary emergencies. *The Nurse Practitioner, 34*(5), 37–44.

Bruce, M. L., & Baril, C. (2008). Save the date: Screening tips and new vaccines for female HPV. *The Nurse Practitioner, 33*(9), 29–33.

Cappelleri, J. C., & Rosen, R. C. (2005). The sexual health inventory for men (SHIM). *International Journal of Impotence Research, 17*, 307–319.

Carcio, H. (2008). Detour around surgery: Tuck and tone to treat pelvic organ prolapse. *Advance for Nurse Practitioners, 16*(10), 61–62, 64, 66.

Cesario, S. K., & Hughes, L. A. (2007). Precocious puberty: A comprehensive review of literature. *Journal of Obstetric, Gynecologic, and Neonatal Nursing, 36*(3), 263–274.

Christensen, T. L., & Andriole, G. L. (2009). Benign prostatic hyperplasia: Current treatment strategies. *Consultant,* 115–117, 120–122.

Cunningham, G. R. (2009). Delivering testosterone replacement in male patients: A comprehensive review of clinicam options. Available at http://cme.medscape.com/viewarticle/709541. Retrieved 10/19/2009.

Day, S. (2008, October). Clear and present danger: Management of women with LCIS. *Advance for Nurse Practitioner,* 49–53.

Diedrich, J., Depke, J., & Engel, J. (2007). What every nurse needs to know about breast cancer. *American Nurse Today, 2*(10), 32–37.

Demir, O., Akgul, K., Akar, Z., Cakmak, O., Ozdemire, I., Bolukbasi, A. et al. (2009). Association between severity of lower urinary tract symptoms, erectile dysfunction and metabolic syndrome. *The Aging Male, 12*(1), 29–34.

Flowers, J. (2008). Uterine fibroids. *Advance for Nurse Practitioners, 16*(10), 36–40.

Frye, D. K., Mahon, S. M., & Palmieri, F. M. (2009). New options for metastatic breast cancer. *Clinical Journal of Oncology Nursing, 13*(suppl 1), 11–18. DOI: 10.1188/09.CJON.S1.11-18.

Greene, M. D. (2009). Diagnosis and management of HPV-related anal dysplasia. *The Nurse Practitioner, 34*(5), 45–47, 49–51.

Greiser, C. M., Greiser, E. M., & Doren, M. (2005). Menopausal hormone therapy and risk of breast cancer: A meta-analysis of epidemiological studies and randomized clinical trials. *Human Reproduction Update, 11*, 561–573.

Guyton, A. C., & Hall, J. E. (2006). *Textbook of medical physiology* (11th ed.). Philadelphia, PA: W.B. Saunders.

Harrington, J. M., & Badger, T. A. (2009). Body image and quality of life in men prostate cancer. *Cancer Nursing, 32*(2), E1–E7.

Helming, M. B. (2009). Genitourinary disorders in children: A review of less common presentations. *Advance for Nurse Practitioners, 17*(3), 24–29.

Hoff, J. (2008). Genital herpes in older women: A silent epidemic. *Journal of the American Academy of Nurse Practitioners, 20*(6), 291–294.

Inman, B. A., St. Sauver, J. L., Jacobson, D. J., McGree, M. E., Nehra, A., Lieber, M. M. et al. (2009). *Mayo Clinic Proceedings, 84*(2), 108–113.

Kaplan, C. (2009). Assessing and managing female sexual dysfunction. *The Nurse Practitioner, 34*(1), 42–49.

Kaplowitz, P. B. (2009). Precocious puberty. *eMedicine Pediatrics*. Retrieved from http://emedicine.medscape.com/article/924002.

Legro, R.S. (2003). Polycystic ovary syndrome and cardiovascular disease: A premature association? *Endocrine Reviews*, 24, 302–312.

Leung-Chen, P. (2008). Syphilis makes another comeback. *American Journal of Nursing*, 108(2), 28–31.

Likes, W. M. (2009). Vulvar cancer in the wake of increasing incidence. *The Nurse Practitioner*, 34(2), 45–47, 49–50.

Lindsey, K., DeCristofaro, C., & James, J. (2009). Anal pap smears: Should we be using them? *Journal of the American Academy of Nurse Practitioners*, 21, 437–443.

Lippert, J., Macchia, R. J., Rothman, I. (2008, August). Recognizing symptoms of an enlarged prostate. *The Clinical Advisor*, 23–26.

Loomis, D. M., Pastore, P. A., Rejman, K., Gutierrez, K. L., & Bethea, B. (2009). Cervical cytology in vulnerable pregnant women. *Journal of the American Academy of Nurse Practitioners*, 21(5), 287–294.

Mahon, S. M., & Palmieri, F. M. (2009). Metastatic breast cancer: The individualization of therapy. *Clinical Journal of Oncology Nursing*, 13(suppl 1), 19–28. DOI: 10.1188/09.CJON.S1.19-28.

Marcum, C. (2008). Dysfunctional uterine bleeding. *Advance for Nurse Practitioners*, 16(7), 57–60.

Marsden, J., & Sturdee, D. (2009). Cancer issues. *Best Practice and Research Clinical Obstetrics and Gynaecology*, 23, 87–107.

Million Women Study Collaborators. (2003). Breast cancer and hormone-replacement therapy in the Million Women Study. *Lancet*, 362, 419–427.

Miner, M. M. (2009). Erectile dysfunction with the "window of curability": A harbinger of cardiovascular events. *Mayo Clinic Proceedings*, 84(2), 102–104.

Mulcahy, N. (2009). Hormone therapy may increase risk for death in men with prostate cancer and heart disease. *Journal of American Medical Association*, 302, 866–873.

O'Sullivan, B., & Savage, E. (2009). Erectile dysfunction and CHD: Related risk factors and implications for nursing practice. *British Journal of Cardiac Nursing*, 4(4), 170–176.

Pitkin, J. (2008). Sexuality and the menopause. *Best Practices and Research Clinical Obstetrics and Gynaecology*, 23, 33–52.

Porth, C. M., & Matfin, G. (2009). *Pathophysiology: Concepts of altered health states* (8th ed.). Philadelphia, PA: Lippincott Williams & Wilkins.

Qualich, S. (2009, July). Determining when men need testosterone. *The Clinical Advisor*, 53–54, 56–58.

Stern, L. (2009). Assessing excessive menstrual bleeding. *The Clinical Advisor*, 25–27, 31, 34, 37.

Takenaka, A., Hara, R., Ishimura, T., Fujii, T, Jo, Y., Nagai, A. et al. (2008). A prospective randomized comparison of diagnostic efficacy between transperineal and transrectal 12-core prostate biopsy. *Prostate Cancer and Prostatic Disease*, 11(2), 134–138.

Tsertsvadze, A., Yazdi, F., Fink, H. A., MacDonald, R., Wilt, T. J., Soares-Weiser, K. et al. (2009). Diagnosis and treatment of erectile dysfunction. Evidence report/technology assessment no.171. Prepared by the University of Ottawa Evidence-based Practice Centre (UO-EPC) under Contract No. 290-02-0021). AHRQ Publication No. 08(09)-E016. Rockville, MD: Agency for Healthcare Research and Quality. May 2009.

Tsilchorozidou, T., Overton, C., & Conway, G. S. (2004). The pathophysiology of polycystic ovary syndrome. *Clinical Endocrinology*, 60, 1–17.

U.S. Preventive Services Task Force (2008). Screening for prostate cancer: U.S. Preventive Service Task Force recommendation statement. *Annals of Internal Medicine*, 149, 185–191.

Wallace, M., Bailey, D. E., & Brion, J. (2009). Shedding light on prostate cancer. *The Nurse Practitioner*, 34(10), 25–33.

Watring, N., & Mason, J. D. (2008). Deciphering dysuria. *Clinician Reviews*, 18(12), 16–22.

Wilt, T., MacDonald, R., Hagerty, K., Schellhammer, P., & Kramer, B. B. (2008). 5-alpha-reductase inhibitors for prostate cancer prevention. *Cochrane Database of Systemic Reviews*, 2. Art. No.: CD007091. DOI: 10.1002/14651858. CD007091.

Zurakowski, T. L. (2010). The genitourinary and renal systems. In P. A. Tabloski (Ed.). *Gerontological nursing* (2nd ed., pp. 538–574). Upper Saddle River, NJ: Pearson.

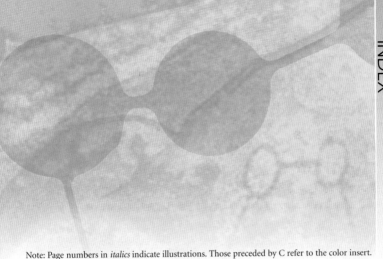

Note: Page numbers in *italics* indicate illustrations. Those preceded by C refer to the color insert. Page numbers followed by t indicate tables.